T0222402

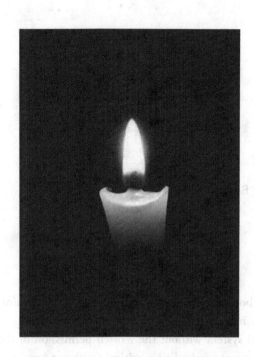

The Little Handbook of Palliative Care

Dr. Tan Seng Beng

PARTRIDGE

To order additional copies of this book, contact
Toll Free 800 101 2657 (Singapore)
Toll Free 1 800 81 7340 (Malaysia)
orders.singapore@partridgepublishing.com

www.partridgepublishing.com/singapore

I would like to dedicate this little handbook to all doctors, nurses and medical students.

May this book be a guide to relieve suffering of palliative care patients and their family caregivers.

May it help all who read it and lead them to the path of enduring happiness.

1

Contents

Foreword, by Professor Dato' Dr Christopher Boey Chiong Meng
Foreword, by Catherine Yee Chiew Huei
Preface

Part I: Introduction to Palliative Care

Part II: Symptom Control – Pain

Part III: Symptom Control – Non-Pain Symptoms

Part IV: Management of Death and Dying

Part V: Psychosocial and Spiritual Care

Part VI: Self-Care

Foreword

by Professor Dato' Dr Christopher Boey Chiong Meng

It is my great honour to write a foreword to this important book on palliative medicine by Dr Tan Seng Beng who has been a friend and colleague for many years.

The dignity and preciousness of life is the fundamental starting point of all effort in medicine. It is essential that practitioners of the art of medicine be well-rounded human beings who are interested in people and not just in pathological processes, and who constantly strive to put themselves in the position of the patients they are caring for. Such a quality is indispensable, especially in palliative care.

The Chinese character for 'benevolence' is a combination of the character for 'person' and the character for the number 'two', and indicates two people in a relationship of friendship and trust. It also means 'to be kind and to feel compassion for'.

Recently, however, there has been concern expressed about the deteriorating quality of doctor-patient relationships. Medical school teachers know that this is an increasingly worrying issue. To reverse this trend is a challenge that we all have to courageously take up.

It is therefore with much expectation that I welcome the publication of this book that contains the wisdom derived from the many years of experience of a dedicated palliative care physician who is trying his best to practice humanistic medicine. I sincerely wish this book the great success that it deserves.

Professor Dato' Dr Christopher Boey Chiong Meng
MBBS DCH MRCP FAMM MD PhD FRCPCH FRCP
Deputy Dean (Postgraduate)
Faculty of Medicine
University of Malaya

15th September 2016

Foreword

by Catherine Yee Chiew Huei

I lost both my parents to cancer, one after the other within a span of three years. When my parents were diagnosed -- first my mother, and later, my father -- I experienced a reversal of our parent-child roles. Despite the roller-coaster of emotions we encountered, I learnt to juggle my new responsibilities as caregiver. I was lost, yet, just like any parent who hoped the best for their child, I was hopeful. At first, I hoped that they would recover and continue what they enjoyed doing daily. As time and the disease progressed, my only hope was to take their pain and suffering away. As I write this foreword, my hope is that they are happy wherever they are.

Over the last three years, I learnt that palliative care is not a miracle cure, but a journey filled with hope, love and care. I still remember the first time we were referred to palliative care's Dr SB Tan. It was back in March 2013. "How do I tell my mom she's dying? Do I tell her how long she has left?", I asked Dr Tan. I had so many questions but I couldn't seem to ask or hear anything. "Practitioners will normally help to break the news," he replied, trying to calm me down. Trying to hold back my tears, I said, "I will tell her but you need to teach me how". And that was my introduction to palliative care. From that day onwards, it was "Dr Tan, I will learn but please teach me how." Little did I know, three years later, I would have to relay this unfortunate news again - this time round, to my dad. Honestly, doing it the second time did not make it any easier. It was actually a lot more difficult.

As unfortunate as the circumstances were, both experiences were truly a blessing. Taking care of them, although extremely painful, brought great joy and wonderful discoveries. I learnt a lot about myself and saw how just being human was extraordinary. Beyond the pain of being vulnerable and fragile is the beauty of our own individuality and the wonders of our adaptability.

Each day was unique and every moment was different. My dad wanted to be pain-free so he could just sleep through the ordeal, whereas my mom fought to stay awake just to enjoy her time with us and do what she liked.

Learning from the doctors how to organise the cocktails of medication and their frequencies was overwhelming. There was never a quiet day, and each day brought new challenges. Whilst cleaning my mom one day I found small blisters on her thigh. The oncologist confirmed the blisters were early signs of shingles and gave her some medication. A week later, as the shingles healed, I discovered pressure sores on her body. I ran to the nearest pharmacy for cream and a ripple bed. The pharmacy was like my local grocery store.

Later, when my dad was bedridden, there were episodes where he soiled himself as a result of the laxatives he was on. Once, while cleaning my dad up, I found some blood stains between his thighs. The skin had cracked and was inflamed. It was back to the pharmacy again. And so it went on.

Many a time I was conflicted by what I wanted for them rather than what they actually needed. In the midst of all the worries, frustrations and tiredness, it was so easy to forget what I was actually doing and more importantly, how they were coping. I constantly reminded myself that my actions were in their best interest - it was for THEM and how THEY would like it at THAT moment. The more aware I was of their feelings and the more I listened to what they wanted, the more I learnt about myself. And I'm sure they learnt about me too. Sometimes, I laughed at the assumptions I made of my parents. My only rule of thumb was to keep them happy and at the same time, not beat myself up when I didn't manage to. I told myself that they would know if I was unhappy. They did not knock their head somewhere, they were just ill. When I learnt to embrace that fluidity, I started truly enjoying each passing moment with them and was thankful for what little time we had left together.

There were bouts of mixed emotions and lots of teeth-grinding moments. There were many questions that I didn't know how to answer. "Why won't you just let me die?", "How did I get this?", "Am I going to get well soon?", "Am I going to die?". Over time, I learnt that it was just them being truly human – it was the frustration of being taken care of by their child instead of them taking care of me; the anger of not being able to do what they enjoyed with me; the sadness of having their future taken away; and not being able to watch my kids grow up. Despite their ordeal, they still tried to be as strong as they could, and I was overwhelmed by the realisation. It made me so proud of them, and never had I been more proud being their daughter than I was then.

Two months have gone by since my dad passed away. As I watched him slowly and peacefully slip away, I remembered Dr Tan's words from three years ago. "Dying is a natural and beautiful process. The body will know when it's dying and will slowly shut down. It will be peaceful if we do not struggle with it." I remember the day my mom passed away just as clearly. I held her hand, repeated Dr Tan's words of advice, and wished her a wonderful journey ahead. She smiled as she drew her last breath.

The journey with palliative care has made my life in this boundless universe more beautiful and meaningful.

"When you want something, all the universe conspires in helping you to achieve it" – Paulo Coelho

In memory of my wonderful father and loving mother.

Thank you Dr Tan for sharing your positive energy with us.

- Catherine Yee Chiew Huei, 2016

Preface

My own first exposure to palliative care happened in November 1998 when I did my elective posting at Hualien Tzu Chi Hospital of Taiwan. With my batchmates, we did a project on types of pain control used in the palliative care ward, also called the Heart Lotus Ward. The ward was named so with the conviction that terminally ill patients can bloom beautifully like lotus flowers from the mud of suffering.

I remember we were asked to do a performance at the hospital three days before Christmas. My batchmates sang a song called Using the Malaysian Weather to Say I Love You. I sang The Heart Sutra, a Buddhist scripture of 260 Chinese characters that describes the experience of liberation from suffering of Avalokiteśvara, the Bodhisattva of Compassion. It was a memorable experience.

We met Master Cheng Yen, the founder of the Tzu Chi Foundation, at the corridor beside the canteen. She said, "You are all from Malaysia. One day you will all become great doctors. Use your heart." We felt very blessed. But I didn't understand what was the exact meaning of 'use your heart'.

In 2006, I joined Hospis Malaysia. During that period, I had my first glimpse of the vast amount of suffering people were going through at their end of life. I was completely unprepared to help them despite my 6 years of experience in medicine. What I learnt in medicine was when and how to treat, but not when and how to stop, and how to continue caring after stopping.

During a hospice home visit, I saw a dying patient lying on a mattress on the floor. She couldn't speak to me. She grabbed my right hand. Eyes fixed on me. I could see her suffering. I didn't say anything. She passed on while she was still holding my hand. It was a deep connection. Although I have seen and related well with many patients during my medical years, I have never felt as deep a connection as that time.

After 5 months in Hospis Malaysia, I went to National Cancer Centre, Singapore to learn palliative medicine under Professor Cynthia Goh, who is one of the pioneers of hospice and palliative care development in Singapore. She taught me many things. But what I remember most is her dedication and compassion towards patients. What I have learnt most from the fellowship is the delicate balance between giving and stopping treatment.

In 2008, I came back to Malaysia to work at University of Malaya Medical Centre. My colleague Dr Loh Ee Chin and I were recruited to set up a palliative care unit in the medical centre. I began writing The Little Handbook of Palliative Care to serve as a reference for myself. With time, the little handbook has become not so little as I added more and more details to it.

Since 2008, I started to have more time for myself. I began to invest more and more time in practicing mindfulness. My favourite book of mindfulness is Present Moment Wonderful Moment written by Vietnamese Zen Master Thich Nhat Hanh. The book contains many mindfulness verses that I use to incorporate mindfulness into my day-to-day life.

I also started to meditate after reading The Joy of Living from Yongey Mingyur Rinpoche. I noticed my stress level reduced to zero after months of meditation practices. I still have breakthrough stress once in a while but it quickly returns to zero once I am aware and once I stop sustaining it. I am able to regulate my stress and emotions much better.

Then, I realized that 'use your heart' means mindfulness. Master Cheng Yen planted the seeds of mindfulness in me during the brief encounter. The seeds grew only after more than a decade! It really has become an indispensable asset for me. Mindfulness protects me from being overwhelmed by the intense emotions in palliative care. It gives me a *psychological holiday*. This is why I never take leave due to exhaustion reasons.

The journey of my learning in medicine has been so: first, I learnt when and how to treat in medicine. Second, I learnt when and how to stop, and how to take care of patients after stopping treatment, a skill grossly deficient in most physicians or surgeons. Third, I learnt the delicate balance between giving and stopping treatment. Last but not least, I learnt how to take care of myself.

I have tried my best to summarize what palliative care is in this book. The sequence of the book is as follows, Part I: Introduction to Palliative Care, Part II and III: Symptom Control, Part IV: Management of Death and Dying, Part V: Psychosocial and Spiritual Care and Part VI: Self-Care.

I pray this book will help you in the alleviation of suffering of terminally ill patients and their family members; and introduce you to the wonderful practices of mindfulness in medicine.

Dr Tan Seng Beng
23rd August 2016

You are like a candle. Imagine you are sending light out around you. All your words, thoughts and actions are going in many directions. If you say something kind, your kind words go in many directions, and you yourself go with them.

Thich Nhat Hanh

True Love

Introduction

Love is the foundation of palliative care. Love is to bring happiness. We may be very good in relieving suffering of patients, but that is not enough. We need to be good in bringing happiness to patients too. Thich Nhat Hanh, a Vietnamese Zen Master described true love as following:

Being there

- Love is being there.
- Love is paying one hundred percent attention to our patients when we are with them.
- To be fully there, we may remind ourselves with the following thought: *Dear one, I am here for you.*
- When we are fully present, we feel real. Patients feel real. And life becomes real in the moment.
- This is the greatest gift we can give to our patients.

Recognizing the presence of others

- We can spend a lot of time with our patients, but if we are not recognizing their presence, we cannot bring happiness to them.
- The second thought can be: *Dear one, I know that you are there and it makes me very happy.*

Deep listening

- The next thing we can do is to listen deeply to our patients without judging them.
- As we listen, we do not say anything. We breathe deeply and open our heart to really listen.

- The third thought: *Dear one, I know you are suffering, that is why I am here to listen.*

Loving speech

- After listening to patients and understanding their situations, we speak in such a way that eases suffering and brings comfort.
- The fourth thought: *Dear one, I am aware that how unkind speech brings hurt and loving speech brings comfort. And I will be mindful of my speech.*

Little experiment

When you meet someone today, think to yourself "Dear one, I am here for you." And truly be there for the person.

Do not think that love, in order to be genuine, has to be extraordinary. What we need is to love without getting tired.

Mother Teresa

Dignity and the Essence of Medicine

Introduction

To reinstate kindness, humanity and respect in patient care, Professor Harvey Max Chochinov, a distinguished Professor of Psychiatry, introduced *ABCD of dignity conserving care*.

A=attitude

- Examine our attitude towards patients. Ask ourselves: How would I be feeling in this situation? Am I aware how my attitude may be affecting patients?
- Make a conscious effort in reflecting these questions in each individual patient.
- Discuss this during ward round and teaching. Make this discussion and teaching a culture within the healthcare setting.

B=behaviour

- Modify our behaviour by changing our attitude.
- Treat contact with patients as we would any important clinical intervention, with respect and kindness.

C=compassion

- Get exposed to human life and experiences by listening to patients' stories, reading novels and watching films on life experiences.
- Cultivate ways to show compassion, such as an understanding look, a gentle touch and communication that acknowledges patients' experiences.

D=dialogue

- Acknowledge the personhood beyond the illness.
- Get to know our patient as a person. Ask: What should I know about you as a person to help me take the best care of you that I can?

Little opinion

One of the key components in developing palliative care is education. Teaching medical students about the ABCD of dignity conserving care is as important as teaching them the ABC of resuscitation.

Palliative Care

Introduction

Palliative care comes from the Latin word pallium, which means a cloak. Palliative care can be likened to providing someone with a cloak when he or she is feeling cold.

Little story

I once gave a blanket to a leukemic patient who was feeling cold at the hematology daycare. He was very grateful and he often mentioned my name when he spoke to others. This led me to think that palliative care is a blanket in the modern setting. We are blanket providers.

WHO Definition of palliative care

Palliative care is an approach that

- *Improves quality of life* of patients and their families facing the problem associated with life-limiting illness
- Through the prevention and *relief of suffering* by means of early identification and impeccable assessment and treatment of pain and other problems, physical, psychosocial and spiritual

Explaining the term 'palliative care' to patients

- Palliative care is a specialized medical care provided by a team of specialists to improve quality of life of patients with serious illnesses through reducing pain and suffering.

Communication caution

Exercise caution while using terms like dying, terminal illnesses or life-threatening illnesses to avoid causing unnecessary distress to patients or their families.

Common conditions requiring palliative care

- Cancer
- Organ failure – heart, lung, liver, kidney
- Neurological conditions – motor neuron disease, Parkinson's disease, multiple sclerosis, stroke
- Geriatric conditions – dementia, frailty
- Human immunodeficiency virus infection
- Intensive care unit patients
- Paediatric illnesses

Important concepts of palliative care

- Palliative care is applicable early in the course of illness, in conjunction with other life-prolonging therapies.
- Palliative care is about helping patients to live.

You matter because you are you,
and you matter to the end of your life.
We will do all we can not only to help you die peacefully,
but also to live until you die.

Cicely Saunders

Little story

My colleague and I once brought a terminally ill child to ride LRT (Light Rail Transit). His wish was to ride a train because he used to stay beside a train station but never had a chance to ride one. We took him out for lunch and drove him to take the LRT from one station to another station. He enjoyed the trip a lot. And he passed away not long after the trip.

The Palliative Care Approach

Introduction

The palliative care approach is a vital part of *all clinical practice*, whatever the illness or its stage, informed by knowledge and practice of palliative care principles and supported by specialist palliative care. (NHS Executive 1996)

Palliative care principles

Palliative care principles should be practised by *all health care professionals:*

- Whole person approach
  - Seeing patient as a person
  - Focusing on quality of life
  - Respecting patient autonomy
  - Emphasizing good communication to patients
- Whole family approach
  - Extending care to family
  - Emphasizing good communication to family
- Whole team approach
  - Emphasizing team cooperation
  - Emphasizing caring of the whole team
  - Emphasizing good communication to colleagues
- Whole journey approach
  - Emphasizing care of the entire journey of illness
  - Emphasizing the practice of nonabandonment

Little summary

4 Ws – whole person, whole family, whole team, whole journey

Little reminder

As health care providers, if we are unable to alleviate the suffering of patients, at least we should not contribute to their suffering. Common suffering caused by health care providers are:

- Lack of attention
- Lack of listening
- Lack of empathy
- Lack of communication
- Lack of hope-giving

Remember, never say "There is nothing more can be done" or "There is no more hope".

Palliative Care Referral

Traditional model of palliative care

Curative or life-prolonging treatment	Palliative care

- The traditional practice is to refer palliative care when nothing more can be done to cure or treat the disease.
- This practice often results in increased suffering and late referral (time from referral to death < 2 months).

Integrated model of palliative care

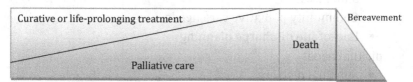

- The integrated model involves palliative care from the start of a life-limiting illness, concurrent with disease-directed care.
- This model is a key to successful patient care. It triggers early referral.
- This model is supported by:
  - World Health Organization (WHO)
  - National Comprehensive Cancer Network (NCCN)
  - American Society of Clinical Oncology (ASCO)
  - European Society for Medical Oncology (ESMO)
- One additional point to decide on referral is whether patient has palliative care needs or not.

Palliative care needs

- Screening question: Is the patient suffering?
- Physical needs
  - Unresolved physical symptoms
  - Complex functional needs
  - Complex nursing needs
- Psychological needs
  - Persistent psychological distress
  - Information needs
  - End-of-life decision-making
  - Advance care planning
- Social needs
  - Caregiver stress
  - Family conflict
  - Staff stress
  - Community palliative care needs
  - End-of-life discharge planning
- Spiritual needs
  - Spiritual distress
  - Existential distress
  - End-of-life discussion
  - End-of-life care
  - Grief and bereavement

Clinical evidence

Temel published a landmark article in New England Journal of Medicine at 2010 reporting improved quality of life and increased median survival of 2.7 months with early palliative care referral in patients with metastatic non-small cell lung cancer.

Palliative Care Assessment

Introduction

A palliative care assessment should focus on finding out the palliative care needs of patients and their family members instead of thinking about our own agenda, such as filling up certain assessment forms.

Physical assessment (symptoms)

- Open-ended questions
    - How are you doing?
    - Are you comfortable?
    - Are there any symptoms that are bothering you?
- Screen for common symptoms
    - Pain
    - Breathlessness
    - Nausea and vomiting
    - Fatigue
    - Constipation
    - Insomnia
- Detailed symptom assessment forms
    - Edmonton Symptom Assessment Scale (ESAS) (10 items) by Eduardo Bruera
    - M.D. Anderson Symptom Inventory (MDASI) (19 items) by Charles Cleeland
    - Memorial Symptom Assessment Scale (MSAS) (32 items) by Russell Portenoy

Physical assessment (functions)

- Open-ended questions
    - What are the things that you do in a day?
    - What are the things that you need help with?
- Screen for problems in performing important activities
    - Bathing
    - Grooming
    - Toileting
    - Ambulating
    - Feeding
    - Shopping
- Assess performance status
    - ECOG score by Oken and Zubrod
    - Barthel index by Mahoney and Barthel
    - Karnofsky Performance Scale by Karnofsky
    - Palliative Performance Scale by Anderson

ECOG (European Cooperative Oncology Group)

- ECOG 0 – asymptomatic
- ECOG 1 – symptomatic but completely ambulatory
- ECOG 2 – symptomatic and <50% in bed during the day
- ECOG 3 – symptomatic and >50% in bed, not bedbound
- ECOG 4 – bedbound
- ECOG 5 – death

Psychological assessment (emotions)

- Open-ended questions
    - How are you feeling today?
    - How are you affected by your emotions?
    - How do you deal with your emotions?
- Screen for distress
    - Distress Thermometer
        - Zero is no distress
        - Ten is extreme distress
- Assess coping mechanisms
    - Problem-focused coping
    - Emotion-focused coping
- Detailed assessment
    - Hospital Anxiety and Depression Scale (HADS) (14 items) by Zigmond and Snaith
    - Mental Adjustment to Cancer Scale (MAC) (40 items) by Watson and Greer
    - Courtauld Emotional Control Scale (CEC) (3 items) by Watson and Greer
    - Cancer Coping Questionnaire (21 items) by Moorey, Frampton and Greer

Psychological assessment (cognitions)

- Open-ended questions to explore ideas, concerns, expectations
    - Are you aware of what is going on?
    - What has the doctor told you about your illness?
    - What are your concerns?
    - What are you hopes?
    - What are your expectations?
- Detailed assessment
    - Cancer Concerns Checklist (14 items)
    - Herth Hope Index (12 items)

- Screen for delirium using Confusion Assessment Method (CAM)
  - Acute onset and fluctuating course
  - Inattention
  - Disorganized thinking
  - Altered level of consciousness

Social assessment (family and friends)

- Open-ended questions
  - Could you tell me about your family?
  - What about your friends?
- Explore
  - Home address for hospice referral
  - Social and cultural background
  - Main caregivers and decision maker
- Draw family tree (genogram)
- Arrange for family meeting
  - Assess family ideas, concerns and expectations
  - Explore caregiver stress and coping
  - Explore family dynamics

Spiritual assessment

- Open-ended questions
  - Could you tell me about your experience of illness?
  - Could you tell me a little about yourself?
  - What is important to you now?
  - How is your quality of life affected by your illness?
  - Could you tell me about your religion?
- Use FICA spiritual history tool
  - F = Tell me about your *faith*
  - I = What *importance* does your faith have in your life?
  - C = Are you part of a spiritual *community*?
  - A = How would you like me to *address* these issues?

- Quality of life assessment forms
    - Short Form 8 (SF-8)
    - Short Form 12 (SF-12)
    - Short Form 36 (SF-36)
    - WHO Quality of Life Assessment Form (WHOQOL)
    - Functional Assessment of Chronic Illness Therapy .– Spiritual Well-being (FACIT-Sp-12)
    - European Organization for Research and Treatment of Cancer – Quality of Life Questionnaire (EORTC-QLQ-C30)
- Palliative care specific quality of life assessment forms
    - McGill Quality of Life Questionnaire (MQOL)
    - Health-related Quality of Life for the dying (HRQOL)
    - Missoula-VITAS Quality of Life Index
    - Schedule for the Evaluation of Individual Quality of Life (SEIQOL)

Peeling the onion

Assessing a palliative care patient can be seen like peeling an onion. The first layer is the physical layer. Second is psychological. Third is social. The innermost is the spiritual core. If patients feel that we care, they will be more willing to allow us to peel their deeper layers of difficulties and suffering. If not, we will only see their surfaces.

Little opinion

It is not uncommon for patients to express their frustration when they are being asked too many questions, especially so when they are already very tired. We may have our personal agendas like filling up certain assessment forms or exploration of psychosocial issues, but the most important thing is to find out what are the agendas of patients, not ours.

Pain Terms

Introduction

Pain is defined by IASP (International Association for the Study of Pain) as an unpleasant sensory and emotional experience associated with actual or potential tissue damage. It is a subjective experience. Margo McCaffrey, an American Pain Management Nurse described pain as what the person says it is.

Background pain

- Constant or continuous pain of long duration, ≥12h/day (Ferrell 1999)
- Also called basal pain, baseline pain or persistent pain
- Treated with around-the-clock (ATC) medication

Breakthrough pain

- A transitory exacerbation of pain experienced by the patient who has relatively stable and adequately controlled baseline pain (Portenoy 2004)
- Also called episodic pain, exacerbation of pain, pain flare, transient pain, transitory pain
- Treated with rescue medication

Types of breakthrough pain (Davis 2005)

- Spontaneous pain (idiopathic pain) – unexpected pain
- Incident pain (precipitated pain) – pain caused by movement
- End-of-dose failure – pain caused by declining analgesic level

Types of incident pain
<ul><li>Volitional – eating, drinking, swallowing, walking, turning</li><li>Non-volitional – coughing, sneezing, urinating, defecating</li><li>Procedural – investigation (blood taking), therapeutic procedures (intravenous line insertion, wound dressing)</li></ul>

Pain terminology

- Nociceptive pain is pain transmitted through a normal nervous system
- Neuropathic pain is pain transmitted through a damaged nervous system
- Sensitization is increased responsiveness of neurons to their normal input
- Allodynia is pain due to a stimulus that does not normally provoke pain
- Hyperalgesia is increased pain from a stimulus that normally provokes pain
- Hyperpathia is a painful syndrome characterized by an abnormally painful reaction to a stimulus

I coined the term 'total pain,' from my understanding that dying people have physical, spiritual, psychological, and social pain that must be treated.

Cicely Saunders

Types of Pain

Introduction

Making an effort to differentiate nociceptive pain from neuropathic pain is important in pain management.

Types of pain

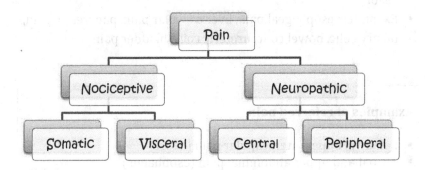

Frequency of cancer pain

- Mixed nociceptive-neuropathic – most common
- Nociceptive – second common
- Neuropathic – third common

Nociceptive pain (superficial somatic pain)

- Pain is usually superficial, sharp and well-localized
- Examples: superficial wound, small pressure sore, cellulitis, abscess, skin metastasis, mucositis and perianal excoriation

Nociceptive pain (deep somatic pain)

- Pain is deep, dull, aching and less well-localized
- Examples: deep wound, huge pressure sore, muscle spasm, chest wall infiltration, psoas infiltration, arthritis, acetabular syndrome, bone metastasis

Nociceptive pain (visceral pain)

- Pain is usually deep, dull and poorly localized
- Associated with referred pain in somatic sites distant from the lesion
- Examples: esophageal pain, liver capsular pain, pancreatic pain, biliary colic, bowel colic, ureteric colic, bladder pain

---

Examples of referred pain

- Left arm, upper interscapular pain (heart)
- Throat and upper abdominal pain (esophagus)
- Epigastric and lower interscapular pain (stomach)
- Back pain (pancreas)
- Right shoulder pain (liver and gallbladder)
- Supraumbilical pain (small bowel)
- Periumbilical pain (appendix)
- Infraumbilical (large bowel)
- Paraumbilical pain (ovary)
- Loin to groin pain (ureter)
- Suprapubic pain (bladder)

Neuropathic pain (central neuropathic pain)

- Pain can be burning, shooting, stabbing, crushing
- Examples: stroke (most common), Parkinson's disease, multiple sclerosis, syringomyelia and cord compression

Neuropathic pain (peripheral neuropathic pain)

- Pain can be burning, shooting, lancinating
- Pain can present as dysesthesia
- Examples: cranial neuropathy, brachial or lumbosacral plexopathy, radiculopathy, peripheral neuropathy (tumour infiltration, chemotherapy like cisplatin, oxaliplatin, vincristine, vinblastine, paclitaxel, thalidomide, post-radiotherapy, post-radical neck dissection, post-mastectomy, post-thoracotomy, post-herpetic neuralgia)

Interesting fact

The brain has no pain receptors. Brain metastasis itself does not cause pain. Headache from brain metastasis is due to pressure on surrounding nerves and blood vessels.

Pain Receptors

Introduction

Pain receptors (nociceptors) transduce noxious stimuli to electrical activities.

Location of nociceptors

- Cutaneous nociceptors are free nerve endings that end at stratum granulosum of epidermis.
- 5 layers of epidermis
  - Stratum corneum
  - Stratum lucidum
  - Stratum granulosum
  - Stratum spinosum
  - Stratum basale

Types of nociceptors (based on conduction)

- Aδ fibers
  - Myelinated fibers
  - Fast conduction at 20m/s
  - Responsible for fast pain or first pain, which is sharp, brief, pricking and well-localized
  - Distributed over body surfaces, muscles and joints
- C fibers
  - Unmyelinated fibers
  - Slow conduction at 2m/s
  - Responsible for slow pain or second pain, which is dull, prolonged, aching, burning and poorly-localized
  - Distributed over most tissues, including visceral tissues, except the brain

Types of nociceptors (based on modalities)

- High threshold mechanoreceptors
  - Aδ fibers
  - Respond to mechanical stimuli only
- Polymodal nociceptors
  - C fibers
  - Respond to multiple modalities
- Silent nociceptors
  - Not respond to any stimuli but may be recruited during tissue injury

Types of nociceptors (based on stimuli)

- Noxious hot stimuli
  - TRPV1-4 (transient receptor potential vanilloid receptor)
- Noxious cold stimuli
  - TRPM8 (transient receptor potential melastatin receptor)
  - TRPA1 (transient receptor potential ankyrin receptor)
- Noxious mechanical stimuli
  - DEG (degenerin receptor)
  - DRASIC (dorsal root acid sensing ion channel receptor)
  - TWIK-1 (tandem pore domain weakly inward-rectifying K channel)
  - TREK-1 (tandem pore domain related K channel)
- Noxious chemical stimuli
  - TRPV1 (transient receptor potential vanilloid receptor)
  - P2X3 (purinoreceptor)
  - ASIC (acid sensing ion channel receptor)
  - DRASIC (dorsal root acid sensing ion channel receptor)

> **Interesting fact:** The spicy sensation of eating chilli is caused by the activation of vanilloid receptors (TRPV1). The pungent sensation of eating wasabi is caused by the activation of ankyrin receptors (TRPA1).

Primary Afferent Neurons

Introduction

Aδ fibers and C fibers are pseudounipolar neurons with cell bodies within dorsal root ganglions. They are primary afferent neurons (first order neurons) which synapse at dorsal horn of spinal cord.

Dorsal horn of spinal cord

- In early 1950s, Bror Rexed identified ten layers of grey matter at the spinal cord.
- They are labelled Rexed laminae I-X.
- The first six laminae are at the dorsal horn.
    - Marginal nucleus (lamina I)
    - Substantia gelatinosa of Rolando (lamina II)
    - Nucleus proprius (lamina III, IV and V)
    - Lamina VI

Synapses of primary afferent neurons

- Aδ fibers
    - Transmit fast pain messages
    - Synapse with second order neuron at lamina I and outer part of lamina II to form neospinothalamic tract
- C fibers
    - Transmit slow pain messages
    - Synapse with interneurons at inner part of lamina II which synapse with second order neurons at lamina V
    - Also synapse with dendrites of second order neurons extending from lamina V
    - Second order neurons form the paleospinothalamic tract

Neurotransmitters

Introduction

Neurotransmitters can be excitatory or inhibitory. The two types of excitatory neurotrasmitters for pain transmission are glutamate and substance P.

Glutamate

- Most common excitatory neurotransmitter
- Major neurotransmitter released from Aδ fibers
- Binds to glutamate receptor:
    - Ionotropic glutamate receptor
        - AMPA receptor
        - NMDA receptor
        - Kainate receptor (role undefined)
    - Metabotropic glutamate receptor

AMPA receptor (AMPAR)

- AMPA: α-amino-3-hydroxy-5-methyl-4-isoxazolepropionic acid
- GluR1, GluR2, GluR3 and GluR4 subunits
- Causes Na^{2+} influx with minimal K^+ efflux
- Generates excitatory post-synaptic potential (EPSP)
- Mediates fast synaptic transmission

NMDA receptor (NMDAR)

- NMDA: N-methyl-D-aspartate
- NR1 and NR2 subunits
- Sufficient depolarization by AMPAR removes Mg^{2+} which blocks the NMDAR
- Causes Na^{2+} and Ca^{2+} influx

- Ca^{2+} influx activates Ca^{2+}/calmodulin-dependent protein kinase II (CaMKII) and protein kinase C (PKC)
- Causes long-term potentiation (LTP) through modifying structure and number of synapses (synaptic plasticity)
- NMDAR also plays a role in glutamate excitotoxicity, where excess Ca^{2+} influx activates calcium-dependent proteases and lipases, degrading proteins and lipids, causing cell death

Metabotropic glutamate receptor

- mGluR1, mGluR2, mGluR3, mGluR4, mGluR5, mGluR6, mGluR7 and mGluR8 subunits
- G-protein-coupled receptor (GPCR)
- Activates phosphoinositol system postsynaptically and increases NMDAR activity or inhibits cyclic AMP system presynaptically and decreases NMDAR activity
- Modulates the activity of NMDAR and regulates neuron vulnerability to glutamate excitotoxicity

Substance P

- Tachykinin neuropeptide
- Major neurotransmitter released from C fibers
- Binds to neurokinin-1 receptor (NK-1), a GPCR which activates the phosphoinositol system
- Integrates pain, stress and anxiety

Little fact

NMDAR plays a crucial role in learning and memory formation.

Ascending Pain Pathways

Introduction

Pain pathway can be ascending or descending. Ascending pain pathways transmit pain impulses to cortex. Descending pain pathways modulate pain transmission.

Projection neurons (Second order neurons)

- Types of projection neurons
    - Nociceptive specific neurons
        - Respond to noxious stimuli only
    - Wide dynamic range neurons (WDR)
        - Respond to all sensory modalities
        - Important in wind-up phenomena
- Cross midline to form lateral and medial pain pathway

Lateral pain pathway (Neospinothalamic tract)

- Fast pain pathway
- A δ fibers synapse with projection neurons at lamina I (marginal nucleus) and outer part of lamina II of dorsal horn
- Cross at anterior white commissure of spinal cord
- Ascend as lateral spinothalamic tract (LST)
- Synapse with third order neurons at ventral posterior lateral (VPL) and ventral posterior inferior (VPI) nuclei of lateral thalamus
- Third order neurons extend from lateral thalamus to primary somatosensory cortex (SI)
- Responsible for sensory-discriminatory component of pain, like location, intensity and quality

Medial pain pathway (Paleospinothalamic tract)

- Slow pain pathway
- C fibers synapse with interneurons at inner part of lamina II (substantia gelatinosa) of dorsal horn
- Interneurons synapse at lamina V
- Cross at anterior white commissure of spinal cord
- Ascend as anterior spinothalamic tract (AST)
- 1/10 of fibers synapse with third order neurons at intralaminar nuclei (parafascicular and centromedian PF-CM complex) of medial thalamus
- Third order neurons extend from medial thalamus to the whole cortex diffusely, notably secondary somatosensory cortex (SII), anterior cingulate cortex and insular cortex
- Responsible for affective-adversive component of pain, like negative emotions and unpleasantness
- Remaining fibers terminate at:
    - Tectum of midbrain (spinotectal tract): turning eyes, head, trunk toward sources of pain (visuospinal effect)
    - Periaqueductal gray of midbrain (spinomesencephalic tract): descending pain inhibition
    - Reticular formation (spinoreticular tract): arousal effect
        - From reticular formation to hypothalamus (spinohypothalamic tract): autonomic effects
        - From reticular formation to limbic system (spinolimbic tract): fear (amygdala)

Face and head

- Trigeminothalamic tract
    - Sends fast discriminative pain messages to ventral posterior medial nucleus (VPM) of lateral thalamus
    - Sends slow affective pain messages to intralaminar nuclei of medial thalamus and reticular formation

Descending Pain Pathways

Introduction

Descending pain pathways can be excitatory or inhibitory. Only inhibitory pathways or antinociceptive pathways are described here.

Reticular formation

- A polysynaptic network in brainstem
- Filters sensory information
- Antinociceptive neurons in reticular formation:
    - Serotonergic neurons
    - Noradrenergic neurons

Serotonergic pathways

- Periaqueductal gray matter (PAG) in midbrain sends excitatory projection to magnus raphe nucleus (MRN) in medulla.
- MRN descends bilaterally as raphespinal tract within the posterolateral tract of Lissauer to end in substantia gelatinosa at all levels of the spinal cord.
- Releases serotonin to excite inhibitory interneurons in dorsal horn – GABAergic and enkephalinergic
- Inhibitory interneurons inhibit pain transmission from first to second order neurons through inhibiting the transmission of impulse from excitatory interneurons to projection neurons of medial pain pathway, presynaptically or postsynaptically.
- This is called gating, which means the control of synaptic transmission from one set of neurons to the next.
- Inhibit slow pain pathway

GABAergic interneurons

- Release gamma-aminobutyric acid (GABA), which is the chief inhibitory neurotransmitter in CNS
- $GABA_A$ receptors – ionotropic receptors that generate inhibitory post-synaptic potentials by causing Cl^- influx
- $GABA_B$ receptors – metabotropic receptors or GPCRs that cause hyperpolarization indirectly by reducing cyclic AMP and directly by expelling K^+ through G-protein inwardly rectifying K^+ channels (GIRK channels)

Enkephalinergic interneurons

- Also called opiate interneurons
- Enkephalin, like endorphin, endomorphin, dynorphin and nociceptin, is an endogenous opioid. It acts on opioid receptor.
- Opioid receptors are GPCRs:
  - Inhibit neurotransmitter release by inhibiting N-type Ca^{2+} channels presynaptically
  - Inhibit adenylate cyclase presynaptically, causing reduction in cAMP and reduction in neurotransmitter release
  - Open voltage sensitive K^+ channels, causing K^+ efflux and postsynaptic hyperpolarization
- Three main opioid receptors – μ, δ and K
- The endogenous ligands of opioid receptors:
  - Enkephalins act on δ opioid receptors.
  - β-Endorphins act on μ and δ opioid receptors.
  - Endomorphins act on μ opioid receptors.
  - Dynorphins act on K receptors.
  - Nociceptins (Orphanin FQ) act on nociceptin receptors (NOP, ORL-1).

Noradrenergic pathways

- For the noradrenergic pathways, cerulean nucleus or locus ceruleus at the floor of fourth ventricle at upper pons descends bilaterally as ceruleospinal tract to end in dorsal horn to inhibit projection neurons of both medial and lateral pain pathways directly.
- Inhibit both fast and slow pain pathways

Differences between nociception and pain

Nociception refers to the processing and transmission of harmful messages to the brain in the form of electrical activities. Pain refers to the complex sensory, psychological, social and spiritual experiencing of such messages. Pain is often magnified by self-cherishing negative thoughts about 'I'. Examples:

- I feel bad.
- I do not want to feel bad.
- I am suffering.
- I do not want to live.

If we are able to remove these thoughts, pain may be reduced to pure nociception. Then we can say, "Nociception is inevitable. Pain is optional."

Miscellaneous Antinociceptive Pathways

Introduction

Apart from the descending pain pathways, pain can also be suppressed by the following pathways.

Tactile-induced analgesia

- Pain relief with rubbing the painful area and TENS
- Aβ fibers give off collaterals to GABA interneurons to inhibit excitatory interneurons which pass pain messages from C fibers to projection neurons

Diffuse noxious inhibitory controls

- Pain relief with acupuncture and pain elsewhere
- Pain elsewhere activates MRN via spinoreticular or trigeminoreticular tract, which in turn inhibits pain

Stress-induced analgesia

- Absence of pain awareness during fight and flight response
- Stress causes hypothalamus to release β-endorphins which disinhibit the inhibitory interneurons of PAG, activating the serotonergic pathways

Thalamic gating

- Serotonergic and noadrenergic afferents send projections to ventral and intralaminar nuclei of thalamus, gating pain transmission in thalamus

Interesting facts

In a study by Zeidan in 2011, practicing mindfulness meditation 20 minutes daily for 4 days reduced pain sensitivity.

fMRI findings:

- Deactivation of primary somatosensory cortex (SI) – sensory discrimination of pain
- Deactivation of thalamus – thalamic gate control of pain
- Activation of anterior cingulate cortex (ACC) – cognitive regulation of pain processing
- Activation of right anterior insula (AI) – interoceptive awareness
- Activation of bilateral orbitofrontal cortex (OFC) – emotional regulation of pain processing

Greatest activation of right AI and bilateral ACC correlates with greatest reduction in pain intensity. Greatest activation of bilateral OFC plus greatest deactivation of thalamus correlate with greatest reduction in pain unpleasantness.

Peripheral Sensitization

Introduction

Repetitive pain transmission can cause structural and functional changes in the neural system, sensitizing the pain pathways and making pain worse.

Pathophysiology

- Peripheral sensitization is caused by sensitization of nociceptors by inflammatory mediators released from damaged tissues and activated immune and inflammatory cells.
- Characterized by spontaneous pain, hyperalgesia and allodynia
- Spontaneous pain is caused by direct activation of specific receptors on nociceptor terminals by inflammatory mediators
- Hyperalgesia and allodynia are caused by:
    - Early post-translational changes of nociceptors
    - Later transcriptional-dependent changes in effector genes

Post-translational changes of nociceptors

- Inflammatory mediators activate intracellular signaling pathways
    - Protein kinase A (PKA)
    - Protein kinase C (PKC)
- Protein kinases phosphorylate membrane receptors
    - TRPV1 receptors
    - Tetrodotoxin-resistant sodium channels (TTXr)

Transcriptional-dependent changes of nociceptors

- Nerve growth factors (NGFs) play a key role
- NGFs bind tyrosine kinase A receptors (TrkA)
- NGF-TrkA complexes are internalized and transported from peripheral terminals to cell bodies of dorsal root ganglion
- Activate transcriptional factors
  - cAMP-responsive element-binding protein (CREB)
    - Also activated by CaMK via calcium influx
  - Mitogen-activated protein kinases (MAPK)
    - Extracellular signal-regulated kinases (ERK)
    - C-Jun N-terminal kinases (JNK)
    - P38 enzymes
- Increase TRPV1 and TTXr at peripheries
- Increase substance P, calcitonin gene-related peptide (CGRP) and brain-derived neurotrophic factor (BDNF) at synapses

---

Interesting facts

Tetrodotoxin is a potent sodium channel blocker produced by pufferfish. Ingestion causes paraesthesia of lips and tongue within 30 minutes, then face and extremities, followed by paralysis of voluntary muscles, including diaphragm, and even death.

Inflammatory Mediators

Introduction

The cardinal features of inflammation described by Aulus Cornelius Celcus, a Roman encyclopaedist, are pain (dolor), redness (rubor), heat (calor) and swelling (tumor). Various plasma-derived and cell-derived inflammatory mediators are involved in peripheral sensitization.

Plasma-derived mediators

- Kinin system (Bradykinin is involved in pain)
- Coagulation system (Thrombin is involved in pain)
- Fibrinolysis system
- Complement system

Cell-derived mediators

- Preformed mediators in secretory granules
  - Histamine
  - Serotonin
- Newly synthesized mediators
  - Eicosanoids
  - Cytokines
  - Nitric oxide

Miscellaneous mediators

- Protons
- Adenosine
- Glutamate
- Substance P
- Nerve growth factor

Bradykinin

- Produced by proteolytic cleavage of kininogen
- Activation of B1 receptors releases prostaglandins
- Activation of B2 receptors sensitizes TRPV1 via PKC

Thrombin

- Produced by proteolytic cleavage of prothrombin
- Activation of PAR1 (proteinase-activated receptors) releases histamine, substance P, calcitonin gene-related peptide (CGRP), cytokines

Histamine

- Released from mast cell by substance P, IL-1, CGRP and NGF
- Produces itch at low concentration
- Produces pain at high concentration
- Activation of H1 receptors increases Ca^{2+} influx and evokes release of neuropeptides and eicosanoids

Serotonin

- Released from platelets by platelet activating factor
- Activation of 5-HT1 receptors decreases K^+ permeability
- Activation of 5-HT2 receptors decreases K^+ permeability
- Activation of 5-HT3 receptors increases Na^+ influx
- Activation of 5-HT4 receptors sensitizes TTXr via PKA

Eicosanoids

- Step 1: Liberation of arachidonic acid from cell membranes by phospholipase A2 (inhibited by steroids)
- Step 2: Metabolism of arachidonic acid to prostaglandin by cyclooxygenase or to leukotriene by 5-lipooxygenase
- Activation of prostaglandin receptors (EP1) by prostaglandin E2 (PGE2) sensitizes TRPV1 via PKC

- Activation of prostaglandin receptors (IP) by prostacyclin (PGI2) sensitizes TTXr via PKA
- Activation of leukotriene B4 receptors (BLTR) by leukotriene B4 releases 8R, 15SdiHETE from leucocytes to sensitize nociceptors

Cytokines

- Polypeptides produced by lymphocytes and macrophages
- TNF-α, IL-1β and IL-6
- Release eicosanoids
- Increase expression of bradykinin and NGF receptors

Nitric oxide (Endothelium-derived relaxing factor EDRF)

- Released from endothelium
- Sensitizes TRPV1 and TRPA1 through S-nitrosylation

Protons

- Released from inflamed tissue
- Low pH sensitizes DRASIC/ASIC-3
- Low pH sensitizes TRPV1

Adenosine and ATP

- Released from inflamed tissue
- Activation of adenosine A2 receptors by adenosine decreases K^+ permeability
- Activation of purinergic receptors (P2X3) by ATP sensitizes nociceptors

Glutamate

- Presence of peripheral glutamate receptors (iGlu and mGlu)
- Role in peripheral sensitization

Substance P

- Released from C fibers
- Activation of NK1 increases prostaglandins

Nerve growth factor

- Produced by fibroblasts and mast cells
- Binds tyrosine kinase A receptor (TrkA)
- Sensitizes TRPV1
- Enhances release of substance P and CGRP
- Increases expression of TRPV1 and TTXr at peripheries
- Increases expression of substance P, CGRP, BDNF at synapses

Little story

I used to aspire to be a neurologist because I love to memorize facts and make difficult diagnoses. But I changed my mind to subspecialize in Palliative Medicine after joining Hospis Malaysia. I noticed the difference between being competent and being caring. The former emphasized knowledge, skills and efficiency (brain). The latter involved love, compassion and spending more time to comfort patients (heart). Both sets of values are important, but I was so moved by my experiences that I chose the latter. I followed my heart.

Intracellular Signaling Pathways

Introduction

Extracellular messages from inflammatory mediators (first messengers) may be propagated intracellularly by second messengers via various intracellular signaling pathways. These pathways include the cAMP pathway, the phosphoinositol pathway, the MAPK pathway and the JAK/STAT pathway.

The cAMP pathway

- Activation of GPCR by first messenger
- Release of G_α subunit to link with GTP
- Conversion of ATP to cAMP with adenylate cyclase
- cAMP is a second messenger
- Activation of protein kinase A (PKA) by cAMP
    - Phosphorylates ion channel
    - Phosphorylates protein
    - Activates transcription factor CREB

The phosphoinositol pathway

- Activation of GPCR by first messenger
- Release of G_α subunit to link with phospholipase C (PLC)
- PLC splits phosphatidylinositol 4, 5-biphosphate (PIP2), a membrane phospholipid, into diacylglycerol (DAG) and inositol 1, 4, 5-triphosphate (IP3)
- DAG and IP3 are second messengers
- Activation of protein kinase C by DAG
    - Phosphorylates ion channel
    - Phosphorylates protein
    - Activates transcription factor via MAPK

- IP3
  - Opens calcium channel
  - Releases Ca^{2+} from smooth endoplasmic reticulum
  - Binds calmodulin
  - Activates Ca^{2+}/calmodulin-dependent protein kinase
  - Activates transcription factor CREB

The MAPK pathway

- Activation of tyrosine kinase receptor by growth factor
- Activation of GTP-binding protein Ras
- Ras-GTP is a second messenger
- Interaction with Raf protein kinase (MAP kinase kinase kinase)
- Raf phosphorylates MEK (MAP kinase kinase)
- MEK phosphorylates ERK (MAP kinase)
- ERK phosphorylates transcription factors
  - C-Myc
  - Elk-1
  - C-Fos
  - C-Jun
- ERK also phosphorylates transcription factor CREB via Rsk2 activation

The JAK/STAT pathway

- Activation of cytokine receptor by cytokine
- Activation of Janus kinase (JAK)
- Activation of signal transducer and activator of transcription (STAT) proteins
- Translocation to nucleus
- Stimulation of transcription of target genes
- No second messenger

Central Sensitization

Introduction

Peripheral sensitization mediates pain hypersensitivity at the injured site (primary hyperalgesia). It continues as long as the peripheral pathology is present. Central sensitization mediates pain hypersensitivity at the uninjured site surrounding the injury (secondary hyperalgesia). It continues even if the peripheral pathology is no longer present.

Pathophysiology

- Central sensitization is caused by sensitization of spinal neurons by neurotransmitters released from C fibers
- Characterized by secondary hyperalgesia and allodynia
- Secondary hyperalgesia and allodynia are caused by:
    - Early post-translational changes of spinal neurons
    - Later transcriptional-dependent changes of spinal neurons

Post-translational changes of spinal neurons

- Repetitive activation of C fibers causes temporal summation of second pain (TSSP), resulting in wind-up phenomena
    - TTSP: each 'second pain' of C fibers becomes stronger and spreads outside the area of injury
    - Wind-up phenomena: like tightening the spring
- Release of neurotransmitters from C fibers
    - Glutamate binds AMPAR – depolarization, Na^+ influx
    - Glutamate binds group I mGluR – activates PKC
    - Substance P binds NK1 – activates PKA and PKC
    - CGRP binds CGRP1 – activates PKA and PKC

- Brain-derived neurotrophic factor (BDNF) binds tyrosine kinase B receptor (TrkB) – activates PKC
- Activation of NMDAR
  - Key step in central sensitization
  - NMDAR is blocked by Mg^{2+} under normal condition
  - Sustained release of glutamate and neuropeptides leads to sufficient depolarization that removes Mg^{2+} block, activating NMDAR
  - Na^+ and Ca^{2+} influx
- Increase in intracellular Ca^{2+}
  - Caused by:
    - Ca^{2+} influx through NMDARs (predominant)
    - Ca^{2+} influx through calcium-permeable AMPARs
    - Ca^{2+} influx through voltage-gated calcium channels
    - Ca^{2+} release from endoplasmic reticulum in response to mGluR-NMDAR coupling (IP3-mediated)
  - Activates protein kinases
    - Calcium/calmodulin-dependent protein kinase II (CaMKII)
    - Protein kinase C (PKC)
    - Mitogen-activated protein kinase/extracellular-signal-regulated kinase (MAPK/ERK) via PKC
- Activated protein kinases
  - Phosphorylate membrane AMPARs and NMDARs
    - PKA (via neuropeptides)
    - PKC
    - CaMKII
    - MAPK
  - Recruit AMPARs to membrane
    - PKA (via neuropeptides)
    - CaMKII
    - MAPK

- Result in increased neuronal excitability

Transcriptional-dependent changes of spinal neurons

- Activated protein kinase MAPK
  - Phosphorylates transcription factors
    - cAMP response element binding (CREB)
    - ELK-1
  - Causes genes transcription
    - Immediate-early genes (IEG)
      - c-Fos
      - Cox-2 – produces prostaglandin for neural and glial cell plasticity (apoptosis, axonal sprouting, new afferent connections)
    - Late-response genes
      - NK1
      - TrkB
      - Dynorphin – increases neuronal excitability
  - Results in increased protein production
    - Synaptic plasticity
      - Modification of structure of synapses
      - Modification of number of synapses
    - Sustained neuronal excitability

Interesting theory

Hebbian theory: Cells that fire together, wire together. Cells that fire out of sync, lose their link.

Pain Assessment

Introduction

A comprehensive pain assessment involves taking a detailed history, performing a targeted examination and ordering relevant investigations.

History taking

- Open-ended question: Could you tell me about your pain?
- Mnemonic: SOCRATES
  - S = Site
  - O = Onset
  - C = Character
  - R = Radiation
  - A = Associated symptoms
  - T = Time
  - E = Exacerbating and relieving factors
  - S = Severity

Determining the type of pain

- Nociceptive pain (superficial somatic pain)
  - Described as superficial, sharp, burning, cutting, pricking, tingling and stabbing pain
  - Well-localized around injured tissues
- Nociceptive pain (deep somatic pain)
  - Described as deep, dull, cramping, aching, throbbing, boring, and crushing pain
  - Less well-localized around injured tissues

- Nociceptive pain (visceral pain)
  - Described as vague, dull, aching, cramping, squeezing, gnawing and pressure pain
  - Poorly-localized in relation to affected organ
  - Presence of referred pain remote from the location of the affected organ
  - Presence of visceral hyperalgesia with pain during normal functioning of affected organ
- Neuropathic pain
  - Described as constant, burning, tingling and numbing in dysesthetic pain
  - Described as episodic, electric-like, shooting, stabbing, lancinating and jabbing in lancinating pain
  - Localized to area innervated by damaged nerves
  - Presence of central sensitization with persistent pain, hyperalgesia and allodynia
  - Presence of neurological symptoms like anaesthesia, paraesthesia, dysesthesia and paralysis

Determining the cause of pain

- Cancer-related pain
  - Bone pain syndromes (most common)
    - Head: skull metastases
    - Chest: rib metastases
    - Back: vertebral metastases
    - Pelvis: acetabular metastases
    - Limbs: pathological fracture
  - Visceral pain syndromes (second common)
    - Head: brain metastases
    - Chest: mediastinal metastases
    - Abdomen: liver metastases, peritoneal metastases, bowel obstruction, ureteric obstruction

- Back: pancreatic cancer, retroperitoneal infiltration
- Pelvis: gynaecological cancer, bladder spasm, rectal spasm, perineal pain
- Neuropathic pain syndromes (third common)
  - Head: leptomeningeal metastases, cranial neuralgias
  - Chest: brachial plexopathy, intercostal neuropathy
  - Abdomen: celiac plexopathy
  - Back: spinal cord compression, radiculopathy
  - Pelvis: lumbosacral plexopathy
  - Limbs: peripheral neuropathy
- Treatment-related pain
  - Chemotherapy-related pain
    - Chemotherapy-induced headache
      - Intrathecal methotrexate meningitic syndrome
      - L-asparaginase-related dural sinus thrombosis
      - Trans-retinoic acid headache
    - Chemotherapy mucositis
    - 5-Fluorouracil-induced angina
    - Post-chemotherapy gynaecomastia
    - Hormonal therapy pain flare
    - Interferon-induced pain
    - Diffuse bone pain from trans-retinoic acid or colony stimulating factor
    - Steroid pseudorheumatism
    - Intravenous steroid-induced perineal discomfort
    - Peripheral neuropathy
    - Intravenous infusion pain
    - Hand-foot syndrome
  - Radiotherapy-related pain
    - Radiation mucositis
    - Radiation brachial plexopathy
    - Radiation enteritis

- Radiation myelopathy
- Radiation cystitis
- Radiation proctitis
- Avascular necrosis
- Surgery-related pain
    - Post-radical neck dissection pain
    - Post-mastectomy pain
    - Post-thoracotomy pain
    - Phantom pain
        - Phantom breast pain
        - Phantom bladder pain
        - Phantom anus pain
        - Phantom limb pain

Determining the pattern of pain

- Background and breaktrough pain
- Fluctuation in location, severity and quality
- Frequency of breakthrough pain
- Aggravating and relieving factors
- Analgesic history, including pain score pre and post-analgesia

Determining the impact of pain

- Activities of daily living
- Instrumental activities
- Leisure activities

Determining the perception of pain

- Ideas, concerns and expectations regarding pain
- Ideas, concerns and expectations regarding analgesia
- Ideas, concerns and expectations of family members
- Associated emotions
- Pain and suffering

Bone Pain Syndromes

Introduction

Cancer-induced bone pain has a nociceptive component caused by skeletal remodelling and inflammatory mediators; and a neuropathic component caused by damage to sensory and sympathetic nerves together with pathological sprouting. Bone pain syndromes caused by skull metastases, rib metastases, vertebral metastases and acetabular metastases will be discussed.

Skull metastases

- Orbital syndrome
    - Metastasis to bony orbit
    - Unilateral supraorbital pain
    - Dull, continuous and progressive
    - Associated features (ipsilateral)
        - Proptosis, chemosis, papilloedema
        - Complete ophthalmoplegia (III, IV, VI)
        - Reduced sensation of V1
- Parasellar syndrome
    - Also called sphenocavernous syndrome
    - Metastasis to petrous apex or sella turcica with secondary extension to cavernous sinus
    - Unilateral frontal pain
    - Dull, continuous and progressive
    - Associated features (ipsilateral)
        - Proptosis, chemosis, papilloedema
        - Hemianopia or quadrantanopia
        - Complete ophthalmoplegia (III, IV, VI)
        - Reduced sensation of V1 and V2

- Middle fossa syndrome
  - Also called Gasserion ganglion syndrome
  - Metastasis to middle fossa
  - Unilateral facial pain
  - Dull, continuous and progressive
  - May have lancinating facial pain (trigeminal neuralgia)
  - Associated features (ipsilateral)
    - Reduced sensation of V2 and V3
    - Weakness of pterygoids and masseters muscles
- Jugular foramen syndrome
  - Metastasis to jugular foramen
  - Unilateral occipital or postauricular headache
  - Exacerbated by movement
  - May have lancinating throat pain (glossopharyngeal neuralgia)
  - Associated features (ipsilateral)
    - Horner's syndrome
    - Hoarseness and dysphagia (IX, X)
    - Neck weakness (XI)
    - Syncope
- Occipital condyle syndrome
  - Metastasis to occipital condyle
  - Unilateral occipital headache or neck pain
  - Exacerbated by neck flexion and rotation
  - Severe, continuous and progressive
  - Associated features (ipsilateral)
    - Neck stiffness
    - Dysarthria and dysphagia due to tongue paresis (XII)
- Clivus syndrome
  - Metastasis to clivus (front of foramen magnum)
  - Vertex headache
  - Exacerbated by neck flexion

- Associated features (ipsilateral, then bilateral)
    - Diplopia (VI)
    - Facial weakness (VII)
    - Hoarseness, dysarthria and dysphagia (IX, X)
    - Neck weakness (XI)
    - Tongue weakness (XII)
- Sphenoid sinus syndrome
    - Metastasis to sphenoid sinus
    - Bifrontal headache and retroorbital pain
    - Radiating to temporal regions
    - Associated features
        - Nasal stuffiness
        - Diplopia (unilateral or bilateral VI)

Rib metastases

- Rib metastasis – no pain or mild pain
- Rib fracture – transient severe chest pain triggered by:
    - Trunk movement (bending, lateral bending and twisting) due to attachment of abdominal muscles to lower ribs
    - Deep breathing
    - Coughing
    - Laughing

Vertebral body syndromes

- Odontoid process syndrome
    - Severe neck pain
    - Radiating to occiput and vertex
    - Exacerbated by neck flexion
    - Progressive sensory and motor involvement beginning in upper limbs

- C7-T1 syndrome
  - Dull lower neck pain
  - Radiating to shoulders and interscapular area
  - May have C7-T1 radicular pain
  - May have C7-T1 percussion tenderness
  - Associated with Horner's syndrome
- T12-L1 syndrome
  - Dull midback pain
  - Radiating anteriorly causing a girdle-like band or to both paraspinal and lumbosacral areas
  - Exacerbated by lying or sitting but relieved by standing
  - May have referred pain to sacroiliac joint and iliac crest
  - May have T12-L1 radicular pain
- Sacral syndrome
  - Localized severe low back pain or coccygeal pain
  - Radiating to buttocks, perineum or posterior thigh
  - Exacerbated by lying or sitting but relieved by walking
  - Lateral extension causes incident hip pain
  - Perianal sensory loss ± bladder and bowel dysfunction
  - May cause impotence

Acetabular or head of femur metastases

- Also called hip joint syndrome
- Localized hip pain
- Radiation to medial thigh or knee
- Exacerbated by hip movement and weight bearing
- May have lumbosacral plexopathic pain from medial extension

Visceral Pain Syndromes

Introduction

Visceral afferents from thoracic and abdominal organs utilize autonomic pathways to reach the central nervous system.

Visceral pain pathways

- Vagal pathway
  - Vagal afferents with cell bodies in nodose ganglion
  - Project to nucleus tractus solitarius
  - Project to thalamus, hypothalamus and limbic system
- Spinal pathway
  - Spinal afferents with cell bodies in dorsal root ganglion
  - Travel alongside:
    - Sympathetic efferents
      - Thoracic splanchnic nerves
        - Greater splanchnic nerve
        - Lesser splanchnic nerve
        - Least splanchnic nerve
      - Lumbar splanchnic nerves
      - Sacral splanchnic nerves
    - Parasympathetic efferents
      - Pelvic splanchnic nerves
  - Terminate in dorsal horn
  - Project to higher centers through:
    - Dorsal column pathways
    - Spinothalamic tracts
    - Spinoparabrachial tracts

Liver metastases

- Innervation of liver capsule (Glisson's capsule)
    - Lower intercostal nerves
    - Phrenicoabdominal branches of phrenic nerve
- Innervation of liver parenchyma
    - Hepatic plexus
        - Sympathetic nerves (from celiac plexus)
        - Parasympathetic nerves (from vagus nerve)
- Liver capsular pain
    - Dull, continuous, aching right hypochondrial pain
    - Exacerbated by movement, pressure and deep inspiration
    - Associated with nausea and anorexia
    - Caused by:
        - Stretching of liver capsule
        - Intrahepatic bleeding
            - Rapidly increasing pain
        - Traction of coronary and falciform ligaments
            - Standing pain
            - Walking pain
        - Distension and compression of biliary tract vessles
        - Diaphragmatic irritation
            - Referred pain to right shoulder, neck, scapula
- Other causes of pain
    - Outward pressure on rib cage
        - Bilateral lower rib cage pain
    - Pinching parietal peritoneum against rib cage
        - Intermittent sharp right hypochondrial pain
    - Pinching abdominal wall
        - Abdominal pain
    - Straining of lumbar spine
        - Back pain

Pancreatic cancer

- Innervation of pancreas
    - Sympathetic (Celiac plexus)
        - Greater splanchnic nerves
    - Parasympathetic (Vagus nerves)
- Pancreatic pain
    - Dull, continuous aching epigastric pain
    - Exacerbated by lying down
    - Eased by bending forward
    - Worse at night
    - Localization of pain
        - Head of pancreas
            - Pain at right of epigastrium
            - Mediated by right splanchnic nerves
            - Associated with jaundice
            - Associated with small bowel obstruction
                - Pain after eating
            - Tumour compression of portal vessels
                - Acute right hypochondrial pain
        - Body of pancreas
            - Pain at mid epigastrium
            - Mediated by bilateral splanchnic nerves
        - Tail of pancreas
            - Pain at left of epigastrium and left upper back
            - Mediated by left splanchnic nerves
    - Radiation of pain to the back
        - Invasion of celiac plexus
        - Similar to midline retroperitoneal syndrome
        - Positive retroperitoneal stretch compared to pain from spinal cord compression

Peritoneal metastases

- Innervation of parietal peritoneum
    - Somatic nerves
    - Anterior abdominal wall
        - Lower six thoracic nerves
        - First lumbar nerves
    - Diaphragmatic peritoneum
        - Lower six thoracic nerves – peripheral
        - Phrenic nerves – central
    - Pelvic peritoneum
        - Obturator nerves (branch of lumbar plexus)
- Innervation of visceral peritoneum
    - Same visceral nerve as the viscera it invests
- Peritoneal pain
    - Pathology of parietal peritoneum
        - Somatic pain
        - Well-localized
        - Lateralized
    - Pathology of visceral peritoneum
        - Visceral pain
        - Poorly localized
        - Midline
        - Associated with referred pain
            - Foregut – epigastrium
            - Midgut – umbilicus
            - Hindgut – suprapubic
- Other causes of pain
    - Ascites – stretching pain
    - Malignant adhesion – colicky pain
    - Malignant bowel obstruction – colicky pain
    - Mesenteric tethering – diffuse abdominal pain or low back pain

Malignant bowel obstruction

- Innervation of gut
    - Foregut (esophagus to duodenum)
        - Sympathetic (Celiac plexus)
            - Greater splanchnic nerves
        - Parasympathetic (Vagus nerves)
    - Midgut (duodenum to proximal 2/3 transverse colon)
        - Sympathetic (Superior mesenteric plexus)
            - Lesser splanchnic nerves
            - Least splanchnic nerves
        - Parasympathetic (Vagus nerves)
    - Hindgut (distal 1/3 transverse colon to anus)
        - Sympathetic (Inferior mesenteric plexus)
            - Lumbar splanchnic nerves
        - Parasympathetic (Pelvic splanchnic nerves)
- Constant pain
    - Abdominal distension
    - Bowel compression by tumour
    - Bowel wall ischemia
    - Mesenteric tension
- Colicky pain
    - Bowel contractions
        - Small bowel obstruction
            - Early onset
            - Periumbilical
            - Intense
            - Short intervals
        - Large bowel obstruction
            - Late
            - Peripheral
            - Less intense
            - Longer intervals

Malignant ureteral obstruction

- Innervation of ureters
    - Ureteric plexus
        - Renal plexus – upper part
        - Superior hypogastric plexus – middle part
        - Inferior hypogastric plexus – lower part
- Usually asymptomatic and detected on imaging
- May present with ureteric colic
    - Unilateral loin pain
    - Radiating to the groin
    - Exacerbated by standing
    - Partially relieved by sitting
    - Colicky breakthrough pain may be induced by:
        - Urination
        - Defecation

Pelvic cancers

- Innervation of pelvic organs
    - Branches of inferior hypogastric plexus
        - Uterus (Uterovaginal plexus)
        - Bladder (Vesical plexus)
        - Prostate (Prostatic plexus)
        - Rectum (Rectal plexus)
    - Inferior hypogastric plexus
        - Sympathetic (Superior hypogastric plexus)
            - Thoracic splanchnic nerves
            - Lumbar splanchnic nerves
        - Sympathetic (Sacral splanchnic nerves)
        - Parasympathetic (Pelvic splanchnic nerves)
- Causes of pain
    - Ovarian mass
        - Paraumbilical pain

- Bladder or uterine mass
  - Suprapubic pain
- Rectal mass
  - Pain on sitting
  - Mild pressure or severe pain till cannot sit down
- Deeper rectal mass with myofascial infiltration
  - No pain on sitting
  - Increasingly severe dragging pain on standing for a few minutes or walking 50-100m
- Lateral pelvic wall invasion
  - Obturator internus muscle infiltration
    - Unilateral iliac fossa pain
  - Iliopsoas muscle infiltration
    - Painful fixed flexion of the hip
    - Exacerbation of pain by passive hip extension (positive psoas test)
    - Pain exacerbated by walking
    - May be bedridden because of pain on walking
- Posterior pelvic wall invasion (presacral mass)
  - Piriformis and coccygeus muscles infiltration
    - Unilateral buttock pain
    - Radiating to posterior thigh (sciatic nerve)
  - Lumbosacral plexopathy
  - Sacral plexopathy
  - T12-L1 syndrome
  - Sacral syndrome

Malignant perineal pain

- Anatomical boundaries of perineum
  - Superior – pelvic diaphragm
  - Anterior – pubic symphysis
  - Posterior – coccyx

- Lateral – inferior pubic rami, inferior ischial rami
- Contents of perineum
  - Urogenital triangle – distal urethra, external genitalia
  - Anal triangle – distal rectum, anus
- Innervation of perineum
  - Visceral nerves (Follow parasympathetic nerves)
    - Sacral nerves (S2, S3, S4)
    - Travel with pelvic splanchnic nerves to inferior hypogastric plexus
    - Supply rectum and upper 2/3 anal canal
  - Visceral nerves (Follow sympathetic nerves)
    - Ganglion impar
    - Supply distal urethra, vagina and rectum; vulva, anus, coccyx and perineum
  - Somatic nerves (Pudendal nerves)
    - Inferior rectal nerve
      - External anal sphincter
      - Lower 1/3 anal canal
    - Perineal nerve
      - Urogenital diaphragm
      - External urethral sphincter
      - External genitalia
    - Dorsal nerve of penis or clitoris
      - Penis (male)
      - Clitoris (female)
- Vague, poorly localized, constant aching pain
- Exacerbated by sitting and standing
- Associated with bladder or rectal tenesmus

Neuropathic Pain Syndromes

Introduction

Neuropathic pain is pain caused by damage to the nervous system. It is mediated by a combination of peripheral and central mechanisms.

Mechanisms of neuropathic pain

- Peripheral sensitization
  - Abnormal ion channel expression
    - Increase in TTXs Na expression
      - Type III TTXs Na channel – NGF-dependent
    - Decrease in TTXr Na expression
      - SNS TTXr Na channel – NGF-dependent
      - NaN TTXr Na channel – GDNF-dependent
    - Translocation of SNS from cell body to neuroma
    - Altered N-type Ca channel expression
    - Decrease in K channel expression
  - Upregulation of nociceptors
    - TRPV1
    - P2X3
  - Neuronal hyperexcitability
    - From abnormal ion channel expression
    - Causes ectopic discharges – spontaneous firing
    - Causes ephaptic conduction – cross-excitation
  - Sprouting of primary afferents into skin – NGF-dependent
  - Coupling between sympathetic and sensory nerves
    - Peripheral sensitization from sympathetic nerves
    - Cross-excitation from sympathetic nerves
    - Sympathetic sprouting into DRG – NGF-dependent

- Central sensitization
  - Spinal cord hyperexcitability
    - Activation of NMDAR
      - Removal of Mg^{2+} block
      - NMDAR phoshorylation
  - Spinal cord reorganization
    - Aβ fibers sprouting into lamina II – NGF-dependent
  - Cortical reorganization
  - Changes in inhibitory pathways

Leptomeningeal metastases

- Meningeal irritation
  - Severe, intractable headache
  - Associated with:
    - Photophobia
    - Nuchal rigidity
    - Nausea and vomiting
- Cerebral involvement
  - Headache
  - Confusion
  - Memory loss
  - Lethargy
  - Behavioural changes
  - Gait disturbances
  - Incontinence
  - Seizures
- Cranial nerve involvement
  - Diplopia – III, IV, VI
  - Facial pain (resembling cluster headache), numbness – V
  - Facial weakness – VII
  - Hearing loss and vertigo – VIII
  - Glossopharyngeal neuralgia – IX

- Spinal nerve root involvement
  - Nuchal rigidity
  - Neck pain
  - Back and radicular pain
  - Weakness and paraesthesia of lower extremities
  - Bowel and bladder dysfunction

Tumour infiltration of cervical plexus

- Cervical plexus
  - Formed from ventral rami of C1-C4
- Severe, deep, constant, boring pain localized to the neck
  - Anterior neck pain – transverse cervical nerves
  - Periauricular pain – great auricular nerve
  - Occipital scalp pain – lesser occipital nerve
  - Shoulder pain – supraclavicular nerve
- May referred to throat, shoulder, face and head
  - Overlap of innervations from cranial nerve V, VII, IX, X
- May have intermittent sharp component or causalgic features
- Exacerbated by neck movement, swallowing, coughing
- Associated with:
  - Horner's syndrome – superior cervical ganglion
  - Dyspnoea – paralyzed hemidiaphragm (phrenic nerve)
  - Shoulder weakness – spinal accessory nerve
  - Head tilt – sternocleidomastoid
- Complication
  - Sharp, severe pain on neck movement
    - Cervical spine involvement
    - Impending epidural extension

Tumour infiltration of brachial plexus

- Brachial plexus
    - Formed from ventral rami of C5-T1
- Lower brachial plexopathy (C8-T1)
    - Tumour infiltrates plexus from below due to anatomy
        - Pancoast syndrome
        - Breast cancer
    - Dull, aching shoulder pain
        - Axillary pain
            - T2 involvement
            - Intercostobrachial nerve
            - Not part of brachial plexus
            - May be the first nerve affected
            - Axilla, anterior chest, medial upper arm pain
        - Pain over medial aspects of arm, elbow and forearm
            - T1 involvement
            - Freezing sensation and hypersensitivity along medial aspect of arm
            - Lancinating pain over elbow
            - Cramp-like, crushing pain over forearm
        - Burning, dysesthetic pain of 4th and 5th fingers
            - C8 involvement
    - Associated with weakness:
        - Small muscles of hand (T1)
        - Finger gripping (C6, C7, C8)
        - Wrist flexion (C6, C7)
        - Wrist extension (C7, C8)
        - Elbow extension (C7, C8)
    - Complication
        - Suspect epidural extension
            - Horner's syndrome
            - Weakness of serratus anterior or rhomboid

- Upper brachial plexopathy (C5-C6)
  - Primary brachial plexus tumour
    - Neurofibromas
    - Schwannomas
  - Breast cancer with supraclavicular node
  - Dull, aching shoulder pain
    - Pain over lateral aspects of arm, elbow and forearm
      - C5 involvement
    - Pain over tips of thumb and 2nd finger
      - C6 involvement
  - Associated with weakness:
    - Shoulder abduction (C5)
    - Elbow flexion (C5, C6)
    - Wrist flexion (C6, C7)
    - Finger gripping (C6, C7, C8)
  - Presence of myokimia on EMG suggests radiation fibrosis rather than tumour infiltration
- Pan brachial plexopathy (C5-T1)
  - Progression from lower plexus infiltration
  - Pain can progress to complex regional pain syndrome
  - Neurological dysfunction can spread from lower to upper plexus, leading to paralysis of entire upper limb
  - Associated with lymphoedema in late stage

Tumour infiltration of lumbosacral plexus

- Lumbosacral plexus
  - Lumbar plexus
    - Formed from ventral rami of L1-L4
    - Received T12 contribution
  - Sacral plexus
    - Formed from ventral rami of S1-S4
    - Received L4-L5 contribution via lumbosacral trunk

- Lower lumbosacral plexopathy (L4-S1)
    - Dull, aching back pain near iliac crest
    - Radiating to buttock and posterior thigh and leg
    - Causes footdrop
    - Associated with weakness:
        - Ankle dorsiflexion (L4, L5), plantar flexion (S1, S2)
        - Knee flexion: hamstrings (L5, S1)
        - Hip abduction (L5, S1), adduction (L3, L4)
    - Associated with:
        - Positive straight leg raising test
        - Absent ankle jerk
        - Sensory loss over posterior thigh and sole
        - Rectal mass
        - Sphincter weakness
- Upper lumbosacral plexopathy (L1-L4)
    - Dull, aching back pain near costovertebral angle
    - Radiating to groin and anteromedial thigh
    - Causes difficulty in climbing stairs
    - Associated with weakness:
        - Hip flexion: iliopsoas (L2, L3, L4)
        - Knee extension: quadriceps (L2, L3, L4)
        - Hip adduction (L3, L4)
    - Associated with:
        - Positive psoas test
        - Absent knee jerk
        - Sensory loss over anterior thigh
- Pan lumbosacral plexopathy (L1-S3)
    - Dull aching back pain
    - Radiating to anterior and posterior thigh and leg
    - Exacerbated by sudden movement or lying supine
    - Relieved by standing and walking (compared to pelvic metastases)

Painful peripheral neuropathies

- Mononeuropathy
    - Nerve compression from bone metastases
        - Ulnar nerve – elbow
        - Radial nerve – humerus
        - Intercostal nerve – ribs
        - Obturator nerve – obturator canal
        - Sciatic nerve – pelvis
        - Peroneal nerve – fibula
    - Entrapment neuropathy from lymphedema
        - Carpal tunnel syndrome
    - Rarely nerve metastasis from breast cancer or melanoma
    - Pain, then sensory and motor loss over distribution of involved nerve
    - Palpable mass compressing the nerve
    - Radiating paraesthesia when nerve is percussed near site of involvement
- Polyneuropathy
    - Chemotherapy-induced polyneuropathies
    - Paraneoplastic polyneuropathies
        - Sensory neuropathy from dorsal root ganglionitis
        - Sensorimotor neuropathy
        - Guillain-Barré syndrome (Rarely)
    - Direct invasion of multiple nerves
        - Lymphomas
        - Leukemias
    - Burning paraesthesias
    - Tingling sensation in the extremities
    - Occasional lancinating and lightning pain
    - May associated with:
        - Sensory ataxia
        - Distal weakness

Pain from Spinal Cord Compression

Introduction

Pain from spinal cord compression could be somatic, visceral or neuropathic.

Somatic pain

- Deep somatic pain from mechanical instability
  - Causes: damaged ligaments or bone fractures
  - Bilateral non-radicular back pain
  - With or without radiation
  - Radiation to buttocks, upper thighs, inguinal, abductors
  - Radiation not below the knees
  - Exacerbated by movement: catch sensation on movement
  - When pain is extreme, patient remains absolutely still
  - Not exacerbated by coughing and straining
  - Full range of spine movement
  - Absence of root tension signs
- Deep somatic pain from muscle spasm
  - Causes: hyperactive stretch reflexes and cutaneomuscular reflexes in spastic muscle groups
  - Triggers: stretching a muscle or stimulating the body below the level of injury
  - Sometimes putting on trousers is enough to produce spasm of the hip and knee flexors
  - Relieved by daily range of motion exercise and treatment of muscle spasm
  - Associated with autonomic effects: sweating, increased blood pressure and urinary incontinence

- Deep somatic pain from secondary overuse syndrome
  - Cause: repetitive microtraumatic injuries
  - Onset: months or years after injury
  - Affects proximal muscles of joints
  - Exacerbated by the use of affected muscles or joints
  - Relieved by proper posture and rest
  - Example: rotator cuff tendinitis in shoulder pain

Visceral pain

- Cause: intact visceral pain pathway post-injury
- Pathology: no obvious visceral pathology
- Onset: delayed after spinal cord injury
- Constantly fluctuating burning or cramping abdominal pain
- Other causes: dysreflexic headache, renal calculus, bowel problems, sphincteric dysfunction

Neuropathic pain

- Complex regional pain syndrome
  - Above-level neuropathic pain – above the level of injury
  - Unilateral throbbing, burning or shooting upper limb pain
  - Presence of hyperalgesia and allodynia
  - Exacerbated by limb movement, dependent position and temperature changes
  - Autonomic dysfunction: skin temperature asymmetries, skin colour changes, oedema, hyper/hypohidrosis
  - Motor dysfunction: weakness, limited movement, tremor, dystonia (rare and late)
  - Trophic changes: disturbed nail and hair growth, palmar or plantar fibrosis, hyperkeratosis, distal osteoporosis

- Compressive mononeuropathy
  - Above-level neuropathic pain
  - Example: carpal tunnel syndrome
- Radicular pain from nerve root compression
  - At-level neuropathic pain
  - Cause: nerve root entrapment
  - Burning, lancinating or stabbing pain
  - Extent: single dermatome unilaterally or bilaterally
  - Exacerbated by spinal movement, coughing and straining
  - Relieved by decompression
- Segmental deafferentation pain
  - At-level neuropathic pain
  - Terms: girdle pain, border pain or transitional zone pain
  - Cause: spinal cord damage at dorsal horn
  - Spontaneous burning or tingling pain
  - Onset: 1st few months post-injury
  - Location: border of normal sensation and anaesthetic skin
  - Extent: 2-4 dermatomes unilaterally or bilaterally
  - Description: half belt or full belt
  - Presence of segmental hyperalgesia and allodynia
  - Stimulus independent
- Syringomyelia
  - At-level neuropathic pain
  - Onset: years post-injury
  - Radicular pain in a cape-like distribution, interscapular pain or central cord pain
  - Dysesthetic pain: burning sensations, pins and needles, stretching of skin
  - Trophic changes: hyperhidrosis, glossy skin, coldness, paleness

- Cauda equina syndrome
  - At-level neuropathic pain
  - Burning pain
  - Location: legs, feet, perineum, genitals and rectum
  - Associated with saddle-shaped loss of sensation and loss of bladder and bowel control
- Deafferentation pain
  - Below-level neuropathic pain
  - Terms: spinal cord injury pain, dysesthetic pain, central dysesthesia syndrome
  - Diffuse, constant, burning, aching or throbbing pain in anaesthetic regions below the level of injury
  - Asscociated with numbness and tingling
  - Exacerbated by infection
  - Not affected by movement or position
  - Usually not relieved by opioids

Pain Assessment Tools

Introduction

Various pain assessment tools can be used to rate the intensity of pain and to document response to pain management.

Numerical rating scale (NRS)

- Pain is rated from 0 to 10
- Ask patient to score his or her pain from 0 to 10
- 0= no pain, 10= worst possible pain
- Clinically significant pain reduction = 2
- Easier to complete than visual analogue scale
- No need to carry the pain ruler

Visual analogue scale (VAS)

- Pain is rated from a 10cm line on a pain ruler
- Ask patient to mark a point that best describes his or her pain
- 0= no pain, 10=worst possible pain
- Clinically significant pain reduction = 2

Categorical rating scale (CRS)

- Pain is rated as mild, moderate or severe
- Ask patient to rate his or her pain as mild, moderate or severe
- Useful in elderly

Wong-Baker faces pain rating scale

- Pain is rated from faces on a Wong-Baker ruler
- Ask patient to point to the face that best matches the type of pain he or she is feeling
- Left end= smiling face, right end= crying face

FLACC scale

- Pain is rated from observing the behaviour of patient
- Originally designed to assess pain in children and babies
- Useful in non-communicative adult patients

Criteria	0	1	2
Face	Normal	Grimace	Clenched jaw
Legs	Normal	Restless	Kicking
Activity	Normal	Squirming	Arched
Cry	Normal	Moaning	Screaming
Consolability	Normal	Reassurable	Nonreassurable

Little story

Once I received a present and a thank you card from a family member of a patient that I could not remember. My boss was a little upset for my forgetfulness. After some effort, I remembered I saw a patient in the haematological ward who was referred to me to find out whether he was in pain. Patient was semi-comatose. I observed him and started him on morphine infusion because he was exhibiting behaviour suggestive of pain. I told his son, "He is in pain. I need to start him on morphine infusion to make him comfortable. Then I asked his son, "How are you?" It was a short encounter. In the thank you card he wrote, "Although I have brought my father to see so many doctors, but I have never come across a doctor who is so kind." The encounter was short. Maybe I was the first doctor who asked about him.

Principle of Pain Management

Introduction

WHO analgesic ladder is a useful guide in cancer pain management. It is 90% effective in pain control.

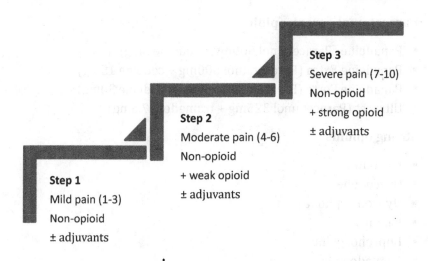

Step 3
Severe pain (7-10)
Non-opioid
+ strong opioid
± adjuvants

Step 2
Moderate pain (4-6)
Non-opioid
+ weak opioid
± adjuvants

Step 1
Mild pain (1-3)
Non-opioid
± adjuvants

Principles

- By the mouth – give orally
- By the clock – give regularly
- By the ladder – give according to ladder
- For the individual – give according to individual
- Attention to details – give with attention to details

Non-opioids

- Paracetamol
- NSAIDs

Weak opioids

- Codeine
- Dihydrocodeine
- Tramadol

Paracetamol + weak opioid

- Panadeine (Paracetamol 500mg + codeine 8mg)
- Panadeine Extra (Paracetamol 500mg + codeine 15mg)
- Panadeine Forte (Paracetamol 500mg + codeine 30mg)
- Ultracet (Paracetamol 325mg + tramadol 37.5mg)

Strong opioids

- Morphine
- Oxycodone
- Hydromorphone
- Fentanyl
- Buprenorphine
- Methadone

Adjuvants

- Steroids
- Antidepressants
- Anticonvulsants
- NMDA receptor blockers
- Muscle relaxants
- Bisphosphonates

Paracetamol

Introduction

Paracetamol is a non-opioid that has been used in the management of mild pain and fever for more than 50 years.

Mechanisms of action

- The exact mechanism is still undefined
- Proposed mechanisms
  - Central COX inhibition (predominantly COX-2)
    - Inhibits PGE2 production from arachidonic acid
      - Activates serotonergic pathway to reduce pain
      - Lowers hypothalamic set point to reduce fever
  - Anandamide uptake inhibition by paracetamol metabolite (N-arachidomoylphenolamine or AM404)
    - Increases endogenous cannabinoids
      - Activates serotonergic pathway
      - Lowers body temperature
  - Direct NMDAR inhibition
  - Inhibition of substance P-dependent synthesis of NO through the L-arginine-nitric oxide pathway

Recommendations

- Typical dose in palliative care: PO Paracetamol 1g tds-qid
  - Timing for qid: 8am, 12pm, 4pm, 8pm
    - Especially if patient is on syrup morphine q4h
  - Timing for qid: 8am, 12pm, 6pm, 10pm
    - Especially if patient is not on syrup morphine q4h
  - Timing for qid: 6am, 12pm, 6pm, 12am
    - 12am dose may affect sleep

- Timing for qid: morning, afternoon, evening, bedtime
    - Especially at home
- PO Paracetamol 1g q4h with morphine q4h (Stockler 2004)
    - Timing: 8am, 12pm, 4pm, 8pm, 12am, 4am
    - Exceeds maximum recommended daily dose of 4g/day
    - Palliative care input recommended
- Syrup Paracetamol
    - Concentration = 125mg/5ml, 250mg/5ml
    - Not suitable for patients who cannot drink ≥20ml
- PR Paracetamol 1g tds-qid
    - 1 paracetamol suppository = 500mg
- IV Paracetamol 1g q6h if >50kg
    - 1 vial = 500mg/50ml
    - Infusion over 15min
    - Maximum 4g/day
- IV Paracetamol 15mg/kg q6h if <50kg
    - Maximum 60mg/kg/day

Additional information

- PO Paracetamol 1g qid is preferred to tds for maximal benefit
- If definite benefit not seen within 2 days after adding paracetamol to strong opioid, discontinue it (Axelsson and Christensen 2003)
- Use of paracetamol ≤4g/day is not contraindicated in stable chronic liver disease (Benson 1983)
- Limit paracetamol use to single dose 1g prn in decompensated chronic liver disease
- Use of paracetamol ≤4g/day is not contraindicated in severe renal impairment with CC<30ml/min
- 5HT3-receptor antagonists may block the analgesic effect of paracetamol completely (Pickering 2006)

Little experience

A patient once complained to me that he was aroused during midnight to take paracetamol. He was unhappy because he felt that it didn't make sense to wake him up for the sole reason of taking paracetamol.

NSAIDs

Introduction

Use an NSAID if it provides better pain relief than paracetamol.

Mechanisms of action

- Peripheral COX inhibition
    - Reduces prostaglandin production from arachidonic acid
        - COX-1 inhibition
            - Reduced cytoprotective prostaglandins
                - Gastrointestinal toxicity
        - COX-2 inhibition
            - Reduced inflammatory prostaglandins
                - Analgesia
            - Reduced renoprotective prostaglandins
                - Renal toxicity
- Central COX inhibition

NNTs from single dose studies (≥50% pain relief)

- Etoricoxib 120mg = 1.6
- Ibuprofen 800mg = 1.6
- Ketorolac 20mg = 1.8
- Diclofenac 100mg = 1.9
- Lumiracoxib 400mg = 2.1
- Diclofenac 50mg = 2.3
- Naproxen 440mg = 2.3
- Ibuprofen 400mg = 2.4
- Celecoxib 400mg = 2.6
- Topical NSAIDs = 3.1
- Celecoxib 200mg = 4.2

Risk of GI bleeding (RR compared to ibuprofen)

- Ibuprofen = 1.0 (lowest risk among nonselective NSAIDs)
- Diclofenac = 1.8
- Naproxen = 2.2
- Indomethacin = 2.4
- Piroxicam = 3.8
- Ketoprofen = 4.2

Risk of UGI bleeding with NSAID ≥ 2 months (Tramer 2000)

- Risk of endoscopic ulcer   1 in 5
- Risk of symptomatic ulcer   1 in 70
- Risk of bleeding ulcer   1 in 150
- Risk of death from bleeding ulcer   1 in 1,300

COX-2 selectivity ratio

- Etoricoxib = 106
- Celecoxib = 7.6
- Diclofenac = 3.0
- Meloxicam = 2.0
- Indomethacin = 0.4
- Ibuprofen = 0.2
- Piroxicam = 0.08

Low gastrointestinal toxicity of ibuprofen

- R(-)-ibuprofen enantiomer is metabolized to active S(+) isomer
- Active S-ibuprofen inhibits prostaglandin synthesis
- Inactive R-ibuprofen masks interaction of S-ibuprofen with COX-1, reducing inhibition of gastric prostaglandin production

Risk factors for GI toxicity

- Age >65 years
- Peptic ulcer disease

- Long term use of NSAIDs
- Serious comorbidity
    - Cancer
    - Diabetes mellitus
    - Hypertension
    - Cardiovascular disease
    - Hepatic impairment
    - Renal impairment
- Concurrent use of steroids, aspirin or anticoagulant
- Concurrent use of SSRI
- Platelet <50 x 10^9/L

Choices of NSAID in palliative care

- PO Ibuprofen 400-800mg tds-qid + GI prophylaxis
- PO Diclofenac 50-100mg tds-qid + GI prophylaxis
- PO Diclofenac SR 75-150mg bd + GI prophylaxis
- PO Naproxen 550-1100mg bd + GI prophylaxis
- PO Etoricoxib 60-120mg daily + GI prophylaxis
- PO Celecoxib 200-400mg bd + GI prophylaxis
- CSCI Diclofenac 75-150mg/24h + GI prophylaxis (PCT advice)
- CSCI Ketorolac 60-90mg/24h + GI prophylaxis (PCT advice)

PCT = palliative care team

GI prophylaxis

- PO Omeprazole 20mg om
- PO Pantoprazole 20mg om
- PO Lansoprazole 30mg om
- PO Ranitidine 300mg bd
- PO Misoprostol 400mcg bd (Rostom 2002)

Additional information

- Limit NSAID use for ≤ 2 months if possible
- For long term NSAIDs, seek palliative care input
- Use of NSAID should be avoided in renal disease unless preservation of renal function is no longer wanted
- Since risk of GI toxicity in palliative care patients is high, consider GI prophylaxis for all palliative care patients
- Consider single dose NSAID for highly selected patients with relative contraindications to NSAID
- Omeprazole and lansoprazole can be given as orodispersible tablets or granules from opening the capsules
- SC Omeprazole 40mg in 100ml normal saline over 3 hours can be used in the symptomatic treatment of GI toxicity when intravenous access is a burden (PCT advice)

Weak Opioids

Introduction

Weak opioids are often used to manage moderate pain in step 2 WHO analgesic ladder. However, step 2 can be skipped. A direct move to third step with small doses of morphine improves pain control compared to traditional three-step strategies (Maltoni 2005). Step 2 is reserved for patients who are not ready to use strong opioids.

Mechanisms of action

- Tramadol: $\mu > \kappa > \delta$
- Codeine and dihydrocodeine: $\mu > \delta > \kappa$
- Additional mechanisms of tramadol
    - Stimulates neuronal release of serotonin
    - Inhibits re-uptake of serotonin and noradrenaline (SNRI)

Pharmacology

- Onset of action
    - Tramadol: 30min
    - Codeine: 30min
    - Dihydrocodeine: 30min
- Duration of action
    - Tramadol: 4h
    - Codeine: 4h
    - Dihydrocodeine: 4h
- Metabolism in liver
    - Tramadol: converted to O-desmethyltramadol (active)
    - Codeine: converted to morphine (active)
    - Dihydrocodeine: converted to dihydromorphine (active)

- Potency
    - Tramadol: 5 times weaker than oral morphine
    - Codeine: 8 times weaker than oral morphine
    - Dihydrocodeine: 10 times weaker than oral morphine
    - Tramadol injection: 2 times weaker than oral tramadol

Doses

- PO Tramadol 50-100mg tds-qid
- PO Codeine 30-60mg tds-qid
- PO Dihydrocodeine 30-60mg tds-qid
- SC Tramadol 50-100mg tds-qid
- CSCI Tramadol 100-600mg/24h (PCT advice)
- CSCI Dihydrocodeine 100-350mg/24h (PCT advice)

Combinations

- Ultracet (Paracetamol 325mg + tramadol 37.5mg)
- Panadeine (Paracetamol 500mg + codeine 8mg)
- Panadeine Extra (Paracetamol 500mg + codeine 15mg)
- Panadeine Forte (Paracetamol 500mg + codeine 30mg)

Combination doses

- PO Ultracet 1-2 tablets tds-qid
- PO Panadeine 1-2 tablets tds-qid
- PO Panadeine Extra 1-2 tablets tds-qid
- PO Panadeine Forte 1-2 tablets tds-qid

Recommendations

- Consider prophylactic antiemetic for first 3-5 days
- Consider regular laxatives
- Consider switching to strong opioid rapidly if pain is uncontrolled or breakthrough analgesia is required

Little experience

Once my boss started a patient on tramadol. After the first dose she went up to the ward to review the patient for pain control and side effects. The patient was so touched that her eyes brimmed with tears. It was not about the tramadol. It was the care and concern that my boss had towards her.

Five Principles of Using Syrup Morphine

Introduction

The five principles of using syrup morphine can serve as an initial guide to manage moderate to severe pain in palliative care.

The five principles

- Prescribe syrup morphine q4h for background pain
- Prescribe syrup morphine prn/q1h for breakthrough pain
- Prescribe regular antiemetic for the first 5 days
- Prescribe regular laxatives
- Provide opioid education

Background pain

- Common error: prescribing syrup morphine prn, on, q6h or q8h for background pain
- Rationale: increasing the interval results in end-of-dose pain because the duration of action of syrup morphine is four hours
- Exception: severe renal failure with CC<30ml/min or severe liver impairment with prolonged prothrombin time

Breakthrough pain

- Common error: not prescribing syrup morphine prn/q1h for breakthrough pain
- Rationale: breakthrough pain needs additional analgesia
- Some centers practice prescribing syrup morphine prn/q2h or prn/q4h for breakthrough pain
- Increasing the interval may result in poorly controlled breakthrough pain

Opioid-induced emesis

- Common error: not prescribing regular antiemetic
- Rationale: some patients refuse to take morphine again once they have vomited even though the chance of vomiting is 25%
- Recommendation: PO Metoclopramide 10mg tds x 5/7 or PO Haloperidol 1.5mg bd x 5/7
- Exception: patients with recent history of using morphine without nausea or vomiting

Opioid-induced constipation

- Common error: not prescribing regular laxatives
- Rationale: opioid-induced constipation is common
- Recommendation: PO Senna 15mg bd ± PO Lactulose 10ml bd
- Exception: patients with diarrhoea or with iliostomy

Opioid education

- Common error: prescribing morphine without explaning about side effects and without addressing fear of morphine
- Rationale: some patients refuse to take morphine due to their fear, some relatives refuse to give patient morphine due to their fear and misconception about morphine
- Recommendation: educate patients and relatives about the common side effects of morphine and address their fear of morphine

---

Opioid teaching

The 5 principles of using syrup morphine is a preliminary guide that we can share with our medical and surgical colleagues on how to start morphine.

Opioid Education

Introduction

The successful use of syrup morphine depends largely on opioid education. The proper amount of information should be communicated to patients and their relatives to improve compliance.

Three common side effects

- Drowsiness
- Nausea and vomiting
- Constipation

Three common fears

- Fear of addiction
- Fear of tolerance
- Fear of using morphine when one is not dying

Opioid-induced drowsiness

- Mild to moderate drowsiness for the first 24 hours of using morphine and during dose increase (Pasero 2011)
- Should be easily arousable to talk and eat as usual
- Drowsiness usually disappears within 3-5 days
- Severe drowsiness needs dose reduction

Opioid-induced emesis

- 1 in 4 will experience nausea or vomiting
- Usually disappears within 3-5 days
- Can be prevented by taking anti-vomiting drug for 3-5 days

Opioid-induced constipation

- Morphine can cause constipation
- Need regular laxatives to assist in bowel opening

Fear of addiction

- Misconception: I don't want to get addicted to morphine
- Explanation: Addiction is extremely uncommon if you are taking morphine to control pain or other symptoms like cough and breathlessness.

Fear of tolerance

- Misconception: If my pain gets worse, there will be nothing left for me to control my pain.
- Explanation: When the pain gets worse, usually it can be controlled by increasing the dose. Besides, there are many alternatives which are stronger than morphine if morphine does not work well for you.

Fear of using morphine when one is not dying

- Misconception: I am not dying yet. Morphine is for the dying.
- Explanation: Morphine is not meant for the dying, but is used when there is a need, even early in the disease. When the pain is controlled, you can continue your daily activities in life.

Little secret

Majority of patients who refuse morphine given by the primary team are willing to take morphine prescribed by the palliative care team after proper information is given to them. The secret is communication.

Opioid Side Effects

Introduction

Opioid can cause a range of side effects. Effective opioid management requires active prevention of common side effects and regular assessment of opioid toxicity.

Drowsiness

- Mild to moderate drowsiness is not a sign of opioid toxicity
- Tolerance develops within first few days
- Persistent drowsiness can be treated with psychostimulants
    - PO Methylphenidate 5-10mg at 8am ± 12pm
    - PO Dextroamphetamine 10-30mg at 8am ± 12pm
    - PO Modafinil 200-400mg at 8am ± 12pm
    - PO Donepezil 2.5-5mg at 8am ± 12pm
- Excessive drowsiness is an early sign of opioid toxicity
    - Causes of excessive drowsiness
        - Opioid naïve
        - Frailty
        - Mild pain
        - Nerve block
        - Acute kidney injury
        - CNS depression
            - CNS depressants
            - Infection
            - Metabolic disturbances
            - Brain metastases
    - Management of excessive drowsiness
        - Opioid dose reduction
        - Opioid rotation

Nausea and vomiting

- Nausea and vomiting occur in 25% of patients
- Tolerance develops within first few days
- High risk group
    - Age < 65 years
    - Female
    - Breast cancer
    - Stomach cancer
    - Gynaecological cancer
- Prescribe prophylactic antiemetic for all patients
    - PO Metoclopramide 10mg tds for 5 days or
    - PO Haloperidol 1.5mg bd for 5 days
- Opioid-induced nausea and vomiting (OINV)
    - Delayed gastric emptying
        - IV/SC Metoclopramide 10mg tds
    - Direct chemoreceptor trigger zone (CTZ) stimulation
        - IV/SC Haloperidol 1.5mg bd for CTZ stimulation
    - Increased vestibular sensitivity
        - IV Promethazine 12.5-25mg tds
        - Scopolamine patch 1.5mg q72h to mastoid
    - Persistent nausea and vomiting
        - IV/SC Dexamethasone 8mg at 8am and 12pm
    - Refractory nausea and vomiting (PCT advice)
        - IV/SC Metoclopramide 10-20mg q4h
        - CIVI/CSCI Metoclopramide 60-120mg/24h

Constipation

- Opioid-induced constipation occurs in 90% of patients
- Tolerance does not develop
- Prescribe prophylactic laxative for all patients unless diarrhoea
    - PO Senna 15mg bd or
    - PO Docusate 100mg bd

- Opioid-induced constipation (OIC)
    - PO Senna 15mg bd + Syrup Lactulose 15ml bd or
    - PO Bisacodyl 10mg bd + Syrup Lactulose 15ml bd or
    - PO Co-danthrusate (Dantron + Docusate) 1-3 cap on-bd
    - PO Co-danthramer (Dantron + Poloxamer) 1-3 cap on-bd
- Education of laxative titration
    - Hard stool: double the dose of stool softener
        - Maximum docusate 400mg qid (4 tablets qid)
        - Maximum lactulose 30ml qid
    - No stool: double the dose of stool pusher
        - Maximum senna 30mg qid (4 tablets qid)
        - Maximum bisacodyl 20mg qid (4 tablets qid)
    - Diarrhoea: stop 3/7, then restart with half the usual dose
- Rectal measures required in 1/3 patients
    - PR Glycerin enema II/II prn if NBO for 3/7 or
    - PR Bisacodyl 10-20mg prn if NBO for 3/7
    - PR Fleet enema I/I prn if still NBO
- Alternative options for OIC
    - PAMORA
        - Peripherally acting μ-opioid receptor antagonists
        - SC Methylnaltrexone 8mg EOD if 40-60kg
        - SC Methylnaltrexone 12mg EOD if 60-120kg
        - PO Naloxegol 25mg om
    - Locally acting chloride channel activator
        - PO Lubiprostone 24mcg bd
- Avoid bulk laxatives for OIC
    - Increase impaction
        - Opioid reduces water in lumen
        - Bulk laxatives draw fluid into lumen

Little knowledge

Drowsiness, nausea and vomiting are side effects that occur during rising serum opioid levels. They tend to resolve as steady state is achieved. Constipation persists despite steady state opioid levels.

Opioid Toxicity

Introduction

Opioid-induced neurotoxicity is a syndrome that includes some or all of the following features: severe drowsiness, respiratory depression, delirium, hallucination, hyperalgesia, allodynia, myoclonus and seizures. The clue to prevent opioid toxicity is frequent review.

Risk factors of opioid toxicity

- Frail patients
- Excessive dose initiation or increment
- Dehydration and renal failure
- Infection
- Pain acutely relieved by procedure like nerve block

Clinical features of opioid toxicity

- Central nervous system depression (inhibitory neurotoxicity)
    - Excessive drowsiness
    - Hypoactive delirium
    - Coma
    - Respiratory depression: respiratory rate <8-10/min
- Central nervous system stimulation (excitatory neurotoxicity)
    - Agitation
    - Hyperalgesia and allodynia
    - Hyperactive delirium
    - Hallucinations and delusions
    - Myoclonus and seizures
    - Coma
    - Respiratory arrest

Excessive drowsiness

- Mild to moderate drowsiness is not a sign of opioid toxicity
- Excessive drowsiness is an early sign of opioid toxicity
- Excessive drowsiness is characterized by poor arousability
- Screen for hypoactive delirium
- Review CNS depressants
- Treat contributory factors
    - Dehydration
    - Infection
    - Hypercalcemia
- Opioid dose reduction
- Opioid rotation

Delirium

- Stable opioid dose does not impair cognition (Bruera 1989)
- Cognitive function improves with pain control
- Median precipitating factors = 3 per episode in palliative care
- Treat precipitating factors
    - Pain
    - Fecal impaction
    - Urinary retention
    - Dehydration
    - Renal failure
    - Infection
    - Hypercalcemia
    - Hypoxia
    - Metabolic encephalopathy
- Rehydration to reduce opioid metabolites
- Opioid dose reduction
- Opioid rotation

- Treat hypoactive delirium with unpleasant hallucinations
    - PO Haloperidol 0.75mg on-bd
    - IV/SC Haloperidol 0.5mg on-bd
- Treat all hyperactive delirium
    - Mild agitation: PO/IV/SC Haloperidol 1.5mg on-bd
    - Moderate agitation: PO/IV/SC Haloperidol 2.5mg on-bd
    - Severe agitation: PO/IV/SC Haloperidol 5mg on-bd

Respiratory depression

- Uncommon in cancer patients with chronic pain
- Does not occur with proper opioid titration (Sykes 2007)
- Risk factors
    - Advanced age
    - Multiple comorbidities
    - Renal failure
    - Morbid obesity
    - Sleep apnoea
    - Nerve block
    - Opioid rotation to methadone
- Naloxone in palliative care (American Pain Society 1992)
    - RR ≥8/min + easily arousable
        - Wait and see
        - Consider opioid dose reduction or omission
    - RR <8/min + poorly arousable
        - Dilute 400mcg (1 ampoule) to 10ml with NS
        - Give 20mcg (0.5ml) q2min IV or q5min SC till RR ≥8/min
        - Further boluses prn if RR<8/min
        - Duration of action of naloxone is 0.5-1.5h
        - Aim for partial reversal, not complete reversal
        - Restart opioid with a lower dose after sustained improvement in consciousness

- Use of naloxone may precipitate a withdrawal syndrome, arrhythmias, seizures and severe pain (Manfredi 1996)

Opioid-induced hyperalgesia (OIH)

- Mechanisms
  - Excitatory opioid metabolites, such as:
    - Morphine-3-glucuronide (M3G)
    - Hydromorphone-3-glucuronide (H3G)
  - Activation of NMDAR
  - Activation of glial cells
  - Alteration in G protein coupling of opioid receptors
    - With G_s rather than G_i or G_o
- Characteristics
  - Worsening pain despite opioid dose escalation
  - Presence of hyperalgesia and allodynia
  - Pain becomes more diffuse, extending beyond area of pre-existing pain
  - Pain of lesser quality and harder to pinpoint
- Management
  - Rehydration to reduce opioid metabolites
  - Rapid opioid dose reduction to 25% of peak dose
  - Switch to an opioid with less risk of OIH
    - Fentanyl (highest risk) > morphine > methadone > buprenorphine (lowest risk)
  - Add paractemol or NSAID
  - Consider neuropathic adjuvant: gabapentin
  - Consider ketamine
  - Consider spinal or epidural opioid
  - Correct hypomagnesemia
  - Consider ultralow doses of opioid antagonist
  - Prescribe benzodiazepine for seizures or distressing myoclonus

Little caution

High index of suspicion is needed to detect opioid excitatory neurotoxicity because these patients may be fully alert. Be cautious when patients are requesting higher and higher doses of opioid without much pain control.

Opioid Concerns

Introduction

It is common for laypeople or healthcare staff to express concerns in using opioids due to various misunderstandings. These misunderstandings can result in undertreatment of pain.

Addiction

- Concern: I don't want to become a drug addict
- Physical dependence
  - Not addiction
  - Patients depend on morphine to reduce pain
- Withdrawal symptoms
  - Not addiction
  - Occur when morphine is stopped abruptly
  - Prevented by reducing morpine gradually
- Psychological dependence
  - Is addiction
  - Presence of mental craving and drug-seeking behaviour in the absence of pain
  - Rare in patient without history of drug abuse: 4 in 12,000 patients (Porter 1980)

Tolerance

- Concern: If the pain gets worse, I will have nothing to use
- Tolerance
  - Requiring higher and higher doses to achieve analgesia
  - Need of increasing dose is due to increasing pain from disease progression, not tolerance
  - Significant tolerance is uncommon

- Broad therapeutic range of morphine allows dose escalation when pain gets worse
- Availability of other strong opioids when morphine fails

Dying

- Concern: I am not dying yet
- Morphine is not used exclusively in dying patients
- Morphine can be used to treat pain in early stages of disease
- Patients can resume their activities when pain is under control

Allergy

- Concern: I am allergic to morphine
- True allergy is rare
- Nausea and vomiting are often mistaken as allergy
- Nausea and vomiting are preventable side effects

Respiratory depression and hastening of death

- Concern of healthcare staff: morphine hastens death
- Proper titration of morphine does not cause clinically significant respiratory depression
- Proper titration of morphine does not hasten death
- Lethal dose of morphine is ≥200mg for opioid naïve patients

---

Little opinion

Misperceptions about opioid are mistaken first impressions about opioid. Misconceptions about opioid are mistaken beliefs about opioid after substantial thinking. The former is easier to rectify than the latter.

Morphine

Introduction

Morphine is named after the Greek God of Dream, Morpheus, because of its sedative effect. It is derived from opium poppy (Papaver somniferum).

Mechanisms of action

- μ opioid receptor agonist
- Presynaptic inhibition of neurotransmitter release at dorsal horn (predominant mechanism)
    - Activation of G_i protein coupled receptors
        - Increased K^+ efflux
            - Hyperpolarization
            - Reduced neurotransmitter release
        - Decreased Ca^{2+} conductance
            - Reduced Ca^{2+} influx
            - Reduced depolarization
            - Reduced neurotransmitter release
        - Inhibition of adenylate cyclase
            - Reduced cAMP dependent cellular processes
            - Reduced neurotransmitter release
- Postsynaptic inhibition of neuron firing at dorsal horn
- Activation of descending pain pathways
    - GABA disinhibition – suppression of GABAergic inputs onto descending pain pathways

Pharmacology

- Metabolites: morphine-6-glucuronide (M6G), morphine-3-glucuronide (M3G)

- Morphine-6-glucuronide (M6G)
  - 10-15%
  - Active metabolite
  - 100x more potent than morphine
  - Less abundant in CNS due to poor penetration of blood brain barrier
  - Activation of opioid receptor: can cause nausea, vomiting, sedation, respiratory depression
- Morphine-3-glucuronide (M3G)
  - 80%
  - Inactive metabolite
  - Indirect activation of NMDAR: excitatory neurotoxicity
- Immediate release oral morphine
  - Bioavailability: 35%
  - Onset of action: 30-45min
  - Plasma half-life: 2-4h
  - Duration of action: 4h

Titration of oral morphine

- Use immediate release oral morphine for titration because the dose can be adjusted up or down rapidly in view of the short half-life
- Starting dose
  - Syrup morphine 2.5mg q4h for moderate pain
  - Syrup morphine 5mg q4h for severe pain
  - Syrup morphine 10mg q4h if on maximum weak opioid
- Breakthrough dose
  - Use 1/6 of oral morphine daily dose (Hanks 2001)
  - Given as frequent as required up to hourly
- Examples of prescription
  - Syrup morphine 5mg q4h
  - Syrup morphine 5mg prn/q1h for breakthrough pain

- Timing of baseline morphine
  - Syrup morphine at 8am, 12pm, 4pm, 8pm, 12am, 4am
- Alternative timing
  - Syrup morphine at 8am, 12pm, 4pm, 8pm
  - Double dose at 12am to avoid waking up for 4am dose
- Titration based on breakthrough doses
  - Titrate the baseline dose if ≥ 3 breakthough doses per day
  - Add the total breakthrough doses to the baseline dose
  - Example
    - Baseline: syrup morphine 5mg q4h
    - Breakthrough: syrup morphine 5mg x 6 doses/day
    - Titration = (5mg x 6) + (5mg x 6) = 60mg/day
    - New baseline: syrup morphine 10mg q4h
    - New breakthrough: syrup morphine 10mg prn/q1h
  - Do not increase the dose <25% (no significant change)
  - Do not increase the dose >100% (higher risk of toxicity)
- Alternative titration based on pain severity
  - Mild pain: increase dose by 25%
  - Moderate pain: increase dose by 50%
  - Severe pain: increase dose by 100%
- Alternative titration based on stepwise increment
  - Increase q4h dose every 24-48h till pain is controlled
  - 5–10–15–20–30–40–60–80–100–130
- Frequency of titration
  - Depends on half-life $(T_{1/2})$ of oral morphine ≈ 2-4h
    - Time to 50% concentration = $1T_{1/2}$
    - Time to 75% concentration = $2T_{1/2}$
    - Time to 90% concentration = $3.3T_{1/2}$
    - Time to steady state ≈ $4T_{1/2}$
  - Time to steady state = 8-16h
- Comparison of plasma half-life of different opioids
  - Immediate release oral morphine: 2-4h

- Immediate release oral oxycodone: 3.5h
- Immediate release oral hydromorphone: 2.5h
- Intravenous morphine: 1.5h
- Fentanyl patch: 0.5-1 day
- Oral transmucosal fentanyl citrate: 6h
- Intravenous fentanyl: 3.5h
- Intravenous sufentanil: 2.5h
- Intravenous alfentanil: 1.5h
- Buprenorphine patch (BuTrans): 0.5-1.5days
- Buprenorphine patch (Transtec): 1-1.5 days
- Sublingual buprenorphine: 1-3 days
- Intravenous buprenorphine: 3-16h
- Oral methadone: 8 hours to 3 days
- Recommended frequency of titration for different opioids
  - Immediate release morphine: q24h
  - Immediate release oxycodone: q24h
  - Immediate release hydromorphone: q24h
  - Sustained release morphine: q48h
  - Sustained release oxycodone: q48h
  - Sustained release hydromorphone: q48h
  - Fentanyl patch: q72h
  - Buprenorphine patch (BuTrans): q72h
  - Buprenorphine patch (Transtec): q72h
  - Methadone: weekly

Preparations of syrup morphine

- Common preparations
  - 1mg/ml
  - 2mg/ml
  - 10mg/ml
- Check with pharmacist regarding available concentration
- Prescribe in mg, not in ml

Sustained Release Morphine Tablets (MST)

Introduction

Convert immediate release oral morphine to sustained release morphine tablets (MST) once the pain is adequately controlled for 2-3 days.

Pharmacology

- Onset of action: 2h
- Half-life: 4h
- Duration of action: 12h

Conversion

- Conversion ratio = 1:1
- Examples of conversion
  - Syrup morphine 5mg q4h ≈ MST 20mg q12h
  - Syrup morphine 10mg q4h = MST 30mg q12h
- Examples of prescription
  - MST 30mg q12h at 8am and 8pm
  - Syrup morphine 10mg prn/q1h for breakthrough pain

Instructions for prescribing MST

- Avoid prescribing 8 hourly dosing (higher risk of toxicity)
- Instruct patient not to chew or crush tablets
- For nasogastric or PEG feeding:
  - Use sustained release morphine granules if available or
  - Change back to immediate release oral morphine or
  - Consider using fentanyl patch

Starting dose for opioid-naïve patients

- Standard opioid titration begins with titration of syrup morphine, then convert to MST once pain is stable
- Consider seeking advice from the palliative care team if you intend to start MST without titrating with syrup morphine
- MST 10mg q12h for breathlessness or moderate pain
    - Syrup morphine 2.5mg prn/q1h for breakthrough pain
- MST 20mg q12h for severe pain
    - Syrup morphine 5mg prn/q1h for breakthrough pain
- MST 30mg q12h if on maximal weak opioid
    - Syrup morphine 10mg prn/q1h for breakthrough pain
- Use 1/6 of oral morphine daily dose as breakthrough doses

Titration of MST

- Mild to moderate pain
    - Titrate MST if ≥ 3 breakthrough doses per day
    - Add total breakthrough doses to baseline dose
    - Frequency of titration is at least 48h
    - Maximal titration: 100%
- Severe pain
    - Retitrate by adding syrup morphine q4h or
    - Retitrate by converting back to syrup morphine q4h

Preparations for q12h dosing (MS Contin)

- MST 10mg = pink
- MST 30mg = purple
- MST 60mg = orange

Preparations for q24h dosing (Kadian, Avinca)

- Kadian 10mg, 20mg, 30mg, 50mg, 60mg, 80mg, 100mg, 200mg
- Avinza 30mg, 60mg, 90mg, 120mg

Fentanyl Patch

Introduction

Fentanyl is an alternative strong opioid. It is a strong μ-opioid receptor agonist. It is highly lipophilic.

Pharmacology

- Onset of action: 12h
- Half-life: 0.5-1 day
- Duration of action: 72h

Indications

- Consider converting immediate release oral morphine to fentanyl patch once the pain is adequately controlled for 2-3 days, in the following conditions:
  - Head and neck cancer
  - Swallowing problem
  - Persistent nausea and vomiting
  - Short bowel syndrome
  - Malignant bowel obstruction
  - PEG feeding

Conversion

- Fentanyl is 100x more potent than oral morphine
- To convert oral morphine mg/day to fentanyl patch mcg/h, divide oral morphine daily dose by 3
- Example of conversion
  - Syrup morphine 5mg q4h = 30mg/day
  - $30 \div 3 = 10 \approx 12$
  - Syrup morphine 5mg q4h = fentanyl patch 12mcg/h/72h

- Example of conversion in details
    - Syrup morphine 5mg q4h = 30mg/day
    - Based on conversion ratio = 1: 100
    - $30 \div 100$ mg/day = $30 \div 100$ x 1000 mcg/day

$$= 30 \div 100 \text{ x } 1000 \div 24 \text{ mcg/h}$$
$$= 30 \div 2.4 \text{ mcg/h}$$
$$\approx 30 \div 3 \text{ mcg/h}$$
$$= 10\text{mcg/h}$$
$$\approx 12\text{mcg/h}$$

Rapid conversion

- Syrup morphine 5mg q4h = fentanyl patch 12mcg/h/72h
- Syrup morphine 10mg q4h = fentanyl patch 25mcg/h/72h
- Syrup morphine 20mg q4h = fentanyl patch 50mcg/h/72h
- Syrup morphine 30mg q4h = fentanyl patch 75mcg/h/72h
- Syrup morphine 40mg q4h = fentanyl patch 100mcg/h/72h

Starting dose for opioid-naïve patients

- Standard opioid titration begins with titration of syrup morphine, then convert to fentanyl patch once pain is stable
- Consider seeking advice from the palliative care team to start fentanyl patch without titrating with syrup morphine
- Fentanyl patch 12mcg/h/72h for moderate to severe pain
    - Syrup morphine 5mg prn/q1h for breakthrough pain
- Fentanyl patch 25mcg/h/72h if on maximal weak opioid
    - Syrup morphine 10mg prn/q1h for breakthrough pain

Titration of fentanyl patch

- Mild to moderate pain
    - Titrate fentanyl patch if ≥ 3 breakthrough doses per day
    - Add total breakthrough doses to baseline dose
    - Frequency of titration is at least 72h

- Maximal titration: 100%
- Examples of titration: 12–25–37–50–62–75–100
- Severe pain
  - Retitrate by adding syrup morphine q4h or
  - Retitrate by converting back to syrup morphine q4h after 12h of patch removal or
  - Retitrate by adding fentanyl infusion or
  - Retitrate by converting to fentanyl infusion after 8h of patch removal

Preexisting analgesia

- Continue pre-existing baseline analgesia for 12 hours because onset of action for fentanyl patch is 12 hours
  - Continue 3 more q4h doses for syrup morphine
  - Continue 1 more q12h dose for MST
  - Continue 8h for morphine infusion

Additional information

- Apply over chest, abdomen and sometimes limbs
- Do not apply at the back
- Do not apply at pain site
- Do not shave body hair, cut it
- Do not cut the patch
- Do not plaster half
- Cover with a transparent plaster like Tegaderm or Opsite
- Label date and time of change with permanent marker pen
- Do not shower hot water over it
- Change the patch every 72 hours
- Dispose by folding it into half with adhesive side inwards and discarding in a sharps container (hospital) or dustbin (home)

Preparations

- Fentanyl patch 12mcg/h/72h
- Fentanyl patch 25mcg/h/72h
- Fentanyl patch 50mcg/h/72h
- Fentanyl patch 100mcg/h/72h

Opioid Review

Introduction

Regular assessment is important during opioid titration. Patients should be assessed for pain control, side effects and opioid toxicity.

	Peak	Steady state
PO Morphine:	15-60min	8-16h
PO Oxycodone:	60-90min	14h
PO Hydromorphone:	60min	10h
PO Methadone:	4h	1.5-12days
PO MST:	1-6h	16h
PO Oxycontin:	3h	18h
SC Morphine:	10-20min	6h
Fentanyl patch:	1-3days	2-4days
OTFC:	20-40min	1day
IV Fentanyl:	4.5min	14h
IV Alfentanil:	1.5min	6h
IV Sufentanil:	2.5min	10h
Buprenorphine patch (BuTrans):	3days	2-6days
Buprenorphine patch (Transtec):	2.5days	4-6days
Sublingual buprenorphine:	1-2h	4-12days

Principles of opioid review

- Risk of opioid toxicity is highest during rising opioid level from onset to peak to steady state
- Risk of opioid toxicity during steady state if:
  - Acute kidney injury
  - Pain is acutely relieved by a procedure like nerve block

Recommended initial review during opioid titration

- Within 12h (Same day)
    - SC/IV Morphine
    - SC/IV Fentanyl
    - SC/IV Alfentanil
    - SC/IV Sufentanil
- Within 24h (Next day)
    - PO Morphine
    - PO Oxycodone
    - PO Hydromorphone
    - PO MST
    - PO Oxycontin
- Within 24h (Next day) and twice-weekly for one week
    - Fentanyl patch
    - Buprenorphine patch
- Within 24h (Next day) and twice-weekly for two weeks
    - PO Methadone

Additional information

- Educate patients and their families regarding opioid toxicity
    - Mild to moderate drowsiness + easy arousability: observe
    - Excessive drowsiness: seek medical advice
    - Poor arousability: seek medical advice

Opioid Switching

Introduction

For opioid switching, first calculate the oral MEDD (morphine equivalent daily dose) of the existing opioid, then convert to the new opioid and consider dose reduction.

Indications for opioid switching

- Uncontrolled pain with dose escalation
- Unacceptable side effects
- Opioid neurotoxicity

Potency of weak opioids

- PO Hydrocodone is 1.5x weaker than PO Morphine
- PO Tramadol is 5x weaker than PO Morphine
- PO Codeine is 8x weaker than PO Morphine
- PO Dihydrocodeine is 10x weaker than PO Morphine
- PO Dextropropoxyphene is 10x weaker than PO Morphine

Switching weak opioid in mg/day to oral MEDD in mg/day

- PO Hydrocodone ÷ 1.5 = oral MEDD
- PO Tramadol ÷ 5 = oral MEDD
- PO Codeine ÷ 8 = oral MEDD
- PO Dihydrocodeine ÷ 10 = oral MEDD
- PO Dextropropoxyphene ÷ 10 = oral MEDD

Potency of strong opioids

- PO Oxycodone is 2x stronger than PO Morphine
- PO Hydromorphone is 5x stronger than PO Morphine
- Fentanyl patch is 100x stronger than PO Morphine

- Buprenorphine patch is 100x stronger than PO Morphine
- SL Buprenorphine is 100x stronger than PO Morphine

Switching oral MEDD in mg/day to other strong opioid

- Oral MEDD ÷ 2 = PO Oxycodone in mg/day
- Oral MEDD ÷ 5 = PO Hydromorphone in mg/day
- Oral MEDD ÷ 3 = Fentanyl patch in mcg/h/72h
- Oral MEDD ÷ 3 = Buprenorphine patch in mcg/h/72h
- Oral MEDD ÷ 100 = SL Buprenorphine in mg/day

Switching to oral hydromorphone

- Syrup morphine 10mg q4h = 60mg/day
- PO Hydromorphone = 60 ÷ 5 = 12mg/day
- Syrup morphine 10mg q4h ≈ PO Hydromorphone 1.3mg q4h

Switching to sublingual buprenorphine

- Syrup morphine 10mg q4h = 60mg/day
- SL Buprenorphine = 60 ÷ 100 = 0.6mg/day
- Syrup morphine 10mg q4h = SL Buprenorphine 0.2mg q8h

Potency of parenteral opioids

- IV/SC Tramadol is 2x weaker than PO Tramadol
- IV/SC Morphine is 2-3x stronger than PO Morphine
- IV/SC Oxycodone is 2x stronger than PO Oxycodone
- IV/SC Hydromorphone is 2x stronger than PO Hydromorphone
- IV/SC Methadone is 2x stronger than PO Methadone
- IV/SC Buprenorphine is 2x stronger than SL Buprenorphine

Switching to parenteral opioid in mg/day

- PO Tramadol x 2 = IV/SC Tramadol
- PO Morphine ÷ 3 = IV/SC Morphine
- PO Oxycodone ÷ 2 = IV/SC Oxycodone

- PO Hydromorphone ÷ 2 = IV/SC Hydromorphone
- PO Methadone ÷ 2 = IV/SC Methadone
- SL Buprenorphine ÷ 2 = IV/SC Buprenorphine

Potency of parenteral fentanyl and fentanyl analogues

- IV/SC Fentanyl is similar potent as fentanyl patch
- IV/SC Fentanyl is 4x stronger than IV/SC Alfentanil
- IV/SC Fentanyl is 10x weaker than IV/SC Sufentanil
- IV/SC Fentanyl is 10x weaker than IV/SC Remifentanil

Switching of parenteral fentanyl

- IV/SC Fentanyl in mcg/h = Fentanyl patch in mcg/h/72h
- IV/SC Fentanyl in mcg/h x 4 = IV/SC Alfentanil in mcg/h
- IV/SC Fentanyl in mcg/h ÷ 10 = IV/SC Sufentanil in mcg/h
- IV/SC Fentanyl in mcg/h ÷ 10 = IV/SC Remifentanil in mcg/h

Switching from parenteral MEDD in mg/day

- Parenteral MEDD = IV/SC Oxycodone in mg/day
- Parenteral MEDD = IV/SC Fentanyl in mcg/h
- Parenteral MEDD ÷ 1.5 = IV/SC Diamorphine in mg/day
- Parenteral MEDD ÷ 5 = IV/SC Hydromorphone in mg/day
- Parenteral MEDD ÷ 15 = IV/SC Alfentanil in mg/day
- Parenteral MEDD ÷ 40 = IV/SC Buprenorphine in mg/day

Switching from parenteral MEDD in mg/day

- Parenteral MEDD ÷ 10 = Epidural morphine
- Parenteral MEDD ÷ 100 = Intrathecal morphine
- Parenteral MEDD ÷ 1000 = Intraventricular morphine

Dose reduction after switching opioid

- Consider palliative care referral for opioid switching unless adequate pharmacological knowledge and clinical experience in using the alternative opioid are available
- Consider dose reduction for incomplete cross tolerance after opioid switching
    - No dose reduction
        - Switching to fentanyl patch
        - Switching for severe uncontrolled pain
    - 30% dose reduction
        - Switching to any opioid except fentanyl/methadone
    - 50% dose reduction
        - Switching to methadone
        - Elderly
        - Severe renal impairment with CC<30ml/min
        - Severe liver impairment with prolonged PT
        - Severe cardiopulmonary disease
    - 75% dose reduction
        - Oral MEDD >2g/day

Alternative Opioids

Introduction

Oral morphine is the first choice opioid in moderate to severe cancer pain. For opioid switching to alternative opioids, referral to palliative care team is *strongly recommended*.

Oxycodone

- Semisynthetic opioid synthesized from thebaine
- Thebaine is an opioid alkaloid found in Persian poppy
- Receptors
    - μ-opioid receptors (less strong than morphine)
    - κ-opioid receptors (animal studies)
- Pharmacology
    - Bioavailability: 75% (morphine: 35%)
    - Onse of action: 20-30min
    - Half-life: 3.5h, 4.5h in renal failure
    - Duration of action: 4h
    - Metabolites: 90% noroxycodone, 10% oxymorphone
- Potency
    - PO Oxycodone is 2x stronger than PO Morphine
    - IV/SC Oxycodone is similar potent to IV/SC Morphine
- Starting dose for opioid-naïve patients
    - Immediate release: PO Oxycodone (Oxynorm) 5mg q4h
    - Modified release: PO Oxycodone (Oxycontin) 10mg q12h
- Starting dose for mild liver impairment or mild to moderate renal impairment
    - Immediate release: Syrup Oxynorm 2.5mg q4h
    - Modified release: PO Oxycontin 5mg q12h

- Starting dose of CSCI for opioid-naïve patients
  - CSCI Oxycodone 5mg/24h (0.2mg/h): breathlessness
  - CSCI Oxycodone 7.5mg/24h (0.3mg/h): moderate pain
  - CSCI Oxycodone 10mg/24h (0.5mg/h): severe pain
  - Review q12h during initial titration
  - Increase 25-50% if pain is uncontrolled
  - Breakthrough dose = 1/6 SC Oxycodone daily dose
  - Breakthrough dose = 4x SC Oxycodone hourly dose
- Example of CSCI prescription
  - CSCI Oxycodone 0.5mg/h
  - SC Oxycodone 2mg prn/q1h for breakthrough pain
- Preparations
  - Immediate release
    - Capsule Oxynorm
      - 5mg: orange/beige
      - 10mg: white/beige
      - 20mg: pink/beige
    - Syrup Oxynorm 1mg/ml
  - Modified release
    - Tablet Oxycontin
      - 5mg: blue round
      - 10mg: white round
      - 20mg: pink round
      - 40mg: yellow round
      - 80mg: green round
    - Tablet Targin (Oxycontin/Naloxone)
      - 5mg/2.5mg: blue oblong
      - 10mg/5mg: white oblong
      - 20mg/10mg: pink oblong
      - 40mg/20mg: yellow oblong
  - Injection
    - 10mg/ml, 1ml amp, 2ml amp

Fentanyl

- Semisynthetic opioid
- Highly lipophilic (morphine: hydrophilic)
    - Suitable for transdermal route
    - Suitable for transmucosal route
    - Less opioid molecules outside CNS
        - Less constipation
        - Less nausea and vomiting
- Sequestrated in body fats
- Strong μ-opioid receptor agonist
- Pharmacology
    - Fentanyl patch
        - Onset of action: 12h
        - Half-life: 0.5-1day
        - Duration of action: 72h
    - Oral transmucosal fentanyl citrate (OTFC)
        - Bioavailability: 50%
        - Onset of action: 5min
        - Half-life: 6h
        - Duration of action: 2h
    - Intravenous fentanyl
        - Onset of action: 1.5min
        - Half-life: 3.5h
        - Duration of action: 1h
    - Metabolites: norfentanyl
- Potency
    - 100x more potent than oral morphine
- Safe in severe renal failure
- Starting dose of fentanyl patch for opioid-naïve patients
    - Fentanyl patch 12mcg/h/72h
      = syrup morphine 5mg q4h
      = syrup oxycodone 2.5mg q4h

- Starting dose of CSCI for opioid-naïve patients
  - CSCI Fentanyl 10mcg/h
  - Review q12h during initial titration
  - Increase 25-50% if pain is uncontrolled
  - Breakthrough dose = 1/24 – 1/12 SC Fentanyl daily dose
  - Breakthrough dose = 1-2x SC Fentanyl hourly dose
- Example of CSCI prescription
  - CSCI Fentanyl 10mcg/h
  - SC Fentanyl 10mcg prn/q1h for breakthrough pain
- OTFC titration for breakthrough pain
  - OTFC 200mcg prn (background oral MEDD ≥ 60mg/day)
  - Rub OTFC around inside of mouth
  - Remove OTFC if patient feels drowsy, nauseated or giddy
  - Repeat OTFC 200mcg after 15min if pain is uncontrolled
  - Increase OTFC to next dose level if pain is uncontrolled with 2 similar doses of OTFC
  - Maximum 4 doses of OTFC per day
  - Dissolve half-used OTFC under hot tap before disposing
- Sublingual fentanyl titration for breakthrough pain
  - For opioid-tolerant patients only
  - Background oral MEDD ≥ 60mg/day
  - Parenteral formulation of fentanyl 50mcg/ml
  - Start with SL Fentanyl 25mcg (0.5ml of 50mcg/ml)
  - Titrate to 50mcg (1ml), then 100mcg (2ml) if necessary
  - Avoid doses >100mcg (>2ml) to ensure absorption
- Preparations
  - Fentanyl patch in mcg/h/72h
    - 12, 25, 50, 100
  - OTFC (Actiq) in mcg
    - 200, 400, 600, 800, 1200, 1600
  - Fentanyl sublingual tablets (Abstral) in mcg
    - 100, 200, 300, 400, 600, 800

- Fentanyl sublingual spray (Subsys) in mcg
  - 100, 200, 400, 600, 800
- Fentanyl buccal tablets (Fentora) in mcg
  - 100, 200, 400, 600, 800
- Fentanyl nasal spray (Lazanda) in mcg
  - 100, 400
- Fentanyl nasal spray (Instanyl) in mcg
  - 50, 100, 200
- Fentanyl injection
  - 50mcg/ml, 2ml amp, 10ml amp

Alfentanil

- Synthetic derivative of fentanyl
- Useful as alternative to fentanyl when volume is a problem
  - Using syringe driver
  - Sublingual administration
- Pharmacology
  - Onset of action: 0.75min
  - Half-life: 1.5h
  - Duration of action: 0.5h
- Potency
  - 4x less potent than fentanyl
- Starting dose for opioid-naïve patients
  - CSCI Alfentanil 0.5-1mg/24h = CSCI Fentanyl 5-10mcg/h
  - Review q12h during initial titration
  - Increase 25-50% if pain is uncontrolled
  - Breakthrough dose = 1/6 SC Alfentanil daily dose
  - Fentanyl breakthrough = 1/40 SC Alfentanil daily dose
- Example of CSCI prescription
  - CSCI Alfentanil 1mg/24h
  - SC Alfentanil 150mcg prn/q1h for breakthrough pain or
  - SC Fentanyl 25mcg prn/q1h for breakthrough pain

- SC Fentanyl is preferred for breakthrough pain because of longer duration of action
- Preparations
  - Injection: 500mcg/ml, 2ml amp, 10ml amp

Sufentanil

- Synthetic derivative of fentanyl
- Useful as alternative to fentanyl when volume is a problem
  - Using syringe driver
  - Sublingual administration
- Pharmacology
  - Onset of action: 1min
  - Half-life: 2.5h
  - Duration of action: 1h
- Potency
  - 10x more potent than fentanyl
- Starting dose for opioid-naïve patients
  - CSCI Sufentanil 15-25mcg/24h
    = CSCI Fentanyl 5-10mcg/h
  - Review q12h during initial titration
  - Increase 25-50% if pain is uncontrolled
  - Breakthrough dose = 1/24 – 1/12 SC Sufentanil daily dose
- Example of CSCI prescription
  - CSCI Sufentanil 25mcg/24h
  - SC Sufentanil 1mcg prn/q1h for breakthrough pain
- Preparations
  - Injection: 50mcg/ml, 1ml amp, 2ml amp, 5ml amp

Hydromorphone

- Semisynthetic opioid
- Strong μ-opioid receptor agonist
- Useful when patient needs high doses of subcutaneous opioid·

- Pharmacology
    - Bioavailability: 30%
    - Onse of action: 30min
    - Half-life: 2.5h
    - Duration of action: 4h
    - Metabolites: hydromorphone-3-glucuronide (H3G)
- Potency
    - 5x more potent than oral morphine
- Starting dose for opioid-naïve patients
    - Immediate release: PO Hydromorphone 1.3mg q4h
      = syrup morphine 10mg q4h
    - Modified release: PO Hydromorphone SR 2mg q12h
      = MST 10mg q12h
- Starting dose of CSCI for opioid-naïve patients
    - CSCI Hydromorphone 2mg/24h
      = CSCI Morphine 10mg/24h
    - Review q12h during initial titration
    - Increase 25-50% if pain is uncontrolled
    - Breakthrough dose = 1/6 SC Hydromorphone daily dose
- Preparations
    - Immediate release: 1.3mg, 2.6mg
    - Modified release: 2mg, 4mg, 8mg, 16mg, 24mg
    - Injection: 10mg/ml, 1ml amp

Buprenorphine

- Semisynthetic derivative of thebaine
- Highly lipophilic
- Receptors
    - μ-receptor partial agnonist
    - κ-receptor antagonist
    - δ-receptor antagonist
    - Nociceptin receptor partial agonist

- Pharmacology
  - Sublingual buprenorphine
    - Onset of action: 15-45min
    - Half-life: 1-3days
    - Duration of action: 8h
  - Buprenorphine patch (BuTrans)
    - Onset of action: 0.5-1day
    - Half-life: 0.5-1.5days
    - Duration of action: 7 days
  - Buprenorphine patch (Transtec)
    - Onset of action: 0.5-1day
    - Half-life: 1-1.5days
    - Duration of action: 4days
  - Intravenous buprenorphine
    - Onset of action: 5-15min
    - Half-life: 3-16h
    - Duration of action: 8h
  - Metabolites: norbuprenorphine
- Potency
  - 100x more potent than oral morphine
- Starting dose for opioid-naïve patients
  - SL Buprenorphine 0.2mg q8h
    = syrup morphine 10mg q4h
- Doses of buprenorphine patch (BuTrans)
  - Buprenorphine patch (BuTrans) 5mcg/h
    = syrup morphine 2.5mg q4h
  - Buprenorphine patch (BuTrans) 10mcg/h
    = syrup morphine 5mg q4h
  - Buprenorphine patch (BuTrans) 20mcg/h
    = syrup morphine 10mg q4h
- Buprenorphine patch (BuTrans)
  - Change patch every 7th day

- Titrate q72h if pain is uncontrolled
- Rest skin site for 3weeks after using
- Doses of buprenorphine patch (Transtec)
  - Buprenorphine patch (Transtec) 35mcg/h
    = SL Buprenorphine 0.2mg q8h
    = syrup morphine 10mg q4h
  - Buprenorphine patch (Transtec) 52.5mcg/h
    = SL Buprenorphine 0.4mg q8h
    = syrup morphine 15mg q4h
  - Buprenorphine patch (Transtec) 70mcg/h
    = SL Buprenorphine 0.4mg q6h
    = syrup morphine 20mg q4h
  - Buprenorphine patch (Transtec) 140mcg/h
    = SL Buprenorphine 0.8mg q4h
    = syrup morphine 40mg q4h
- Buprenorphine patch (Transtec)
  - Change patch every 3rd day
  - Titrate q72h if pain is uncontrolled
  - Allow 12-24h for maximum effect
  - Allow 12-24h post patch removal for effect to wear off
- Opioid switching to SL Buprenorphine/Naloxone (Suboxone)
  - Useful for opioid-tolerant patients with opioid-induced hyperalgesia (OIH)
  - Background oral MEDD ≥ 60mg/day
  - Stop all opioids
  - SL Suboxone 2mg prn/q6h for breakthrough pain or withdrawal symptoms
  - Maximum dose: 8mg q6h
- Preparations
  - BuTrans: 5mcg/h, 10mcg/h, 20mcg/h
  - Transtec: 35mcg/h, 52.5mcg/h, 70mcg/h
  - Sublingual tablets (Subutex): 0.4mg, 2mg, 8mg

- Sublingual tablets (Temgesic): 0.2mg, 0.4mg
- Sublingual buprenorphine/naloxone (Suboxone) tablets
  - 2/0.5mg (hexagonal orange tablets)
  - 8/2mg (hexagonal orange tablets)
- Sublingual buprenorphine/naloxone (Suboxone) films
  - 2/0.5mg (green box)
  - 4/1mg (purple box)
  - 8/2mg (blue box)
  - 12/3mg (orange box)
- Injection: 0.3mg/ml, 1ml
- Instructions to use suboxone film
  - Not to eat immediately before dosing
  - Take sip of water to moisten mouth
  - Dry hands
  - Hold film by its edge
  - Place under tongue one at a time
  - For multiple films, place two under tongue on either side of frenulum, place the rest onto inside of cheeks
  - Do not move the film after placement
  - Do not chew or swallow
  - Wait until it dissolves in 2-5min
  - Recommended supervision time: <1min because film adheres to mucous membranes within seconds

Methadone

- Synthetic strong opioid
- Lipophilic
- Receptors
  - μ-opioid receptor agonist
  - δ-opioid receptor agonist
  - NMDA receptor blocker
  - Serotonin re-uptake presynaptic blocker

- Pharmacology
  - Bioavailability: 80%
  - Onset of action: < 30min
  - Half-life: 8 hours to 3 days
  - Duration of action: 8-12h with repeated doses
- Potency
  - 10x more potent than oral morphine when oral MEDD <1000mg/day
  - 20x more potent than oral morphine when oral MEDD 1000-2000mg/day
  - 30x more potent than oral morphine when oral MEDD >2000mg/day
- Starting dose for opioid-naïve patients
  - Syrup methadone 5mg q12h and prn/q3h
  - Syrup methadone 2.5mg q12h and prn/q3h for elderly
  - Titrate weekly if necessary
  - Keep the same breakthrough doses
  - If syrup methadone ≥30mg q12h, increase breakthrough dose to 1/10 – 1/6 of the daily dose

Opioid switching to syrup methadone

- Morley-Makin method
  - Stop previous opioid
  - Start syrup methadone as 1/10 of oral MEDD prn/q3h
  - Maximum starting dose 30mg prn/q3h
  - Day 6 (steady state): use average total methadone daily dose used on day 4 and 5 as divided dose q12h
  - Breakthrough: 1/6 of total methadone daily dose prn/q3h
- Modified Morley-Makin method
  - Stop previous opioid
  - Give stat dose of syrup methadone 1/10 of oral MEDD
  - Then start syrup methadone 1/30 of oral MEDD prn/q3h

- Maximum starting dose 30mg prn/q3h
- Day 6 (steady state): use average total methadone daily dose used on day 4 and 5 as divided dose q12h
- Breakthrough: 1/6 of total methadone daily dose prn/q3h
- Titrate weekly if ≥ 2 doses of prn per day
- Reduce dose 30-50% if excessively drowsy
- Give prn/q1h of previous opioid to control withdrawal symptoms or moderate to severe pain < 3h
- Give paracetamol to control mild pain < 3h
- Example for modified Morley-Makin method
  - Stop syrup morphine 50mg q4h (300mg/day)
  - Give stat dose of syrup methadone 30mg
  - Then start syrup methadone 10mg prn/q3h
  - Day 6: if total methadone dose on day 4 and 5 is 60mg, then prescribe syrup methadone 30mg/day = 15mg q12h
  - Breakthrough = 5mg prn/q3h
- Friedman method
  - Oral MEDD (<1000mg/day + age<65) ÷ 10
  - Oral MEDD (<1000mg/day + age>65) ÷ 20
  - Oral MEDD (1000-2000mg/day + any age) ÷ 20
  - Oral MEDD (>2000mg/day + any age) ÷ 30
- Ripamonti method
  - Oral MEDD (30-90mg/day) ÷ 4
  - Oral MEDD (90-300mg/day) ÷ 6
  - Oral MEDD (>300mg/day) ÷ 8
- Mercadante method
  - Oral MEDD (30-90mg/day) ÷ 4
  - Oral MEDD (90-300mg/day) ÷ 8
  - Oral MEDD (>300mg/day) ÷ 12
- Ayonrinde method
  - Oral MEDD (<100mg/day) ÷ 3
  - Oral MEDD (100-300mg/day) ÷ 5

- Oral MEDD (300-600mg/day) ÷ 10
- Oral MEDD (600-800mg/day) ÷ 12
- Oral MEDD (800-1000mg/day) ÷ 15
- Oral MEDD (>1000mg/day) ÷ 20

Rapid switch versus 3-day switch to methadone

- Rapid switch
  - Stop previous opioid and start equianalgesic methadone in 3 daily divided doses
  - Success 77%
  - Side effects 7%
    - Sedation 4%
    - Respiratory depression 0.4%
- Ad libitum switch
  - Morley-Makin or modified Morley-Makin
  - Success 93%
  - Side effects 2%
- 3-day switch
  - Day 1: replace 30% previous opioid with equianalgesic dose of methadone in 3 daily divided doses
  - Day 2: replace 60% previous opioid with equianalgesic dose of methadone in 3 daily divided doses
  - Day 3: replace 100% previous opioid with equianalgesic dose of methadone in 3 daily divided doses
  - Success 93%
  - Less side effects compared to rapid switch

Recommended switch

- Outpatient switch
  - Use modified Morley-Makin method
  - Dose reduce 50% for incomplete cross tolerance

- Review after one week instead of D6 to get the average total methadone daily dose based on previous 2 days
- Breakthrough: 1/6 total daily methadone dose prn/q3h
- Inpatient switch
  - Use Friedman method
  - Dose reduce 50% for incomplete cross tolerance
  - Use 3-day switch
  - Breakthrough options
    - Use previous short-acting opioid prn/q1h
    - Use alternative equianalgesic short-acting opioid prn/q1h if neurotoxic with previous opioid
    - Use 1/6 total daily methadone dose prn/q3h

Tapendatol

- Centrally acting opioid of benzenoid class
- Receptors
  - μ-receptor agonist
  - Noradrenaline reuptake inhibitor
- Pharmacology
  - Bioavailability: 30%
  - Onset of action: 30min
  - Half-life: 4h
  - Duration of action: 4-6h
  - No active metabolites
- Potency
  - 2x more potent than oral tramadol
  - 2.5x less potent than oral morphine
- Conversion
  - Oral Tramadol ÷ 2 = Oral Tapendatol
  - Oral Morphine x 2.5 = Oral Tapendatol
- Dosage
  - Immediate release: 50-100mg q4-6h

- Modified release: 50-250mg q12h
- Preparations
    - Immediate release
        - Nucynta 50mg , 75mg, 100mg
    - Modified release
        - Nucynta ER 50mg, 100mg, 150mg, 200mg, 250mg

Pethidine

- Avoid using pethidine in cancer pain
- Disadvantages of pethidine
    - Excitatory neurotoxicity with chronic use
    - Due to accumulation of toxic metabolite: norpethidine
        - Tremors
        - Multifocal myoclonus
        - Agitation
        - Seizures
    - Ceiling effect due to neurotoxicity
    - Short duration of action 2-3h
    - More emetogenic
    - Contraindicated in renal failure
    - Usually prescribed as intramuscular injection which is painful

Pain Control in Renal Failure

Introduction

The presence of renal failure affects the pharmacokinetics and pharmacodynamics of many drugs. Special precautions are needed before initiating analgesics in renal failure.

Not recommended in renal failure

- Codeine
    - Do not use in renal failure
    - Cumulation of C6G, M6G, M3G
    - Reports of serious side effects
- Dihydrocodeine
    - Do not use in renal failure
    - Cumulation of DHC6G, DHM6G, DHM3G
- Morphine
    - Do not use in renal failure
    - Cumulation of M6G (inhibitory), M3G (excitatory)
    - Opioid toxicity can occur even with small doses
    - Use temporarily only if no other strong opioid available
        - Use immediate release
        - Do not use modified release
        - Do not use infusion
        - Breakthrough: prn/q6h

Dosage reduction recommended by Bunn and Ashley 1999

Morphine	% normal dose	Dose (mg)	Interval
CC20-50	75	5	q6h
CC10-20	50	2.5	q8h
CC<10	25	2.5	q12h

Use cautiously in renal failure

- Tramadol
    - First line weak opioid in renal failure
    - Use with dose reduction in severe renal failure
    - Metabolites: O-desmethyltramadol
    - Use immediate release
    - CC<10: PO Tramadol 50mg tds (on dialysis)
    - CC<10: PO Tramadol 50mg bd (not on dialysis)

Tramadol	% normal dose	Dose (mg)	Interval
CC20-50	100	50-100	q6h
CC10-20	50	50-100	q8h
CC<10	50	50	q12h

- Oxycodone
    - Use with dose reduction and careful monitoring
    - Metabolites: noroxycodone, oxymorphone
    - Case report of CNS-depressant effect in renal failure
    - Use temporarily only if hydromorphone is unavailable
        - Use immediate release in the form of syrup
        - Use in low doses only
        - Do not use modified release
        - Do not use infusion
        - Breakthrough: prn/q6h

Oxycodone	% normal dose	Dose (mg)	Interval
CC20-50	50	2.5-5	q6h
CC10-20	25-50	2.5-5	q8h
CC<10	25-50	2.5-5	q12h

- Hydromorphone
    - First line oral strong opioid in renal failure
    - Use with careful monitoring

- Metabolites: H3G (excitatory)
- Use if oral strong opioid is needed in renal failure
    - Use immediate release
    - Do not use modified release
    - Do not use infusion
- Dose: PO Hydromorphone 1.3mg q4h and prn/q4h
- Keep the total daily dose low by using fentanyl patch when >12mg/day

Fentanyl patch (mcg/h/72h)	PO Hydromorphone prn/q4h (mg)
12	No data
25	1.3
50	2.6
75	5.2
100	7.8
125	9.1

Generally safe with close monitoring in renal failure

- Fentanyl
    - First line strong opioid in renal failure
    - Metabolites: norfentanyl (inactive)
    - Titrate with oral hydromorphone or fentanyl infusion
    - Then convert to fentanyl patch once pain is stable
    - Dose
        - CSCI Fentanyl 5mcg/h for breathlessness
        - CSCI Fentanyl 10mcg/h for moderate/severe pain
        - Breakthrough: 1-2x the hourly dose prn/q1h
- Alfentanil
    - Drug of choice for use in syringe driver
    - Metabolites: noralfentanil (inactive)
    - Use when CSCI Fentanyl > 25mcg/h or 600mcg/24h
    - Not recommended for titration due to short duration of action: 30min

- Dose
  - CSCI Alfentanil 0.5mg/24h for breathlessness
  - CSCI Alfentanil 1mg/24h for moderate/severe pain
  - Breakthrough: 1/10 – 1/6 total daily dose prn/q1h
- Sufentanil
  - Safe with close monitoring
  - Metabolites: N-desalkylsufentanil, O-desmethylsufentanil
  - Dose
    - CSCI Sufentanil 15mcg/24h for breathlessness
    - CSCI Sufentanil 25mcg/24h for pain
    - Breakthrough: 1/24 – 1/12 total daily dose prn/q1h
- Remifentanil
  - Safe with close monitoring
  - Metabolized by esterases
  - Metabolites: remifentanil acid (inactive)
- Buprenorphine
  - Safe with close monitoring
  - Metabolites: norbuprenorphine
    - Does not cross blood-brain barrier
    - Little central effect
- Methadone
  - Safe with close monitoring
  - Metabolites: methadone pyrrolidine (inactive)
  - Pyrrolidine is excreted in feces
  - Some recommend 50% dose reduction when CC<10

Pain Control in Liver Impairment

Introduction

Most opioids are metabolized by liver through phase 1 reactions by cytochrome P450 enzymes 2D6 and 3A4. Some are through phase 2 glucuronidation. Liver impairment may lead to increased risk of opioid toxicity because the parent drug is not adequately converted to metabolites for elimination.

- CYP2D6: O-demethylation
- CYP3A4: N-demethylation

Not recommended in severe liver impairment

- Codeine
    - Do not use in severe liver impairment
    - Not converted to active metabolite morphine
- Dihydrocodeine
    - Do not use in severe liver impairment
    - Not converted to active metabolite dihydromorphine
- Methadone
    - Do not use in severe liver impairment
    - Methadone is highly protein-bound: 80-90%
    - Increased free-drug level due to reduced albumin and α-1-acid glycoprotein production in liver impairment
- Buprenorphine
    - Do not use in severe liver impairment
    - Buprenorphine is highly protein-bound: 96%
    - Increased free-drug level due to reduced albumin and α-1-acid glycoprotein production in liver impairment

Dose adjustment in severe liver impairment (prolonged PT)

- Tramadol
    - PO Tramadol 50mg bd (maximum dose)
    - Use immediate release
    - Do not use modified release
- Morphine, oxycodone, hydromorphone
    - Parent drug may not be converted to metabolites
    - Use oral
    - Use immediate release
    - Do not use modified release
    - Reduce dose 50%
        - PO Morphine 2.5-5mg q8h
        - PO Oxynorm 5mg q8h
        - PO Hydromorphone 1.3mg q8h
- Alfentanil
    - Accumulate in severe liver impairment
    - Reduce dose 50%

Generally safe with close monitoring in severe liver disease

- Fentanyl, sufentanil and remifentanil
    - First line strong opioids in severe liver impairment
    - Pharmacokinetics unaffected by severe liver impairment
    - Fentanyl is affected by reduced hepatic blood flow
    - No dosage adjustment needed
    - Close monitoring for precipitation or aggravation of hepatic encephalopathy

Pain Crisis

Introduction

Pain crisis is a palliative care emergency. Patient needs to be attended immediately.

Definition

- Pain score ≥7
- Patient is in acute distress because of the pain

Rapid parenteral opioid titration

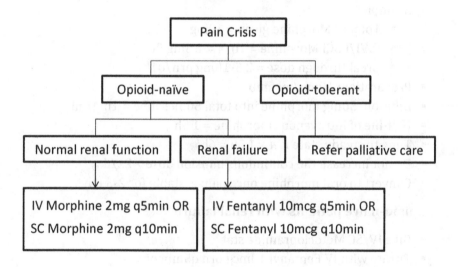

Definitions

- Opioid-tolerant
    - Patients who are taking oral morphine ≥ 60mg/day or an equianalgesic dose of another opioid for a week or longer

- Opioid-naïve
    - Patient who are not taking any opioid
    - Patients who do not meet the definition of opioid-tolerant

Opioid-naïve patients with normal renal function

- Give IV/SC Metoclopramide 10mg stat
- Titrate with IV Morphine 2mg q5min or
- Titrate with SC Morphine 2mg q10min if no IV access
- Check respiratory rate (RR) before each titration
- Titrate till patient is in less distress or pain score <4
- Calculate the total morphine dose given during titration
- Divide the total dose by 4 to get the hourly infusion dose
- Breakthrough: 1-4x hourly dose prn/q1h
- Example:
    - Total IV Morphine given = 10mg
    - CIVI/CSCI Morphine = 10/4 = 2.5mg/h
    - Breakthrough dose = 2.5-10mg prn/q1h
- Preparation: 10mg/ml amp
- Dilution: 50mg morphine into total 50ml saline = 1mg/ml
- Half-life of intravenous morphine = 1.5h
- Time to steady state is 4 x 1.5h = 6h
- Do not increase the continuous infusion dose > 2x/day
- Convert to oral morphine once pain is stable for 2-3 days

Opioid-naïve patients with renal failure

- Give IV/SC Metoclopramide stat
- Titrate with IV Fentanyl 10mcg prn q5min or
- Titrate with SC Fentanyl 10mcg prn q10min if no IV access
- Check respiratory rate (RR) before each titration
- Titrate till patient is in less distress or pain score <4
- Calculate the total fentanyl dose given during titration
- Divide the total dose by 2 to get the hourly infusion dose

- Breakthrough: 1-2x hourly dose prn/q1h
- Example:
    - Total IV Fentanyl given = 50mcg
    - CIVI/CSCI Fentanyl = 50/2 = 25mcg/h
    - Breakthrough dose = 25-50mcg prn/q1h
- Preparation: 100mcg/2ml amp
- Dilution: 500mcg into total 50ml saline = 10mcg/ml
- Half-life of intravenous fentanyl = 3.5h
- Time to steady state is 4 x 3.5h = 14h
- Do not increase the continuous infusion dose > 2x/day
- Convert to fentanyl patch once pain is stable for 2-3 days

"1 + 1" titration method for hydromorphone

- IV Hydromorphone 1mg stat, then 1mg prn 15min later
- Adequate analgesia within 1h in 96% (Chang 2009)

Opioid-tolerant patients

- Refer palliative care team for advice
- Use the breakthrough dose as bolus for rapid titration
- Example:
    - Syrup morphine 30mg q4h
    - Oral morphine breakthrough dose = 30mg
    - Parenteral morphine breakthrough dose = 10mg
    - IV Morphine 10mg q5min or SC Morphine 10mg q10min

Patient controlled analgesia (PCA)

- Opioid-naïve patients
    - PCA IV Morphine
        - Strength: 1mg/ml
        - Dose: 1-3mg
        - Lockout: 10min
        - Total dose over 4h ÷ 4 = infusion rate in mg/h

- New PCA dose = 50% hourly infusion rate
- Max PCA doses/hour = 3-5x estimated required dose
- PCA IV Hydromorphone
  - Strength: 0.2mg/ml
  - Dose: 0.2-0.4mg
  - Lockout: 10min
- PCA IV Fentanyl
  - Strength: 10mcg/ml
  - Dose: 10-20mcg
  - Lockout: 10min
- Opioid-tolerant patients
  - PCA IV Morphine
    - Continuous infusion rate in mg/h
    - PCA dose = 50% hourly infusion rate

Dosage increase and opioid toxicity

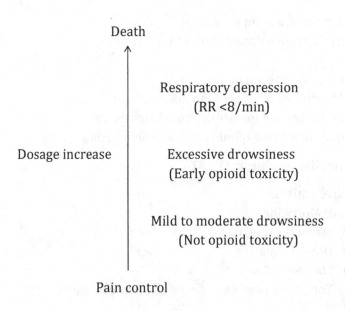

Death

Respiratory depression
(RR <8/min)

Dosage increase

Excessive drowsiness
(Early opioid toxicity)

Mild to moderate drowsiness
(Not opioid toxicity)

Pain control

Monitoring in the hospital

- Pain control
  - Numerical pain score q4h
  - End point
    - Patient is less distressed by the pain or
    - Pain score <4
    - Do not reduce pain to 0 during rapid titration to minimize the risk of opioid toxicity
  - Give breakthrough dose if pain score ≥4
- Drowsiness
  - Pasero Opioid-induced Sedation Scale (POSS) q4h
    - S = Sleep, easily arousable
    - 1 = Awake and alert
    - 2 = Slightly drowsy, easily arousable
    - 3 = Frequently drowsy, arousable, drifts off to sleep during conversation
    - 4 = Somnolent, minimal or no response to verbal and physical stimulation
  - S, 1, 2: increase opioid dose if pain is uncontrolled
  - 3: decrease 25-50% opioid dose
  - 4: decrease 50% opioid dose if RR≥8/min; give naloxone 20mcg prn q2min IV or q5min SC if RR<8/min
- Respiratory depression
  - Check RR q1h for first 24h, then q4h
  - Count 1min
  - Give naloxone if RR<8/min
    - Dilute 400mcg (1 ampoule) to 10ml with NS
    - Give 20mcg (0.5ml) q2min IV or q5min SC till RR ≥8/min

Neuropathic Pain Management

Introduction

Neuropathic pain is pain caused by damage to the somatosensory system. The damage is associated with somatosensory signs and symptoms that can be picked up using various neuropathic pain screening tools.

Neuropathic pain screening tools

- LANSS (Leeds Assessment of Neuropathic Symptoms and Signs)
- DN4 (Douleur Neuropathique 4)
- NPQ (Neuropathic Pain Questionnaire)
- PainDETECT
- ID Pain

LANSS (Bennett 2001)

- Does your pain feel like strange, unpleasant sensations in your skin? Words like pricking, tingling, pin and needles might describe these sensations. (5 marks) *Dysesthetic pain*
- Does your pain make the skin in the painful area look different from normal? Words like mottled, looking more red or pink might describe the appearance. (5 marks) *Skin appearance*
- Does your pain make the affected skin abnormally sensitive to touch? Getting unpleasant sensations when lightly stroking the skin, or getting pain when wearing tight clothes might describe the abnormal sensitivity. (3 marks) *Allodynia*
- Does your pain come on suddenly and in bursts for no apparent reason when you are still? Words like electric shocks, jumping and bursting describe these sensations. (2 marks) *Lancinating pain*

- Does your pain feel as if the skin temperature in the painful area has changed abnormally? Words like hot and burning describe these sensations. (1 mark) *Skin temperature*
- Unpleasant sensations like tingling and nausea while lightly stroking cotton wool across painful area. (5 marks) *Allodynia*
- No sensation, reduced sensation or very painful sensation during pinprick examination on painful area. (3 marks) *Anaesthesia, hypoesthesia or hyperalgesia*
  - Score <12: neuropathic mechanisms are unlikely
  - Score ≥12: neuropathic mechanisms are likely
  - Sensitivity 80%, specificity 85%

NNTs of neuropathic agents (Finnerup 2005, 2007)

Antidepressants	NNT
Tricyclic antidepressants (TCAs)	2-3
▪ Balanced SNRIs	2.1
▪ Amitriptyline	
▪ Imipramine	
▪ Clomipramine	
▪ Predominantly NRIs	2.5
▪ Nortriptyline	
▪ Desipramine	
▪ Maprotiline	
Serotonin-noradrenaline reuptake inhibitors (SNRIs)	5.1
▪ Duloxetine	
▪ Venlafaxine	
Dopamine-noradrenaline reuptake inhibitors (DNRIs)	1.6
▪ Bupropion	
Selective serotonin reuptake inhibitors (SSRIs)	7
▪ Paroxetine	
▪ Citalopram	
▪ Fluoxetine	

Anticonvulsants	NNT
Gabapentin (all doses)	5.1
Gabapentin 800mg tds	3.8
Pregabalin 150-300mg bd	3.7
Sodium valproate 400mg tds	2.5
Phenytoin	2.1
Carbamazepine	2.0
Lamotrigine 400mg dly	4.9
Topiramate	7.4

NNTs of opioids

- Morphine   2.5
- Oxycodone   2.6
- Tramadol   3.9

NNTs of miscellaneous agents

- Topical lignocaine   4.4
- Topical capsaicin   6.7

Choices of neuropathic medications in palliative care

- Step 1: strong opioid ± NSAID/steroid
- Step 2: tricyclic antidepressant or anticonvulsant
- Step 3: tricyclic antidepressant and anticonvulsant
- Step 4: ketamine
- Step 5: spinal opioid

Tricyclic antidepressant titration

- Standard titration
    - Day 1: PO Amitriptyline 25mg on
    - Day 3: PO Amitriptyline 50mg on
    - Week 2: PO Amitriptyline 75mg on

- Week 2: PO Amitriptyline 100mg on
- Week 3: PO Amitriptyline 150mg on (often unnecessary)
- Frail elderly
  - Day 1: PO Amitriptyline 10mg on
  - Day 3: PO Amitriptyline 25mg on
  - Week 2: PO Amitriptyline 50mg on
  - Week 4: PO Amitriptyline 75mg on
  - Week 6: PO Amitriptyline 100mg on
  - Week 8: PO Amitriptyline 150mg on (often unnecessary)
- Amitriptyline
  - Mechanism: serotonin-noradrenaline reuptake inhibitor
  - Analgesic effect: after 3-7 days
  - Antidepressant effect: after 2-4 weeks
  - Contraindicated in significant heart disease
  - Taken at night
  - Taken 2h pre-bed if early morning drowsiness
  - Significant blood level indicated by dry mouth
  - Stop if <50% pain reduction despite reasonable doses
  - Length of trial: 4-6 weeks
  - Stop gradually over 2-3 weeks
  - When switching from one antidepressant class to another, overlap the gradual stopping of old antidepressant with the gradual introduction of new antidepressant over 2-3 weeks

Other antidepressants

- Second generation TCAs
  - Secondary amines
  - First line antidepressant for neuropathic pain
  - Recommended by NeuPSIG of IASP
  - NeuPSIG: Neuropathic Pain Special Interest Group
  - Less adverse effect than first generation TCAs

- PO Nortriptyline 25-150mg on
- PO Desipramine 25-150mg on
- First generation TCAs
  - Tertiary amines
  - First line antidepressant for neuropathic pain
  - Recommended if secondary amines are not available
  - More analgesic property than second generation TCAs
    - PO Amitriptyline 25-150mg on
    - PO Imipramine 25-150mg on
- PO Duloxetine (Cymbalta)
  - Second line antidepressant for neuropathic pain
  - Mechanism: serotonin-noradrenaline reuptake inhibitor
  - Week 1: 30mg on
  - Week 2: 60mg on (more nausea if initiate at 60mg dly)
  - Week 2: 60mg bd (more analgesia and more side effects)
  - Optimal dose: 60mg on
  - Contraindicated if CC<30ml/min
  - Stop if no benefit despite maximum dose
  - Length of trial: 4 weeks
  - Stop gradually over 2-3 weeks
- PO Venlafaxine (Effexor)
  - Second line antidepressant for neuropathic pain
  - Mechanism: serotonin-noradrenaline reuptake inhibitor
  - Week 1: 37.5mg dly
  - Week 2: 37.5mg bd
  - Week 4: 75mg bd
  - Optimal dose: 75mg bd
  - May increase systolic BP ≥10mm with 75mg bd
  - Contraindicated if CC <10ml/min or PT>18s
  - Stop if no benefit despite maximum dose
  - Length of trial: 4-6 weeks
  - Stop gradually over 2-3 weeks

- PO Venlafaxine MR (Effexor XL)
  - Week 1: 37.5mg dly
  - Week 2: 75mg dly
  - Week 4: 150mg dly
- PO Bupropion (Wellbutrin)
  - Mechanism: serotonin-noradrenaline reuptake inhibitor, dopamine reuptake inhibitor
  - Psychostimulant properties
  - Starting dose: 75mg bd
  - Average dose: 100-150mg bd
  - Maximum dose: 300mg bd (risk of seizure)
- PO Citalopram (Celexa)
  - Mechanism: selective serotonin reuptake inhibitor
  - Starting dose: 10mg om
  - Average dose: 20-40mg om
  - Maximum dose: 60mg om
  - Taper gradually
- PO Paroxetine (Paxil)
  - Mechanism: selective serotonin reuptake inhibitor
  - Starting dose: 10mg on
  - Average dose: 20-40mg on
  - Maximum dose: 60mg on
  - Taper gradually

Gabapentin titration in normal renal function

- Rapid titration
  - Day 1: PO Gabapentin 300mg on
  - Day 2: PO Gabapentin 300mg bd
  - Day 3: PO Gabapentin 300mg tds
  - Day 6: PO Gabapentin 600mg tds
  - Day 9: PO Gabapentin 800-900mg tds
  - Day 12: PO Gabapentin 1200mg tds (often unnecessary)

- Slow titration in frail elderly
    - Week 1: PO Gabapentin 300mg on
    - Week 2: PO Gabapentin 300mg tds
    - Week 3: PO Gabapentin 600mg tds
    - Week 4: PO Gabapentin 800-900mg tds
    - Week 5: PO Gabapentin 1200mg tds (often unnecessary)

Gabapentin titration in renal impairment

CC in ml/min	Starting dose	Maximum dose
>80	300mg tds	800mg tds
50-80	200mg tds	400mg tds
30-50	300mg on	300mg bd
15-30	300mg EOD	300mg on
<15	300mg EOD	300mg EOD
After 4h HD	200-300mg stat	

- Gabapentin (Neurontin)
    - First line anticonvulsant in neuropathic pain
    - Mechanism: $\alpha2\delta$ subunit calcium channel blocker
    - GABA analogue but no activity at GABA receptor
    - Analgesic effect: from immediate to 1-2 weeks
    - Maximum analgesic effect: 2 months
    - Synergism: Gabapentin 600mg tds+nortriptyline 50mg on
        - More effective than either drug alone at high doses
        - Without significant side effects
    - Drowsiness in 50%: resolves in 7-10 days
    - Capsule can be opened
    - Contents can be mixed with water or fruit juice
    - Stop if no benefit despite ≥800mg tds
    - Length of trial: 8 weeks
    - Stop gradually over 1-2 weeks

Pregabalin titration in normal renal function

- Standard titration
    - Day 1: PO Pregabalin 75mg bd
    - After 3-7 days: PO Pregabalin 150mg bd
    - After 3-7 days: PO Pregabalin 225mg bd
    - After 3-7 days: PO Pregabalin 300mg bd
- Slow titration in frail elderly
    - Day 1: PO Pregabalin 75mg on
    - Increase cautiously every week if necessary

Pregabalin titration in renal impairment

CC in ml/min	Starting dose	Maximum dose
>60	75mg bd	300mg bd
31-60	25mg tds	150mg bd
15-30	25-50mg on	150mg on
<15	25mg on	75mg on
After 4h HD	25mg stat	150mg stat

- Pregabalin (Lyrica)
    - First line anticonvulsant in neuropathic pain
    - Mechanism: α2δ subunit calcium channel blocker
    - GABA analogue but no activity at GABA receptor
    - Analgesic effect: <24h
    - Maximum analgesic effect: 2 weeks
    - Compared to gabapentin
        - More rapid onset of pain relief
        - Linear pharmacokinetics: less individual variability
        - Less dose-related side effects: faster titration
        - Twice daily dosing
        - Maximum benefit at 2 weeks (gabapentin 2 months)

- Stop if no benefit despite 300mg bd
- Length of trial: 8 weeks
- Stop gradually over 1-2 weeks

Other anticonvulsants

- PO Sodium valproate (Epilim)
    - Mechanism: GABA reuptake inhibitor, GABA transaminase inhibitor, sodium channel blocker
    - Week 1: 200mg tds
    - Week 2: 400mg tds
    - Week 3: 600mg bd
- PO Phenytoin (Dilantin)
    - Mechanism: sodium channel blocker
    - 100mg tds
- PO Carbamazepine (Tegretol)
    - Mechanism: sodium channel blocker
    - Starting dose: 100-200mg bd
    - Titration: 200mg increment every 1-2 weeks
    - Maximum dose: 600mg bd
- PO Lamotrigine (Lamictal)
    - Mechanism: sodium channel blocker
    - Starting dose: 25-50mg on
    - Titration: 50mg increment every 2 weeks
    - Maximum dose: 400mg on
- PO Topiramate (Topamax)
    - Mechanism: sodium channel blocker, GABA potentiation
    - Starting dose: 50mg on
    - Titration: 50mg increment every 2 weeks
    - Maximum dose: 200mg bd
- PO Levetiracetam (Keppra)
    - Mechanism: calcium channel blocker
    - Starting dose: 500mg bd

- Titration: 1000mg increment every 2 weeks
- Maximum dose: 1500mg bd
- PO Zonisamide (Zonegran)
  - Mechanism: sodium channel blocker, calcium channel blocker, GABA release
  - Starting dose: 100mg dly for 2 weeks
  - Titration: 200mg increment every week
  - Maximum dose: 200mg bd

Miscellaneous neuropathic agents

- PO/SC/IV Dexamethasone
  - Dexamethasone 4-8mg om for plexus or root compression
  - Dexamethasone 12-16mg om for spinal cord compression
  - Trial of 5-7 days
- PO Ketamine
  - Mechanism: NMDAR blocker
  - Day 1: 10mg tds-qid
  - Day 2: 20mg tds-qid
  - Day 3: 40mg tds-qid
  - Day 4: 60mg tds-qid
  - Day 5: 80mg tds-qid
  - Day 6: 100mg tds-qid
  - Consider the following:
    - 30-50% opioid dose reduction at the beginning
    - Further opioid dose reduction during titration
    - PRN/tds ketamine equivalent to regular dose
    - Q4h dosing for end-of-dose pain
    - Smaller doses and q4h dosing for neuropsychiatric side effects or drowsiness despite opioid reduction
    - Prevention of neuropsychiatric side effects
      - PO Haloperidol 1.5-3mg on
      - PO Diazepam 2.5-5mg on

- Lignocaine patch 5% (Lidoderm)
  - Useful in localized neuropathic pain
  - 1-3 patches daily
  - 12h on, 12h off: to avoid tachyphylaxis (acute tolerance)
  - Applied to intact skin to cover the most painful area
- Capsaicin patch 8% (Qutenza)
  - Useful in localized neuropathic pain
  - 1-4 patches every three months
  - Application techniques
    - Wear gloves
    - Mark painful area
    - Wash the area with mild soap and water
    - Dry thoroughly
    - Anaesthetize skin with topical LA
    - Wash and dry the area
    - Cut patch to fit area
    - Leave patch in place
      - 30min for feet
      - 60min for other locations
    - Remove patch by gently rolling it inward
    - Apply cleansing gel to area for 1 minute
    - Wash the area with mild soap and water
    - Dry thoroughly
  - Side effects in 5%: redness, pain, itching, papules
- Capsaicin cream 0.075%
  - Useful in localized neuropathic pain
  - Applied to painful area tds-qid
  - Causes severe burning sensation
  - Stop if no benefit after 1 week
- EMLA cream
  - Useful in localized neuropathic pain
  - Eutectic mixture of LA: prilocaine and lignocaine

Neuropathic pain crisis

- Step 1: rapid parenteral morphine titration or IV PCA opioid
- Step 2: parenteral opioid switching
- Step 3: parenteral lignocaine or ketamine
- Step 4: spinal opioid

Parenteral lignocaine

- Mechanism: sodium channel blocker
- Standard dose: IV Lignocaine 5mg/kg over 30-60min
    - <250mg: dilute with 100ml D5
    - ≥250mg: dilute with 500ml D5
    - Maximum dose: 900mg
- Low dose: IV Lignocaine 1mg/kg over 30min
- Syringe driver dose
    - CSCI Lignocaine 1-2mg/kg/h or
    - CSCI Lignocaine 500-1000mg/24h
    - Useful for patients who require frequent IV Lignocaine

Parenteral ketamine

- Mechanism: NMDAR blocker
- Standard titration of subcutaneous ketamine infusion
    - Day 1: CSCI Ketamine 50mg/24h (2mg/h)
    - Day 2: CSCI Ketamine 100mg/24h (4mg/h)
    - Day 3: CSCI Ketamine 200mg/24h (8mg/h)
    - Day 4: CSCI Ketamine 300mg/24h (12mg/h)
    - Day 5: CSCI Ketamine 400mg/24h (16mg/h)
    - Day 6: CSCI Ketamine 500mg/24h (20mg/h)
    - Day 7: CSCI Ketamine 600mg/24h (25mg/h)
    - Consider the following:
        - Starting at 25mg/24h (1mg/h) for frail elderly
        - Loading dose of 10mg in 1ml NS
        - 50-100% q8h titration in severe uncontrolled pain

- 30-50% opioid dose reduction at the beginning
- Further opioid dose reduction during titration
- Prevention of neuropsychiatric side effects
  - CSCI Haloperidol 1.5-3mg/24h
  - CSCI Midazolam 5-10mg/24h
- Burst ketamine
  - Day 1: CSCI Ketamine 100mg/24h
    - Effective: continue for 3 days, then stop
    - Ineffective: titrate
  - Day 2: CSCI Ketamine 300mg/24h
    - Effective: continue for 3 days, then stop
    - Ineffective: titrate
  - Day 3: CSCI Ketamine 500mg/24h
    - Effective: continue for 3 days, then stop
    - Ineffective: stop
- Preparation: 50mg/ml in 10ml vial
- Conversion to oral ketamine
  - Oral ketamine is metabolized by CYP3A4 to norketamine
  - Norketamine
    - 1/3 as potent as parenteral ketamine as anaesthetic
    - Equipotent to parenteral ketamine as analgesia
  - Switch to oral ketamine q6h with 1:1 conversion

Miscellaneous parenteral neuropathic agents

- IV Dexmedetomidine 0.2-0.6mcg/kg/h over 50min
- IV Phenytoin 600mg over 24h
- IV Phenytoin 15mg/kg over 2h
- IV Sodium valproate 200-400mg tds
- IV Ondansetron 8mg once
- IV Magnesium sulfate 30mg/kg over 30min

Bone Pain Management

Introduction

Optimal management of bone metastases needs integration of opioid and non-opioid analgesia, bone-targeted agents, cancer-directed treatment and sometimes orthopaedic surgery.

Clinical features of bone pain

- Dull and constant pain
- Increases gradually with time
- May be aggravated by movement or weight-bearing
- Progresses to spontaneous pain with time
- Spontaneous pain can be acute, severe and unpredictable

Mechanisms of cancer-induced bone pain

- Nociceptive component
    - Inflammatory mediators
    - Skeletal remodelling
- Neuropathic component
    - Damage to sensory and sympathetic nerves
    - Pathological sprouting

Analgesia

- Use WHO analgesic ladder
    - Paracetamol
    - NSAIDs: reduce inflammatory mediators
    - Steroids: reduce inflammatory mediators
    - Opioid
    - Neuropathic agents: target neuropathic component

Bone-targeted agents

- Biphosphonates
    - Osteoclast inhibitor
    - Target skeletal remodelling
    - Benefits
        - Reduce frequency of skeletal-related events (SREs)
        - Reduce bone pain
        - Reduce hypercalcemia
    - Onset of analgesia: 2 weeks
    - NNT for pain control: 11 at 4 weeks, 7 at 12 weeks
    - Long term use ≥6 months reduces new SREs in breast cancer, prostate cancer and myeloma
    - Non-nitrogen containing bisphosphonates
        - Clodronate and etidronate
        - Converted intracellularly into methylene-containing ATP analogue
        - Accumulate in macrophages and osteoclasts
        - Cause direct apoptosis
    - Nitrogen containing bisphosphonates
        - Pamidronate, zoledronate, ibandronate
        - Also inhibit farnesyl diphosphate synthase (rate-limiting enzyme of mevalonate pathway)
            - Prevent protein prenylation of small GTPase (Ras, Rho, Rab): important signalling proteins that regulate osteoclast survival
    - Indications
        - Breast cancer with symptomatic bone mets
        - Hormone-resistant prostate cancer with bone mets
        - Myeloma requiring chemotherapy ± bone mets
    - Dosages
        - IV Pamidronate (Aredia) 90mg over 4h monthly
        - IV Zoledronate (Zometa) 4mg over 15min monthly

- Avoid in renal failure
- Side effect: osteonecrosis of the jaw
  - Long term pamidronate 4%
  - Long term zoledronate 10%
- Stop if declining performance status
- Denosumab
  - RANK-L antibody
  - Osteoclast inhibitor
  - Superior over zoledronate in preventing SREs
  - Dosage: SC Denosumab (XGEVA) 120mg monthly
  - No need dose adjustment in renal failure

External beam radiotherapy

- For localized bone metastases
- Pain relief within 4-6 weeks
  - 60%: partial pain relief
  - 30%: complete pain relief
  - 10%: pain flare during first few days
- Single fraction 8Gy as efficacious as 5 fractions 20Gy
- Single fraction: re-treatment rate 2.5x higher

Radiopharmaceuticals

- For widespread painful bone metastases
- Response rate: 40-95%
- Strontium-89 or samarium-153
- Side effect: bone marrow suppression (mild, reversible)

Spinal cord compression

- Combined surgery and radiotherapy for fit patients
  - Superior to radiotherapy alone in functional outcome
- Radiotherapy alone
  - For unfit patients with poor prognosis

Miscellaneous treatment

- Radiofrequency ablation (RFA)
- High intensity focused ultrasound (HIFU)
- Vertebroplasty
- Surgical fixation of pathological fracture or impending pathological fracture

---

Interesting facts

Chronic pain can be unlearned through 6 weeks of visualization based on neuroplasticity because neurons that fire together wire together, neurons that fire apart wire apart. The techniques are summarized in the acronym MIRROR (Moskowitz 2013).

- **M**otivation: Stay motivated to change the brain even without immediate success.
- **I**ntention: Focus on changing the brain to stop persistent pain.
- **R**elentlessness: Counter-stimulate every pain intrusion using thoughts, images, sensations, memories, soothing emotions, movement and beliefs.
- **R**eliability: Count on the brain to make positive change.
- **O**pportunity: Use pain intrusions as an opportunity to practice neuroplastic treatment approaches to stop pain.
- **R**estoration: Disconnect expanded pain map to its important role of sounding and alarm about danger.

Incident Pain Management

Introduction

Incident pain is pain caused by a specific event like movement.

Types of breakthrough pain (BTP)

- Spontaneous pain
- Incident pain
    - Volitional: movement, sitting, eating, drinking
    - Non-volitional: cough, micturition, defecation
    - Procedural: wound dressing
- End-of-dose failure

Simple measures

- Movement-related pain
    - Make use of a draw sheet correctly
    - Turn patient gently
    - Pay attention to facial expression or vocalization of pain
- Cough-related pain
    - Give cough suppressant
    - Advise to reduce smoking if appropriate
    - Advise to reduce food or drink which aggravates cough
- Meal-related pain
    - Treat oral candidiasis
    - Use lignocaine viscous or coating agent for mucositis
    - Consider alternative feeding route like NG feeding
- Micturition-related pain
    - Rapid response to request for help
    - Urinary catheter for urinary retention
    - Rapid diaper change for perianal excoriation

- Defecation-related pain
  - Rapid response to request for help
  - Laxatives for constipation
  - Local anaesthetic for haemorrhoids
  - Rapid diaper change for perianal excoriation
- Procedure-related pain
  - Explanation about the procedure
  - Distract patient by talking if appropriate
  - Stop immediately if requested
  - Local anaesthetic before procedure

Analgesics and onset of analgesia

- Onset of analgesia ≤5min
  - IV Alfentanil: 0.75min
  - IV Sufentanil: 1min
  - IV Fentanyl: 1.5min
  - IV Morphine: 5min
- Onset of analgesia ≤10min
  - SL Sufentanil: 4-6min
  - SL Alfentanil: 5-10min
  - SL Fentanyl: 5-10min
  - IN Fentanyl: 5-10min
  - OTFC: 5-10min
  - SC Morphine: 10min
  - IN Ketamine: 10min
- Onset of analgesia ≤30min
  - Neb Fentanyl: 15min
  - SL Buprenorphine: 15-30min
  - SC Ketamine: 15-30min
  - Syrup Morphine: 20-30min
  - PO Methadone: 30min
  - PO Ketamine: 30min

Sedatives and onset of sedation

- Nitrous oxide: <1min
- IV Midazolam: 2-3min
- SC Midazolam: 5-10min
- SL Lorazepam: 5min
- PO Lorazepam: 10-15min
- Buccal Midazolam: 15min

Characteristics of BTP

- Rapid onset BTP (ROBTP)
    - Peaks within 5min
    - Fades within 15min
- Gradual onset BTP (GOBTP)
    - Peaks within 15-30min
    - Fades within 1h

	ROBTP	Syrup morphine	OTFC
Onset	Immediate	20-30min	5-10min
Peak	5min	40-60min	20min
Duration	15min	4h	1-2h

Management of GOBTP and ROBTP

- Triple opioid therapy (TOT)
    - Baseline pain: long acting opioid
    - GOBTP: short acting opioid
    - ROBTP: rapid onset opioid
- Rapid onset opioids
    - OTFC
    - SL Fentanyl
    - IN Fentanyl
    - SL Alfentanil
    - SL Sufentanil

Management of non-volitional incident pain

- Step 1: SL Fentanyl 25mcg
- Step 2: SL Fentanyl 50mcg
- Step 3: SL Sufentanil 12.5mcg or SL Alfentanil 0.5mg
- Step 4: SL Sufentanil 25mcg or SL Alfentanil 1mg
- Step 5: SL Sufentanil 50mcg or SL Alfentanil 2mg

Management of volitional incident pain and procedural pain

- Step 1: PO Analgesia ± PO Sedative
  - PO Analgesia 60min before incidence/procedure
    - PO Diclofenac 50-100mg or
    - PO Dihydrocodeine 30-60mg or
    - PO Tramadol 50-100mg or
    - Syrup morphine 1/6 total oral daily dose
  - PO Sedative 60min before incidence/procedure
    - PO Lorazepam 0.5-1mg or
    - PO Diazepam 5mg
- Step 2: SL/SC Analgesia ± SL/SC Sedative
  - SL/SC Analgesia 30min before incidence/procedure
    - OTFC (Actiq) 200mcg or
    - Fentanyl buccal tablet (Effentora) 100mcg or
    - Fentanyl sublingual tablet (Abstral) 100mcg or
    - Fentanyl intranasal spray (Lazanda) 100mcg or
    - Fentanyl sublingual solution 50-100mcg or
    - Alfentanil sublingual solution 250-500mcg or
    - Sufentanil sublingual solution 12.5-25mcg or
    - SC Morphine 1/6 total SC daily dose
  - SL/SC Sedative 30min before incidence/procedure
    - SL Lorazepam 0.5-1mg
    - SL Alprazolam 0.25-0.5mg
    - SC Midazolam 2.5-5mg
    - Buccal Midazolam 2.5-5mg

- Step3: IV Analgesia ± IV Sedative
  - IV Analgesia 5min before incidence/procedure
    - IV Morphine 1/6 total IV daily dose
    - IV Fentanyl 1/12 total IV daily dose
    - IV Ketamine 25-50mg
      - Give 5mg q1min till sedation
  - IV Sedative 5min before incidence/procedure
    - IV Midazolam 2.5-5mg
      - Give 0.5mg q1min till sedation

Cautions

- Health care providers must be competent in:
  - Opioid and sedative titration
  - Airway management
  - Reversal of analgesia and sedation
    - Benzodiazepine reversal
      - IV Flumazenil 0.2mg prn/q1min
      - Maximum 4 doses
      - Repeat after 20min if re-sedation
      - Benzodiazepine tolerance
        - Aim: partial reversal
        - Endpoint: RR≥8/min
    - Opioid reversal
      - IV Naloxone 20mcg prn/q2min
      - Opioid tolerance
        - Aim: partial reversal
        - Endpoint: RR≥8/min

Anaesthetic Procedure in Pain Control

Introduction

Interventional pain management is considered 'step 4' in WHO analgesic ladder. (Miguel 2000)

Neuraxial infusions

- Indications
    - Unacceptable side effects with systemic opioids
    - Poor pain control with systemic opioids
    - Unsuccessful opioid switching
- Epidural opioid infusion
    - Short term use ≤ 3 weeks
    - Higher rate of catheter migration and occlusion
    - Divide parenteral morphine daily dose by 10 to get the epidural morphine daily dose
- Intrathecal opioid infusion
    - Long term use 3 weeks to 3 months
    - Lower rate of catheter migration and occlusion
    - Divide parenteral morphine daily dose by 100 to get the intrathecal morphine daily dose
    - Consider an implantable pump system if:
        - Long term use ≥ 3 months
        - Able to afford the implant pump
        - Diffuse pain from widespread metastases
        - Access to pump refill/reprogramming capabilities
        - Favourable response to intrathecal trial with >50% pain relief

- Absence of severe incident pain requiring frequent patient-controlled doses
    - Absence of the need for an epidural infusion which requires a higher volume
- Implantable pump system
    - Fixed rate pump
        - 0.5ml/day or 1ml/day
        - Titration based on changing concentration
        - Refillable drug reservoir up to 60ml
    - Programmable rate pump
        - Titration based on programming the pump
        - Refillable drug reservoir 20-40ml

Intrathecal analgesia

- Step 1: morphine/hydromorphone
- Step 2: morphine/hydromorphone + bupivacaine
- Step 3: morphine/hydromorphone + bupivacaine + clonidine
- Switch to fentanyl/sufentanil if side effects or lack of analgesia

Equianalgesic opioid switching in mg

Opioid	Parenteral	Epidural	Intrathecal
Morphine	100	10	1
Hydromorphone	20	2	0.25
Fentanyl	1	0.01	0.001

Maximum long term IT drug concentrations and doses

- Proposed to minimize risk of catheter tip granuloma

Drug	Max concentration (mg/ml)	Maximum daily dose (mg)
Morphine	20	15
Hydromorphone	10	4
Bupivacaine	40	30
Clonidine	2	1

Spinal drugs

- Morphine and hydromorphone
  - First line spinal opioids
  - Hydrophilic
  - Penetrate spine effectively
  - Slow redistribution
- Fentanyl and sufentanil
  - Second line spinal opioids
  - Hydrophobic
  - Penetrate spine less effectively
  - Rapid redistribution
  - Lower risk of catheter tip granuloma
- Bupivacaine
  - Concentration
    - 0.125% = 1.25mg/ml (pain relief)
    - 0.25% = 2.5mg/ml (pain relief)
    - 0.375% = 3.75mg/ml (sensory/motor block)
    - 0.5% = 5mg/ml (sensory/motor block)
  - Epidural (ED) Bupivacaine 2-6ml/h
  - Intrathecal (IT) Bupivacaine 0.5-2ml/h
  - Side effects: dose-dependent sensory/motor block
  - Sensory/motor block: dose ≥15mg/day
- Clonidine
  - ED Clonidine 150-300mcg/24h
  - IT Clonidine 15-30mcg/24h
  - Side effects: dose-dependent hypotension, bradycardia

Breakthrough pain for spinal analgesia

- Oral or SC Morphine prn
- Oral or SC Ketamine 10-25mg prn

Nerve blocks

- Esophageal visceral pain
  - Interpleural block
- Upper abdominal visceral pain
  - Coeliac plexus block
- Pelvic visceral pain (except ovarian pain)
  - Superior hypogastric block
- Perineal visceral pain
  - Ganglion impar block
- Perineal and perianal pain
  - Saddle block

Peripheral nerve blocks

- Peripheral nerve blocks with proven success rate
  - Gasserian block for trigeminal neuralgia
  - Intercostal block for chest wall or rib metastases
  - Paravertebral block for radicular pain
- Infusion rate
  - Peripheral infusion of lignocaine 1-2% 3-8ml/h
  - Peripheral infusion of bupivacaine 0.125-0.25% 3-8ml/h
  - Peripheral infusion of ropivacaine 0.2-0.3% 3-8ml/h

Breathlessness

Introduction

Breathlessness is a subjective experience of breathing discomfort. It is caused by a mismatch between the need of breathing and the work of breathing.

Sensory information on the need of breathing

- Chemoreceptors
    - Central chemoreceptors
        - Ventrolateral surface of medulla oblongata
            - Detect CSF pH, not plasma pH
                - CO_2 crosses blood-brain barrier
                - Reacts with H_2O
                - Becomes carbonic acid
                - Reduces pH
                - Stimulates central chemoreceptors
            - Cannot detect plasma pH
                - H^+ cannot cross blood-brain barrier
    - Peripheral chemoreceptors
        - Carotid bodies
            - At common carotid arteries
            - Detect blood O2, CO2 and pH
            - By type I glomus cell
            - To carotid sinus nerve
            - To glossopharyngeal nerve
            - To medulla oblongata
        - Aortic bodies
            - At aortic arch
            - Detect blood O2 and CO2

- By type I glomus cell
- To vagus nerve
- To medulla oblongata
- Cold receptors at upper airway
  - Innervated by vagus nerve
  - Detect change in temperature of upper airway
  - Stimulation reduces dyspnoea
- Juxtacapillary receptors (J receptors)
  - Also called pulmonary C-fiber receptors
  - Located within alveolar wall
  - In juxtaposition to pulmonary capillaries of the lung
  - Innervated by vagus nerve
  - Detect increase in pulmonary interstitial volume
    - Due to pulmonary oedema
  - Detect physical engorgement of pulmonary capillaries
    - Due to left heart failure
- Stretch receptors
  - Slowly adapting stretch receptors (SARs)
    - Located at smooth muscle of larger airway
    - Myelinated afferent fibers of vagus
    - Detect increase in airway wall tension
    - Rhythmic discharge during normal breathing
      - Increased discharge during inspiration
      - Reduced discharge during expiration
    - Stimulation of SARs decreases dyspnoea
  - Rapidly adapting stretch receptors (RARs)
    - Located throughout the respiratory tract
    - Thin myelinated afferent fibers of vagus
    - Detect mechanical and chemical irritant stimuli
    - Irregular discharge
    - Stimulations of RARs causes dyspnoea, cough, bronchospasm, secretion

- Chest wall receptors
  - Muscle spindles in chest wall
  - Detect stretch and tension of respiratory muscles

Motor control on the work of breathing

- Medullary respiratory center
  - Primary respiratory control
  - Groups of respiratory neurons
    - Dorsal respiratory group (DRG)
      - Nucleus tractus solitarius (NTS)
      - Inspiratory neurons
        - Activate phrenic nerve neurons
        - Control diaphragm
        - Control inspiration
        - Inhibit expiratory neurons in VRG, PRG
    - Ventral respiratory group (VRG)
      - Nucleus ambiguous (NA)
        - Inspiratory neurons
          - Supply external intercostal muscles
          - Supply accessory muscles
      - Nucleus retroambigualis (NRA)
        - Rostral NRA: inspiratory neurons
        - Caudal NRA: expiratory neurons
          - Supply internal intercostal muscles
          - Supply abdominal muscles
          - Control voluntary forced expiration
          - Inhibit inspiratory neurons
    - Pre-Botzinger complex (pre-BotC)
      - Pacemaker neurons
    - Botzinger complex (BotC)
      - Nucleus retrofacialis (NRF)
        - Expiratory neurons

- Pontine respiratory center
  - Pneumotaxic center
    - Expiratory neurons
      - Medial parabrachial nucleus
    - Inspiratory neurons
      - Lateral parabachial nucleus
      - Kolliker-Fuse nucleus
    - Inhibits DRG
    - Shortens inspiration
    - Causes phase switching
      - More breaths within a given time
      - Increases respiratory rate
  - Apneustic center
    - Believed to stimulate DRG
    - Not found
- Control of breathing
  - Inspiration
    - 1-2s during normal quiet breathing (eupnoea)
    - Inspiratory neurons in DRG and rVRG send signals to diaphragm and external intercostal muscles
    - Diaphragm pulls downward
    - External intercostals pull ribs upward and outward
  - Expiration (passive)
    - 2-3s
    - Expiratory neurons in BotC terminate inspiration by inhibiting inspiratory neurons
    - Inspiratory muscles relax
    - Ribs return to relaxed position due to compliance
    - Expiratory neurons in cNRA are responsible for forced expiration
    - Send signals to internal intercostal muscles and abdominal muscles

Measuring Breathlessness

Introduction

Unidimensional tools are suitable for the rapid assessment of breathlessness and treatment response. Multidimensional tools are best reserved for quality of life assessment.

Definition of dyspnoea

A subjective experience of breathing discomfort that is comprised of qualitatively distinct sensations that vary in intensity. (American Thoracic Society 1999)

Unidimensional tools

- Numerical rating scale (NRS)
    - Scores breathlessness from 0 to 10
    - 0 = breathlessness
    - 10 = worst possible breathlessness
    - Types of NRSs
        - NRS0: breathlessness score right now
        - NRS24 average: average score last 24h
        - NRS24 best: best score last 24h
        - NRS24 worst: worst score last 24h
- Visual analogue scale (VAS)
    - Scores breathlessness from a 10cm line on a ruler
    - 0 = no breathlessness
    - 10 = worst possible breathlessness
    - Ask patient to mark a point that best describes his or her breathlessness
    - VAS24: average score last 24h
    - ESAS: combined VAS and NRS from 0 to 10

- Modified Borg scale
  - Categorical scale with ratio properties
  - Can be used over the phone
  - Nothing at all = 0
  - Very, very slight (just noticeable) = 0.5
  - Very slight = 1
  - Slight = 2
  - Moderate = 3
  - Somewhat severe = 4
  - Severe = 5
  - Very severe = 7
  - Very, very severe (almost maximal) = 9
  - Maximal = 10

Multidimensional tools

- Breathlessness-specific
  - Modified MRC Dyspnoea Scale
  - Baseline/Transition Dyspnoea Index
  - Feinstein's Index of Dyspnoea
- Disease-specific
  - Cancer Dyspnoeic Scale
  - MND Dyspnoeic Rating Scale
  - Clinical COPD Questionnaire

Treating Causes of Breathlessness

Introduction

Disease-directed management can be helpful in the management of breathlessness. Decision making should be based on autonomy, risk-benefit proportionality, performance status, prognosis and quality of life.

Specific treatment of causes of breathlessness

- Upper airway obstruction
    - Steroids
    - Tracheostomy
    - Stenting
    - Radiotherapy
    - Brachytherapy
    - Laser treatment
- Bronchospasm
    - Bronchodilators
    - Steroids
- Pneumonia
    - Antibiotics
    - Steroids if infective exacerbation of COAD
- Heart failure
    - Diuretics
    - Nitrates
    - Digitalis
    - ACE inhibitors
- Lung cancer
    - Radiotherapy
    - Chemotherapy

- Pleural effusion
  - Pleural drainage
  - Pleurodesis
- Lymphangitis carcinomatosis
  - Steroids
  - Bronchodilators
  - Diuretics
- Pulmonary embolism
  - Low molecular weight heparin
- SVCO
  - Steroids
  - Stenting
  - Radiotherapy
  - Chemotherapy
- Anemia
  - Blood transfusion
  - Erythropoietin

Non-pharmacological Management of Breathlessness

Introduction

Focus more on non-drug approach in the early part of illness. Recognize the increasing role of drug approach as disease progresses.

Breathing environment

- Fan
    - To increase airflow
    - Reduces sensation of breathlessness via trigeminal nerve
    - Types
        - Ceiling fan
        - Table fan
        - Stand fan
        - Hand-held fan
    - Tailor distance, airflow direction, speed and duration according to preferences
    - Could be small battery-operated hand-held or clip-on fan from the night market
- Cool temperature
    - Reduces sensation of breathlessness via trigeminal nerves and thoracic nerves
    - Types
        - Air-conditioner
        - Hand-held small portable air-conditioner
        - Cooling mask for eyes
        - Cold cucumber slices for eyes

- Open space
    - Near-window bed
    - Open window if appropriate
    - Draw curtain according to preferences
    - Avoid overcrowding of visitors
- Loose comfortable clothing

Breathing positions

- Ask patients for their most comfortable positions
- Common positions
    - Lying position
        - High lying: lying supine with more pillows
        - High side lying: lying laterally with more pillows
    - Sitting position
        - Upright: sitting upright
        - Leaning forward: arms supported by a cardiac table
        - Leaning backward: back supported by pillows
    - Standing position
        - Leaning forward: arms supported by a ledge
        - Leaning backward: back against the wall

Breathing techniques

- Educate patients about different breathing techniques
- Deep breathing
    - Breathe in as much air as possible slowly
    - Breathe out as much air as possible slowly
- Pursed-lip breathing
    - Breathe in through the nose
    - Breathe out through partially closed lips
- Abdominal breathing
    - Breathe in and feel the rising of abdomen
    - Breathe out and feel the falling of abdomen

Supportive therapy

- Three main components of supportive therapy
    - Open-ended questions
    - Active listening
    - Empathy
- Explore the breathlessness experience
    - Tell me a little about your experience of breathlessness
    - What are the things that make it better?
    - What are the things that make it worse?
    - What are your feelings when you are breathless?
    - What are your thoughts when you are breathless?
    - How is your breathlessness affecting your daily life?
- Common negative emotions
    - Fear
    - Panic attack
    - Anxiety
    - Sadness
- Common negative thoughts
    - I will suffocate to death
    - I will choke to death
    - I am going to die
- Communicate empathy verbally and non-verbally
    - Acknowledge the experience
    - Validate the experience
    - Normalize the experience

Cognitive-behavioural therapy

- Cognitions
    - Address negative automatic thoughts, eg:
        - Filtering: focusing on the negative
        - Magnifying: exaggerating the negative
        - Catastrophizing: overestimating negative outcome

- Cognitive restructuring
    - Filtering: help patient to focus on the positive
    - Magnifying: help patient to see the reality as it is
    - Catastrophizing: help patient to understand that it is very unlikely to suffocate to death
    - Tell patient that fear, anxiety and panic can make the breathlessness worse
- Behaviours
    - Relaxation
        - Teach patient how to relax during breathlessness
            - Mindful breathing
            - Body scan
            - Visualization
            - Progressive muscular relaxation
    - Panic management
        - Give patient a plan of action in advance of the attack
            - Non-pharmacological plan
            - Pharmacological plan
        - Write down the instructions step by step
    - Goal setting
        - Set a realistic goal for the patient
        - Work with the patient to achieve it
        - Indoor activities: talking, eating, drinking, dressing, walking, bathing, toileting
        - Outdoor activities: gardening, strolling, exercising, shopping, travelling
    - Activity pacing
        - Change routine to suit energy level
        - Sit down while dressing, bathing, toileting if possible
        - Reserve energy for important activities
        - Rest more after certain activities

Supporting the family

- Explore understanding of the situation
    - Give proper information about the situation
- Explore thoughts and emotions
    - Empathic communication
    - Address fear and anxiety
    - Address negative thoughts
    - Cognitive restructuring
    - Teach family to relax
    - Teach family to help patient to relax
- Explore coping skills
    - Remind family of self-care
        - Eat
        - Sleep
        - Relax
    - Involve family in:
        - Relaxation
        - Panic management
        - Goal setting
        - Activity pacing

Little teaching from Thich Nhat Hanh

In Vietnam, there are many people, called boat people, who leave the country in small boats. Often the boats are caught in rough seas or storms, the people may panic, and boats may sink. But if even one person aboard can remain calm, lucid, knowing what to do and what not to do, he or she can help the boat survive.

Pharmacological Management of Breathlessness

Introduction

This chapter focuses on the symptomatic management of breathlessness irrespective of the pathology.

Oxygen

- Hypoxic patients are not necessarily breathless
- Breathless patients are not necessarily hypoxic
- Benefits of oxygen therapy
  - Improves resting and exertional hypoxia, hence reducing the need of breathing
  - Produces a facial or nasal cooling effect, hence reducing breathlessness, even in normoxic patient
  - May act as a placebo in reducing breathlessness
- Harms of oxygen therapy
  - Not comfortable for some patients
  - Costly in certain settings
  - Patients may become psychologically dependent
  - Blocks communication
  - Makes eating and drinking difficult
  - Dries the nasal mucosa
  - Causes pressure sores over the face or the ears
- Normoxic patients
  - Breathless: cooling hand-held or electrical fan
  - Still breathless: oxygen nasal prong 2-3L/min for 15min
    - Improvement: continue and reassess after 24h
    - No improvement: stop oxygen

- Hypoxic patients SaO2 <90%
  - Baseline: oxygen nasal prong 2-3L/min for 15min
    - Improvement: continue and reassess after 24h
    - No improvement: stop oxygen
  - Breakthrough: oxygen face mask ± reservoir
    - During acute attack of breathlessness
      - Incident breathlessness
      - Acute pneumonia
      - Acute bronchospasm
      - Acute pulmonary oedema
      - Acute pulmonary embolism
- Dying patients
  - Many dying patients do not need oxygen
  - Many semi-comatose patients do not tolerate oxygen via face mask or even nasal prong
  - Consider a cooling fan before prescribing oxygen
  - Some do not tolerate even a cooling fan
  - Use oxygen only if there is hypoxia and an absolute improvement in comfort after instituting it
  - Use oxygen nasal prong 2-3L/min prn
  - Take off the continuous saturation monitoring
  - Check saturation prn if really necessary
  - Do not restrain patients when they attempt to pull away the delivery device
  - Stop if patients are not tolerating the device
  - Focus on pharmacological management of breathlessness like opioid or benzodiazepines

Opioids in breathlessness

- Use of opioid in cancer and non-cancer breathlessness is supported by systematic review (Jennings 2002)

- Opioid reduces the sensation of breathlessness and associated anxiety
- Breathlessness improves with doses that do not cause clinically significant respiratory depression
  - Bruera 1990, 1993
  - Mazzocato 1999
  - Abernethy 2003
  - Allen 2005
  - Clemens 2008
- Breathlessness in opioid-naïve patients
  - Mild breathlessness NRS 1-3
    - PO Dihydrocodeine 30-60mg tds-qid or
    - Syrup morphine 2.5mg prn/q1h
  - Moderate breathlessness NRS 4-6
    - Syrup morphine 2.5mg q4h and
    - Syrup morphine 2.5mg prn/q1h for breakthrough
  - Severe breathlessness NRS 7-10
    - Syrup morphine 5mg q4h and
    - Syrup morphine 5mg prn/q1h for breakthrough
- Breathlessness in opioid-tolerant patients
  - Mild breathlessness NRS 1-3
    - Give 25% of the q4h analgesic dose
  - Moderate breathlessness NRS 4-6
    - Give 50% of the q4h analgesic dose
  - Severe breathlessness NRS 7-10
    - Give 100% of the q4h analgesic dose
  - Consider increasing baseline opioid dose by 25-50%
- Breathlessness in patients who are too breathless to swallow
  - No renal failure
    - Stat: SC/IV Morphine 2.5mg
    - Infusion: CSCI/CIVI Morphine 0.5mg/h
    - Breakthrough: SC/IV Morphine 2.5mg prn/q1h

- Renal failure
  - Stat: SC/IV Fentanyl 10mcg
  - Infusion: CSCI/CIVI Fentanyl 10mcg/h
  - Breakthrough: SC/IV Fentanyl 10mcg prn/q1h
- Breathlessness crisis
  - When breathlessness is severe (NRS ≥7) and patient is acutely distressed, consider rapid parenteral opioid titration, like in pain crisis
- Nebulized opioid
  - Evidence does not support the use of nebulized morphine (Jennings 2002)
  - Nebulized morphine 10-20mg in 5ml normal saline q4h
  - Nebulized fentanyl 25-50mcg in 5ml normal saline q4h

Phenothiazines in breathlessness

- Second line agents
- Use in persistent breathlessness despite opioid titration
- Benefits
  - Reduce breathlessness
  - Reduce anxiety
  - Reduce secretions
  - Reduce nausea
- Dose
  - PO Promethazine 12.5-25mg tds-qid (Viola 2008)
  - PO Chlorpromazine 12.5-25mg tds-qid (McIver 1994)
  - PO Levomepromazine 6-12mg on
  - SC Levomepromazine 6.25-12.5mg on
- Side effects
  - Sedation
  - Hypotension
  - Dysphoria
  - Extrapyramidal side effects

Anxiolytics in breathlessness

- Benzodiazepines
    - No direct anti-breathlessness effect
    - Mechanism of action: bind benzodiazepine receptors between α and γ subunits of GABA-A receptors, enhance GABA effect
    - Benefit: reduce anxiety
    - Indications
        - Short-term relief (2-4 weeks) of severe anxiety
        - Panic attack
    - Consider non-pharmacological approaches first
        - Supportive therapy
        - Cognitive-behavioural therapy
    - Types of benzodiazepines
        - Short acting: half-life <12h
            - PO Midazolam 7.5-15mg prn/tds
            - Buccal Midazolam 2.5-5mg prn/tds
        - Intermediate acting: half-life 12-24h
            - PO/SL Alprazolam 0.25-0.5mg prn/tds
            - PO/SL Lorazepam 0.5-1mg prn/tds
        - Long acting: half-life >24h
            - PO Diazepam 2.5-5mg on
            - PO Clonazepam 0.5-1mg on
    - Selection of benzodiazepines
        - Sustained anxiety: long acting
        - Episodic anxiety: intermediate acting
- Buspirone
    - 5-HT1A receptor partial agonist
    - Reduces anxiety, but not panic attack
    - No sedative or respiratory depressant effect
    - Anxiolytic effect after 2-4 weeks
    - PO Buspirone 5mg tds, up to 10-20mg tds

Steroids in breathlessness

- Indications
    - Multiple lung metastases
    - Upper airway obstruction
    - Lymphangitis carcinomatosis
    - Superior vena cava obstruction
    - Bronchospasm
    - Radiation pneumonitis
- Dose: PO/SC/IV Dexamethasone 8-12mg om for 7 days
- Prescribe dexamethasone as a single daily dose in the morning
- Dexamethasone dose in bd or tds is best avoided in palliative care to prevent insomnia
- Stop dexamethasone abruptly if no improvement in 7 days
- Taper dexamethasone gradually if breathlessness improves

Bronchodilators in breathlessness

- Indication: bronchospasm
- Consider metered-dose inhaler (MDI) with an aerochamber if patient cannot tolerate nebulizer
- Types of bronchodilators and doses
    - Short-acting β_2-agonists (SABA)
        - MDI Salbutamol 100mcg/puff
            - Acute breathlessness: 4-6 puffs prn/q10min
            - Stable breathlessness: 2-4 puffs prn/qid
        - Nebulized Salbutamol
            - Acute breathlessness: 2.5-5mg prn/q30min
            - Stable breathlessness: 2.5-5mg prn/qid
    - Long-acting β_2-agonists (LABA)
        - MDI Salmeterol 1 puff (75mcg) daily
        - DPI Salmeterol 1 puff (50mcg) bd
        - DPI Formoterol 1 puff (12mcg) bd
        - MDI Indacaterol 1 puff (75mcg) daily

- Nebulized Arformoterol 15mcg bd
- Short-acting muscarinic antagonist (SAMA)
  - MDI Ipratropium 20mcg/puff
    - Acute breathlessness: 4-6 puffs prn/q10min
    - Stable breathlessness: 2-4 puffs prn/qid
  - Nebulized Ipratropium
    - Acute breathlessness: 0.25-0.5mg prn/q30min
    - Stable breathlessness: 0.25-0.5mg prn/qid
- Long-acting muscarinic antagonist (LAMA)
  - DPI Tiotropium 1 puff (18mcg) daily
  - Nebulized Tiotropium 0.5mg tds-qid
- Combination agents
  - MDI Combivent (Salbutamol + Ipratropium)
    - Acute breathlessness: 4-6 puffs prn/q10min
    - Stable breathlessness: 2-4 puffs prn/qid
  - Nebulized Combivent
    - Acute breathlessness: 3ml prn/q10min
    - Stable breathlessness: 3ml prn/qid
  - MDI Berodual (Fenoterol + Ipratropium)
    - Acute breathlessness: 4-6 puffs prn/q10min
    - Stable breathlessness: 2-4 puffs prn/qid
  - MDI Stiolto Respimat (Olodaterol + Tiotropium)
    - 2 puffs daily
  - DPI Seretide (Salmeterol + Fluticasone)
    - 1 puff bd
- Methylxanthines
  - PO Theophylline SR 150-300mg bd
  - IV Aminophylline
    - In severe bronchospasm with RR ≥25/min
    - Cannot complete sentence in one breath
    - 250mg in 500ml normal saline over 4h
    - May repeat prn/tds

Diuretics in breathlessness

- Indication: breathlessness due to acute heart failure
- Parenteral loop diuretics are preferred initially because of poor oral absorption from bowel oedema
- Initial doses
    - IV/SC Frusemide 20-80mg om-tds
    - IV/SC Bumetanide 0.5-1mg om-tds
- Continuous infusion in advanced chronic kidney disease
    - CIVI/CSCI Frusemide 5-20mg/h
    - CIVI/CSCI Bumetanide 0.5-2mg/h
- Oral maintenance doses
    - PO Frusemide 20-80mg om
    - PO Bumetanide 0.5-2mg om
- Oral maintenance doses in advanced chronic kidney disease
    - PO Frusemide 80-120mg bd-tds
    - PO Bumetanide 2-5mg bd
- Conversion
    - IV/SC Frusemide = PO Frusemide
    - IV/SC Frusemide 40mg = IV/SC Bumetanide 1mg
- Nebulized Frusemide
    - Reduces breathlessness without causing diuresis
        - Kohara 2003
        - Shimoyama 2002
        - Stone 1994
    - Reduces cough
        - Ventresca 1990
    - Nebulized frusemide 20mg qid

Nitrates in breathlessness

- Indication: breathlessness due to acute heart failure
- Contraindication: hypotension
- Can be combined with diuretic

206

- Sublingual glyceryl trinitrate (GTN)
    - 0.5mg prn/q5min
- Oral nitrates
    - PO Isosorbide dinitrate (Isordil) 10-40mg tds-qid
    - PO Isosorbide mononitrate (Imdur) 30-240mg om
    - PO Isosorbide mononitrate (Elantan Long) 50-100mg om
- Parenteral nitrates
    - IV Nitroglycerin (GTN) 0.5-2mg/h, max 6mg/h
    - IV Isosorbide dinitrate (Isoket) 1-2mg/h, max 10mg/h

Mucolytics in loosening thick respiratory tract secretions

- Indication: thick mucous secretions
- Useful for those who can expectorate
- PO N-Acetylcysteine (NAC) 200mg bd-tds
- PO N-Acetylcysteine (NAC) 600mg bd for COPD patients
- Nebulized acetylcysteine 10% 6-10ml tds-qid
- Nebulized saline 2.5-5ml prn/qid
- Steam inhalation tds

Anticholinegics in reducing respiratory tract secretions

- Indication: respiratory tract secretions
- Useful for those who cannot expectorate
- SC Glycopyrrolate 0.2-0.4mg stat
    - Then CSCI Glycopyrrolate 0.6-1.2mg/24h
- SC Hyoscine hydrobromide 0.4mg stat
    - Then CSCI Hyoscine hydrobromide 1.2-2.4mg/24h
- SC Hyoscine butylbromide 20mg stat,
    - Then CSCI Hyoscine butylbromide 60-120mg/24h

Cannabinoid in breathlessness

- Consider cannabinoid if opioid is contraindicated
- PO Nabilone 0.1-0.2mg bd-qid (Ahmedzai 1997)

Chest wall vibration in breathlessness (Sibuya 1994)

- In-phase chest wall vibration reduces breathlessness
- Out-of-phase chest wall vibration increases breathlessness

Retrosternal block in breathlessness (Barak 2005)

- Lignocaine 1% 35-50ml
- 5cm long needle bent at its middle to create a 60° angle
- Direction in very close relation to the manubrium sterni
- As anterior as possible behind the sternum
- Improves breathlessness within minutes
- Bilateral vocal cord palsies reported when needle position was too posterior behind the sternum

Management of Incident Breathlessness

Introduction

Incident breathlessness is breathlessness which occurs during movement or activity. Most incident breathlessness resolves rapidly with rest.

Indications of treatment

- The movement or activity is prolonged
- The incident breathlessness is distressing or incapacitating

Management of incident breathlessness

- Palliative care referral recommended
- Sublingual use of parenteral formulations
- Maximum sublingual volume = 2ml
- Titrate according to the following steps:

Steps	Fentanyl 50mcg/ml		Alfentanil 0.5mg/ml		Sufentanil 50mcg/ml	
	mcg	ml	mg	ml	mcg	ml
Step 1	25	0.5	0.1	0.2	2.5	Too small
Step 2	50	1	0.2	0.4	5	0.1
Step 3	125	Too big	0.5	1.0	12.5	0.25
Step 4	250	Too big	1.0	2.0	25	0.5
Step 5	500	Too big	2.0	Too big	50	1.0
Step 6	1000	Too big	4.0	Too big	100	2.0

Terminal Breathlessness

Introduction

Terminal breathlessness is breathlessness during the terminal phase.

Diagnosis of terminal breathlessness

- Patient is terminally ill
- Patient is breathless
- Patient has respiratory failure
- Patient is not a candidate for ventilation

Communication

- Drowsiness or coma in dying patients (Morita 1998)
  - 1 week before death: 50%
  - 1 day before death: 70%
  - 6 hours before death: 90%
- Opioids in terminal breathlessness
  - Opioids can increase drowsiness in dying patients
  - Patients may not have enough time to develop tolerance
- Sedatives in terminal breathlessness
  - Sedatives can sedate patients
  - Patients may not be able to communicate with family
- Endpoints of titration of opioid or benzodiazepine
  - Primary: dosage is just enough to relieve breathlessness
  - Secondary: dosage is low enough to maintain a reasonable level of consciousness (may not be achieved in all cases)
- Progression of terminal breathlessness
  - Drowsiness or reduced consciousness may happen even in the absence of opioids or sedatives

Opioids in terminal breathlessness (PCT input)

- Opioid-naïve patients without renal failure
    - Consciousness is important
        - CSCI/CIVI Morphine 0.2mg/h
        - SC/IV Morphine 1mg prn/q1h for breakthrough
    - Consciousness is not an issue
        - SC/IV Morphine 2.5mg stat
        - CSCI/CIVI Morphine 0.5mg/h
        - SC/IV Morphine 2.5mg prn/q1h for breakthrough
- Opioid-naïve patients with renal failure
    - Consciousness is important
        - CSCI/CIVI Fentanyl 5mcg/h
        - SC/IV Fentanyl 10mcg prn/q1h for breakthrough
    - Consciousness is not an issue
        - SC/IV Fentanyl 25mcg stat
        - CSCI/CIVI Fentanyl 10mcg/h
        - SC/IV Fentanyl 25mcg prn/q1h for breakthrough

Sedatives in terminal breathlessness (PCT input)

- Add a sedative if breathlessness persists despite opioid
- Midazolam
    - Consciousness is important
        - CSCI/CIVI Midazolam 0.2-0.5mg/h
        - SC/IV Midazolam 1mg prn/q1h for breakthrough
    - Consciousness is not an issue
        - CSCI/CIVI Midazolam 1mg/h
        - SC Midazolam 2.5mg prn/q1h for breakthrough
        - Avoid IV Midazolam boluses
- Alternative benzodiazepines suitable for home administration
    - Sublingual lorazepam 0.5mg tds and prn/tds or
    - Rectal diazepam 5mg on and prn/tds

- If benzodiazepine fails to calm patient down or fear is present, add SC Levomepromazine 12.5-25mg on and prn/bd
- If levomepromazine is unavailable, give rectal chlorpromazine 25mg tds and prn/tds

Nausea and Vomiting

Introduction

Nausea and vomiting affect 30% of palliative care patients. The number increases to 60% at last weeks of life and 70% at last days.

Definitions

- Nausea is an unpleasant sensation experienced over the pharynx or stomach with an urge to vomit
- Vomiting is the forceful expulsion of gastric or gut contents through the mouth or nasal cavity
- Retching is the attempt to vomit without bringing anything up
- Regurgitation is an effortless expulsion of gastric contents through the mouth or nasal cavity

Causes of nausea and vomiting (N & V)

- Gastrointestinal causes
    - Nausea and vomiting are associated with **FOOD**
        - Oropharyngeal candidiasis
            - Vomiting from pharyngeal irritation
            - With or without odynophagia
            - Contents: phlegm
        - Esophageal obstruction
            - Vomiting immediately after swallowing
            - With or without dysphagia
            - Contents: undigested food
    - Gastric stasis
        - Large volume vomiting
        - Low pressure vomiting

- Infrequent vomiting
- Symptoms relieved by vomiting
- Contents
    - Undigested or partially digested food
    - Gastric juices (yellowish fluid)
- Squashed stomach syndrome
    - Small volume vomiting
    - Low pressure vomiting
    - Symptoms relieved by vomiting
    - Contents
        - Undigested or partially digested food
        - Gastric juices (yellowish fluid)
- Proximal bowel obstruction
    - Large volume vomiting
    - High pressure vomiting
    - Symptoms relieved by vomiting
    - Contents
        - Undigested or partially digested food
        - Gastric juices ± bile (greenish fluid)
- Bowel obstruction
    - Abdominal distension
        - May be absent
            - Proximal obstruction
            - Peritoneal carcinomatosis
    - Abdominal colic
    - Constipation
    - Contents
        - Gastric juices in gastric outlet obstruction
        - Bile in small bowel obstruction
        - Feces in large bowel obstruction

- Constipation
    - Nausea is prominent
    - Vomiting is less prominent
    - Symptoms relieved by defecation
- Intracranial causes
    - Causes: brain tumour, brain or meningeal metastases
    - Early **MORNING** nausea and vomiting
    - Worse with head movement
    - Associated with headache
    - Associated with empty retching and regurgitation
- Vestibular causes
    - Causes: cerebellar metastases, opioid, ENT problems
    - Nausea and vomiting are associated with **MOVEMENT**
    - Positional
    - Associated with vertigo or other ENT symptoms
- Chemical causes
    - Drugs
        - Opioids
        - Chemotherapy
        - Antibiotics
        - SSRIs
    - Toxins
        - Infection
        - Organ failure
    - Electrolyte problems
        - Hypercalcemia
        - Hyponatremia
    - **CONSTANT** nausea
    - Not always relieved by vomiting
    - Variable vomiting
    - Temporal relationship with the chemicals

- Emotional causes
  - **WAVES** of nausea
  - Worse during anxiety or fear
  - Temporal relationship with emotional distress
  - May be triggered by sight, smell or thoughts
  - Relieved by distraction

Mechanisms of nausea and vomiting

- Central pathways
  - Vomiting center
    - Site: medulla oblongata
    - Contents
      - Reticular formation
      - Nucleus of tractus solitarius
    - Input from 4 principal areas
      - Higher centers
        - Cerebral cortex (GABA, 5HT)
        - Thalamus
        - Hypothalamus
        - Higher brainstem
      - Vestibular system
      - Chemoreceptor trigger zone
      - Gastrointestinal tract (5HT3)
        - Vagus nerves
        - Splanchnic nerves
    - Output to 3 principal areas
      - Upper GIT via 5, 7, 9, 10, 12 cranial nerves
      - Lower GIT via 10 and sympathetic nerves
      - Diaphragm and abdominal muscles via spinal nerves
    - Activation produces the vomiting reflex

- Principal receptors
  - Muscarinic cholinergic receptors (M1)
  - Histamine receptors (H1)
- Other receptors
  - Serotonin receptors (5HT3, 5HT2)
  - Neurokinin receptors (NK1)
- Chemoreceptor trigger zone (CTZ)
  - Site: medulla oblongata
  - Specific site: area postrema, floor of fourth ventricle
  - No blood-brain barrier
  - Input
    - Input in bloods
    - Vagus nerve
  - Output
    - Vomiting center
  - Principal receptors
    - Dopamine receptors (D2)
  - Other receptors
    - Muscarinic cholinergic receptors (M1)
    - Histamine receptors (H1)
    - Serotonin receptors (5HT3)
    - Neurokinin receptors (NK1)
    - Opioid receptors
  - Activation stimulates vomiting center
- Afferent pathways
  - Descending fibers from higher centers
  - Vestibular system (H1, M1)
  - Vagus nerves
  - Glossopharyngeal nerves
  - Splanchnic nerves
  - Sympathetic ganglias

The act of vomiting

- Inputs
    - Toxins and drugs activate CTZ (D2, 5HT)
        - CTZ activates vomiting center (H1, M1)
    - Motion sickness activates vestibular nuclei (H1, M1)
        - Vestibular nuclei activate CTZ
        - CTZ activates vomiting center
    - Chemotherapy activates gut (5HT3)
        - Vagal afferents activate vomiting center and CTZ
    - Pain, anxiety, sight and smell activate higher centers
        - Higher centers activate vomiting center
- Parasympathetic output
    - Increases salivation to protect tooth enamel from acid
    - Retroperistalsis pushes contents of small intestines to stomach through relaxed pyloric sphincter
- Motor output
    - Contraction of inspiratory muscles
        - Lowers intrathoracic pressure
        - Deep breathing to prevent aspiration
        - Coordination with abdominal contraction to retch
    - Contraction of abdominal muscles
        - Increases abdominal pressure
        - Expels stomach contents into esophagus and mouth through relaxed esophageal sphincter
- Sympathetic output
    - Sweating
    - Palpitation

Feeling good after vomiting

- Release of abdominal pressure
- Release of endorphins

Non-pharmacological Management of Nausea and Vomiting

Introduction

Non-pharmacological management of nausea and vomiting includes simple measures to modify the sensory inputs and the autonomic and motor outputs of the vomiting center.

Simple measures to modify the sensory inputs

- Sight: keep visual inputs of nausea away from the sight of patient, such as food, vomitus and other repulsive sight
- Hearing: keep auditory inputs of nausea away from the hearing of patient, such as food talk, noise and other repulsive sound
- Smell: keep olfactory inputs of nausea away from the smell of patient, such as food smell, vomitus and other repulsive odour
- Touch: keep tactile triggers of nausea away from the body of patient, such as tight fitting clothing and abdominal pillow
- Feeling: address the fear and anxiety of patient and family, establish a calm environment with fresh air
- Thoughts: address automatic negative thoughts which worsen the symptoms of nausea and vomiting

Dietary modifications

- Follow patient as the lead in eating and drinking
- Patient can eat and drink whatever he or she can tolerate
- Small, frequent meals
- Avoid fatty food
- Avoid overly sweet food
- Avoid favourite food during nausea

- Certain food or drink that can be offered:
    - Bland food at room temperature
    - Salty food
    - Sour food
    - Clear soup
    - Flavoured gelatin
    - Cold, carbonated drink
    - Popsicles and ice cubes
    - Dairy product
    - Sandwiches
    - Fruits
- Separate eating time and drinking time if appropriate
- Eat and drink slowly
- Stop eating and drinking when the feeling of nausea arises
- Sit up for 1-2h after meals if appropriate

Alternatives

- Body scan
- Progressive muscular relaxation
- Guided imagery
- Systematic desensitization
- Hypnosis
- Music
- Acupuncture or acupressure

Simple measures to modify the motor outputs

- Avoid retching
- Hold abdomen while vomiting
- Prepare the 3 essential items for vomiting
    - A vomit container
    - Water for gargling
    - Tissues

Attending to a vomiting episode

- Urgent attention
- Calm presence
- Supply the 3 essential items of vomiting
- Institution of anti-emetics
- Immediate cleaning and changing of stained clothes and bed-sheet

Antiemetics

Introduction

Narrow spectrum antiemetics act on single or limited receptors of vomiting. Broad spectrum antiemetics act on multiple receptors.

Antiemetics and receptor affinities

Drugs	D2	H1	M1	α1	5HT2	5HT3	5HT4
Levomepromazine	-	-	-	-	-		
Olanzapine	-	-	-	-	-	-	
Risperidone	-	-		-	-		
Quetiapine	-	-		-	-	-	
Chlorpromazine	-	-	-	-	-		
Promethazine	-	-	-	-			
Prochlorperazine	-	-		-			
Cyclizine		-	-				
Diphenhydramine		-	-				
Metoclopramide	-					-	+
Domperidone	-						+
Cisapride							+
Haloperidol	-			-			
Hyoscine			-				
Ondansetron						-	
Mirtazapine					-	-	

- Antagonist   + Agonist

Narrow spectrum antiemetics

- Prokinetics
- Haloperidol
- Antihistamines
- 5HT3 antagonists

Broad spectrum antiemetics

- Phenothiazines
- Atypical antipsychotics

Prokinetics

- Metoclopramide
    - Commonly used antiemetic
    - Works on stomach and proximal small bowel
    - Little effect on colonic motility
    - Mechanisms of action
        - 5HT4 agonist at GIT: prokinesis
        - D2 antagonist at GIT
        - D2 antagonist at CTZ
        - 5HT3 at CTZ and GIT at high doses
- Domperidone
    - Does not cross blood-brain barrier
    - Negligible risk of extrapyramidal side effects
    - Antiemetic of choice for Parkinson's disease
    - Mechanisms of action
        - D2 antagonist at GIT
        - D2 antagonist at CTZ
- Cisapride
    - More potent than metoclopramide
    - Increases motility of entire length of GIT
    - Can induce arrhythmia due to class III antiarrhythmic properties
    - Mechanism of action
        - Pure 5HT4 agonist at GIT
- Erythromycin
    - Most potent prokinetic when given intravenously
    - Effective after subtotal gastrectomy
    - Not effective after total gastrectomy

223

- Not effective for postoperative ileus
- Mechanism of action
  - Motilin receptor agonist at upper GIT
- Levosulpiride
  - Superior to metoclopramide in one RCT (Corli 1995)
  - Effective in 80% of patients
  - Mechanism of action: D2 antagonist

Butyrophenone

- Haloperidol
  - Potent antiemetic
  - Causes less drowsiness compared to chlorpromazine
  - >5mg/day: higher risk of extrapyramidal side effects
  - Mechanism of action: D2 antagonist at CTZ
  - No RCT reported in a Cochrane review (Perkins 2009)

Antihistamines

- Phenothiazines
  - Promethazine
- Piperazines
  - Buclizine
  - Cyclizine
  - Cinnarizine
  - Meclizine
- Monoethanolamines
  - Diphenhydramine
  - Dimenhydrinate
- Mechanisms of action
  - H1 antagonist at vomiting center and vestibular system
  - M1 antagonist at vomiting center and vestibular system
- No RCT reported (Keeley 2008)

Anticholinergics

- Mechanism of action
  - M1 antagonist at vomiting center and GIT
    - Hyoscine hydrobromide
  - M1 antagonist at GIT
    - Hyoscine butylbromide
    - Glycopyrrolate

5HT3 antagonists

- Examples
  - Ondansetron
  - Granisetron
  - Tropisetron
  - Dolasetron
  - Palonosetron
- Mechanism of action
  - 5HT3 antagonist at CTZ, vomiting center and GIT
- Sources of excess 5HT3
  - Enterochromaffin cells after gut mucosa damage
    - Chemotherapy
    - Radiotherapy
    - GI Surgery
  - Enterochromaffin cells because of bowel distension
    - Malignant bowel obstruction
  - Leaky platelets
    - Uremia
  - Raphe nucleus
    - Head injury
    - Brainstem radiotherapy
    - Multiple sclerosis affecting brainstem
- Side effects: headache, giddiness, constipation
- High level of evidence in chemotherapy-induced emesis

Phenothiazines

- Chlorpromazine, prochlorperazine and levomepromazine are broad spectrum antiemetics
- Second or third line antiemetics in palliative care
- Levomepromazine
    - Acts on most receptors involved in vomiting
    - Has analgesic effect
    - Mechanisms of action
        - D2 antagonist at CTZ and GIT
        - H1 antagonist at vomiting center and vestibular sys
        - M1 antagonist at vomiting center and vestibular sys
        - 5HT2 antagonist at vomiting center
        - α1-Adrenergic receptors at CTZ

Atypical antipsychotics

- Olanzapine, risperidone and quetiapine are broad spectrum antiemetics
- Second or third line antiemetics in palliative care
- Olanzapine
    - Mechanisms of action
        - D2 antagonist at CTZ and GIT
        - H1 antagonist at vomiting center and vestibular sys
        - M1 antagonist at vomiting center and vestibular sys
        - 5HT2 antagonist at vomiting center
        - 5HT3 antagonist
        - α1-Adrenergic receptors at CTZ
    - 100% effective in prevention of nausea and vomiting caused by moderate to highly emetogenic chemotherapy when combined with palonosetron and dexamethasone (Navari 2007)

Miscellaneous antiemetics and mechanisms of action

- Dexamethasone
    - Reduces permeability of blood-brain barrier at CTZ
    - Reduces GABA in brainstem
    - Reduces leu-enkephalin release in brainstem
    - Reduces cerebral oedema
    - Reduces tumoral oedema
    - Reduces obstruction at GIT
- Aprepitant (neurokinin 1 receptor antagonist)
    - NK1 antagonist at vomiting center, CTZ, cortex, GIT
- Nabilone (cannabinoids)
    - Cannabinoid receptor agonist (CB1)
- Benzodiazepines
    - GABA$_A$ receptor agonist
- Octreotide
    - Somatostatin receptor agonist
- Propofol
    - GABA$_A$ receptor agonist
        - Inhibits 5HT3 at CTZ

Five Principles of Using Antiemetics

Introduction

The five principles of using antiemetics can serve as an initial guide to manage nausea and vomiting in palliative care.

The five principles

- Prescribe antiemetic regularly for baseline N&V
- Prescribe antiemetic for breakthrough N&V
- Prescribe antiemetic based on the causes of N&V
- Prescribe parenteral antiemetic
- Provide antiemetic education

Baseline N&V

- Prescribe antiemetic regularly, not prn
- Examples
    - SC/IV Metoclopramide 10mg tds
    - SC/IV Haloperidol 1.5mg bd

Breakthrough N&V

- Prescribe antiemetic for breakthrough N&V
- Examples
    - SC/IV Metoclopramide 10mg prn/tds
    - SC/IV Haloperidol 1.5mg/tds

Choice of antiemetics

- Prescribe antiemetic based on the likely causes of N&V
- Step 1: narrow spectrum antiemetic
- Step 2: combination of narrow spectrum antiemetics
- Step 3: broad spectrum antiemetics

- Step 1
  - Narrow spectrum antiemetic ± dexamethasone
    - Gastroparesis: metoclopramide
    - Chemicals: haloperidol
    - Vestibular: antihistamine
    - Chemotherapy: 5HT3 antagonist
  - Increase dose if improvement in 24h
  - Increase step if no improvement in 24h
- Step 2
  - 2 narrow spectrum antiemetics ± dexamethasone
  - Choose combination with additive actions
    - Prokinetic + haloperidol
    - Prokinetic + antihistamine
    - Haloperidol + antihistamine
  - Avoid combination with antagonism
    - Prokinetic + anticholinergic
  - Increase dose if improvement in 24h
  - Increase step if no improvement in 24h
- Step 3
  - Broad spectrum antiemetic ± dexamethasone
    - Phenothiazine: levomepromazine
    - Atypical antipsychotic: olanzapine

Route of antiemetics

- Prescribe parenteral antiemetic
- Oral antiemetic is indicated in:
  - Nausea per se
  - No vomiting
  - No bowel obstruction
  - No swallowing difficulties
- Switching from parenteral to oral antiemetic is recommended only after 72 hours of good control with parenteral antiemetic

Antiemetic education

- Information
    - Causes of N&V
    - Baseline and breakthough N&V
    - Baseline and breakthrough antiemetic prescription
    - Timing of antiemetic with meals
    - Common side effects of prescribed antiemetic
    - Conversion to oral antiemetic after 72h emetic control
    - Aim for complete control of nausea
    - Aim for partial control of vomiting if mechanical causes

Management of Nausea and Vomiting

Introduction

Two different approaches are available in the management of nausea and vomiting: the mechanistic approach (antiemetic selection based on causes of N&V) and the empirical approach (antiemetic selection based on physician preference). Mechanistic approach is practiced in most palliative care settings. However, no study has directly examined the effectiveness of one approach over the other.

Gastrointestinal causes

- Oropharyngeal and esophageal candidiasis
  - Non-pharmacological
    - Mouth care
      - Prevention: drink water immediately after food
      - Treatment: brush teeth and dentures with soft toothbrush and rinse with water
      - Dying patients: swab with gauze dipped in sodium bicarbonate
      - Moisturize mouth regularly with water
      - Consider artificial saliva for dry mouth
  - Pharmacological
    - Antifungals
      - Syrup Nystatin 100,000-500,000 unit qid
      - Treat for 7-14 days
      - Swish and swallow
      - Paint over tongue and mouth if cannot swallow
      - Can make small popsicles with toothpicks to suck on

- Triazole antifungals
  - Indications
    - Resistant infection
    - Esophageal involvement
    - Laryngeal involvement
  - PO Fluconazole 150mg single dose
  - PO Fluconazole 100mg daily
  - PO Itraconazole 100mg bd: with food
  - Syrup Itraconazole 100mg bd: empty stomach
  - Short prognosis: treat with a single dose
  - Longer prognosis: treat for 7-14 days
- Parenteral antifungals for systemic infections
  - IV Fluconazole 100mg daily for 7-14 days
  - IV Itraconazole 100mg bd 7-14 days
- Antiemetics
  - Antihistamines
- Gastric stasis
  - Non-pharmacological
    - Small, frequent meals (4-6x/day)
    - Low fat diet
    - Low fiber diet
    - Liquid diet in severe cases
    - Stop eating once feeling uncomfortable
  - Pharmacological
    - First line prokinetics (30min pre-meals for tds dose)
      - SC/IV/PO Metoclopramide 10-20mg tds
      - CSCI/CIVI Metoclopramide 30-120mg/24h
      - PO Domperidone 10-20mg tds
    - Second line prokinetics
      - IV/PO Erythromycin 250-500mg tds
      - PO Cisapride 10-20mg tds
      - PO Levosulpiride 25mg tds

- Alternative antiemetics to reduce nausea
  - Prochlorperazine
  - Antihistamines
- Antisecretory agents to reduce emetic volume
  - H2 antagonists
  - PPIs
  - SC Octreotide 50-100mcg on
- Anti-foaming agent to reduce bloatedness
  - Syrup Simethicone (Maalox Plus) 10-20ml tds
  - PO Simethicone (Maalox Plus) 2-4 tablets tds
- Antidepressants in refractory cases
  - PO Mirtazapine 15mg on
  - PO Amitriptyline 25-50mg on
  - PO Nortriptyline 25-50mg on
- Interventions for refractory cases
  - Venting nasogastric tube
  - Venting gastrostomy
  - Feeding jejunostomy
  - Botulinum toxin injection into pyloric sphincter
  - Gastric electrical stimulation
- Constipation
  - Refer to chapter of constipation
- Malignant bowel obstruction
  - Refer to chapter of malignant bowel obstruction

Chemical causes

- Opioid-induced nausea and vomiting (OINV)
  - CTZ stimulation
    - Constant nausea during rising opioid level
    - SC/IV/PO Haloperidol 1.5-5mg bd
    - CSCI/CIVI Haloperidol 1.5-20mg/24h

- Gastric stasis
  - Associated with post-prandial stomach fullness >2h
  - SC/IV/PO Metoclopramide 10-20mg tds
  - CSCI/CIVI Metoclopramide 30-120mg/24h
- Increased vestibular sensitivity
  - Associated with vertigo
  - IV/PO Promethazine 25-50mg tds
  - CSCI Promethazine 50-150mg/24h
- Constipation
  - Treat constipation
- Anticipatory nausea and vomiting
  - Associated with sight, smell and thoughts of opioid
  - PO Alprazolam 0.25-0.5mg prn/tds
  - PO Lorazepam 0.5-1mg prn/tds
- Refractory nausea and vomiting
  - IV/SC Dexamethasone 8mg at 8am and 12pm
  - IV/PO Granisetron 1mg bd
  - CSCI Granisetron 1-3mg/24h
  - SC Levomepromazine 6.25-25mg on-bd
  - CSCI Levomepromazine 6.25-50mg/24h
  - PO Levomepromazine 6-25mg on-bd
  - IV/PO Chlorpromazine 25-50mg tds
  - SL Olanzapine 2.5-10mg on
- Chemotherapy-induced nausea and vomiting (CINV)
  - Types of CINV
    - Acute: within first 24h after chemotherapy
      - Serotonin release from enterochromaffin cells
    - Delayed: 1-5 days after chemotherapy
      - Substance P-mediated disruption of blood-brain barrier, GI motility and adrenal hormone
    - Anticipatory: prior to chemotherapy
      - Classical conditioning

- Highly emetogenic chemotherapy HEC (>90%)
  - AC/FAC/FEC combinations for breast cancer
  - Anthracycline + cisplatin combinations
  - Carmustin
  - Cisplatin 5 days regimen
  - Cyclophosphamide >1500mg/m^2
  - Dactinomycin
  - Streptozocin
- Moderately emetogenic chemotherapy MEC (30-90%)
  - CHOP/CHOMP/BEACOPP/ABVD for lymphoma
  - FOLFOX/FOLFIRI/XELOX/XELIRI
  - Carboplatin/oxaliplatin
  - Cyclophosphamide <1500mg/m^2
  - Ifosfamide
  - Oral etoposide/imatinib/temozolomide/vinorelbine
  - Methotrexate
- Low emetogenic chemotherapy LEC (10-30%)
  - Capecitabine
  - Catumaxomab/cetuximab/panitumumab
  - Docetaxel/paclitaxel
  - Fluorouracil
  - Gemcitabine
  - IV Etoposide
  - Pemetrexed
  - Topotecan
- Minimally emetogenic chemotherapy (<10%)
  - Alemtuzumab/bevacizumab/gemtuzumab
  - Erlotinib/gefitinib/sorafenib/sunitinib
  - Hydroxyurea
  - IV Vinorelbine
  - Lenalidomide/thalidomide
  - Vinblastine/vincristine

- Prevention of acute CINV
  - HEC: 5HT3 antagonist + NK1 antagonist + dexa
  - MEC: 5HT3 antagonist + dexa
  - LEC: dexa
  - Minimal: no routine prophylaxis
- Prevention of delayed CINV
  - HEC: NK1 antagonist + dexa
  - MEC: no routine prophylaxis
  - LEC: no routine prophylaxis
  - Minimal: no routine prophylaxis
- Prevention of anticipatory CINV
  - Psychological techniques
  - Low dose benzodiazepine before chemotherapy
- Doses of prophylactic antiemetics
  - 5HT3 antagonists at D1 for HEC and MEC
    - PO Ondansetron 24mg (HEC), 16mg (MEC)
    - IV Ondansetron 8mg
    - PO Granisteron 2mg
    - IV Granisetron 1mg
    - PO/IV Tropisetron 5mg
    - PO/IV Dolasetron 100mg
    - PO Palonosetron 0.5mg
    - IV Palonosetron 0.25mg
  - Dexamethasone
    - PO Dexamethasone 12mg at D1 (HEC, MEC)
    - PO Dexamethasone 8mg at D2-4 (HEC)
    - PO Dexamethasone 8mg at D1 (LEC)
  - NK1 antagonists
    - PO Aprepitant 125mg at D1 (HEC)
    - PO Aprepitant 80mg at D2-3 (HEC)
    - IV Fosaprepitant 150mg at D1 only (HEC)

- Radiotherapy-induced nausea and vomiting (RINV)
  - High risk
    - Total body irradiation
    - 5HT3 antagonist prophylaxis + dexamethasone
  - Moderate risk
    - Upper abdomen
    - 5HT3 antagonist prophylaxis
  - Low risk
    - Brain, head and neck, lower thorax, spine, pelvis
    - 5HT3 antagonist rescue
  - Minimal Risk
    - Breast, extremities
    - D2 antagonist or 5HT3 antagonist rescue
- Toxin-induced nausea and vomiting
  - Causes
    - Drugs: opioids, chemo, antiepileptics, antibiotics
    - Metabolic: hypercalcemia, hyponatremia, uremia
    - Toxin: bacterial toxins, tumour necrosis
  - Antiemetics
    - Block D2 receptors at CTZ
      - SC/IV/PO Metoclopramide 10-20mg tds
      - CSCI/CIVI Metoclopramide 30-120mg/24h
      - SC/IV/PO Haloperidol 1.5-5mg bd
      - CSCI/CIVI Haloperidol 1.5-20mg/24h
    - Block H1, M1 receptors at vomiting center
      - Antihistamines
    - Block multiple receptors
      - SC Levomepromazine 6.25-25mg on-bd
      - CSCI Levomepromazine 6.25-50mg/24h
      - PO Levomepromazine 6-25mg on-bd
      - IV/PO Chlorpromazine 25-50mg tds
      - SL Olanzapine 2.5-10mg on

- Increased intracranial pressure
  - Antiemetics
    - First line: reduce vasogenic cerebral oedema
      - SC/IV/PO Dexamethasone 12mg om 1/52
    - Second line: block H1, M1 at vomiting center
      - IV/PO Cyclizine 50-100mg tds
      - CSCI Cyclizine 150-300mg/24h
      - IV/PO Promethazine 25-50mg tds
      - CSCI Promethazine 50-150mg/24h
    - Third line: block multiple receptors
      - SC Levomepromazine 6.25-25mg on-bd
      - CSCI Levomepromazine 6.25-50mg/24h
      - PO Levomepromazine 6-25mg on-bd
      - SL Olanzapine 2.5-10mg on
- Vestibular causes
  - Antiemetics
    - Antihistamines
      - SC boluses can cause tissue necrosis
      - IV boluses have to be given slowly
      - IV/PO Cyclizine 50-100mg tds
      - CSCI Cyclizine 150-300mg/24h
      - IV/PO Promethazine 25-50mg tds
      - CSCI Promethazine 50-150mg/24h
      - IV/PO Diphenhydramine 25-50mg tds
      - IV/PO Dimenhydrinate 50-100mg tds
    - Anticholinergics
      - SC/SL Hyoscine hydrobromide 0.2-0.4mg tds
      - CSCI Hyoscine hydrobromide 1.2-2.4mg/24h
      - Scopolamine patch 1.5mg q72h to mastoid
    - Phenothiazines
      - IV Prochlorperazine 5-10mg tds slow bolus
      - PO Prochlorperazine 5-10mg tds

- Psychogenic causes
  - First line: non-pharmacological treatment
    - Body scan
    - Progressive muscular relaxation
    - Guided imagery
    - Systemic desensitization
    - Hypnosis
    - Music
  - Second line: benzodiazepines
    - PO/SL Alprazolam 0.25-0.5mg prn/tds
    - PO/SL Lorazepam 0.5-1mg prn/tds
    - PO Diazepam 2.5-5mg on
- Intractable nausea and vomiting
  - Step 1: 2 narrow spectrum antiemetics ± dexamethasone
  - Step 2: 1 broad spectrum antiemetic ± dexamethasone
  - Step 3: intravenous propofol (Lundström 2005)
    - IV Propofol 0.5mg/kg/h
    - Titrate 0.25-0.5mg/kg/h q30-60min till better
    - Optimal dose: 0.5-1.0mg/kg/h for most patients
    - Sedation may happen with doses >1mg/kg/h
    - Monitor sedation and RR at 1, 2, 6, 12h, then bd
    - Stop 2-3min if too drowsy, then restart at lower dose
    - Reduce dose within 24h if patient is better
  - Alternative
    - ABHR suppositories
      - Lorazepam (Ativan) 0.5mg
      - Diphenhydramine (Benadryl) 12.5mg
      - Haloperidol (Haldol) 0.5mg
      - Metoclopramide (Reglan) 10mg

Constipation

Introduction

Constipation is difficulty in passing motion. It is fundamentally defined by the patient.

Characteristics of constipation (≥1 of the following)

- Hard stools
- Infrequent bowel movement
- Difficult bowel movement with excessive straining
- Painful bowel movement
- Absent bowel movement
- A sense of incomplete evacuation

Assessment of constipation (3Ds)

- Diet history
    - Daily dietary history
    - Fibre intake
    - Water intake
    - Coffee, tea and alcohol ingestion
    - Milk products
- Drug history
    - Opioids
    - Laxatives
    - Anticholinergics
    - 5HT3 antagonists
    - Antidepressants
- Defecation history
    - Explore the whole defecation process, from the intention to move bowels till completion and back to activities

- Need of assistance
- Site of defecation
    - Toilet
    - Commode
    - Bedpan
    - Diapers
- Process of defecation
    - Effort in defecation
    - Manoeuvres in facilitating defecation
    - Excessive straining
    - Pain during or after defecation
    - Incomplete evacuation
    - Duration of defecation
    - Frequency of defecation
- Stool characteristics
    - Consistencies
    - Volume
    - Shape
    - Colour
    - Odour
- Patient's expectation of bowel movement

Examination of constipation

- Hydration status
- Abdominal examination
    - Signs of bowel obstruction
    - Signs of constipation: left-sided indentable fecal masses
    - Bowel sounds
- Rectal examination
    - Perianal excoriation
    - Haemorrhoids or fissures
    - Anal tone

- Stool consistencies
- Stool colour
- Ballooned rectum: suggesting higher impaction
- Steps in performing a rectal examination for constipation
  - Step 1: preparation of gloves and lubricant
  - Step 2: positioning of patient
  - Step 3: inspection of perianal area
  - Step 4: touch the anus with lubricated gloved finger
  - Step 5: wait for the anus to relax
  - Step 6: advance the finger slowly following the curve
  - Step 7: circumferential palpation of rectal vault
  - Step 8: remove the finger and inspect stools
- Avoid rectal examination
  - Refusal
  - Neutropenic sepsis
  - Abdominoperineal resection

Bristol stool chart

- Type 1: separate hard lumps – constipation
- Type 2: sausaged-shaped, lumpy – constipation
- Type 3: sausaged-shaped, cracked surface – normal
- Type 4: sausaged-shaped, smooth surface – normal
- Type 5: soft blobs – diarrhoea
- Type 6: mushy – diarrhoea
- Type 7: watery – diarrhoea

Investigations

- Abdominal x-ray in suspected malignant bowel obstruction

Mechanisms of Constipation

Introduction

Normal intenstinal function depends on the control of intestinal motility and fluid handling by neural, endocrine and paracrine factors.

Neural control of intestinal activity

- Enteric nervous system (ENS): the second brain
    - 100 million neurons
    - Embedded in GI lining from esophagus to anus
    - Comprises 2 interconnected networks
        - Myenteric ganglia (Auerbach's plexus)
            - Within muscular layer
            - Parasympathetic and sympathetic input
            - Innervate muscular layer: inner and outer
            - Regulate GI motility
            - 30% sensory neurons (myenteric IPANs)
                - IPAN = intrinsic primary afferent neurons
                - Detect intraluminal chemistry
                - Mediate GI reflexes
        - Submucosal ganglia (Meissner's plexus)
            - Within submucosal layer
            - Parasympathetic input only
            - Derived from Auerbach's plexus
            - Regulate fluid and electrolyte transport
            - 14% sensory neurons (submucosal IPANs)
                - Detect intraluminal chemistry
                - Mediate mucosally driven peristaltic and secretory reflexes

- Autonomic nervous system (ANS)
  - Parasympathetic nervous system
    - Vagus: innervates ENS
      - Foregut: celiac plexus
      - Midgut: superior mesenteric plexus
    - Pelvic splanchnic nerves: innervate ENS
      - Hindgut: inferior mesenteric plexus
    - Stimulates GI motility and secretion
  - Sympathetic nervous system
    - Inhibits GI motility and secretion

Neurotransmitters

- Excitatory neurotransmitters
  - Acetylcholine (primary)
    - Binds muscarinic receptors (GPCR)
    - Increases cytosolic Ca^{2+}
    - Causes secretion and smooth muscle contraction
  - Substance P
    - Binds neurokinin 1 receptors (NK1)
    - Causes secretion of saliva and pancreatic enzymes
    - Causes smooth muscle contraction
    - Promotes inflammation and tissue repair
  - Serotonin
    - 95% of body's serotonin is found in the gut
    - Source: enterochromaffin cells
    - 5HT1P
      - Stimulates submucosal IPANs
      - ↑ peristalsis and secretion
      - Agonist: causes diarrhoea
      - Antagonist: causes ileus
      - Not the best target for treatment of GI motility compared to 5HT4

- 5HT3
  - Stimulates extrinsic sensory nerves and sends sensory signals like N&V to CNS
  - Stimulates myenteric IPANs
  - ↑ reflexes such as giant migratory contractions, but not peristaltic and secretory reflexes
  - 5HT3 antagonists
    - Reduce CINV
    - Reduce visceral hypersensitivity of IBS, particularly bloating sensation
    - Cause constipation
    - Do not paralyze bowels
- 5HT4
  - Stimulates submucosal IPANs presynaptically
  - Enhances release of acetylcholine and CGRP
  - Promotes transmission in prokinetic pathways
  - Depends on natural stimuli to evoke peristaltic and secretory reflexes
  - Will not induce overwhelming motility
  - But not effective if damaged enteric nerves
  - 5HT4 agonists: safe compared to 5HT1P
- Inhibitory neurotransmitters
  - Nitric oxide
    - Binds NO receptors
    - Increases cGMP
    - Causes smooth muscle relaxation
  - ATP
    - Causes smooth muscle relaxation
  - Vasoactive intestinal peptide (VIP)
    - Binds VIP receptors (GPCR)
    - Increases cytosolic Ca^{2+}
    - Causes secretion and smooth muscle relaxation

Endocrine control of intestinal activity

- Gastrin
    - Source: G cells of stomach
    - Receptors: CCK-B receptors
    - Function: ↑ acid secretion from parietal cells
- Cholecystokinin (CCK)
    - Source: I cells of duodenum and jejunum
    - Receptors: CCK-A receptors
    - Function: ↑ pancreatic enzyme secretion
- Secretin
    - Source: S cells of duodenum
    - Receptors: secretin receptors
    - Function: ↑ pancreatic and biliary HCO_3^- secretion
- Glucose dependent insulinotropic peptide (GIP)
    - Source: K cells of duodenum and jejunum
    - Receptors: GIP receptors
    - Function: ↑ insulin secretion from pancreatic β cells

Paracrine factors

- Histamine
    - Source: enterochromaffin cells of stomach
    - Receptors: H2 receptors
    - Function: ↑ acid secretion from parietal cells
- Somatostatin
    - Source: D cells of stomach
    - Receptors: somatostatin receptors
    - Function: inhibits gastrin secretion from G cells

Intestinal motility

- Small intestine motility
    - Peristalsis
        - Pattern of intestinal motility after meals

- Forward movement of small intestine contents
- Orad smooth muscle contraction via acetylcholine
- Caudad smooth muscle relaxation via NO, ATP, VIP
  - Segmentation
    - Pattern of intestinal motility after meals
    - Mixing of small intestine contents
  - Migrating motor complexes
    - Pattern of intestinal motility in between meals
    - A wave of peristalsis from stomach to ileum
    - Initiated by motilin from duodenum
    - Occur every 1.5-2 hours
    - Clear stomach and small intestines of residue
    - Reduce bacterial growth
    - Responsible for rumbling when hungry
- Large intestine motility
  - Segmentation and haustral migration
    - Mixing of large intestine contents
    - Facilitate water absorption
    - Move feces gradually to rectum
  - Mass movement
    - 1-3/day
    - High-amplitude propagated contractions
    - Stimulated by gastrocolic and duodenocolic reflexes after food
    - Pushes feces into rectum

Intestinal fluid handling

- Dynamic state of secretion and absorption
  - Secretion
    - Secreted intestinal fluid: 7L/day
      - Saliva: 1.5L/day
      - Gastric secretions: 2L/day

- Pancreatic juices: 1.5L/day
- Bile: 0.5L/day
- Small intestine secretions: 1.5L/day
- Dietary fluid: 2L/day (8 x 8 ounces glasses)
- Absorption
  - Small bowel transit: 2-4 hours
  - Large bowel transit: 1-2 days
  - Small bowel absorption 8.5L/day
  - Large bowel absorption 0.4L/day
  - Fecal excretion 0.1L/day
- Gut fluid balance
  - In: 9L/day
  - Out: 9L/day
  - Normal stool: 75% water (100ml)
  - Diarrhoea: >85% water
  - Constipation: <65% water

Defecation

- Feces stored in rectal ampulla
- Distension of rectum
- Stimulation of stretch receptors
- Reflex contraction of rectum
- Relaxation of internal anal sphincter
- Urge to defecate
- Relaxation of external anal sphincter
- Defecate

Common causes of constipation in cancer patients

- Chemotherapy (neurotoxicity)
  - Platinum compounds
  - Vinca alkaloids
  - Taxanes

- Thalidomide/lenalidomide
- Bortezomib
- 5HT3 antagonists
- Opioids
  - Motility: prevent integration needed for propulsive contractions by inhibiting enteric interneurons
  - Fluid handling: increase water absorption by slowing of passage of luminal contents, reduce secretion by inhibiting secretomotor neurons
  - Defecation: precipitate fecal impaction by reducing sensations of rectal distention
  - Opioids that are less constipative
    - Fentanyl
    - Alfentanil
    - Buprenorphine
    - Methadone
    - Tramadol
- Drugs with anticholinergic effects
  - Anticholinergics
  - Antihistamines
  - Tricyclics
  - Neuroleptics
- Direct tumour effect
  - Invasion of gut wall
  - Infiltration of enteric nerves
  - Compression of extrinsic nerves
  - Spinal cord compression
- Paraneoplastic constipation
  - Small cell lung cancer
  - Carcinoid tumour
- Hypercalcemia of malignancy
- Age-related loss of enteric neurons (>65 years old)

- Agre-related reduction in rectal sensitivity
- Reduced mobility
- Reduced dietary fluid intake

Five Principles of Using Laxatives

Introduction

There is no one single correct way in using laxatives in palliative care.

5 principles

- Rule out bowel obstruction
- Regular oral laxatives based on mechanisms
- PRN Rectal laxatives for fecal impaction
- PAMORA for unsuccessful laxation in OIC
- Laxatives and lifestyle education

Rule out bowel obstruction

- Most laxatives are not suitable in bowel obstruction
- Risk of worsening obstruction with bulk-forming laxatives
- Risk of worsening colic with stimulant laxatives
- Risk of perforation with stimulant laxatives
- Use softening laxatives if in doubt

Regular oral laxatives based on mechanisms

- Prescribe softening laxatives for hard stools
- Prescribe stimulating laxatives for no bowel movement
- Often a combination of both is necessary

PRN Rectal laxatives for fecal impaction

- Prescribe rectal softeners for hard impaction
- Prescribe rectal pushers for soft impaction
- Prescribe high enema for high impaction
- Consider manual evacuation for unsuccessful disimpaction

PAMORA for unsuccessful laxation in OIC

- Prescribe peripherally acting μ-opioid receptor antagonists for unsuccessful laxation in OIC
- Use PAMORA to clear accumulation of stool
- Then restart conventional laxatives and establish new regime

Laxatives and lifestyle education

- Laxatives education
    - Types
    - Actions
        - Softening laxatives: soften stools
        - Stimulating laxatives: move stools
    - Titration
    - Rectal measures
- Lifestyle education
    - Target cortex
        - Ensure time, privacy and favourable environment
    - Target intestinal fluid handling
        - Encourage adequate fluid intake as preferred
        - Encourage dietary fiber if appropriate
        - Drink barley – fiber
    - Target gut motility
        - Encourage regular toilet habits
            - Recognize urge of defecation
            - Do not ignore the urge
            - Make use of gastrocolic reflex
                - Toilet sitting after meals
        - Encourage exercise and mobility as preferred
        - Encourage gentle abdominal massage
        - Drink prune juice – mild stimulant laxative

Laxatives

Introduction

Laxatives can be divided into predominantly softening laxatives and predominantly stimulating laxatives.

Classification

- Stool lubricants   Predominantly softening
- Bulk-forming agents
- Macrogols
- Stool surfactants
- Osmotic agents
- Saline laxatives
- Anthranoids
- Phenolics   ↓   Predominantly stimulating

Stool lubricants

- Seldom used in palliative care
- Types
    - Mineral oil
    - Liquid paraffin
    - Liquid paraffin + magnesium hydroxide (Milpar)
- Doses
    - Mineral oil 10-20ml pre-breakfast and pre-bed
    - Liquid paraffin 10-20ml pre-breakfast and pre-bed
    - Milpar 10-20ml pre-breakfast and pre-bed
- Mechanisms
    - Lubricate stool surface
    - Soften stool

- Onset of action: 1-3 days
- Side effects
  - Leakage of oily fecal material
  - Perianal irritation
  - Lipoid pneumonia – not with Milpar

Bulk-forming agents

- Not suitable for most palliative care patients
  - Need to drink 200-300ml of water each time
  - Unpalatable
- Types
  - Wheat bran
  - Psyllium or Ispaghula (Fybogel)
  - Methylcellulose (Celevac)
  - Sterculia (Normacol)
  - Malt soup extract (Maltsupex)
- Doses
  - Wheat bran 10g bd with 250ml water after meals
  - Fybogel 1 sachet bd with 150ml water after meals
  - Celevac 3-6 tablets bd with 250ml water after meals
  - Normacol 1-2 sachets bd with 250ml water after meals
  - Maltsupex 15ml bd with 250ml water after meals
- Mechanisms
  - Normalizers: soften hard stool, make loose stool firmer
  - Increase stool bulk: shorten transit
  - Fermentation: shorten transit
- Onset of action: 2-4 days
- Side effects
  - Inadequate water intake
    - Form viscous mass
    - Obstruct bowels

Macrogols

- Polyethylene glycol
- Short term use in palliative care to flush bowels
- Brand names
    - Forlax
    - Movicol
    - Fortrans
    - Others: MiraLAX, SoftLAX, ClearLAX, GoLYTELY etc
- Doses in constipation
    - Forlax 2 sachets dly-bd in 250ml water
    - Movicol 2 sachets dly-bd in 250ml water
- Doses in fecal impaction
    - Forlax 8 sachets dly in 1L water
    - Movicol 8 sachets dly in 1L water
    - Fortrans 1 sachet dly in 1L water
- Mechanisms
    - Osmotic laxative
    - Non-absorbable polymer solution
    - Soften stool
    - Accelerate transit
- Onset of action: 1-3 days
- Side effects
    - Abdominal distension
    - Abdominal pain
    - Diarrhoea

Stool surfactants (emollients)

- Useful stool softeners in partial bowel obstruction
- Combinations: laxatives of choice in many palliative centers
- Types
    - Docusate sodium (Coloxyl tablets)
    - Poloxamer (Coloxyl drops)

- Doses
  - Docusate sodium 100-200mg bd
  - Coloxyl drops: for infants
- Mechanisms
  - Reduce surface tension of stool
  - Increase water penetration of stool
  - Soften stool
  - Stimulate secretion
  - Stimulate peristalsis at higher doses
- Onset of action
  - Coloxyl tablets: 12-72h
  - Coloxyl drops: 12-24h
- Side effects
  - Abdominal cramps
  - Diarrhoea
  - Nausea

Osmotic agents

- Lactulose is a common osmotic agent used in palliative care
- Useful for those who can drink ≥ 2L of water per day
- With less water, it ferments and causes bloating and colic
- Types
  - Lactulose
  - Sorbitol
  - Mannitol
- Doses
  - Syrup lactulose 10-30ml bd, max 30ml qid
  - Syrup sorbitol 10-30ml bd
  - Syrup mannitol 10-30ml bd
- Mechanisms
  - Osmotic laxatives: small bowel flushers
  - Non-absorbable sugars

- Increase water in intestinal lumen
- Soften stool
- Fermentation produces acetic, formic, lactic acids that stimulate peristalsis
- These acids are absorbed so the osmotic effect does not extend throughout the colon
- Onset of action: 1-2 days
- Side effects
  - Sweet taste (does not affect diabetic control)
  - Flatulence
  - Colic
- Contraindication
  - Anuria (risk of fluid overload)

Saline laxatives

- Last option in palliative care because of strong purgative action
- Types
  - Magnesium hydroxide (Milk of Magnesia)
  - Magnesium sulphate (Epsom salt)
  - Magnesium citrate (Citroma)
  - Sodium phosphate (Fleet Phospho-Soda solution)
- Doses
  - Milk of Magnesia 15-30ml bd
  - Epsom salt 2-4 teaspoons in 8oz water bd
  - Citroma 150-300ml single dose with 8oz water
  - Fleet solution 45ml stat, then 45ml 6h later
- Mechanisms
  - Osmotic laxatives: small and large bowels
  - Osmotic influence throughout the gut
  - Soften stool
  - Increase secretion
  - Stimulate peristalsis

- Onset of action: 1-6h
- Side effects
  - Sudden passage of offensive liquid feces
- Contraindications
  - Chronic kidney disease
  - Heart failure (sodium phosphate)

Anthranoids

- Senna is a common anthranoid used in palliative care
- Types
  - Dantron – small and large bowel pusher
  - Senna – large bowel pusher
  - Cascara sagrada – large bowel pusher
  - Casanthranol – large bowel pusher
- Doses
  - Dantron 50-150mg bd
  - Senna 15-30mg bd, max 30mg qid
  - Cascara sagrada 300mg dly ($\geq$ 1/52: hepatotoxicity risk)
  - Casanthranol: available in combination with docusate
- Senna
  - Derived from plants
  - Inactive glycosides
  - Hydrolyzed by bacterial glycosidases in large bowel to active aglycone compound
  - Effect on large bowel but no effect on small bowel
- Dantron
  - Synthetic anthranoid
  - Direct action on small and large bowel
- Mechanisms
  - Stimulant laxatives: stool pushers
  - Stimulate Meissner's plexus: ↑ secretion
  - Stimulate Auerbach's plexus: ↑ motility

- Onset of action: 6-12h
- Side effects
  - Abdominal cramp
  - Diarrhoea
  - Red urine (Dantron)
  - Perianal excoriation (Dantron)
  - Pseudomelanosis coli with chronic use
    - Reversible in 12 months after stopping laxative
    - Association with colon cancer not established

Phenolics

- Bisacodyl is a common phenolic used in palliative care
- Types
  - Bisacodyl – small and large bowel pusher
  - Sodium picosulphate – large bowel pusher
  - Phenolphthalein – withdrawn from market
- Doses
  - Bisacodyl 10-20mg on-bd, max 20mg qid
  - Sodium picosulphate 5-10mg on, max 15mg bd
- Bisacodyl
  - Hydrolyzed to active metabolites by intestinal esterases
  - Acts on small and large bowels
- Sodium picosulphate
  - Hydrolyzed to active metabolites by colonic bacteria
  - Acts on large bowel
- Mechanisms
  - Similar laxative effect to anthranoids
  - Stimulant laxatives: stool pushers
- Onset of action: 6-12h
- Side effects
  - Abdominal cramp
  - Diarrhoea

Miscellaneous oral and parenteral laxatives

Ricinoleic

- Vegetable oil obtained from seeds of Ricinus communis
- Type: Castor oil – small bowel pusher
- Dose: Castor oil 15-30ml daily
- Mechanisms
    - Hydrolysed by lipase in small bowel to ricinoleic acid
    - Release of neurotransmitters from enterochromaffin cells
    - Inhibits water absorption
    - Increases mucosal permeability
    - Stimulates motility
- Onset of action: 2-6h
- Side effects
    - Cramp
    - Severe diarrhoea

Chloride channel activator

- Bicyclic fatty acid derived from PGE1
- Type: Lubiprostone (Amitiza)
- Dose: Lubiprostone 24mcg bd
- Mechanisms
    - Acts on type 2 chloride channels on apical surface of luminal epithelium
    - Increases secretion without affecting serum Na^{2+} and K^+
    - Accelerates small and large bowel transits
- Onset of action: within 24h
- Side effects
    - Nausea
    - Diarrhoea
    - Headache
    - Flatulence

Prokinetics

- Use: constipation with intestinal hypomotility or gastroparesis
- Types
    - Metoclopramide
    - Domperidone
    - Cisapride
    - Tegaserod
    - Neostigmine
- Doses
    - Metoclopramide 10-20mg tds before meals
    - Domperidone 10-20mg tds before meals
    - Cisapride 10-20mg tds before meals
    - Tegaserod 6mg bd before meals
    - SC Neostigmine 0.5mg prn/tds
- Mechanisms
    - 5HT4 agonists
        - Metoclopramide
        - Domperidone
        - Cisapride
        - Tegaserod
    - Acetylcholinesterase inhibitor
        - Neostigmine
- Onset of action
    - Metoclopramide: 15-60min
    - Domperidone: 30min
    - Cisapride: 30-60min
    - Tegaserod: within 4 weeks
    - Neostigmine: minutes to 10h
- Side effects
    - Extrapyramidal effects (Metoclopramide, domperidone)
    - Cardiac arrhythmias (Cisapride)
    - Heart attack or stroke (Tegaserod)

Peripherally acting μ-opioid receptor antagonists (PAMORA)

- Use: opioid-induced constipation (OIC)
- Types
    - Oral naloxone
    - Methylnaltrexone
    - Alvimopan
    - Naloxegol
- Doses
    - PO Naloxone 0.8mg bd
        - Double the dose q2-3 day
        - Till bowel movement or adverse effect
    - SC Methylnaltrexone 8mg EOD if 40-60kg
    - SC Methylnaltrexone 12mg EOD if 60-120kg
    - PO Alvimopan 0.5-1.5mg dly, max 12mg bd
    - PO Naloxegol 25mg om
- Onset of action
    - Methylnatrexone: 30-60min
    - Alvimopan: 4-7h
    - Naloxegol: 1-3h
- Side effects
    - Diarrhoea
    - Cramp
    - Nausea and vomiting
    - Opioid withdrawal symptoms

Combination laxatives

- Benefits: dual mechanisms, compliance
- Types
    - Liquid paraffin and magnesium hydroxide (Milpar)
    - Docusate sodium and casanthranol (Peri-Colace)
    - Docusate sodium and senna (Senna-Plus)
    - Dantron and docusate (Co-Danthrusate)

- Dantron and poloxamer (Co-Danthramer)
- Doses
  - Milpar 10-20ml bd
  - Peri-Colace 2-4 cap on-bd
  - Senna-Plus 2-4 tab on-bd
  - Co-Danthrusate 2-4 cap on-bd
  - Co-Danthramer 2-4 cap on-bd

Rectal laxatives

- Indications
  - Unsuccessful oral laxatives
  - Cannot swallow oral laxatives
  - Cannot tolerate oral laxatives
  - Fecal impaction
  - Neurogenic bowel
- Stool lubricants
  - Arachis oil enema (peanut oil) 130ml prn
  - Olive oil enema 250ml prn
  - Mineral oil enema 100ml prn
  - Give overnight for hard stools
  - Then give stool flusher enema next day
  - Can give as high enema for ballooned rectum
- Stool softener
  - Docusate sodium (Norgalax micro-enema) 1 tube prn
  - Onset: 15-30min
- Stool flushers
  - Glycerin enema (Ravin enema) 2 tubes prn
  - Sodium citrate enema 2 tubes prn
  - Sodium phosphate enema (Fleet enema) 133ml prn
  - Tap water enema 500ml prn: risk of fluid overload
  - Onset: 15-30min (glycerin), 5-15min (sodium citrate), 2-5min (sodium phosphate)

- Fleet enema: can give as high enema for ballooned rectum
- Stool pusher
  - Bisacodyl suppository 10-20mg prn
  - Onset: 20-60min
  - Contact: rectal mucosa
  - Converted by colonic flora to desacetyl form
  - Stimulates colonic peristalsis

Malignant Bowel Obstruction

Introduction

In the past, surgery was the treatment of choice for malignant bowel obstruction. In 1985, Baines and colleagues reported in Lancet the first successful medical management of 38 patients with malignant bowel obstruction without surgery or NG tube. Since then, medical palliation of symptoms of malignant bowel obstruction was increasingly reported in the literature.

Survival of patients with malignant bowel obstruction (MBO)

- Median survival
    - 1 month (Woolfson 1997)
    - 2 months (Chan 1992)
    - 3 months (Jong 1995)
    - 6 months (Lau 1993)
- Median survival according to ECOG (Wright 2010)
    - ECOG 0-1: 7 months
    - ECOG 2: 2 months
    - ECOG3-4: 1 month
- Surgical vs medical Rx: no survival difference (Woolfson 1997)

Good surgical candidates

- Good performance status
- Good nutritional status
- Ascites <3L
- Unifocal obstruction
- Absence of palpable abdominal or pelvic masses
- Options of future disease-modifying treatments
- Life expectancy > 2months

Absolute contraindications to surgery (EAPC 2001)

- Recent laparotomy demonstrated inoperability
- Previous abdominal surgery showed diffuse metastatic cancer
- Involvement of proximal stomach
- Intraabdominal carcinomatosis demonstrated radiologically
- Diffuse palpable intra-abdominal masses
- Massive ascites which rapidly recurred after drainage

Relative contraindications to surgery (EAPC 2001)

- Advanced age with cachexia
- Poor performance status
- Poor nutritional status
- Previous abdominal or pelvic radiotherapy
- Symptomatic extra-abdominal metastases
- Asymptomatic extensive extra-abdominal metastases

Candidates for stenting

- Unifocal obstruction
- Advanced metastatic disease
- Poor surgical candidate
- Patients for surgery once medically optimized

Traditional conservative management

- Drip and Suck Therapy
    - Not suitable in the palliative care setting
    - Vigorous hydration
        - ↑ bowel secretions
        - ↑ bowel oedema
        - ↑ peripheral oedema
        - Best replaced with judicious hydration PRN
        - Hydration for comfort and preference
        - Example: SC hydration 5-10ml/h, max 20ml/h

- Nasogastric (NG) tube insertion (Pictus 1988)
    - Nasopharyngeal irritation
    - Nasal cartilage erosion
    - Occlusion necessitating flushing or replacement
    - Spontaneous expulsion
    - Best replaced with temporary PRN NG for symptoms
    - Temporary NG insertion for large volume vomiting
    - Aim to remove NG as soon as possible

Palliative management

- Medical resolution
    - Spontaneous resolution occurs in 1/3 within 48h
    - Medical resolution if no spontaneous resolution in 5 days
    - Steroids
        - Shrink bowel oedema
        - SC Dexamethasone 8-16mg om for 1/52 or
        - CSCI Dexamethasone 8-16mg/24h for 1/52
        - NNT = 6 (Cochrane Review 2000)
        - Statistically non-significant trend in resolution
    - Metoclopramide
        - Pushes bowel contents
        - SC Metoclopramide 10-20mg tds
        - CSCI Metoclopramide 30-120mg/24h
        - Can worsen colic
        - Combined with opioid to control colic
        - Contraindicated in complete bowel obstruction
        - Risk of perforation with complete obstruction
- Symptomatic management
    - Pain
    - Nausea and vomiting
    - Constipation
    - Abdominal distension

Pain management

- Treat abdominal pain according to WHO ladder
- Prescribe parenteral opioid during initial titration
- Opioid-naïve patients
    - CSCI/CIVI Morphine 0.5mg/24h
    - SC/IV Morphine 2.5mg prn/q1h for breakthrough pain
- Opioid-naïve patients with renal failure CC<30ml/min
    - CSCI/CIVI Fentanyl 10mcg/h
    - SC/IV Fentanyl 20mcg prn/q1h for breakthrough pain
- Switch to fentanyl patch once pain is stable for 2-3 days
- Stop opioid infusion 8h after application of fentanyl patch
- Fentanyl and methadone may have less constipating effects in comparison with morphine
- Non-opioids for additional analgesia
    - IV Paracetamol 1g over 15min q6h
    - CSCI Dclofenac 75-150mg/24h
    - CSCI Ketorolac 60-90mg/24h
- Anticholinergics for colic
    - Use breakthrough opioid as first line analgesia for colic
    - Use anticholinergic as second line
    - SC/IV Hyoscine butylbromide 20mg prn/q1h for colic
    - CSCI/CIVI Hyoscine butylbromide 60-120mg/24h if ≥3 doses/day + irreversible bowel obstruction

Management of nausea and vomiting

- Targets
    - Complete relief of nausea
    - Partial relief of vomiting (1-2 vomit/day)
- Steps
    - Step 1: haloperidol or metoclopramide
    - Step 2: step 1 + antihistamine
    - Step 3: broad spectrum antemetic

- Haloperidol
  - Antiemetic of choice in complete bowel obstruction
  - SC/IV Haloperidol 1.5-5mg bd or
  - CSCI/CIVI Haloperidol 1.5-10mg/24h
  - Partial response to 10mg/24h : titrate to max 20mg/24h
  - No response to 10mg/24h: add antihistamine
- Metoclopramide
  - Antiemetic of choice in functional or partial obstruction
  - Avoid in the presence of colic
  - Avoid combining with hyoscine butylbromide because they antagonize each other
  - SC/IV Metoclopramide 10-20mg tds
  - CSCI/CIVI Metoclopramide 30-120mg/24h
  - Stop if patient develops colic
- Antihistamines
  - SC boluses can cause tissue necrosis
  - IV boluses have to be given slowly
  - CSCI is the preferred route of administration
  - Dilute with water for injection (WFI), not saline
  - Stop if patient complains of burning
  - SC Cyclizine 50-100mg tds
  - CSCI Cyclizine 150-300mg/24h
  - SC Promethazine 25-50mg tds
  - CSCI Promethazine 50-150mg/24h
  - SC Diphenhydramine 25-50mg tds
  - SC Dimenhydrinate 50-100mg tds
- Broad spectrum antiemetics
  - SL Olanzapine 2.5-10mg on
  - SC Levomepromazine 6.25-25mg on-bd
  - SC Levomepromazine 6.25-50mg/24h
- 5HT3 antagonists
  - Consider adding a 5HT3 antagonist after step 3

- SC/IV Granisetron 1mg dly-bd
- SC/IV Ondansetron 8mg dly-tds
- CSCI/CIVI Ondansetron 8-24mg/24h
- Neostigmine
  - Functional obstruction despite metoclopramide
  - SC Neostigmine 1-2.5mg test dose
  - Then CSCI Neostigmine 5-20mg/24h if tolerated
- Rectal antiemetics
  - No access to parenteral medications
  - ABHR suppositories tds
    - Lorazepam (Ativan) 0.5mg
    - Diphenhydramine (Benadryl) 12.5mg
    - Haloperidol (Haldol) 0.5mg
    - Metoclopramide (Reglan) 10mg
  - Gralla suppositories tds
    - Diphenhydramine 25mg
    - Dexamethasone 5mg
    - Metoclopramide 20mg
  - PR Prochlorperazine 25mg tds
  - PR Chlorpromazine 50-100mg tds
- Venting nasogastric tube
  - Use: large volume vomiting or proximal obstruction
  - Remove NG when vomitus <100ml/day
  - Use antisecretory agents to expedite removal
- Venting gastrostomy
  - Use: long term decompression
  - 84% had symptom resolution and return of ability to consume liquids or soft food for a median of 74 days (Campagnutta 1996)
  - Contraindications
    - Significant ascites
    - Tumour infiltration of stomach

Management of constipation

- Rectal measures
    - Options
        - Glycerin enema 2 tubes prn
        - Fleet enema 133ml prn
        - Olive oil enema 250ml prn
    - High fleet enema may be tried with special care with the gentle insertion of urinary catheter and instillation of fleet enema with or without olive oil
    - Enema may be given through stoma with care
- Oral laxatives
    - Complete bowel obstruction
        - Little role
        - Can worsen the situation
    - Partial bowel obstruction
        - Liquid paraffin or sodium docusate may be used
        - Osmotic and stimulant laxatives
            - Used with extreme care if no colic
            - Osmotic: lactulose
            - Stimulant: senna
            - Stop if colic or no response

Management of abdominal distension

- Food
    - Fasting is usually unnecessary
    - Patients will stop eating if they are very uncomfortable
    - Allow orally as tolerated
    - Inform patients that vomiting may occur
    - Liquid-based low fiber diet is preferred
    - Juices are preferred for vegetables and fruits
    - Balance between QOL and symptom control as decided by patients

271

- Temporary venting NG tube for large volume vomitus
- Parenteral nutrition may be useful for selected MBO patients with good performance status ECOG1-2 who are unable to take oral or enteral nutrition adequately
- Fluid
  - Oral fluid few ml prn/q1-2h as tolerated
  - Small ice cube if cold fluid is preferred
  - IV/SC fluid 250-1000ml/day prn
  - Regular review for peripheral oedema
  - Anticholinergics for high volume vomitus
    - CSCI Hyoscine butylbromide 60-120mg/24h
    - CSCI Hyoscine hydrobromide 1.2-2.4mg/24h
  - Octreotide for high volume vomitus
    - Very expensive
    - Onset of action: 24-48h
    - Use: failed maximal dose of anticholinergics
    - Starting dose: CSCI Octreotide 100-300mcg/24h
    - Usual dose: CSCI Octerotide 300-600mcg/24h
    - Maximal dose: CSCI Octreotide 900mcg/24h
    - Diluent: normal saline
  - Depot injection
    - Use: favourable response to octreotide
    - Octreotide (Sandostatin LAR)
      - Deep IM 10-30mg monthly
    - Lanreotide (Somatuline LA)
      - IM 30mg every 2 weeks
    - Lanreotide (Somatuline Autogel)
      - Deep SC 60-120mg every 28 days
  - PPI and H2 antagonists for gastric secretions
- Air
  - Simethicone: coalesces air bubbles
    - Syrup Maalox Plus 10-20ml tds

- PO Maalox Plus 2-4 tablets tds
- Carbonated drinks: induce burping
  - Coke or 100 Plus
  - May increase air inside bowels

3-step protocol for inoperable MBO (Laval 2006)

- Step 1: symptomatic management for 5 days
  - Corticosteroids
  - Antiemetics
  - Anticholinergics
  - Analgesics
  - IV fluids
  - ± NG tube
- Step 2: somatostatin analogue for 3 days if vomiting persists
  - Stop corticosteroids
  - Start octreotide for 3 days
  - Response: find lowest effective dose of octreotide
- Step 3: definitive procedure if vomiting persists
  - Venting gastrostomy or stenting
- Symptom control
  - Step 1: 62%
  - Step 1 + 2: 76%
  - Step 1 +2 + 3: 90%

Sleep

Introduction

Sleep is a naturally recurring state with reduced consciousness and diminished sensory and muscular activities.

Two-process model of sleep regulation

- Two main processes involved in sleep regulation
- Process C (Circadian rhythm)
    - Function: regulates alertness level by circadian clock
    - Site: suprachiasmatic nucleus (SCN) in hypothalamus
    - Reset: using Zietgebers (environmental cues)
    - Most important Zietgeber: daylight
    - Coordinated with day-night cycle
    - Hormone: melatonin from pineal gland
    - Control of timing of sleep
    - Independent of amount of preceding sleep or wakefulness
    - Peripheral clock: heart, lung, liver, kidneys, intestines etc
- Process S (Sleep homeostasis)
    - Function: regulates sleepiness level by homeostatic sleep drive due to accumulation of hypnogenic substances
    - Best known hypnogenic substance: adenosine
    - Adenosine: byproduct of using energy ATP
    - Control of sleep duration and intensity
    - Correlate of sleep intensity: slow-wave sleep
    - Dependent on amount of preceding sleep or wakefulness: sleep debt
    - Adenosine antagonists
        - Caffeine in tea, coke, coffee
        - Theophylline in tea, chocolate

Neurological mechanisms of sleep

- Sleep center
    - Site: anterior hypothalamus (VLPO)
    - VLPO
        - Ventrolateral preoptic nucleus
        - Sleep switch
        - Neurotransmitters: GABA and galanin
        - Function: inhibits arousal systems
- Arousal systems (wakefulness center)
    - Site: brainstem, hypothalamus, basal forebrain
    - Reticular activating system (RAS) of brainstem
        - Cholinergic system
            - Pedunculopontine nucleus (PPT)
            - Laterodorsal tegmental nuclei (LDT)
        - Serotonergic system
            - Dorsal raphe nuclei (DR)
            - Median raphe nuclei (MR)
        - Noradrenergic system
            - Locus coeruleus (LC)
        - Dopaminergic system
            - Ventral periaqueductal gray matter (vPAG)
    - Orexinergic system of lateral hypothalamus
        - Perifornical region
    - Histaminergic system of posterior hypothalamus
        - Tuberomammillary nucleus (TMN)
    - Cholinergic system of basal forebrain
        - Magnocellular nuclei (basal nuclei of Meynert)
- Flip-flop switch model of sleep
    - Mutual inhibition between VLPO and arousal systems
    - Either sleep neurons or arousal neurons are active
    - No intermediate state
    - Similar to the electrical flip-flop circuit

- Wakefulness
  - Monoaminegic systems inhibit VLPO
    - TMN inhibits VLPO
    - LC inhibits VLPO
    - DR inhibits VLPO
  - Orexinergic system reinforces monoaminergic tone
    - Stabilizes the switch
    - No direct inhibition of VLPO
- Sleep
  - VLPO inhibits monoaminergic systems
  - VLPO inhibits orexinergic system
- Reciprocal interaction model of NREM-REM cycle
  - Interaction between REM-ON and REM-OFF neurons
  - Anticholinergic mechanisms: REM-OFF
  - Cholinergic mechanisms: REM-ON
  - REM-OFF: LC/DR inhibits PPT/LDT
  - REM-ON: PPT/LDT inhibits LC/DR

Types of sleep

- Non-rapid eye movement sleep (NREM)
  - Synchronized sleep
  - R&K scoring (Rechtschaffen and Kales 1968)
    - Stage 1: light sleep
    - Stage 2: medium sleep
    - Stage 3: deep sleep
    - Stage 4: deep sleep
  - AASM stages (American Academy of Sleep Medicine 2004)
    - N1: stage 1
    - N2: stage 2
    - N3: stage 3 and 4
- Rapid eye movement sleep (REM)
  - Unsynchronized sleep

Stages of sleep (R&K scoring)

- Alert awake state
  - Gamma waves: 30-40Hz
    - Fastest brainwaves
    - Smallest amplitude
    - Occurrence
      - Extreme focus
      - Ecstasy
      - Compassion meditation
  - Beta waves: 12-30Hz
    - Dominate normal waking state
    - Called awake waves
    - Fast and small
    - Occurrence
      - Focused mental activity
      - Problem solving
      - Decision making
      - Judgment
    - Types
      - High beta waves: 20-30Hz
      - Beta waves: 16-20Hz
      - Low beta waves: 12-16Hz
- Relaxed state with eyes closed
  - Alpha waves: 8-12Hz
    - Predominantly from occipital area
    - Called drowsy waves
    - Occurrence
      - Drowsiness
      - Daydreaming
      - Mindfulness meditation
  - Hypnagogic hallucination and myoclonic jerk may occur

- Stage 1 sleep
  - Light sleep
  - Theta waves: 4-8Hz
  - Called light sleeping waves
  - Slower frequency, greater amplitude
  - 5-10min
  - Conscious awareness of external environment reduces
- Stage 2 sleep
  - Medium sleep
  - Sleep spindles
    - Sigma waves
    - Short burst of 12-14Hz brain activity
    - Lasting 0.5s
    - Produced by thalamic reticular nucleus (TRN)
      - Phenomena: oscillation
      - Spontaneous burst-firing of TRN neurons
      - Surround inhibition of thalamocortical neurons
  - K-complexes
    - Short negative high-voltage peak
    - Followed by a slower positive complex
    - Then a final negative peak
    - Lasting 1-2min
    - Often followed by bursts of sleep spindles
  - Sleep spindles and K complexes
    - Protect sleep
    - Suppress cortical arousal in response to stimuli
  - 20min
  - Conscious awareness of external environment disappears
- Stage 3 sleep
  - Deep sleep or slow-wave sleep (SWS)
  - Delta waves: 0.5-4Hz
  - Called deep sleeping waves

- Slowest frequency, greatest amplitude
- Initiated in the preoptic area
- 20-50% delta waves
- Most restful form of sleep
- Important in declarative memory (conscious memory)
- Stage 4 sleep
  - Deep sleep or slow-wave sleep (SWS)
  - >50% delta waves
  - 30min
  - Combined with stage 3 in AASM stages
  - Parasomnias: night terror, sleep walking, sleep talking and bed wetting occur during the end of this period
- REM sleep
  - Dreaming sleep, active sleep or paradoxical sleep
  - Very similar to awake brain with beta waves
  - Fast, small, random with sawtooth waves
  - Body is paralyzed with atonia
  - Most dreams occur during this stage
  - Important in procedural memory (unconscious memory)

Sleep cycles

- Frequency: 4-5 sleep cycles per night
- Duration for first cycle: 90min
- Duration for subsequent cycles: 100-120min
- 1-2-3-4-3-2-REM-2-3-4-3-2-REM-2-3-4-3-2-REM-2-3-2-REM
- Best illustrated by hypnogram (not shown)
- Characteristics:
  - Light to deep sleep, then deep to light sleep, then REM
  - Stage 1: only in the beginning
  - Duration of deep sleep reduces with each cycle
  - Duration of REM sleep increases with each cycle

Sleep Terms

Introduction

Sleep disorders can be primary or secondary.

Primary sleep disorders

- Dyssomnias
    - Insomnia is difficulty in initiating or maintaining sleep
        - Early insomnia (sleep-onset insomnia)
            - Also called initial insomnia
            - Difficulty in falling asleep
            - Increase in sleep latency
            - Association: anxiety
        - Middle insomnia (sleep-maintenance insomnia)
            - Difficulty in maintaining sleep
            - Decrease in sleep efficiency
            - Fragmented unrestful sleep
            - Frequent awakening during sleep
            - Association: medical illness, pain, depression
        - Late insomnia (end-of-sleep insomnia)
            - Also called terminal insomnia
            - Early morning awakening
            - Inability to return to sleep
            - Association: major depression
    - Hypersomnia is excessive daytime sleepiness
- Parasomnias
    - Sleep disorders that occur during sleep or arousal
        - Sleep transition disorders
            - Hypnic jerks (at sleep onset)
            - Sleep talking (during sleep)

- Nocturnal leg cramps (during sleep)
  - Arousal disorders
    - Sleep walking (during deep sleep)
    - Sleep terrors (sudden arousal from deep sleep)
    - Confusional arousal (arousal from deep sleep)
- REM parasomnias
  - Nightmares
  - Sleep paralysis

Secondary sleep disorders

- Associated with psychological disorders
- Associated with neurological disorders
- Associated with other medical disorders

Sleep terminology

- Sleep onset: the transition from awake to sleep
- Sleep latency: the duration of time from bedtime to sleep onset
- Sleep fragmentation: repetitive interruptions of sleep by arousals or awakenings
- Sleep efficiency: the ratio of total sleep time to time in bed
- Early morning awakening: early termination of sleep, accompanied by an inability to return to sleep
- Arousal: an abrupt change from a deeper stage of NREM sleep to a lighter stage, or from REM to wakefulness, with the possibility of awakening as the final outcome
- Awakening: the return to the awake state
- Sleep inertia: feeling groggy after abrupt awakening
- Sleep hygiene: the conditions and practices that promote continuous and effective sleep
- Zeitgeber: an environmental cue, such as sunlight, noise, social interaction, that usually helps an individual entrain to the 24-hour day

Sleep Assessment

Introduction

A comprehensive sleep assessment is necessary before managing sleep disorders.

Determining the type of sleep disorders

- Early insomnia: difficulty falling asleep
- Middle insomnia: difficulty staying asleep
- Late insomnia: early morning awakening
- Non-restorative sleep: sleep with poor quality
- Parasomnia: abnormal behaviour during sleep

Determining the risk factor of sleep disorders

- Predisposing factors
    - Young cancer patients
    - Female
    - History or family history of insomnia
    - History of anxiety or depressive disorders
    - Medical comorbidities
- Precipitating factors
    - Physical symptoms
        - Pain
        - Breathlessness
        - Cough
        - Nausea and vomiting
        - Diarrhoea
        - Urinary frequency
        - Fever
        - Delirium

- Psychological reactions to bad news
    - Anxiety
    - Depression
    - Fear
    - Anger
    - Automatic negative thoughts
- Cancer treatment
    - Surgery
    - Radiotherapy
    - Chemotherapy
    - Hormonal therapy
- Diet
    - Caffeine
    - Nicotine
    - Alcohol
- Drugs
    - Steroids
    - Bronchodilators
    - Psychostimulants
    - Antihypertensives
        - Methyldopa
        - Propranolol
    - Antidepressants
        - Fluoxetine
        - MAOIs
        - Protriptyline
        - Bupropion
- Hospitalization
    - Unfamiliar environment
    - Change of pre-sleep routine
    - Lighting at night
    - Noise from other patients

- Noise from healthcare staff
- Noise from beeping machines
- Night time vital signs checking
- Night time medication dispensing
- Perpetuating factors
  - Cognitive distortions about sleep
  - Maladaptive sleep behaviours
    - Poor sleep hygiene
      - Irregular sleeping time
      - Lying on bed during the day
      - Frequent nap during the day
      - Spending time on bed other than sleeping

Taking a sleep history

- Daytime activities
- Afternoon nap
- Sleep hygiene
- Pre-sleep routine and changes
- Pre-sleep emotions and thoughts
- Sleep environment
- Sleep partner
- Sleep time
- Sleep latency
- Sleep duration
- Sleep efficiency
- Nocturnal awakening
- Reasons of difficulty falling asleep
- Reasons of nocturnal awakening
- Aggravating and relieving factors
- Dreams
- Freshness after waking up
- Impact of sleep disorder on patient or caregivers

Sleep Architecture

Introduction

Various factors influencing sleep architecture are mentioned here.

Age

- Sleep latency: ↑
- Light sleep: ↑
- Deep sleep: ↓
- REM sleep: ↓
- Nocturnal awakening: ↑
- Circadian rhythm: phase advance (sleep and wake up earlier)

Pain

- Light sleep: ↑
- Deep sleep: ↓
- REM sleep: ↓
- Nocturnal awakening: ↑
- Alpha waves intrusion into SWS: fibromyalgia

Depression

- Deep sleep: ↓
- REM latency: ↓ (biological marker of depression)
- REM sleep: ↑ in early night
- Nocturnal awakening: ↑

Anxiety

- Sleep latency: ↑
- Light sleep: ↑
- Deep sleep: ↓

- Nocturnal awakening: ↑
- REM parasomnia: nightmares

Delirium

- Circadian rhythm: reversed

Opioids (Studies based on healthy subjects not in pain)

- Sleep latency: ↓ (chronic use)
- Deep sleep: ↓
- REM sleep: ↓ (initial use)
- Nocturnal awakening: ↑

Benzodiazepines

- Sleep latency: ↓
- Light sleep: ↑
- Deep sleep: ↓ (especially long-acting benzodiazepines)
- REM latency: ↑
- REM sleep: ↓ (especially long-acting benzodiazepines)
- Nocturnal awakening: ↓
- Benzodiazepine-induced sleep is not as restful as natural sleep
    - Reduction of slow-wave sleep
    - Reduction in REM sleep
        - Reduced daytime performance
            - REM sleep: learning and memory
        - Reduced sleep quality
            - REM sleep: resting of all muscles except eyes
- Hangover effect: sleepiness and reduced cognitive performance during the next day

Non-benzodiazepines

- Longer SWS compared to benzodiazepines
- Less hangover effect compared to benzodiazepines

Non-pharmacological Management of Sleep Disorders

Introduction

Cognitive-behavioural therapy (CBT) is the mainstay of non-pharmacological intervention for sleep disorders.

CBT components

- Cognitive therapy
    - Address dysfunctional thoughts
        - My sleep problem will get worse and worse
        - If I cannot sleep, my cancer will progress faster
        - I am going to die with a lot of suffering
    - Cognitive restructuring
        - My sleep problem will improve if I worry less
        - I know poor sleepers who are in remission
        - My suffering can be relieved
- Sleep hygiene education (American Sleep Association 2007)
    - Maintain a regular sleep routine
    - Avoid naps if possible
    - Do not stay in bed awake for more than 5-10minutes
    - Do not drink caffeine inappropriately
    - Do not watch TV or read in bed
    - Avoid substances that interfere with sleep
    - Exercise regularly
    - Have a quiet, comfortable bedroom
    - If you are a "clock-watcher" at night, hide the clock
    - Have a comfortable pre-bedtime routine

- Stimulus control therapy
  - Behavioural therapy to reassociate stimulus and sleep
  - Goal: establish regular circadian sleep-wake rhythm
  - Stimulus: bed
  - Use bed for sleep only
  - No reading, eating, watching TV, listening to radio on bed
  - Go to bed only when sleepy
  - Get out of bed if cannot sleep within 15-20min
  - Return to bed only when sleepy
  - Avoid napping during the day
- Sleep restriction therapy
  - Behavioural therapy to curtail the time in bed to the actual sleep time
  - Goal: create mild sleep debt
  - Restrict total time spent in bed to actual amount of time asleep based on completed sleep diaries
  - Avoid fixing sleep window <5 hours
  - Adjust bedtime weekly according to sleep efficiency
    - Sleep efficiency >85%: sleep 30min earlier
    - Sleep efficiency 80-85%: keep similar bedtime
    - Sleep efficiency <80%: sleep 30min later
- Relaxation therapy
  - Progressive muscular relaxation
  - Guided imagery
  - Hypnosis
  - Body scan
  - Meditation

Pharmacological Management of Sleep Disorders

Introduction

Benzodiazepine and nonbenzodiazepine hypnotics are standard medications of choice for insomnia.

Benzodiazepine hypnotics

- Mechanism of action: bind benzodiazepine receptors between α1 and γ2 subunits of GABA-A receptors, increase Cl⁻ influx, hyperpolarize neurons, enhance GABA effect

Drugs	Onset	Half-life
Short acting		
PO Triazolam	Intermediate	1-5h
PO Midazolam	Fast	2-5h
Intermedate acting		
PO Oxazepam	Slow	5-15h
PO Alprazolam	Intermediate	6-20h
PO Bromazepam	Fast	10-20h
PO Temazepam	Fast	10-20h
PO Lorazepam	Intermediate	10-20h
Long acting		
PO Nitrazepam	Fast	24h
PO Clonazepam	Intermediate	20-40h
PO Clobazam	Fast	36-42h
PO Quazepam	Fast	29-73h
PO Chlordiazepoxide	Intermediate	3-100h
PO Flurazepam	Fast	47-100h
PO Diazepam	Fast	24-120h

- Onset of action of benzodiazepines
  - Fast onset = <15min
  - Intermediate onset = 15-30min
  - Slow onset = 30-60min
- Duration of action of benzodiazepines
  - Short acting: half-life <12h
  - Intermediate acting: half-life 12-24h
  - Long acting: half-life >24h
- Doses of short acting benzodiazepines
  - PO Triazolam 0.25-0.5mg on
  - PO Midazolam 7.5-15mg on
- Doses of intermediate acting benzodiazepines
  - PO Oxazepam 15-30mg on
  - PO Alprazolam 0.25-0.5mg on
  - PO Bromazepam 1.5-12mg on
  - PO Lorazepam 0.5-2mg on
  - PO Temazepam 7.5-30mg on
- Doses of long acting benzodiazepines
  - PO Nitrazepam 5-10mg on
  - PO Clonazepam 0.5-2mg on
  - PO Clobazam 20-30mg on
  - PO Quazepam 7.5-15mg on
  - PO Chlordiazepoxide 5-10mg on
  - PO Flurazepam 15-30mg on
  - PO Diazepam 5-10mg on
- Short acting benzodiazepines
  - Best used for sleep-onset insomnia
  - Least hangover effect
  - Suitable for active person and elderly
  - Highest risk for rebound insomnia
  - Highest risk for tolerance and dependence
  - For short term use: < 1 week

- Intermediate acting benzodiazepines
  - Best used for sleep-maintenance insomnia
  - More hangover effect
  - Less rebound insomnia
  - Less tolerance and dependence
  - For short term use: < 1 month
- Long acting benzodiazepines
  - Best used for insomnia with concomitant daytime anxiety
  - May be effective for 2 nights or more
  - Accumulation of active metabolites is most problematic in elderly and in those with impaired liver function
  - Most hangover effect
  - Least rebound insomnia
  - Least tolerance and dependence
- Using benzodiazepines in insomnia
  - Fast onset is preferred
  - Intermediate acting is preferred
  - First line: bromazepam, temazepam, lorazepam
  - Second line: nitrazepam, flurazepam, diazepam
  - Half the recommended doses in elderly
  - Sublingual administration can be used in palliative setting
- Stopping benzodiazepine
  - Reduce dose gradually within several weeks or months, or eliminate doses at certain nights, such as Friday and Saturday night
- Switching benzodiazepine to nonbenzodiazepine
  - Overlap with administration of non-benzodiazepine
  - Reduce benzodiazepine dose gradually within 10 days

Nonbenzodiazepine hypnotics

- Mechanism of action: benzodiazepine receptor agonists with selectivity for α1 subunit of GABA-A benzodiazepine-1 receptor

- Promote physiological sleep
- Sleep latency: ↓
- Deep sleep: ↑
- Nocturnal awakening: ↓ except zaleplone (no change)
- Total sleep time: ↑ except zaleplone (no change)
- Little hangover effect
- Little rebound insomnia except eszopiclone
- Less tolerance and dependence
- For short term use: < 1 month except eszopiclone
- Action can be reversed by flumazenil
- Zolpidem (Stilnox)
    - Class: imidazopyridine
    - Onset: <30min
    - Half-life: 2-3h
    - Use: sleep-onset insomnia
    - Dose: 10mg on, 5mg on (elderly)
    - For short term use: < 1 month
- Zaleplone (Sonata)
    - Class: pyrazolopyrimidine
    - Onset: <30min (faster than zolpidem)
    - Half-life: 1h
    - Use: sleep-onset insomnia, breakthrough awakening
    - Dose: 10-20mg on, 5mg on (elderly)
- Zopiclone (Imovane)
    - Class: cyclopyrrolone
    - Onset: <30min
    - Half-life: 3-5h
    - Use: sleep-onset and sleep-maintenance insomnia
    - Dose: 7.5-15mg on, 3.75mg on (elderly)
- Eszopiclone (Lunesta)
    - S-enantiomer of zopiclone
    - Class: cyclopyrrolone

- Onset: <30min
- Half-life: 6h
- Use: sleep-onset and sleep-maintenance insomnia
- Dose: 1-3mg on
- Potential hangover effect with 2-3mg
- Potential rebound insomnia
- For use up to 6 months

Melatonin receptor agonist

- Ramelteon
    - Mechanism: binds MT1 and MT2 receptors in SCN
    - Sleep latency: ↓
    - Total sleep time: ↑
    - Onset: 30min
    - Half-life: 1-2h
    - Use: sleep-onset insomnia, delayed sleep phase syndrome
    - Dose: 8mg on
    - No hangover effect
    - No rebound insomnia
    - No tolerance and dependence
    - Approved for long term use

Clomethiazole

- Also called chlormethiazole
- Positive allosteric modulator at barbiturate/picrotoxin site of GABA-A receptor, and glycine receptor
- Enhances both GABA effect and glycinergic effect
- Onset: rapid
- Half-life: 3-5h
- Best used for insomnia in elderly
- Dose: 192-384mg on
- Little hangover effect

- Rebound insomnia
- Tolerance and dependence
- Limit use to <9 days to avoid dependence

Chloral hydrate

- Enhances GABA effect
- Modest short term efficacy
- Onset: 20-60min
- Half-life: 8-12h (metabolites)
- Dose for adult: 0.5-1g on
- Dose for children: 25-50mg/kg on
- More toxic than benzodiazepines
- Hangover effect
- Tolerance and dependence

Antidepressants with sedative effects

- Trazodone 25-100mg on
    - Sedating heterocyclic antidepressant
    - Serotonin antagonist and reuptake inhibitor (SARI)
    - Milder anticholinergic side effects than TCA
    - Onset: 30-60min for insomnia
    - Half-life: 7h, shorter than most TCA
    - Best used for insomnia with depression
    - Can be administered over a longer period for insomnia
- Amitriptyline 25-100mg on
    - Sedating tricyclic antidepressant (TCA)
    - Serotonin and noradrenaline reuptake inhibitor (SNRI)
    - Onset: 20-45min for insomnia
    - Half-life: 9-25h (metabolite nortriptyline 15-39h)
    - Best used for insomnia with pain or depression
    - Dose for insomnia per se: 10-50mg on
    - Side effects: anticholinergic effects, daytime sedation

- Mirtazapine 15-30mg on
    - Sedating tetracyclic antidepressant
    - Noradrenergic and specific serotonergic antidepressant
    - NaSSA
    - Sleep latency: ↓
    - SWS: ↑ (5HT2A/C antagonism)
    - REM sleep: unchanged
    - Total sleep time: ↑
    - Onset: 2 weeks
    - Half-life: 20-40h
    - Best used for insomnia with depression
    - Hangover effect in 10% with rapid tolerance

Antipsychotics with sedative effects

- Best used for insomnia with delirium
- Haloperidol 1.5-5mg on (useful for unpleasant dreams)
- Olanzapine 2.5-10mg on
- Risperidone 0.5-2mg on
- Quetiapine 25-100mg on

Antihistamines with sedative effects

- Best used for insomnia with pruritus or cough
- Chlorpheniramine (Piriton) 4-8mg on
- Hydroxyzine (Atarax) 25-50mg on
- Diphenhydramine (Benadryl) 25-50mg on
- Promethazine (Phenergan) 25-50mg on

Barbiturates

- Bind GABA-A receptors
- Enhance GABA effect
- Effective hypnotics
- Onset: 20-60min for phenobarbital

- Half-life: 2-6 days for phenobarbital
- Dose: PO Phenobarbital 100-200mg on
- Hangover effect
- Rapid development of tolerance after about 2 weeks
- Risk of dependence
- Serious or fatal consequences with overdose, esp with alcohol
- Gradual withdrawal recommended

Medication adjustment to avoid insomnia

- Give steroid as a single morning dose
- Give diuretic as a single morning dose
- Give fluoxetine as a single morning dose
- Give sertraline as a single morning dose
- Give methylphenidate at 8am and 12pm

Delirium

Introduction

Delirium is a syndrome of acute brain failure characterized by disturbances in consciousness. The disturbances can be a change in the content of consciousness (attention), a change in the level of consciousness (arousal), or both.

Types of delirium

- Hyperactive delirium (agitated delirium): patient is agitated, restless and confused
- Hypoactive delirium (lethargic delirium): patient is lethargic, withdrawn and confused
- Mixed delirium: patient has a mixture of hyperactive and hypoactive delirium

Causes of delirium

- Check for simple reversible causes of delirium before thinking about the complicated ones
- Symptom distress: pain, breathlessness, nausea and vomiting, acute urinary retention, fecal impaction, insomnia, fatigue
- Psychosocial distress: fear of pain, fear of dying, fear of being alone, witnessing death of another patient
- Hospital causes: blood-taking, nasogastric tube insertion, urinary catheter insertion, continuous vital sign monitoring, physical restraint, change of bed, soiled bed sheets, folded bed sheets, uncomfortable bed
- Organ failure causes: respiratory failure, cardiac failure, liver failure, renal failure, brain failure (brain metastases, stroke, encephalopathy)

- Metabolic and toxin causes: hypoglycaemia, hyponatremia, hypercalcemia, septic encephalopathy
- Drug causes: opioid, steroid, benzodiazepine, anticholinergic, antihistamine, antidepressant, antipsychotic, anticonvulsant
- Antibiotic causes: penicillin, cephalosporin, fluoroquinolone, sulfonamide, metronidazole
- Chemotherapy causes: asparaginase, bleomycin, carmustin, cisplatin, cytarabine, 5-fluorouracil, gemcitabine, ifosfamide, methotrexate, procarbazine, vincristine, vinblastine

Delirium assessment

- Confusion Assessment Method (CAM)
    - Acute onset and fluctuating course
    - Inattention
    - Disorganized thinking
    - Altered level of conscious
- Memorial Delirium Assessment Scale (MDAS)
    - Reduced level of consciousness
    - Disorientation
    - Short-term memory impairment
    - Impaired digit span
    - Reduced ability to maintain and shift attention
    - Disorganized thinking
    - Perceptual disturbance
    - Delusions
    - Decreased or increased psychomotor activity
    - Sleep-wake cycle disturbance

Pathophysiology of delirium

- Multifactorial
- Not fully understood
- Decreased cerebral oxidative metabolism

- Neuroanatomical structures
  - Level of consciousness (Arousal)
    - Ascending reticular activating system (ARAS)
      - Dorsal mesencephalic reticular formation
      - Mesencephalic nucleus
      - Locus ceruleus and raphe nuclei
      - Thalamic intralaminar nucleus
      - Dorsal hypothalamus
      - Tegmentum
      - Basal forebrain
  - Content of consciousness (Attention)
    - Alerting network: maintaining alertness
      - Same areas for arousal: ARAS
      - Main neurotransmitter: noradrenergic system of locus ceruleus
    - Orienting network: orienting to sensory information
      - Pulvinar
      - Superior colliculus
      - Superior parietal lobe
      - Temporoparietal junction
      - Frontal eye field
      - Main neurotransmitter: cholinergic system of basal forebrain
    - Executive network: resolving conflicts between multiple competing attention cues
      - Anterior cingulate gyrus
      - Dorsolateral prefrontal cortex (DLPRC)
      - Main neurotransmitter: dopamine system of mesocortex
- Neurotransmitters
  - Acetylcholine-dopamine hypothesis
    - Acetylcholine insufficiency

- Dopamine excess
- Other neurotransmitters
  - Serotonin, noradrenaline, histamine, hypocretin, glutamate, endorphins, GABA
- Cytokines: IL-1, IL-6, IL-8, IFN, TNF
- Chronic hypercortisolism

Non-pharmacological management of delirium

- Environmental interventions
  - Avoid over and understimulation
  - Visual interventions
    - Adequate lighting during daytime
    - Minimal lighting during night-time
    - Huge calender and clock
    - Make the environment familiar
      - Photographs
      - Personal objects
  - Auditory interventions
    - Keeping a quiet environment
    - Silent monitoring
    - Slow music if appropriate
    - Slow electronic chanting if appropriate
  - Physical interventions
    - Familiar objects
    - Home pillows and blankets
    - Bed sheet rearrangement
    - Avoid restraints
    - Avoid continuous vital signs monitoring
    - Minimize tubes and lines
  - Social interventions
    - Family staying in
    - Familiar staff if possible

- Sleep interventions
    - Facilitate normal sleep
    - Exposure to sunlight during daytime
    - Encourage activities during daytime
    - Keep room dark during night-time
    - Minimize interruption during night-time
    - Avoid vital signs checking at night if appropriate
- Patient support
    - Maintain communication
    - Active listening
    - Explore patient's ideas, concerns and expectations
    - Explore patient's emotions
    - Explore reasons behind hallucination or delusion
    - Explore reasons behind patient's behaviour
    - Explain to patient about each procedure and intervention
- Family support
    - Taking care of a delirious patient is stressful
    - Do not forget to support the family member
    - Give simple explanation of the nature of delirium
    - Explore family's ideas, concerns and expectations
    - Acknowledge family distress
    - Educate family in consoling patient
    - Educate family in re-orientating patient
    - Facilitate the linking of the content of hallucination and delusion with past experiences
    - Provide respite care if needed

Pharmacological management of delirium (PCT input)

- Review of meditations
    - Stop deliriogenic drugs if appropriate
    - Consider opioid rotation for opioid neurotoxicity
    - Consider steroids for brain metastases

- Typical antipsychotics
  - Haloperidol
    - Gold standard treatment for delirium
    - Onset: 1h (PO), 10-15min (SC)
    - Half-life: 0.5-1.5 days
    - Duration: 24h
    - Less sedating compared to chlorpromazine
    - Less anticholinergic effect
    - Extrapyramidal effect more likely when ≥ 7.5mg/day
    - Mild delirium (10 < MDAS score ≤ 15)
      - PO Haloperidol 0.75-1.5mg bd
      - SC Haloperidol 0.5-1.5mg bd
    - Moderate delirium (15 < MDAS score ≤ 22)
      - PO Haloperidol 2.5-5mg bd
      - SC Haloperidol 2.5-5mg bd
    - Severe delirium (MDAS score > 22)
      - PO Haloperidol 5-10mg bd
      - SC Haloperidol 5-10mg bd
    - Rapid titration of haloperidol for severe agitation
      - PO/SL/SC Haloperidol 0.5-2.5mg prn/q1h
      - Administer until delirium is controlled in 24h
    - 30-minute haloperidol titration schedule
      - 0.5, 0.5, 0.5, 1, 1, 1, 2, 2, 2, 5, 5, 5mg prn
      - Administer q30min
    - Maximum reported dose 50mg/day
  - Chlorpromazine
    - Onset: 30-60min (PO), 15-30min (SC)
    - Half-life: 1.25 days
    - Duration: 4-6h
    - PO/SC/PR Chlorpromazine 12.5-50mg q4-6h
    - Risk of skin irritation with SC
    - Preferred in agitated delirium (sedation)

- Levomepromazine
  - Onset: 30min
  - Half-life: 0.5-1.25 days
  - Duration: 12-24h
  - PO Levomepromazine 5-25mg bd
  - SC Levomepromazine 6.25-25mg bd
  - Preferred in agitated delirium (sedation)
- Atypical antipsychotics
  - Less extrapyramidal side effects
  - PO Olanzapine 2.5-10mg on, max 20mg bd (agitation)
  - PO Quetiapine 12.5-100mg bd, max 200mg bd (agitation)
  - PO Risperidone 0.25-1mg bd, max 3mg bd
  - PO Ziprasidone 10-40mg bd, max 80mg bd
  - PO Aripiprazole 5-30mg dly, max 30mg dly
- Benzodiazepines
  - Second line treatment of agitated delirium
  - Usually added if haloperidol dose has reached 20mg/day
  - SC Midazolam 2.5mg prn/q1h
  - CSCI Midazolam 0.5-1mg/h
  - SL Lorazepam 1-2mg prn/q1h
  - SC Lorazepam 0.5-2mg prn/q4h
  - CSCI Lorazepam: risk of precipitation
  - CIVI Lorazepam 4mg/24h
  - Risk of paradoxical reactions: < 1% (Mancuso 2004)
- Miscellaneous agents
  - Trazodone
    - Sedating heterocyclic antidepressant
    - Serotonin antagonist and reuptake inhibitor (SARI)
    - Less anticholinergic effects than TCA
    - PO Trazodone 25-50mg tds or 25-100mg on
    - Maximum dose: 300mg/day
    - Maximum use: 7 days

- Mianserin
  - Tetracyclic antidepressant
  - Noradrenergic and specific serotonergic antidepressant (NaSSA)
  - Use: delirium in elderly
  - Dose: PO Mianserin 10-30mg on
  - Effects
    - Controls behavioural symptoms
    - Improves sleep
    - Reduces hallucinations
    - No change in cognition
- Clomethiazole (Chlormethiazole)
  - GABA-A and glycine agonist
  - Use: restlessness in elderly
  - Dose: PO Clomethiazole 192mg tds or 192-384mg on
  - Maximum use: 7 days
- Psychostimulants
  - PO Methylphenidate 5-10mg at 8am and 12pm
  - PO Modafinil 100-200mg om
  - Use: hypoactive delirium
  - Evidence: case reports
- Cholinesterase inhibitors
  - PO Donepezil 5-10mg on
  - PO Rivastigmine 1.5-6mg bd
  - Rivastigmine patch 4.6, 9.5, 13.3mg q24h
  - Evidence: no evidence from RCT

Terminal Delirium

Introduction

Terminal delirium is delirium that occurs in some patients during their last few days of life.

Communication with patients and family members

- Involve palliative care specialists
- Initiate discussion with family members and patient (if patient has lucid moments)
- Discuss goals of care
- Discuss palliative sedation
  - Level of sedation
    - Conscious sedation: partially responsive
    - Deep sedation: unresponsive
  - Temporal
    - PRN sedation
    - Night sedation
    - Respite sedation
    - Continuous sedation
  - Goals of sedation
    - Palliate symptoms
    - Not hastening of death
- Elicit wishes and concerns
  - Wish to maintain consciousness
  - Wish to reverse sedation
  - Address concern about reversibility of sedation
  - Address concern about hastening of death
- Shared decision making
- Respect dignity and values of patient and family

Management of terminal delirium in palliative care

- Wait-and-see approach
    - Hypoactive or lethargic delirium
    - Pleasant confusion
    - Pleasant hallucinations or delusions
    - Natural part of the dying process
    - Anticipatory prescription for agitation
        - SC Haloperidol 1-2mg prn/q1h
        - SC Midazolam 2.5-5mg prn/q1h
- Pharmacological interventions
    - Hyperactive or agitated delirium
    - Synonyms
        - Terminal restlessness
        - Terminal agitation
        - Terminal anguish
        - Pre-death restlessness
    - Clinical features
        - Restlessness
        - Fidgeting
        - Purposeless movements
            - Pulling tubes and lines
            - Snatching the air
            - Plucking bedsheets
            - Taking off clothes
            - Getting out of the bed
            - Pacing to and fro
            - Going to toilet repetitively
    - First line treatment for terminal restlessness
        - Benzodiazepines
        - Goal: sedation just enough to palliate restlessness
        - Also useful for delirium with seizures
        - Risk of paradoxical agitation, esp elderly

- Midazolam
  - SC Midazolam 2.5-5mg stat, then 1-2.5mg/h
    - Titrate up to 5mg/h if necessary
  - SC Midazolam 2.5-5mg stat, then 30-60mg/24h
    - Titrate up to 120mg/24h if necessary
  - Maximum reported midazolam dose: 50mg/h
- Alternative benzodiazepines
  - SL Lorazepam 1-2mg q4-6h
  - SC Lorazepam 1-2mg q4-6h
  - CSCI Lorazepam: risk of precipitation
  - CIVI Lorazepam 4-20mg/24h
  - SL Clonazepam 1-4mg q12h
  - CSCI Clonazepam 2-8mg/24h
  - PR Diazepam 10-20mg q6-8h
  - IV Diazepam 5-10mg q6-8h
- Rapid titration
  - IV Midazolam 0.5mg q5min till settled
  - SC Midazolam 1mg q15min till settled
  - SL Lorazepam 1-2mg q1h till settled
    - Usual dose: 2-10mg/day
    - Up to 20-50mg/day for extreme agitation
- Second line treatment for terminal restlessness
  - Neuroleptics
  - Add haloperidol if CSCI Midazolam 1.5mg/h fails or
  - Add haloperidol if paradoxical agitation with benzo
  - SC Haloperidol 2.5-5mg stat, then 10-30mg/24h
  - Alternative neuroleptics
    - PR Chlorpromazine 25-50mg q4-6h
      - Max dose 200mg q4h
    - SC Levomepromazine 12.5-25mg stat
      - Then 50-75mg/24h
      - Max dose 300mg/24h

- Rapid titration
  - IV Haloperidol 0.5-2mg q10min till settled
  - SC Haloperidol 0.5-2mg q30min till settled
  - PR Haloperidol 0.5-2mg q60min till settled
    - Then give total dose at night or
    - Divide total dose by 4 for q6h dosing
  - IV/SC Chlorpromazine 12.5-25mg q30min
  - PO/PR Chlorpromazine 12.5-25mg q60min
    - Then give total dose at night or
    - Divide total dose by 4 for q6h dosing
- Third line treatment for terminal restlessness
  - Failed CSCI Midazolam 60-120mg/24h +
    - Failed CSCI Haloperidol 30mg/24h or
    - Failed CSCI Levomepromazine 200mg/24h
  - Phenobarbital (single agent)
    - Onset: 5min (IV)
    - Half-life: 2-6 days
    - Duration: 4 hours to 2 days
    - Concentration: 200mg/ml
    - Do not mix with another drug
    - Local necrosis: SC bolus or IV extravasation
    - IM Phenobarbital 100-200mg undiluted stat or
    - IV Phenobarbital 100-200mg with 10ml WFI in rate of 50mg/min
    - Then CSCI Phenobarbital 600-1600mg/24h
    - Max 2400mg/24h
    - Dilute 1ml phenobarbital with 10ml WFI
      - Phenobarbital 600mg with 30ml WFI
      - Phenobarbital 800mg with 40ml WFI
      - Phenobarbital 1200mg with 60ml WFI
      - Phenobarbital 1600mg with 80ml WFI
      - Phenobarbital 2400mg with 120ml WFI

- Propofol (single agent)
  - Onset: 0.5min
  - Half-life: 3-12h
  - Duration: 3-10min
  - Concentration: 10mg/ml (1%), 20mg/ml (2%)
  - Aim: conscious sedation (open eyes to call)
  - IV Propofol 1mg/kg/h via forearm vein
  - Increase 0.5mg/kg/h q5-10min till sedation
  - Usual dose 1-2mg/kg/h
  - Max dose 4mg/kg/h
  - Bolus: 1mg/kg/min for 2-5min
  - RR and sedation assessment q1h for 24h
  - Then q12h review
  - No response to call or RR<8/min: stop 2-3min, restart at lower dose
  - Replenish infusion immediately once empty
  - No response to 4mg/kg/h: add CSCI Midazolam
  - No analgesic property: continue analgesia
- Dexmedetomidine (Precedex)
  - α2 agonist with analgesic properties
  - Onset: <5min
  - Half-life: 2h
  - Duration: 4h
  - Dilute 400mcg in 100ml normal saline
  - IV Dexmedetomidine 0.2mcg/kg/h
  - Increase 0.1mcg/kg/h q30min till sedation
  - Usual dose 0.2-0.7mcg/kg/h
  - Max dose 1.5mcg/kg/h
  - RR and sedation assessment q1h for first 24h
  - Then q12h review
  - Side effects: hypotension, bradycardia
  - Reduce opioid dose gradually during titration

Prognostication

Introduction

Prognostication is the act of predicting how much time is left for a patient to live.

Benefits of prognostication

- Clinical decision making
- Advance care planning
- Prioritization in life
- Preparation for dying

Components of prognostication (Lamont, Christakis 1999)

- Foreseeing: formulating a prognosis
- Foretelling: communicating prognosis

The optimism of physicians

- Physicians tend to overestimate life expectancy by a factor of 5 on average (Christakis 1996)

Little thoughts

First sign of dying: when we were born

Second sign of dying: when we are told of having a life-limiting illness

Third sign of dying: when we see the palliative care team

Fourth sign of dying: when we see distant relatives coming back to see us

Fifth sign of dying: when we hear people saying prayers around our bed

---

Clinical Prediction of Survival (CPS)

- Overly optimistic: 3-5x actual survival
- Actual survical: 30% shorter than CPS
- Horizon effect: more accurate for shortest survival
- Most effective when added to other prognostic tools

Foreseeing prognosis of months

- GSF Prognostic Indicator Guidance 2011
- Step 1: surprise question
    - Ask ourself the one year surprise question
    - Would you be surprised if patient dies within one year?
    - Not surprised: prognosis < 1 year
    - Sensitivity 69%, specificity 84% (Moroni 2014)
- Step 2: general indicators of poor prognosis
    - Functional decline
    - Comorbidities
    - Increasing symptom burden
    - Decreasing response to treatment
    - Repeated crisis admissions
- Step 3: specific indicators of poor prognosis
    - Cancer
        - Metastatic cancer
        - ECOG 3-4
    - Heart failure
        - NYHA Class III/IV
        - Difficult symptoms despite optimal therapy
        - Multiple admissions for heart failure
    - Chronic obstructive pulmonary disease
        - FEV1 <30%
        - Breathless after 100m or house-bound
        - On LTOT
        - Multiple admission for COPD exacerbation

- Renal failure
    - Stage 4/5 CKD
    - Symptomatic renal failure
    - Difficult symptoms despite optimal therapy
    - Withholding or withdrawal of dialysis
- Neurological diseases
    - Progressive functional and cognitive decline
    - Difficult symptoms despite optimal therapy
    - Speech and swallowing problems
- Geriatric diseases
    - Poor functional and cognitive status
    - Multiple comorbidities
    - Multiple symptoms
    - Recurrent infections
- HIV disease (not in GSF)
    - Age > 65
    - ADL dependent
    - Poor performance status
    - HAART withdrawal

Foreseeing prognosis of weeks to short months

- Eastern Cooperative Oncology Group (ECOG)
    - ECOG 3 (>50% bed-ridden): prognosis < 3 months
    - ECOG 4 (total bed-ridden): prognosis < 1 month
- Karnofsky Performance Scale (KPS)
    - KPS 30-40 (total dependence): prognosis < 2 months
    - KPS 10-20 (very sick): prognosis < 2 weeks
- Palliative Performance Scale (PPS)
    - PPS 50 (total dependence): prognosis < 2 months
    - PPS 30-40 (reduced oral intake): prognosis < 1 month
    - PPS 10-20 (sips or no oral intake): prognosis < 2 weeks

- Palliative Prognostic Score (PaP) (Pirovano 1999)
    - Prognosis < 1 month
    - Score 0-17.5
    - Higher score = higher likelihood for prognosis < 1 month
        - CPS < 1 year
        - KPS 10-20
        - Dyspnoea
        - Anorexia
        - Leucocytosis
        - Lymphocytopenia
- Palliative Prognostic Index (PPI) (Morita 1999)
    - Prognosis < 3-6 weeks
    - Score 0-15
    - PPI >4 = prognosis < 6 weeks
    - PPI ≥6 = prognosis < 3 weeks

Palliative Prognostic Index	
Prognostic factors	Score
Performance status	
• PPS 10-20	4
• PPS 30-50	2.5
• PPS > 50	0
Oral intake	
• Mouthfuls or less	2.5
• Moderately reduced	1
• Normal	0
Edema	1
Dyspnoea at rest	3.5
Delirium	4

- 3-Variable Model for Advanced Cancer (Chow 2002)
    - 1 risk factor = prognosis < 14 months
    - 2 risk factors = prognosis < 5 months
    - 3 risk factors = prognosis < 3 months

- Risk factors
  - Non-breast cancer
  - Non-bone metastases
  - KPS ≤ 60

Foreseeing prognosis of days

10 Clinical signs of impending death within 7 days (Hui 2014)	Prognosis (days)	Frequency* (%)
Liquid dysphagia	7	90
Reduced consciousness	7	90
PPS ≤ 20	4	93
Peripheral cyanosis	3	59
Cheyne-Stokes breathing	2	41
Urine output<100ml in 12h	1.5	72
Apnoea periods	1.5	46
Respiration with mandibular movement	1.5	56
Death rattle	1.5	66
Pulselessness of radial artery	1	38

7 Clinical signs of impending death within 3 days (Hui 2015)	Prognosis (days)	Frequency* (%)
Decreased response to visual stimuli	3	70
Hyperextension of neck	2.5	46
Drooping of nasolabial fold	2.5	78
Non-reactive pupil	2	38
Decreased response to verbal stimuli	2	69
Grunting of vocal cords	1.5	54
Inability to close eye lids	1.5	57

*Frequency of sign in last 3 days of life

Foretelling prognosis

- Please refer to the chapter of communicating prognosis

Dying trajectories

Introduction

While prognostication deals with the "when" of dying, dying trajectory deals with the "how" of dying.

Dying trajectories (Lynn 2003)

Sudden death trajectory

Function

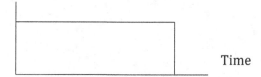

Time

- Little or no time to help the patient
- Intense bereavement support for the family

Cancer trajectory

Function

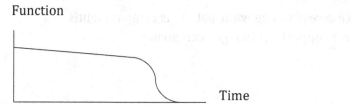

Time

- Rapid functional decline during last few months of life
- Anticipatory grief support for the patient and family

Organ failure trajectory

Function

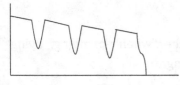

Time

- Sine-waving
- Not sure which dip is final
- Advance care planning

Frailty trajectory

Function

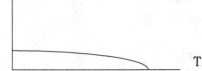

Time

- Lingering death
- Advance care planning while patient is compos mentis
- Caregiver support – prolonged caregiving

Symptom Management in the Last Days of Life

Introduction

The most important step in the management of patients in their last days of life is to recognize dying. If dying is unrecognized, patients will continue to receive useless treatment.

Diagnosing dying

- The process of dying can be seen as a process of deterioration of the different organ systems of a person
- The sequence of deterioration depends on the dynamic process of ongoing multiple organ failure
- Pre-active phase of dying (days to short weeks before death)
  - Musculoskelatal system
    - Rapidly increasing weakness and fatigue
    - Difficulty getting out of bed or sitting up
    - Bed-ridden
    - Total dependent in activities of daily living
  - Gastrointenstinal system
    - Rapid decline in oral intake
    - Reduced or absence of hunger or thirst
    - Fecal incontinence
  - Cardiovascular system
    - Tachycardia
    - Low blood pressure
  - Renal system
    - Peripheral oedema
    - Urinary incontinence

- Neurological system
    - Limited attention span
    - Delirium
    - Restlessness
    - Sleepy most of the time
    - Loss of interest in surroundings
- Respiratory system
    - Reduced communication
    - Grunting or moaning
- Active phase of dying (hours to short days before death)
    - Gastrointenstinal system
        - Inability to swallow tablets
        - Inability to swallow fluid
    - Cardiovascular system
        - Peripheral mottling or cyanosis
        - Pulselessness of radial artery
        - Cold extremities
    - Renal system
        - Reduced urine output
        - Anuria with urine output <100ml in 12h
    - Neurological system
        - Reduced consciousness
        - Reduced or absent response to call
        - Inability to close eyelids
        - Reduced or no blinking
    - Respiratory system
        - Inability to speak
        - Death rattle
        - Abnormal respiratory patterns
            - Cheyne-Stokes breathing
            - Apnoea periods
            - Respiration with mandibular movement

Communicating the diagnosis of dying

- Assess patient's ability to communicate
- Assess insight into situation
- Involve family members
- Provide relevant information sensitively
- Explain the significance of signs and symptoms of dying
- Allow time for digestion of the information
- Provide support for emotional and cognitive reactions
- Respect all psychological reactions, including non-acceptance
- Explore what is important to patient and family at this time
- Discuss goals of care
- Discuss management plan
- Explore preference of place of dying if appropriate
- Allow time and space for patient and family to grieve
- Encourage family and friends to talk to patient
- Tell them patient may still be hearing even though unconscious
- Encourage expressions of intimacy
- Tell them patient may still be feeling
- Encourage family to stay with patient if possible
- Discuss the process of dying if appropriate
- Discuss what to do after death if appropriate
- Address spiritual needs

Little story

I was stopped by my boss as I attempted to rush through a crowd of family members to see a dying patient. My boss asked me to wait. After a while the family moved aside spontaneously. It was a beautiful experience. Remember. The most important person at the deathbed is the patient, not us. Second is the family.

Stopping unnecessary investigations and treatments

- Do no harm
- Stop monitoring of vital signs
- Stop all unnecessary blood-taking
- Stop all unnecessary investigations
- Stop all unnecessary medications
- Stop all unnecessary medical and nursing interventions
- Review the need of artificial hydration and nutrition
- Deactivate implantable cardiac defibrillator if present
- Document Do Not Resuscitate (DNR) order

Symptom management of a dying patient

- Continue essential symptom medications
    - Analgesics
    - Antiemetics
    - Anxiolytics
- Continue some symptom medications as PRN if appropriate
    - Anticonvulsants
    - Antibiotics
    - Insulin
- Convert to an appropriate route
    - Subcutaneous
    - Intravenous
    - Sublingual
    - Suppository

Anticipatory prescriptions for symptoms

- SC Morphine 2.5mg prn/q1h for pain or breathlessness
- SC Hyoscine butylbromide 20mg prn/q1h for secretions
- SC Haloperidol 1.5mg prn/q1h for nausea and vomiting
- SC Midazolam 2.5mg prn/q1h for sleeplessness or agitation

Pain and breathlessness

- Misconception: pain will increase at the end of life
- Reality: pain may increase, stabilize or decrease (Sykes 2003)
- Conscious patient: assess symptoms by asking patient
- Unconscious patient: assess pain by using FLACC scale

FLACC scale

Criteria	0	1	2
Face	Normal	Grimace	Clenched jaw
Legs	Normal	Restless	Kicking
Activity	Normal	Squirming	Arched
Cry	Normal	Moaning	Screaming
Consolability	Normal	Reassurable	Nonreassurable

- Unconscious patient: assess breathlessness by looking for signs of respiratory distress, such as RR ≥ 25 breaths/min, laboured breathing
- Pain or breathlessness in opioid-naïve patient
    - CSCI Morphine 0.5mg/h
    - SC Morphine 2.5mg prn/q1h for breakthrough symptoms
- Pain or breathlessness in opioid-naïve renal failure patient
    - CSCI Fentanyl 10mcg/h
    - SC Fentanyl 25mcg prn/q1h for breakthrough symptoms
- Pain or breathlessness in opioid-tolerant patient
    - Consult palliative care team for opioid conversion
- Alternative drugs
    - SL Morphine: moribund patients at home
    - SL Buprenorphine: moribund patients at home
    - SL Methadone: moribund patients at home
    - SL Dextromoramide 5-20mg prn/q3h: procedural pain
    - Fentanyl patch: stable pain
    - Buprenorphine patch: stable pain

Respiratory tract secretions

- Death rattle: gurgling noise from secretions during last days
- Median prognosis: 1.5 days
- Patients are usually unconscious
- Type I death rattle (true death rattle)
  - Secretions from salivary glands
  - Failure of swallowing reflex
  - During final hours
  - Responsive to anticholinergics
- Type II death rattle (pseudo death rattle)
  - Secretions from bronchial glands
  - Failure of cough reflex
  - Less responsive to anticholinergics
- Victoria Respiratory Congestion Scale (VRCS)
  - 0 = inaudible
  - 1 = audible only very close to patient
  - 2 = clearly audible from end of bed in quiet room
  - 3 = audible at 9.5m or at door of room
- VRCS 0-1: reassurance
- VRCS 2-3: positioning + antisecretory agents
- Antisecretory agents
  - SC Glycopyrrolate 0.2-0.4mg q4h or
    - CSCI Glycopyrrolate 0.6-1.2mg/24h
  - SC Hyoscine hydrobromide 0.4-0.6mg q4h or
    - CSCI Hyoscine hydrobromide 1.2-2.4mg/24h
  - SC Hyoscine butylbromide 20mg q4h or
    - CSCI Hyoscine butylbromide 60-120mg/24h
- Alternative drugs
  - SL Atropine eyedrops 1% 3-4 drops tds-qid
  - Scopolamine patch 1.5-4.5mg q72h to mastoid
    - Onset: 8h after application
    - Effect: continues 12h after removal

Nausea and vomiting (N&V)

- Determining the precise cause of N&V can be difficult
- Treat N&V empirically
- Antiemetics
    - SC Haloperidol 1.5-5mg bd or
        - CSCI Haloperidol 1.5-20mg/24h
    - SC Metoclopramide 10-20mg tds or
        - CSCI Metoclopramide 30-120mg/24h
    - IV Promethazine 25-50mg tds or
        - CSCI Promethazine 50-150mg/24h
    - SC Levomepromazine 6.25-25mg on-bd or
        - CSCI Levomepromazine 6.25-50mg/24h
- Do not combine metoclopramide and antisecretory agents
- Alternative drugs
    - SL Olanzapine 2.5-10mg on
    - PR Chlorpromazine 50-100mg tds
    - ABHR suppositories tds
        - Lorazepam (Ativan) 0.5mg
        - Diphenhydramine (Benadryl) 12.5mg
        - Haloperidol (Haldol) 0.5mg
        - Metoclopramide (Reglan) 10mg

Sleeplessness

- Most patients will sleep more during their final days
- Some may experience reversal of sleep pattern
- Treatment of insomnia in last days of life
    - SC Midazolam 2.5-5mg on or
        - CSCI Midazolam 1-2.5mg/h during nighttime
- Alternative drugs
    - SL Lorazepam 1-2mg on
    - PR Diazepam 10-20mg on

Agitation or restlessness

- Common
- Sometimes can be reversed by simple measures
  - Breakthrough medications for symptoms
  - Re-positioning for positional discomfort
  - Urinary catheter insertion for retention of urine
  - Fecal disimpaction for retention of feces
- Treatment of agitation or restlessness
  - CSCI Midazolam 1-2.5mg/h
    - SC Midazolam 2.5mg prn/q1h for agitation
  - CSCI Haloperidol 10-30mg/24h
    - SC Haloperidol 2.5-5mg prn/q1h for agitation
  - CSCI Levomepromazine 50-75mg/24h
    - SC Levomepromazine 12.5-25mg prn/tds
- Alternative drugs
  - SL Lorazepam 1-2mg tds
  - PR Diazepam 10-20mg tds
  - PR Chlorpromazine 50-100mg tds

Nursing care for a dying patient

- Oral care
  - Keep the mouth moist
    - Frequent sips of water, ice chips, pineapple chunks
    - Artificial saliva
    - Moisturizing gel with aloe vera
    - Cooking oil for lips
  - Keep the mouth clean
    - Soft toothbrush and bland toothpaste if able to rinse
    - Soft-cotton or sponge-tipped swabs moistened with a solution of water and baking powder
    - Gentle swabbing q30-60min prn for comfort
  - Encourage family participation in oral care

- Skin care
    - Ripple mattress
    - Gentle turning with a draw sheet
    - Reduce turning to bd-tds
    - Incident pain: SC Morphine 30min before turning
    - Re-position prn for comfort
    - Smoothen bed surface and draw sheet
    - Moisturize the skin
- Eye care
    - Artificial tears for dry eyes
    - Gentle swabbing with moistened cotton
- Feeding
    - Explain reduced to no eating and drinking at final days
    - Explain reduced to no sensation of hunger and thirst
    - Discuss natural dehydration in the dying process
    - Benefit of endorphin release in natural dehydration
    - Discuss futility of artificial hydration and nutrition
    - Risks of secretions, ascites and oedema
    - Respect individual and sociocultural beliefs
    - Allow orally as tolerated
    - Consider sips or droplets of oral feeding prn
- Bladder and bowel care
    - Urinary catheter if appropriate
    - Incontinence pad if appropriate
    - Change pad immediately after soiling
    - Switch oral laxatives to glycerin enema prn

Psychosocial and spiritual care

- Ensure supportive physical environment
- Ensure well-being of family or caregiver
- Address psychosocial and spiritual needs of patient and family
- Regular review irrespective of patient's situation

Care after death in the hospital

- Confirm death
- Notify family member gently
- Allow time for family to come to see patient
- Allow time for family to grieve
- Respect spiritual or religious rites and rituals
- Perform last office according to policy when family is ready
- Explain to family what to do next
- Notify primary team or community hospice if appropriate

Hydration and Nutrition at the End-of-life

Introduction

One of the most difficult issues to deal with at the end of life is hydration and nutrition. Patients will consume less and less up to a stage when they consume near-nothing or nothing. Witnessing this diminishing of oral intake can be a hard time for the family.

Goals of hydration and nutrition

- Sustain life by provision of calories, nutrients and water
- Sustain function
- Alleviate suffering by reducing thirst and hunger
- Enhance pleasures in life
- ·Enhance social activities: nurturing and being nurtured

Types of feeding

- Natural feeding (basic care)
  - Unassisted
  - Assisted
    - Spoon-feeding
    - Syringe-feeding
- Artificial feeding (medical treatment)
  - Artificial hydration
    - Subcutaneous hydration
    - Intravenous hydration
  - Artificial nutrition
    - Tube feeding
    - Parenteral nutrition

Tube feeding

- Prevention of aspiration pneumonia
  - Benefit
    - Non-bedridden stroke
  - No benefit
    - Bedridden stroke
    - Other neurological disorders
    - Advanced dementia
    - Aspiration risk demonstrated with videofluoroscopy
    - Cancer
- Prevention of pressure sores
  - No benefit
    - Advanced dementia
    - Nursing home residents
- Prolongation of life
  - Benefit
    - Non-bedridden head & neck cancer with dysphagia
    - Non-bedridden malignant proximal GI obstruction
    - Proximal GI cancer receiving chemo or radiotherapy
    - Reversible illness in catabolic state: eg acute sepsis
    - Motor neuron disease
    - Nursing home residents < 40 years
    - AIDS with wasting syndrome
  - No benefit
    - Advanced cancer except above conditions
    - Advanced dementia
- Quality of life
  - Benefit
    - True hunger and thirst: eg proximal GI cancer
  - No benefit
    - Active dying
    - Dry mouth

Hunger in terminal illnesses (McCann 1994)

- 64% did not experience hunger
- 34% experienced hunger only initially
- 3% experienced hunger throughout their stay
- When hunger was reported, it was ameliorated by providing small amounts of food

Tube feeding and harm

- Denied pleasure of eating if kept nil by mouth (NBM)
- Distress of NG tube insertion
- Nasopharyngeal discomfort
- Nausea and vomiting
- Delirium
- Restraint
- Aspiration
- Complications of PEG/PEJ

Weissman's triad of a dying patient in the hospital

- Triad: feeding tube, restraints and pulse oximetry
- Death spiral
    - Hospital admission
    - Poor oral intake
    - Swallowing evaluation
    - Feeding tube placement
    - Increased agitation
    - Self-removal of feeding tube
    - Restraint
    - Re-insertion of feeding tube
    - Aspiration pneumonia
    - Intravenous antibiotics and pulse oximetry
    - Few cycles of release-remove-restraint-reinsert
    - Death

Recognition of dying

- Poor or no oral intake in the setting of a chronic life-limiting illness and declining function: marker of the dying process

Golden rule of eating at the end of life

- Let the patient be the lead
    - When to eat
    - What to eat
    - What amount to eat

Artificial hydration

- Benefit
    - Delirium
    - Opioid toxicity, esp in renal failure
- No benefit
    - Thirst
- Harm
    - ↑ respiratory tract secretions
    - ↑ ascites
    - ↑ oedema
    - Inhibits mobility further
    - Impedes family involvement
    - Medicalization of death

Treatment of thirst or dry mouth at the end of life

- Regular mouth care
- Small amounts of fluids
- Ice chips
- Small pineapple chunks
- Artificial saliva
- Moisturizing mouth gel

Natural dehydration

- Benefit
    - ↓ cerebral oedema: more lucid
    - ↓ respiratory secretions: less cough, choking, rattles
    - ↓ GI secretions: less vomiting
    - ↓ peritumoural oedema: less pain
    - ↑ endorphins: less pain

Summary of hydration and nutrition at the end of life

- Conventional nutritional care
    - Earlier stages of illness
    - Allows patient to cope with illness and treatment
- Palliative nutritional care
    - Later stages of illness
    - Focuses on symptom control and quality of life
    - Supplementation as appropriate
    - Relaxes dietary restriction
    - Emotional support
    - Family support

Communication

- Family: He is not eating. He is getting weaker.
- Staff: You are right. It is common for patients to eat less and less as the disease progresses. Someday they eat a little; someday they eat a bit more. But overall their interest in food will gradually decline. They may even reach a stage of eating nothing. It can be difficult for family to see them eating so little.
- Family: He is going to starve to death.
- Staff: We need to continue offering him small amounts of food as he wishes. Most of the time the sensation of hunger will gradually disappear when the disease progresses.

- Family: What can we do to help him?
- Staff: At this stage, it is common for family to encourage them to eat more. Some even force them to eat, resulting in a so-called "food battle". Patient may then suffer more or vomit. The best thing you can do for him is to let him be the lead. Let him choose when to eat, what to eat and what amount to eat. You can offer him his favourite food but do not pressurize him too much.

Withholding and Withdrawal of Life-Sustaining Treatment

Introduction

Withholding and withdrawal of life-sustaining treatment are medical procedures. All healthcare staff should be equipped with the knowledge and skills in the practice of withholding and withdrawal of medical treatment.

Clinical situations (mostly in ICUs)

- Refusal of treatment
  - Patient has a right to refuse treatment provided:
    - Patient has intact decision-making capacity
    - Patient is fully informed of the risks and benefits of the treatment, and the consequences of refusing it
- Medical futility
  - Medical futility refers to medical treatment which is extremely unlikely to benefit patients
    - Quantitative futility: the likelihood of a medical treatment to benefit patient is extremely unlikely
    - Qualitative futility: the quality of the benefit produced by a medical treatment is extremely poor

Decisional capacity assessment (Appelbaum & Grisso 1988)

- The ability to EXPRESS a choice
- The ability to UNDERSTAND the relevant information
- The ability to APPRECIATE a situation and its consequences
- The ability to REASON rationally

Diagnosing medical futility

- Quantitative definition
  - Physicians conclude that in the last 100 cases a medical treatment has been useless (Schneiderman 1990, 1996)
    - Through personal experiences
    - Through experiences shared with colleagues
    - Through consideration of reported empirical data
  - Objective outcome predictions in ICU
    - Multiple Organ Dysfunction Score
    - MOD >20 = 100% mortality
      - PaO_2/FiO_2 ratio
        - <300 (1 point)
        - <225 (2 points)
        - <150 (3 points)
        - <75 (4 points)
      - Platelet count
        - <120 (1 point)
        - <80 (2 points)
        - <50 (3 points)
        - <20 (4 points)
      - Serum bilirubin
        - >20 (1 point)
        - >60 (2 points)
        - >120 (3 points)
        - >240 (4 points)
      - Pressure adjusted heart rate (HR x CVP/MAP)
        - >10 (1 point)
        - >15 (2 points)
        - >20 (3 points)
        - >30 (4 points)

- Glasgow Coma Scale
  - <15 (1 point)
  - <13 (2 points)
  - <10 (3 points)
  - <7 (4 points)
- Serum creatinine
  - >100 (1 point)
  - >200 (2 points)
  - >350 (3 points)
  - >500 (4 points)
- Qualitative definition (Schneiderman 2011)
  - The unacceptable likelihood of achieving an effect that the patient has the capacity to appreciate as a benefit
  - None of the effects is a benefit unless the patient has at the very least the capacity to appreciate it, a circumstance that is impossible if the patient is permanently unconscious

Principles of withholding and withdrawal of treatment

- The intention is to remove useless treatment
- The intention is not to hasten death
- Even though hastening of death can be foreseen
- The intention to hasten death is ethically impermissible
- The intention to hasten death is legally impermissible
- Withholding and withdrawal of treatment are ethically similar
- If withholding of treatment is justified, withdrawal is justified
- Withdrawal of treatment is a medical procedure
- Any medical treatment can be withdrawn
- Basic care cannot be withdrawn

The decision-making hierarchy

- Fully informed patient with intact decisional capacity
- Legally appointed surrogate decision maker
- Advance decision to refuse treatment (ADRT)
- Substituted judgment from close family members
    - Patient's previous statement of wishes and preferences
    - Patient's possible wishes and preferences based on values and beliefs if patient is presumed to understand current condition and prognosis
- Best interest of patient
    - Represented by close family members with careful weighing of the risk-benefit explained by the physician
    - Represented by physician if family is unable to represent patient's best interest

The decision-making process

- The first step is to arrive at the decision. If no clear consensus within the health care team, time should be taken to resolve disagreement. Ethical principles and outcome data should be applied rather than personal values and biases.
- If the decision has been made to withdraw treatment by the patient or the senior clinician responsible for the care of the patient, doctors or nurses who have a conscientious objection to the decision may withdraw from the care of patient, with the arrangement of a replacement to take over his or her role.
- Informed consent is needed before withdrawal of treatment. Physician is not obliged to provide futile intervention requested by family but effort should be made to reach an agreement.
- Useful ways include open and sensitive communication, exploration and sensitive handling of misunderstanding, and responding to emotions.

- If family insists on intervention after open communication, then the primary physician should make a decision whether to withdraw treatment, withhold further treatment or to allow a time-limited trial.

Communication with colleagues

- Before discussing with the patient or family, it is crucial for different teams to meet and discuss about patient's prognosis and plan. If there is any difference in opinion, a general consensus needs to be achieved.
- Sometimes it is not uncommon for a clinician to remain hopeful even in the most drastic situation. Giving time for the clinician to accept the situation may be the best solution if condition allows.
- On the other hand, clinician may give up hope early even though there may be a reasonable chance of recovery. Then we should communicate our opinion in a non-confrontational manner.

Communication with patient

- Most patients for withdrawal of treatment are semi-comatose or comatose. If patient is mentally sound, every effort needs to be made to discuss the situation with the patient. Sometimes this will require a long time, especially if the patient has difficulty in communication.

Communication with family members

- Find out the decision maker in the family. If decision making is shared within the family, then try to involve those who can represent the patient.

- Discussion of withdrawal of treatment needs a gentle explanation of patient's condition and prognosis. Discuss prognosis in a way that is meaningful to the family.
- Then, ask the family to focus on what the patient would want, not what the family wants.
- Explain the reasons of withdrawal of treatment. The treatment cannot reverse the disease process. Stopping it allows the disease to take it natural course. Comfort care and nursing care will be continued.
- Respond to family's emotion and thoughts. If family is in denial, allow time for them to sink in if possible.
- If family is ready, explain the steps of withdrawal and what will likely happen after the withdrawal. Explain agonal breathing and respiratory tract secretions and steps in palliation.
- Stress to family that withdrawal of treatment is a medical decision, not a family decision. This is to reduce any feeling of guilt for making this difficult decision.
- Mention organ donation if appropriate.

Little information

Although hastening of death can be foreseen in withdrawal of life-sustaining treatment. The intention to hasten death is wrong. Caution needs to be taken to avoid misunderstanding.

- Allow time for reaching a consensus
- Allow time-limited trial for the lack of consensus
- Consider compassionate continuation of futile treatment for family's non-acceptance if appropriate
- Administer drugs just enough to make patient comfortable
- Continue palliative care if patient survives the withdrawal

Checklist for ventilation withdrawal

- The multidisciplinary team has agreed to withdraw ventilation, and one or more of the following may apply
  - Continuing ventilation has a very small chance of benefiting patient
    - Patient is dying
    - Patient has progressive irreversible multi-organ failure despite intensive treatment
    - Patient is diagnosed to have brainstem death or impending brainstem death
  - Continuing ventilation produces an exceedingly poor quality of benefit
    - Patient is in a coma, persistent vegetative state or minimally conscious state
    - Patient has advanced metastatic cancer with poor prognosis
  - Advance decision of refusal of ventilation or presumed refusal of ventilation
    - Patient has legal document in ADRT
    - Patient has appointed a legal surrogate decision maker for refusal of consent
    - Presumed refusal of ventilation based on substituted judgment from the family, complemented by adequate value history of patient
- Consensus on withdrawal of ventilation has been achieved from ALL of the following
  - The multidisciplinary team
  - Patient (if intact decisional capacity)
  - Family members

- Information on ventilation withdrawal has been communicated
    - Family is aware that decision of ventilation withdrawal is a medical decision
    - Family is aware that ventilation cannot reverse the underlying disease process
    - Family is aware that ventilation withdrawal allows the natural course of the disease to take place
    - Family is aware that ventilation withdrawal is not euthanasia, but the removal of useless treatment
    - Family is aware that palliative care will be continued to ensure patient's comfort
    - Family is aware of the procedures after death
- Discussion of organ or body donation if appropriate
- Family preferences have been elicited in terms of the following
    - Family presence during ventilation withdrawal
    - Time of ventilation withdrawal
    - Place of ventilation withdrawal: hospital or home
    - Religious practices and rituals before, during and after
- Documentation of decision making process and communication has been done
    - Indication of ventilation withdrawal
    - Consensus on ventilation withdrawal
    - Communication on ventilation withdrawal
    - Family preferences
    - Do not resuscitate (DNR) order
- Facilitation of practices that support family grief
    - Ensure privacy if possible
    - Liberalize visitation
    - Ensure access to patient by lowering the side rails
    - Allow family to perform last rites or rituals
    - Allow family to grief
    - Encourage family to speak to patient

- Procedures of ventilation withdrawal
  - Discontinue unnecessary monitoring and treatment, such as cardiac monitoring, inotropes, feeding tubes
  - Initiate or maintain opioid and sedative infusion
    - Ensure patency of intravenous line by flushing
    - Initiate opioid infusion: IV Morphine 2.5-5mg/h
    - Initiate sedative infusion: IV Midazolam 2.5-5mg/h
  - Ensure adequate analgesia and sedation
    - Assess pain with FLACC scale
    - Aim pain score 0 with IV Morphine 2.5-5mg prn
    - Assess sedation with Riker Sedation-Agitation Scale
    - Aim sedation scale 1 with IV Midazolam 2.5-5mg prn
      - Riker Sedation-Agitation Scale
        - 7 = dangerous agitation
        - 6 = very agitated
        - 5 = agitated
        - 4 = calm and cooperative
        - 3 = sedated
        - 2 = very sedated
        - 1 = unarousable
    - Ensure adequate time for patient to has sufficient motor activity for pain and sedation assessment after stopping any paralytic drug
  - Sequential reduction of ventilation settings
    - Titrate FiO2 down to 21% and PEEP to 0 in 5min
    - Titrate PS down to 5 in 5-10min
    - Titrate IMV rate down to 5 in 5-10min
    - Give IV Morphine 5mg and IV Midazolam 5mg for any slightest sign of distress
    - Explain to family about potential secretions sounds
    - Extubate patient
    - Give IV Morphine 5mg and IV Midazolam 5mg prn

- Care after withdrawal of ventilation
  - IV Morphine 5mg prn/q15min for distress
  - IV Midazolam 5mg prn/q15min for distress
  - Reassure family if patient is comfortable
  - Allow family to stay with patient
- Document the steps of withdrawal in the medical notes

Do Not Resuscitate (DNR)

Introduction

Cardiopulmonary resuscitation (CPR) is a life-saving technique useful in many emergencies. But when death is inevitable, CPR negates the possibility of a peaceful death.

Do not resuscitate (DNR)

- Also called "no code"
- A legal order written either in the hospital or on a legal form to respect the wishes of a patient not to undergo CPR or ACLS if their heart were to stop or they were to stop breathing

History of CPR and DNR

- 1960: first introduction of CPR (Kouwenhoven 1960)
- 1970s: implementation of DNR policies in US (Fosbinder 1980)
- 1993: proposal of formal DNR guidelines (Doyal 1993)
- 1989: introduction of DNAR (Hadorn 1989)
- 2005: introduction of AND (Knox 2005)

Differences between DNR, DNAR and AND

- DNR
  - Do not resuscitate
  - Gives misimpression that the attempt is likely to succeed
  - Patients think they are deciding whether to live or die, even though they are in an end-of-life situation
- DNAR
  - Do not attempt resuscitation
  - Indicates a resuscitation attempt
  - Does not indicate that it is likely to succeed

- AND
    - Allow natural death
    - Affirms that patients want nature to take its course
    - Without CPR or ACLS

Variety of terms

- Do not attempt CPR (DNACPR): specific
- Do not intubate (DNI): specific
- Not for active resuscitation (NAR): non-specific
- Best supportive care (BSC): non-specific
- Maximal medical management (MMM): non-specific

CPR statistics

- Outcomes
    - Reversal of spontaneous circulation (ROSC)
    - Survival to discharge: more meaningful
- CPR success rate on television (Diem 1996)
    - Chicago Hope: 36% survival to discharge
    - ER: not applicable (events in emergency room only)
    - Rescue 911: 100% survival to discharge
    - CPR success rate on TV shows was over-optimistic
- National Registry of CPR (Peberdy 2003)
    - 14, 720 resuscitation attempts from 2000-2002
    - ROSC: 44%
    - Survival to discharge: 17%
- Meta-analysis of CPR outcomes (Ebell 1998)
    - 49 publications
    - 9,838 patients
    - ROSC: 41-44%
    - Survival to discharge: 13-15%

- CPR success rate in cancer patients (Reisfield 2006)
  - Meta-analysis of 42 studies
  - Localized cancer: 9.1% survival to discharge
  - Metastatic cancer: 7.8% survival to discharge
- CPR success rate in dialysis patients (Hijazi 2003)
  - 14% survival to discharge
  - 3% survival to 6 months
- CPR success rate in elderly (Kim 2000)
  - < 80 years: 19% survival to discharge
  - 81-90 years: 9% survival to discharge
  - > 90 years: 4% survival to discharge
- In-hospital CPR success rate of different countries
  - UK: 17% survival to discharge
  - Canada: 16% survival to discharge
  - US: 15% survival to discharge
  - Other European countries: 14% survival to discharge
  - Iran: 12%
  - Malaysia: 10% survival to discharge
- Factors which predict a failure to survive to discharge
  - Sepsis the day prior to the CPR event
  - Serum creatinine >130µmol/l
  - Metastatic cancer
  - Dementia
  - Dependent status
- CPR success rate with 0% success rate (O'Keefe 1991)
  - Metastatic cancer ECOG3-4
  - Pneumonia
  - Creatinine >150µmol/l
  - Shock
  - PaO2 <6kPa

DNR facts

- DNR = withholding CPR (+ ACLS + intubation)
- DNR ≠ withholding treatment of reversible causes
- DNR ≠ withholding of artificial hydration and nutrition
- DNR preferences ≠ other end-of-life preferences
- DNR ≠ agreeing to giving up hope
- DNR ≠ agreeing to abandonment
- DNR ≠ agreeing to termination of life

The problems in DNR discussion

- Too little and too late
  - 76% occurred when incapacitated (Bedell 1986)
  - 2-3 days before death (Baker 2003)
- Lack of information for informed consent (Tulsky 1995)
  - 4% residents discussed survival rate
  - Discussion length: 10min
  - Doctors: 8min talking
  - Patients: 2min talking
- Incorrect knowledge (Adams 2006)
  - Assumption of CPR survival rate >50% in 80%
- Depersonalized discussion (Deep 2008)
  - Should we try to restart your heart?
  - Should we shock you, press on your chest?
  - Should we not do anything?
  - Did not discuss values and goals
- Extrapolation of DNR to limit other treatments
  - Withholding blood products in 43%
  - Withholding antibiotics in 32%
  - Withholding diagnostic tests
  - Withholding other life-sustaining treatments

The reasons for the problems in DNR discussion (Yuen 2011)

- Technological-driven medical culture
- Inadequate hospital DNR policies
- Insufficient communication skills training
- Profit-driven

CPR Preferences (Murphy 1994)

- >60 years old and healthy
  - Before learning success rate: 41% wanted CPR
  - After learning success rate: 22% wanted CPR
- >60 years old with chronic illness with life expectancy < 1 year
  - Before learning success rate: 11% wanted CPR
  - After learning success rate: 5% wanted CPR

Decision-making

- Futile CPR
  - Doctors are not obliged to offer futile treatment
  - Sensitive communication is needed
- Not futile
  - Intact decisional capacity: patient can refuse
  - Impaired decisional capacity
    - Legally appointed surrogate decision maker
    - Advance decision to refuse treatment (ADRT)
    - Substituted judgment from the family
    - Best interest

DNR discussion

- DNR discussion is not necessary if
  - CPR is futile
  - Patient does not want to discuss
  - Patient may be excessively distressed by the discussion
  - Patient lacks capacity

- How to discuss DNR
    - Explore insight into illness and prognosis
    - Discuss values
        - Tell me a little about what is important to you now
        - What is your current view about your quality of life?
    - Discuss goals of care
        - What are your preferences in terms of treatment?
        - Explore priority
            - Survival
            - Function
            - Comfort
    - Discuss DNR
        - Futile CPR
            - Discuss end-of-life preferences sensitively
            - Explain futility of CPR if appropriate
            - Respond to emotions
        - Not futile
            - Discuss advance care planning
            - Explore CPR preferences if appropriate
            - Discuss CPR success rate
                - In-hospital: 15% (1 in 6)
                - Out-of-hospital: 5% (1 in 20)
                - Terminal illness: 0%

Palliative Sedation

Introduction

Palliative sedation is a final resort in the relief of refractory suffering. It is an important and necessary medical intervention in selected terminally ill patients with refractory suffering.

Definitions of palliative sedation

- Intentional administration of sedative drugs in dosages and combinations required to reduce the consciousness of a terminal patient as much as necessary to adequately relieve one or more refractory symptoms. (Broeckaert 2002)
- The use of sedative medications to relieve intolerable and refractory distress by the reduction in patient consciousness. (Morita 2002)
- The monitored use of medications intended to induce varying degree of unconsciousness, but not death, for relief of refractory and unendurable symptoms in imminently dying patients. (Hospice and Palliative Nurses Association 2003)
- The use of sedating medications to decrease a patient's level of consciousness to mitigate the experience of suffering, but not to hasten the end of life. (The American Academy of Hospice and Palliative Medicine 2003)
- The primary intention of deliberately inducing a temporary or permanent light-to-deep sleep, but not deliberately causing death, in patients with terminal illness and specific refractory symptoms. (Paul Rousseau 2004)
- The use of specific sedative medications to relieve intolerable suffering from refractory symptoms by a reduction in patient consciousness, using appropriate drugs carefully titrated to the cessation of symptoms. (De Graeff 2007)

- The monitored use of medications intended to induce a state of decreased or absent awareness (unconsciousness) in order to relieve the burden of otherwise intractable suffering in a manner that is ethically acceptable to the patient, family and health-care providers. (European Association of Palliative Care 2009)

Important points from the definitions

- Patient is imminently dying
- Patient has refractory symptoms or suffering not relieved by standard palliative care treatment
- The use of sedative medications is monitored
- The intention is to relieve refractory suffering by reducing consciousness, but not to cause death
- The level of sedation varies from light to deep
- The duration of sedation can be temporary or permanent
- The intervention should be done in an ethically acceptable manner, to patient, family and healthcare providers

Determining intractable or refractory suffering

- All possible treatments have failed, or it has been determined by team consensus, based on repeated and careful assessment by skilled experts, that there is no method for alleviation within the time frame and risk-benefit ratio that the patient can tolerate. (Cherny 1994, Morita 2002, Levy 2005)
- To determine the refractoriness of physical suffering, palliative care consultation is strongly recommended
- To determine the refractoriness of psychoexistential suffering, palliative care consultation is a MUST
- Determined on basis of patient evaluation if possible
- Determined by proxy judgments in collaboration with families and staff if patient evaluation is impossible

Adverse effects of palliative sedation

- Patients
    - Impairment or loss of ability to interact
    - Paradoxical agitation
    - Small risk of hastening of death
        - Respiratory depression
        - Aspiration
        - Hemodynamic compromise
    - Although there are data indicating that palliative sedation does not hasten the death of patients overall, a small risk of hastened death for individual patient exists
    - Prognosis hours to days
        - The risk may be judged to be trivial relative to the goal of relieving otherwise intolerable suffering
    - Longer prognosis
        - The risk of hastened death may have significant, or even catastrophic, consequences
        - Risk-reducing precautions may be indicated
            - Vital sign monitoring and antidotes availability
- Distress among family members or healthcare staff
    - Inability to interact with patient
    - Disagreement regarding the indication for sedation
    - Perception that decision to sedate is precipitous
    - Perception that decision to sedate is delayed
    - Perception that sedation hastens death

Problems of palliative sedation (EAPC 2009)

- Abuse of palliative sedation (illegal practices)
    - The deliberate use of deep sedation in patients without refractory symptoms
    - The deliberate use of high doses of sedation that far exceeds that which is necessary to provide comfort

- Injudicious use of palliative sedation
  - Reversible causes of distress are not being addressed
  - Palliative care experts are not being engaged
  - Decision of sedation affected by frustration in caring of a complex symptomatic patient
  - Sedation is requested by the family, not the patient
- Injudicious withholding of palliative sedation
  - To avoid difficult end-of-life discussion
  - Exaggerated concern of hastening death
- Substandard clinical practice of palliative sedation
  - Inadequate consultation with the patient, family members or staff to ensure understanding of the indication for the intervention, the goals of care, the anticipated outcomes and potential risks
  - Inadequate assessment of psychosocial-spiritual factors
  - Inadequate monitoring of symptom distress and relief
  - Inadequate monitoring of adverse effects
  - Inappropriately rapid dose escalation
  - Inadequate support to family and distressed staff

EAPC framework for palliative sedation 2009

- Pre-emptive discussion of the role of sedation in EOL care
  - Discuss goals of care
  - Discuss end-of-life care preferences
  - Discuss the use of sedation if clinically appropriate
    - In refractory symptoms
    - In catastrophic events: eg terminal bleeding
  - Document outcome of discussion
- Describe the indications of palliative sedation
  - Refractory physical symptoms
    - Agitated delirium
    - Breathlessness

- Pain
- Seizures
- Refractory psychoexistential suffering in rare cases
- Continuous deep sedation only if prognosis hours to days
- Transient or respite sedation may be indicated earlier
- Describe the necessary evaluation and consultation procedures
  - Multi-professional palliative care input
  - Medical evaluation for reversible causes of deterioration
  - Psychosocial-spiritual evaluation
  - Prognostic evaluation
  - Decisional capacity evaluation
  - Document the following:
    - Indication of sedation
    - Decision-making process
    - Aim of sedation
    - Planned depth and duration of sedation
- Specific consent requirement
  - Discuss condition and prognosis
  - Discuss rationale for sedation
  - Discuss aim of sedation
  - Discuss method of sedation
    - Sedative
    - Depth or planned sedation
    - Duration of planned sedation
  - Discuss anticipated outcomes
    - Reduced consciousness
    - Communication impairment
    - Effects on oral intake
  - Discuss potential uncommon risks
    - Paradoxical agitation
    - Delayed or inadequate relief
    - Small risk of hastening of death

- Discuss continuation of palliative and nursing care
- Discuss expected outcome without sedation
- Discuss commitment to the patient's well-being and provision of best possible care irrespective of patient treatment choices
- Involve family members in the discussion if possible
- Documentation of the discussion
- In the care of the terminally ill patients who have no advanced directive and no healthcare proxy and who are in severe distress whilst actively dying, provision of comfort measures (including, if necessary, the use of sedation) is the 'standard of care' and should be the default strategy for clinician treatment decisions
- Indicate the need to discuss the decision-making with family
  - Explain patient's condition and suffering
  - Explain the rationale and aim of sedation
  - Address differences in opinion
  - Support families to relieve them of factors that contribute to conflicts, such as grief and guilt
- Selection of sedation method
  - The level of sedation should be the lowest necessary to provide adequate relief of suffering
  - Mild intermittent sedation should be attempted first unless in emergency situations
  - Down-titration to re-establish lucidity after an agreed interval should be considered and discussed to re-evaluate patient's preferences regarding sedation and for pre-planned famly interactions, with the understanding of the possibility of failure to restore lucidity or the re-appearance of refractory symptoms before death
  - Deep sedation should be adopted when mild sedation is ineffective

- Deep continuous sedation should be selected first if
  - The suffering is intense
  - The suffering is definitely refractory
  - Death is anticipated within hours or a few days
  - The patient's wish is explicit
  - Terminal catastrophic events
    - Massive bleeding
    - Asphyxia
- Present direction for dose titration, monitoring and care
  - Q20min review till adequate sedation
  - Then TDS review
  - Monitor severity of suffering
  - Monitor level of sedation
  - Monitor adverse effects of sedation
    - Paradoxical agitation
    - Aspiration
  - Consider vital signs monitoring for longer prognosis
  - Continue nursing care
- Decision regarding hydration and nutrition and medications
  - The decision about artificial hydration and nutrition is independent of the decision about sedation
  - Comprehensive evaluation of of the patient's wishes and the estimated benefits-harms in palliation of suffering
  - Medications for palliation should be continued
- Care and information needs of family
- Care for healthcare professionals

Level of sedation (Claessens 2011)

- Mild intermittent sedation
  - Intermittent
  - Mild reduction in consciousness
  - Still reacts to stimuli

- Mild continuous sedation
  - Continuous
  - Mild reduction in consciousness
  - Still reacts to stimuli
- Deep intermittent sedation
  - Intermittent sedation to unconsciousness
    - Acute: to treat an acute refractory symptom
    - Non-acute: to treat a non-acute refractory symptom
- Deep continuous sedation
  - Continuous sedation to unconsciousness
    - Acute: to treat an acute refractory symptom
    - Non-acute: to treat a non-acute refractory symptom

Monitoring the severity of suffering

FLACC scale

Criteria	0	1	2
Face	Normal	Grimace	Clenched jaw
Legs	Normal	Restless	Kicking
Activity	Normal	Squirming	Arched
Cry	Normal	Moaning	Screaming
Consolability	Normal	Reassurable	Nonreassurable

Monitoring the level of sedation

- Riker Sedation-Agitation Scale
  - 7 = dangerous agitation
  - 6 = very agitated
  - 5 = agitated
  - 4 = calm and cooperative (easily arousable)
  - 3 = sedated (arousable with verbal stimuli)
  - 2 = very sedated (arousable with physical stimuli)
  - 1 = unarousable

Drugs used for palliative sedation

- Midazolam (IV/SC)
  - Starting dose: 0.5-1mg/h
  - Usual effective dose: 1-20mg/h
  - Boluses: 1-5mg prn/q1h
- Lorazepam (IV)
  - Starting dose: 4mg/h
  - Usual effective dose: 4-20mg/24h
  - Boluses: 0.5-2mg prn/q2h
- Flunitrazepam (IV/SC)
  - Starting dose: 0.2-0.5mg/h
  - Boluses: 1-2mg prn
- Levomepromazine (IV/SC)
  - Starting dose: 50-75mg/24h
  - Maximum dose: 300mg/24h
  - Boluses: 12.5-25mg prn/q1h
- Chlorpromazine (IV/IM/PR)
  - Starting dose
    - 12.5mg q4-12h (IV/IM)
    - 3-5mg/h (IV)
    - 25-100mg q4-12h (PR)
  - Usual effective dose
    - 12.5-50mg q8h (IV/IM)
    - 25-100mg q8h (PR)
- Phenobarbital (IV/IM/SC)
  - Starting dose: 600mg/24h (SC)
  - Usual effective dose: 600-1600mg/24h (SC)
  - Maximum dose: 2400mg/24h (SC)
  - Dilute 1ml phenobarbital with 10ml WFI
    - Phenobarbital 600mg with 30ml WFI
    - Phenobarbital 800mg with 40ml WFI
    - Phenobarbital 1200mg with 60ml WFI

- Phenobarbital 1600mg with 80ml WFI
  - Phenobarbital 2400mg with 120ml WFI
- Boluses
  - IM Phenobarbital 100-200mg undiluted prn/q4-8h
  - IV Phenobarbital 100-200mg with 10ml WFI in rate of 50mg/min prn/q4-8h
- Propofol (IV)
  - Starting dose: 0.5mg/kg/h via forearm vein
  - Increase 0.5mg/kg/h q5-10min till sedation
  - Usual dose 1-2mg/kg/h
  - Max dose 4mg/kg/h
  - Bolus: 1mg/kg/min for 2-5min prn

Palliative sedation for refractory psychoexistential suffering

- Problems
  - Difficult to establish true refractoriness
  - Severity of suffering may be dynamic and idiosyncratic
  - Standard approaches have low intrinsic morbidity
  - Presence of symptoms does not necessarily indicate a far advanced state of physiological deterioration
- Special guidelines
  - Reserved for patients with advanced terminal illness
  - Diagnosis of refractory symptoms
    - By clinicians skilled in psychological care who have established relationship with patient and family
    - Following a period of repeated assessment
    - Trials of routine approaches for anxiety, depression and existential distress
  - Multidisciplinary case conferences, including psychiatry, chaplaincy, ethics, nurses, family members
  - Initiated on a respite basis for 6-24h, then down-titration
  - Continuous sedation after repeated respite sedation trials

Physician-Assisted Suicide and Euthanasia

Introduction

Physician-assisted suicide and euthanasia are illegal practices in Malaysia. However, it is important to understand these practices to avoid confusion with withdrawal of life-sustaining treatment and palliative sedation.

Physician-assisted suicide (PAS)

- Physician-assisted suicide occurs when a physician provides the means, usually a prescription for a large dose of oral barbiturates, by which a patient can ingest by him or herself to end his or her life.
- The practice of PAS is legal in the following country:
    - Colombia
    - Luxembourg
    - Netherlands
    - Switzerland
    - United States (California, Oregon, Vermont, Washington)

Voluntary active euthanasia (VAE)

- Voluntary active euthanasia occurs when a physician administers lethal injections at a patient's request.
- The physician injects a combination of drugs, eg
    - Sodium thiopental to induce coma
    - Pancuronium to paralyze respiratory muscles
    - Potassium chloride to stop the heart
- The practice of VAE is legal in the following country:
    - Belgium
    - Colombia

- Luxembourg
- Netherlands

Intentionality

- In PAS and VAE, the intention of the physician is to relieve suffering by killing or hastening of death.
- In withdrawal of life-sustaining treatment, the intention of the physician is to remove futile treatment to allow natural death. Hastening of death can be foreseen, but not intended. In the unusual event where patient continues to survive, continued support is necessary.
- In palliative sedation, the intention of the physician is to relieve refractory suffering, but not hastening of death. Sedative is titrated to a level just enough to relieve suffering, but no further once suffering is relieved.

Ethics in Palliative Care

Introduction

In the palliative care setting, it is not uncommon for one to face ethical dilemma in decision-making. Therefore, it can be useful for us to know some of the major ethical theories which we can use to analyse a situation and to help us in the decision-making.

Deontological ethics (duty ethics)

- The morality of an action is judged based on the duties of the healthcare professionals
- Deon = duty in Greek
- The term deontology was coined by Charlie Dunbar Broad
- Deontology formulated by Immanuel Kant
- Immanuel Kant described:

Nothing in the world – indeed nothing beyond the world – can possibly be conceived which could be called good without qualification except a good will.

- Duties as identified by William David Ross
  - Duty of beneficence
  - Duty of non-maleficence
  - Duty of justice
  - Duty of self-improvement
  - Duty of reparation
  - Duty of gratitude
  - Duty of promise keeping
- Principlism is the main deontological approach
  - Four basic principles from Beauchamp and Childress
  - Foundation of current medical decision-making

The four principles or duties of biomedical ethics

Autonomy = respect patient autonomy

- Latin: *Voluntas aegroti suprema lex*
- Meaning: free will of the patient is the supreme law
- Secondary principles
    - Shared decision making
    - Informed consent
        - Information
        - Comprehension
        - Voluntariness
    - Informed refusal
    - Advance decision to refuse treatment (ADRT)
    - Truth-telling
    - Confidentiality

Non-maleficence = do no harm

- Latin: *Primum non nocere*
- Meaning: first, do no harm
- Secondary principles
    - Do not kill
    - Do not cause needless pain
    - Do not incapacitate others
- Negligence
    - The professional must have a duty to the patient
    - The professional must breach the duty
    - The patient must experience a harm
    - The harm must be caused by the breach of duty

Beneficence = do good

- Latin: *Salus aegroti suprema lex*
- Meaning: well-being of the patient is the supreme law

- Secondary principles
    - Do no harm
    - Prevent harm
    - Remove harm
    - Do good

Social justice = do justice

- Distributive justice
- Meaning: fair distribution of limited medical resources
- Secondary principles
    - Use medical factors to determine fair distribution
        - Likely benefit to the patient
            - Cure
            - Prolongation of survival
            - Improvement in quality of life
            - Improvement in function
        - Urgency of need
        - Duration of benefit
    - Do not use non-medical factors
        - Age
        - Gender
        - Race
        - Lifestyle
        - Social status or social worth
        - Contribution to society
        - First come first served basis
        - Random pick
- Caveats of deontology
    - Emphasis on rules and duties: inflexibility in applying the rules may do harm
    - Duties ≠ intention: one may not intend to do good, but may act merely out of the duty of doing good

Consequentialism

- The morality of an action is judged based on the consequences
- The term consequentialism was coined by Elizabeth Anscombe
- Utilitarianism is the main consequentialism approach
    - Founder: Jeremy Bentham
    - Expanded by John Stuart Mill
    - Utility = happiness, pleasure, satisfaction
    - Utilitarian calculus (felicific or hedonic calculus)
      = greatest happiness for the greatest number
    - The morality of an action is judged based on its usefulness in maximizing utility or minimizing negative utility among everyone
- The judged consequences
    - The positive and negative consequences of an action
    - The positive and negative consequences of other options
    - The consequences of such decision on patients, families, friends, healthcare professionals, health care institution and society
- Caveats of consequentialism
    - Emphasis on consequences and outcome
        - Character of the person can be bad
        - Intention of the person can be bad

Virtue ethics

- The morality of an action is judged based on the characters of healthcare professionals
- Emphasizes the character of the person performing the action
- Influence: Plato and Aristotle
- Eudaimonism is the main virtue ethics approach
    - Eudaimonia = happiness, well-being, human flourishing
    - Happiness is achieved through virtue
    - In order to act rightly, one should be a virtuous person

- Caveats of virtue ethics
  - Emphasis on the character of the moral agent
    - A kind person may still do harm to patients

Casuistry

- Casuistry = case-based reasoning
- Casus = case in Latin
- Relies on analysis of individual cases versus paradigm cases
- Useful especially when conflicting rules occur
- Caveats of casuistry
  - Emphasis on individual cases
  - Needs a paradigm case to compare

Doctrine of double effect (DDE)

- Origin: Summa Theologiae written 1265-1274
- Author: Thomas Aquinas
- To judge an action which is intended to achieve a good effect but with the potential of giving rise to an unintended bad effect
- The action must satisfy 4 conditions to be morally permissible
  - The nature-of-the-act condition: the action must be either morally good or indifferent
  - The means-end condition: the bad effect must not be the means by which one achieves the good effect
  - The right-intention condition: the intention must be the achieving of only the good effect, with the bad effect being only an unintended side effect
  - The proportionality condition: the bad effect must not be disproportionate to the good effect
- DDE in pain management of terminally ill patients
  - Irrelevant in most cases
  - Appropriate use of opioids does not hasten death in terminally ill patients (Fohr 1998)

- Use of high dose opioids in terminally ill patients does not hasten death (Morita 2001)
- Deaths during opioid titration are related to disease progression in most patients, not to the use of opioids (Manfredi 1998)
- DDE is not needed to justify the use of high dose opioids in pain management of terminally ill patients
- DDE in sedation of terminally ill patients
  - Irrelevant in most cases
  - Appropriate use of sedatives does not hasten death in terminally ill patients (Morita 2001)
  - Palliative sedation used to relieve refractory symptoms does not hasten death (Maltoni 2009)
  - DDE is not needed to justify the use of sedation in the palliative care setting
- DDE in special cases
  - In rare circumstances when very high doses of opioids or sedatives are needed in a rapidly escalating manner to relieve suffering in terminally ill patients, with the risk of hastening death foreseen but unintended, DDE may be invoked to justify its use

Psychosocial Care

Introduction

The relief of suffering in palliative care patients needs a combination of good symptom control and psychosocial care.

Definition of psychosocial care

- Care concerned with the psychological and emotional well-being of the patient and their family/carers, including issues of self-esteem, insight into and adaptation to the illness and its consequences, communication, social functioning and relationships. (The National Council for Hospice and Specialist Palliative Care Services 1997)

The 5 components of psychosocial care (Tan 2015)

Presence

- Definitions
    - A mode of being available or open in a situation with the wholeness of one's unique being, a gift of self which can only be given freely, invoked or evoked (Paterson 1976)
    - A mode of being available in a situation with the wholeness of one's unique individual being; a process resulting in exchange of authentic meaningful awareness, essence linking, and thus more being (Hines 1991)
    - The physical "being there" and the psychological "being with" a patient with the purpose of meeting the patient's healthcare needs (Gardner 1985)
    - The state achieved when one moves within oneself to an inner reference of stability of being in the moment (Dossey 1995)

- The first and foremost requisite for a therapeutic relationship
- Types of presence (Stiles 1997)
  - Physical presence
    - Being there
    - Body to body contact
    - Skills: seeing, examining, touching, hugging
    - Requisite: recognizing patient as a person, empathy
    - Barrier: rushing, excessively task-orientated
  - Psychological presence
    - Being with
    - Mind to mind contact
    - Skills: listening, communicating, caring, connecting
    - Requisite: attention, empathy
    - Barrier: lack of concern
  - Spiritual presence
    - Therapeutic presence, transcendent presence
    - Spirit to spirit contact
    - Whole being to whole being
    - Skills: meditating, at-one-ment, openness, loving,
    - Requisite: inner quietude, mindfulness
    - Barrier: cognitive and emotional reactivity

Listening

- A crucial component of communication skills
- Goal: to understand the thoughts and feelings of a person
- Active listening
  - Originated from person-centered therapy of Carl Rogers
  - 3 core concepts of person-centered therapy
    - Congruence
      - Relating to another genuinely
      - Not hiding behind a professional façade

- Unconditional positive regard
  - Accepting another as who he or she is
  - Listening without judgment
- Empathy
  - Communicating the desire to understand and appreciate another's perspective and feelings
- Techniques of active listening
  - Encourage expression of thoughts and feelings
    - Use open-ended questions
    - Use silence
    - Use facilitations such as nodding and fillers
    - Pay attention to speech and body language
  - Check for understanding
    - Clarifying
    - Repeating
    - Paraphrasing
    - Summarizing
    - Reflecting
  - Avoid reacting
    - Avoid interrupting
    - Avoid judging
    - Avoid explaining reactively
    - Avoid advising prematurely
    - Avoid blocking of expression

Empathy

- Etymology
  - Empatheia: in passion (Greek)
  - Einfühlung: into feelings (German) by Lipps in 1903
  - Empathy: coined by Edward B. Titchener in 1909 as a "translation" from Einfühlung

- Definitions
  - Empathy means entering the private perceptual world of the other and becoming thoroughly at home in it. It involves being sensitive, moment to moment, to the changing felt meanings which flow in this other person, to the fear or rage or tenderness or confusion or whatever, that he or she is experiencing. It means temporarily living in his or her life, moving about in it delicately without making judgment, sensing meanings of which he or she is scarcely aware... It includes communicating your sensing of his or her world as you look with fresh and unfrightened eyes at elements of which the individual is fearful. It means frequently checking with him or her as to the accuracy of your sensing, and being guided by the responses you receive... to be with another in this way means that for the time being you lay aside the views and values you hold for yourself in order to enter another world without prejudice. (Carl Rogers 1975)
  - The capacity to think and feel oneself into the inner life of another person (Kohut 1984)
  - The ability to understand another's situation, perspective and feelings (Coulehan 2000)
- Types of empathy
  - Emotional empathy: the capacity to respond with an appropriate emotion to another's mental states
  - Cognitive empathy: the capacity to understand another's perspective or mental state
- Stages of empathy
  - Empathic understanding
    - Perceptions
    - Emotions
    - Cognition: beliefs, concerns, hope and meaning

370

- Communicated empathy
  - Acknowledgment
  - Validation
  - Normalization
- Perception of empathy from patients and families
- Exquisite empathy
  - A highly present, intimate, and heartfelt interpersonal connection in the therapeutic relationship with clients, without fusing or losing sight of the clinician's own perspective (Harrison 2009)
- Sympathy, pity and emotional contagion
  - Pity and sympathy: feeling sorry
  - Emotional contagion: the tendency to automatically mimic and synchronize expressions, vocalizations, postures, and movements with those of another person's and, consequently, to converge emotionally

Compassion

- Definitions
  - The sincere wish to alleviate the suffering of another. The desire to alleviate another's pain includes not only their present experience of discomfort but also the cause of their suffering, the underlying reasons they are not well. (Nyima 2006)
  - The feeling that arises when witnessing another's suffering and that motivates a subsequent desire to help (Goetz 2010)
- Types of compassion (Nyima 2006)
  - Conceptual compassion
    - Arises from concepts
    - Deliberate
    - Requires conscious effort

- Unstable
- Selective
- Situational
- Goal-orientated
- Fatigable
- Non-conceptual compassion
  - Arises from a concept-free state of mind
  - Natural
  - Effortless
  - Stable
  - Non-selective: embraces everyone without prejudice
  - Non-situational
  - Process-orientated
  - Non-fatigable
- Developing a compassionate attitude (Nyima 2006)
  - On waking up, make the first thought a noble one – a very sincere and strong thought of doing good
  - Remind ourselves of that noble thought every so often throughout the day
  - Before falling asleep, make the final thought a noble one
- Steps to becoming more compassionate (Nyima 2006)
  - Reduce negative habits: judgment of others
  - Increase positive habits: being kind and helpful to others
  - Free oneself from clinging to concepts

Boundary awareness

- The mutually understood, unspoken, physical, and emotional limits of the relationship between the trusting patient and the caring physician or provider (Farber 1997)
- Examples of potential boundary issues
  - Receiving gifts from patients
  - Giving out phone number to patients

- Socializing with patients outside of the clinical setting
- Revealing excessive personal information to patients
- Examples of definite boundary issues
  - Accepting money from a patient or family member
  - Attending to patient to fulfil a personal need
  - Attempting a deathbed conversion
  - Giving in to request for futile treatment
  - Giving in to request for hastening of death
- Although sometimes crossing boundaries can enhance patient care, boundary awareness is essential to avoid boundary issues that are harmful to the therapeutic relationship and boundary violation

Communication

Introduction

Communication is an indispensable component of psychosocial care. To communicate effectively, first, make a connection.

Making a connection (Dalai Lama & Howard Cutler 2009)

- Contemplating our basic human nature
  - Recognize that every person is basically a social person
  - Cultivate a deep appreciation of this basic human nature, which is to connect with each other and to cooperate together in improving the situations
- Contemplating our interconnectedness
  - Reflect on how human beings depend on each other for survival in the society
  - Reflect on how our welfare is closely connected to the welfare of others
- Contemplating our common humanity
  - Reflect on the fact that human beings share the same basic wish to be happy and free from suffering
  - Cultivate an empathic attitude towards others
  - Connect with others on a human-to-human level, based on our common humanity, our basic wish
- Connecting with others
  - Interact exactly the same with every person
  - Exhibit the same level of interest and warmth
  - Give every person the same level of full attention
  - Speak with every person as if they are the most important person in the world at that moment, as if they are the only person

The three crucial components of communication

- Non-verbal communication
  - Body language (kinesics)
    - Microkinesics
      - Oculesics: study of eye behaviour
      - Facial kinesics: study of facial expressions
    - Macrokinesics
      - Appearance
      - Artifacts
      - Postures
      - Gestures
      - Body movement
  - Paralanguage: study of non-lexical component of speech
  - Haptics: study of touch
  - Proxemics: study of space and distance
  - Chronemics: study of time
- Listening
  - Language
  - Paralanguage
- Empathy
  - Diagnostic empathy
  - Therapeutic empathy

Comparison of verbal and non-verbal communication

Verbal communication	Non-verbal communication
- $\approx 35\%$	- $\approx 65\%$
- By words	- By cues
- Conveys information	- Conveys feeling
- Intermittent	- Continuous
- Unichanneled	- Multichanneled
- May not be reliable	- More reliable

Non-verbal communication

Emotional recognition from oculesics (Straker 2008)

- Anger: eyes wide open and staring
- Disgust: eyes turned away rapidly
- Fear: eyes wide or looking downward, or closed
- Anxiety: eyes wet, blinking more
- Sadness: eyes looking downward, possibly wet with tears
- Happiness: eyes sparkling

Signs of crying

First sign: a sudden pause in communication
Second sign: eyes shiny
Third sign: tears lining lower eyelids (silver line sign)
Fourth sign: tears filling medial canthus
Fifth sign: tears falling

Emotional recognition from facial expressions (Paul Ekman 2003)

- Anger
  - Lowered and drawn-together brows
  - Raised upper eyelids: the glare
  - Tightened upper and lower eyelids
  - Pressed lips or open in square or rectangular shape
  - Red margin of lips becomes narrower
  - Lips become thinner
  - Clenched jaw
  - Jaw thrust forward
  - Exposed teeth

- Disgust and contempt
  - Lowered brows
  - Pushed up lower eyelids
  - Crow's-feet wrinkles
  - Raised cheeks
  - Deepened nasolabial folds: inverted U
  - Nose wrinkling
  - Raised upper and lower lips
  - Slightly protruding lower lips
  - Asymmetry: contempt
- Surprise and fear
  - Raised and drawn together eyebrows
  - Raised upper eyelids
  - Tensed lower eyelids: fear
  - Horizontally stretched lips toward ears: fear
  - Jaw dropped down: surprise
  - Pulled back chin
- Sadness
  - Angling upward of the inner corners of the eyebrows (triangulation of inner brows): the sad brows
  - Vertical wrinkle between the brows
  - Drooping of upper eyelids
  - Tensing of lower eyelids
  - Downward gaze
  - Raised cheeks, sometimes causing a false grin
  - Horizontal stretching of lips
  - Pushing up of lower lips
  - Pulling down of lip corners
  - Opening of mouth
  - Chin pouting

- Happiness
    - Raised lip corners: smile
    - Raised cheeks
- Accuracy of facial emotional recognition
    - Happiness 100%
    - Sadness 80%
    - Anger 80%
    - Fear 80%
    - Disgust 80%

Emotional recognition from bodily expression (Darwin 1965)

- Anger
    - Head erect
    - Shoulders squared
    - Arms rigidly suspended by the sides
    - Elbows squared
    - Fist clenched and shaking
    - Intends to push or strike
    - Purposeless or frantic gestures
    - Chest well expanded
    - Whole body trembles
    - Feet planted firmly on the grounded
    - Pacing up and down
- Disgust and contempt
    - Spitting
    - Shoulders raised as when horror is experienced
    - Arms pressed close to the sides
    - Gestures as if to push away or to guard oneself
    - Turning away of the whole body: contempt
    - Snapping one's fingers: contempt

- Fear
  - Head sinks between shoulders
  - Shoulders raised
  - Arms bent and pressed closely against sides or chest
  - Arms thrown wildly over the head
  - Arms violently protruded as if to push away
  - Hands clenched and opened alternately with twitching
  - Whole body often turned away or shrinks
  - Motionless or crouches down
- Sadness
  - Head hangs on contracted chest
  - Motionless
  - Passive
- Shame
  - Turning away the whole body
  - Face averted, bent down
  - Ackward
  - Nervous movement
- Joy
  - Head upright
  - Head nods to and fro while laughing
  - Various purposeless movement
  - Clapping of hands
  - Body held erect
  - Whole body is thrown backward and shakes or almost convulsed during excessive laughter
  - Stamping
  - Jumping
  - Dancing for joy
- Pride
  - Head and body held erect

Listening

- Language
    - Expression of physical complaints
    - Expression of thoughts
        - Ideas
        - Concerns
        - Hope and expectation
    - Expression of emotions
    - Expression of relationships and social interactions
    - Expression of spirituality
- Paralanguage (paralinguistics)
    - Non-verbal elements of speech
    - Not related to content or verbal message
    - Pitch: the degree of highness or lowness of a tone
    - Rate: the speed of speaking
    - Volume: the loudness of a voice
    - Prosody: the rhythm, stress and intonation of a speech
        - Rhythm: the flow of speech produced from the variation of pitch, rate and volume
        - Stress: making a syllable prominent
        - Intonation: pitch variation not to distinguish words
        - Inflection: pitch variation to distinguish words
        - Pause: a break while speaking
    - Articulation: the act of speaking clearly
    - Pronunciation: the act of speaking a word correctly
    - Quality: the unique vocal characteristics of every person
    - Tone of voice: the feelings added while speaking
    - Paralinguistic respirations
        - Gasp: sudden sharp inhalation through mouth
        - Sigh: deep, audible exhalation through mouth/nose
    - Side sounds
        - Laughter, cry, scream, cough

Speech emotional recognition: (Juslin & Laukka 2003)

- Anger: higher mean pitch, higher pitch variation, upward pitch inflection, faster voice onsets, faster speech rate, higher volume, higher volume variation, more high frequency spectral energy, higher first formant, higher precision of articulation, less pauses
- Disgust: lower mean pitch, downward pitch inflection, faster voice onsets, more high frequency spectral energy, higher first formant
- Fear: higher mean pitch, lower pitch variation, upward pitch inflection, faster speech rate, higher volume, higher volume variation, lesser high frequency spectral energy than anger, lower first formant, variable precision of articulation, less pauses
- Anxiety: higher mean pitch, lower pitch variation, lesser high frequency spectral energy than anger
- Sadness: lower mean pitch, lower pitch variation, downward pitch inflection, slower speech rate, lower volume, lower volume variation, longer voicing duration, least high frequency spectral energy, lower first formant, lower precision of articulation, more pauses
- Happiness: higher mean pitch, higher pitch variation, upward pitch inflection, faster speech rate, higher volume, higher volume variation, more high frequency spectral energy, higher precision of articulation, less pauses
- Accuracy of speech emotional recognition (Scherer 1991)
  - Sadness   72%
  - Anger   68%
  - Joy   59%
  - Fear   52%
  - Disgust   28%

Empathy

- Diagnostic empathy
    - A state of being conscious or aware of another person's feeling or perspective through observing the person and the body language, listening to the voice and experiences, and imagining oneself in his or her position
- Therapeutic empathy
    - A caring response to another's mental state, verbally or non-verbally, that causes the person to feel better

Therapeutic non-verbal empathy

- Oculesics
    - Maintain good eye contact
    - Maintain a kind look
    - Sit down at same eye level
- Facial kinesics
    - Face the person
    - Smile if appropriate
- Body kinesics
    - Kind first impression
    - Open posture: no crossed arms or legs
    - Leaning forward to show genuine interest
    - Mirror the body language during rapport building
    - Minimize unintentional body movements or gestures
- Paralanguage
    - Speak with a gentle voice
    - Articulate clearly to show confidence
    - Match the vocal cues of the person
    - Follow their pitch, volume, rate and rhythm if appropriate
    - Adjust your pitch, volume, rate and rhythm if appropriate
        - Higher pitch, higher volume, faster rate: motivating
        - Lower pitch, lower volume, slower rate: calming

- Haptics
  - Be aware of cultural or gender sensitivity to touch
  - Touch shoulder or elbow if appropriate
- Proxemics
  - Be aware of a comfortable distance
  - Be aware of arrangement of sitting position
  - No barrier: medical notes, side rails
- Chronemics
  - Proper communication of appointment time
  - Punctuality
  - Avoid rushing
  - State time limitation politely if time is a constraint

Smile in palliative care

- Smile is a very important facial expression
- Smile releases the following "feel good" neurotransmitters:
  - Endorphins
  - Serotonin
  - Dopamine
- Smile is contagious
- Smile lifts our mood as well as the mood of those around us
- A calm and genuine smile is appropriate in most situations
- A barely noticeable, calm and genuine smile can be appropriate even in the setting of angry or sad atmosphere

12 Muscles of smiling	11 Muscles of frowning
• Orbicularis oculi (2)	• Corrugator supercilii (2)
• Zygomaticus major (2)	• Orbicularis oculi (2)
• Zygomaticus minor (2)	• Procerus (1)
• Levator labii superioris (2)	• Orbicularis oris (1)
• Levator anguli oris (2)	• Depressor anguli oris (2)
• Risorius (2)	• Mentalis (1)
	• Platysma (2)

Types of smile

- True smile (Duchenne smile)
    - Involves eyes and lips
    - Orbicularis oculi muscles narrow eyes
    - Zygomatic major muscles raise lip corners
    - Timing matches with stimulus
    - Slow onset
    - Short apex duration, usually <5s
    - Smooth offset
    - Symmetrical
- Social smile (fake smile, botox smile, Pan American smile)
    - Involves lips only
    - Zygomatic major muscles raise lip corners
    - Timing too early or too late compared to stimulus
    - Abrupt onset
    - Long apex duration
    - Abrupt offset
    - Slightly asymmetrical

Therapeutic verbal empathy

- The key expression of empathy is to "ALLOW"
- Allow patients or family to talk about their experiences
- Allow patients or family members to express their thoughts
- Allow patients or family to express their emotions
- The primary obstacle of expressing empathy is to "BLOCK"
- Do not block the expression of thoughts and emotions:
    - Interrupting the conversation
    - Deviating away from the topic
    - Giving explanation prematurely
    - Giving advice prematurely
    - Focusing on the biomedical aspect of the person
    - Giving tissues as a signal for patient to stop crying

- Express empathy verbally once the catharsis is complete:
  - Acknowledging the emotion: talk about the emotion
  - Validating the emotion: tell patient it is ok or normal
  - Normalizing the emotion: tell patient you or others would feel the same too given the same situation

---

Little experience

Once I was standing at the bedside of a breast cancer patient. She was accompanied by her family on the other side of the bed. Her pain had been well controlled. I asked her, "Is there anything else you would like me to do for you?" She said, "Can you give me a hug?" I was completely unprepared and her family hugged her instead. The next day she passed away. I felt sorry about that. Then I started to accept hugging from patients and families. I was quite stiff in the beginning but now I have improved a lot. Hugging is often a sign of gratitude in palliative care. So next time if your patient wants to hug you, go for it and hug him or her with all your body, heart and spirit.

Breaking Bad News

Introduction

Breaking bad news, done poorly, can cause devastating effects on patients, family members as well as health care providers. There is no one simple way to break bad news. The aim of this chapter is to provide a short introduction to what is bad news and describe how to apply the SPIKES strategy in delivering bad news.

Definition (Buckman 1984)

- Bad news can be defined as any information that seriously and adversely changes a person's view of his future

Cleopatra's syndrome

- The bearer of the bad news is blamed for the bad news itself

  No one loves the messenger who brings bad news. Sophocles

SPIKES (Walter 2000)

- S = Setting
  - Set up the interview
  - Get all the facts ready before the discussion
  - Switch your handphone to silent or vibration mode
  - Arrange for a quiet room if possible
  - Sit down with the patient or family
- P = Perception
  - Assess patient's perception
  - Find out what is known or suspected
  - Examples
    - How much do you know about your situation?
    - What have you been told by the other doctors?

- What do you think is going on?
- Have you been suspecting anything serious?
- I = Invitation
  - Obtain permission to share the information
  - Examples
    - Would you like me to tell you about your results?
    - How much would you like to know?
    - Are you the kind of person who would like to know everything in details?
- K = Knowledge
  - Consider giving a warning shot
  - Example: I am afraid the news is not good
  - Give information following patient's pace
  - Give information in small pieces
  - Avoid medical jargons
  - Be honest but sensitive
  - Be mindful of emotional cues
- E = Emotions
  - Address patient's emotions with empathy
    - Pick up emotional cues
    - Allow patient to express emotion
    - Be comfortable with silence
    - Do not block emotional expression
      - Continuing to talk about medical facts
      - Diverting from the conversation
      - Asking patient to stop crying
      - Explaining away patient's anger
  - Acknowledge the emotion
  - Validate the emotion
  - Normalize the emotion
  - Imagine yourself in the situation and see whether you can find out what patient wants you to say or do

- Never say "there is nothing more can be done"
- Never say "there is no more hope"
- S = Strategy
    - Summarize the discussion when patient is ready
    - Give a plan when patient is ready
    - Give hope: refer to the "Hope" chapter

Little opinion

Strictly speaking, all news is neutral in its own sense. There is no such thing as bad news. It is the perception of the patient that makes it good or bad. This is why some patients are hardly affected by the so-called "bad" news but some can be devastated by it. So, as physicians, we have to be mindful of our own perception too.

Communicating Prognosis

Introduction

Foreseeing is the science of formulating a prognosis. Foretelling is the art of communicating it. Majority of patients want to know about their prognosis, but how we communicate it to them may affect how they live the rest of their lives.

Doctor, how much time do I have?

- Be mindful of what you are going to say when you hear this
- This is a common question in palliative care
- Great sensitivity is needed in answering it
- How we answer may give a long-lasting impact on patients

What is the reason patient asks this question?

- Find out the reason behind the question
- Is there anything that the patient wants to do?
- Is patient expecting some important event?
- Knowing this can help us a lot

Does the patient have the answer?

- Find out how much time does the patient think he or she has
- Patient may have been told about their prognosis by others
- Patient may know deep inside how much time is left

How long does the patient want to live?

- It is prudent to find out patient's expectation
- This gives us a clue how ready they are to know their prognosis
- This can help us on how to answer

Is it appropriate to answer without answering?

- For some patients, they are aware of their prognosis
- We may not need to answer their question about prognosis

Is it appropriate to answer without giving the prognosis?

- For some patients, they don't really want to know if it is short
- We may say doctors do not know the actual prognosis

Is it appropriate to answer without giving the duration?

- For some patients, they are asking because they want to know whether they have enough time to complete certain unfinished business or celebrate certain important event
- If it is a yes, we may tell them the likehood of being able to do it or celebrate the event
- If it is a no, think of what the patient wants us to say when the likelihood is low

Is it appropriate to answer without giving the time range?

- For some patients, they just want to know whether it is short
- If it is long, we can tell them that they still have time
- We can tell them that time is running short only when they are completely bed-ridden and no longer conscious
- If it is short, we may tell them: I am afraid time could be short

Is it appropriate to answer based on functional decline?

- If one is getting weaker and weaker every month, then the time could be in months
- If one is getting weaker and weaker every weeks, then the time could be in weeks
- If one is getting weaker and weaker every days, then the time could be in days

Is it appropriate to give the estimated time range?

- If nothing happens suddenly, the time could be:
  - Months to years
  - Weeks to months
  - Days to weeks
  - Hours to days

Is it appropriate to give an exact number?

- No
- Do not give exact number
  - You have 3 months to live
  - You have 2 weeks to live
- These are death sentences
- Don't be a judge; be a doctor

What is next after communicating prognosis?

- Communicate empathy: refer to the "Communication" chapter
- Communicate hope: refer to the "Hope" chapter

End-of-life Discussion

Introduction

End-of-life discussion is one of the most important conversations in the care of the dying. A skilled physician can help patients to slowly come to terms to what is happening so that they can make the most out of their remaining time.

Insight and acceptance

- Assess patient's insight into his or her illness and prognosis
- Assess patient's acceptance towards illness and prognosis

Goals of care

- Assess patient's goals of care
  - Survival: to live as long as possible
  - Function: to live as independent as possible
  - Comfort: to live as comfortable as possible

Readiness

- Ready: discuss end of life and preferences
- Not ready: discuss advance care planning (ACP)
- Not ready to discuss ACP: give time

Preferred information

- Assess what patient wants to know
- Assess how much patient wants to know

Communicating information

- Communicate information according to patient's wish
- Communicate information according to patient's pace

- Illness
- Prognosis
- Realistic goals
- Disease trajectories
- Clinical features of dying if appropriate
- Potential medical problems during dying if appropriate

Hope and preferences

- Assess hope
  - Hope regarding their illness
  - Hope regarding their life
    - Things to complete
    - Things to do
    - Things to see
    - Things to say
      - Ask for forgiveness from someone
      - Express forgiveness to someone
      - Express love to someone
      - Express thank you to someone
      - Express farewell to someone
  - Hope after death if appropriate
  - Consider helping patients to fulfil their hope if possible
- Preferences
  - Place of care
  - Place of dying if appropriate
  - Ritual and ceremonies if appropriate

Suffering of Palliative Care Patients

Introduction

The importance of suffering has been highlighted in the 2002 WHO definition of palliative care: Palliative care is an approach that improves the quality of life of patients and their families facing the problem associated with life-threatening illness, through the prevention and relief of **_SUFFERING_** by means of early identification and impeccable assessment and treatment of pain and other problems, physical, psychosocial and spiritual.

Definitions of suffering

- A state of severe distress associated with actual or perceived threat to the intactness of a person (Eric Cassell 1982)
  - A simplified description of a person
    - A person cannot be reduced to their parts
    - A person has a past
    - A person has a family
    - A person has a cultural background
    - A person has roles
    - A person has a relationship with himself or herself
    - A person is a political being
    - A person does things
    - A person has an unconscious component
    - A person has regular behaviour
    - A person has a body
    - A person has a secret life
    - A person has a perceived future
    - A person has a transcendent dimension
- Suffering is experienced by person, not bodies (Cassell 1991)

- A perceived threat to the integrity of the self, helplessness in the face of the threat, and exhaustion of psychosocial and personal resources of coping (Chapman 1993)
- An aversive emotional experience characterized by the perception of personal distress that is generated by adverse factors that undermine the quality of life (Cherny 1994)
- An experience of distress and disharmony caused by loss or threatened loss of what we most cherish (Coulehan 2012)

The biopsychosocial-spiritual model of suffering

- Based on the concept of total pain (Saunders 1983)
- Suffering has four dimensions
- Physical suffering, such as
  - Pain
  - Breathlessness
  - Nausea and vomiting
  - Constipation
- Psychological suffering, such as
  - Anxiety
  - Depression
  - Delirium
  - Insomnia
- Social suffering, such as
  - Loss of employment and income
  - Loss of social connections or roles
  - Concerns about family
  - Distress related to healthcare services
- Spiritual suffering, such as
  - Hopelessness
  - Meaninglessness
  - Fear of death
  - Why me?

The existential-experiential model of suffering (Tan 2014)

- Suffering is an unpleasant existential experience
- Suffering can be seen from two perspectives
    - Existential suffering: the view of suffering from the perspective of the events that make one suffer
    - Experiential suffering: the view of suffering from the perspective of the inner experiences of the person
- Existential suffering
    - Loss-related events
        - Loss and change
            - Loss of function
            - Loss of independence
            - Loss of freedom
            - Loss of sense of control
            - Loss of job and income
            - Loss of role
            - Loss of normality
            - Loss of quality of life
            - Loss of future
            - Loss of hope
            - Loss of confidence
            - Loss of fighting spirit
            - Anticipated loss
        - Dependence on others
            - Dependence on family
            - Dependence on friends
            - Dependence on healthcare providers
            - Perceived burdening of others
            - Perceived uselessness
            - Embarrassment of dependence
            - Loss of self-image due to dependence
            - Anticipated dependence

- Witnessing family suffering
  - Witnessing physical exhaustion of family
  - Witnessing emotional exhaustion
  - Witnessing helplessness
  - Witnessing family grief
  - Lack of self-concern in family
  - Concerns about family future
- Gain-related events
  - Facing terminal disease and death
    - Diagnosis of a terminal illness
    - Disease progression
    - Multiple recurrences
    - Multiple complications
    - Fear of dying
    - Fear of suffering
    - Fear of the unknown
    - Near-death experiences
    - Short estimated life span
    - Dying young
    - Unfinished business
  - Unpleasant healthcare encounter
    - Lack of full attention
    - Lack of immediate attention
    - Lack of listening
    - Lack of empathy
    - Lack of information
    - Different information from different teams
    - Poor communication
    - Hearing "nothing more can be done"
    - Perceived lack of competency
    - Lack of efficiency
    - Lack of coordination of different teams

- Unpleasant hospital stay
  - Hospital confinement
  - Mobility restriction from tubes and lines
  - Boredom in hospital
  - Loneliness in hospital
  - Noisy hospital environment
  - Unpalatable hospital food
  - Witnessing suffering of other patients
  - Witnessing death in the hospital
- Experiential suffering
  - Physical experience
    - Various physical symptoms
    - Impact of symptoms
      - Physical functions
      - Mental functions
      - Routines
      - Social activities
      - Employment
      - Sleep
      - Family
    - Sense of impending death due to intense symptoms
    - Desire to die due to refractory symptoms
  - Emotional experience
    - Shock
    - Surprise
    - Worry
    - Fear
    - Anger
    - Frustration
    - Boredom
    - Sadness
    - Loneliness

- Regret
- Cognitive experience
  - Hope-hopelessness spectrum
    - Hope for cure
    - Hope for survival
    - Hope for function
    - Hope for comfort
    - Hope for peace
    - Hope for sooner death
    - Hopelessness
  - Denial-acceptance spectrum
    - Complete denial
    - Partial acceptance
    - Choiceless acceptance
- Spiritual experience
  - Unanswered questions
    - Reason of having the disease
    - Reason of having to suffer
    - Reason of having to die
    - Contribution of past actions
    - Time of death
    - The unknown after death
  - Loss of faith
  - Religious doubts
  - Spiritual loneliness

Psychological processes of suffering (Tan 2016)

- Although patients have unique suffering experiences at their end of life, the psychological processes follow 5 set patterns
  - Perceptions: becoming aware of the sources of suffering through the senses

- Cognitive appraisals: interpretation of the sources of suffering
- Hope and the struggles with acceptance: the cognitive processes that occur when patients are relating with the sources of suffering
- Emotions: the subjective experiences of perceptions, cognitive appraisals, hope and acceptance that move patients to fight with or run away from the sources of suffering
- Clinging: the fixation on the suffering experiences and the difficulty to move forward

Perceptions (seeing, hearing, feeling, knowing)

- Experiencing loss of function
- Experiencing loss of ability to do things
- Experiencing loss of ability to walk far
- Experiencing loss of ability to go out
- Experiencing loss bit by bit
- Experiencing loss of confidence
- Experiencing loss of faith while in pain
- Experiencing loss of social engagement
- Experiencing dependence on others
- Experiencing pain
- Experiencing pain all of a sudden
- Experiencing pain all the time
- Experiencing pain everywhere
- Experiencing pain for the whole day
- Experiencing pain from injections
- Experiencing worst pain in life
- Experiencing sleeplessness
- Experiencing other symptoms
- Experiencing side effects of treatment

- Experiencing impoliteness of medical staff
- Experiencing hospital confinement
- Seeing family crying
- Seeing family feeling scared
- Seeing family getting stressed
- Seeing family not getting enough sleep
- Seeing the corpse trolley
- Seeing death in the hospital
- Hearing 'I have seen worse cases than you' from the doctors
- Knowing that the disease is incurable
- Knowing that death is imminent
- Knowing that death is inevitable
- Knowing that death is unpredictable
- Knowing that no one else can die for you
- Knowing that one is troubling the family
- Knowing that family is stressed

Cognitive appraisals

Interpreting

- Interpreting loss of ability to do many things as worst suffering
- Interpreting loss of ability to do enjoyable things as no life
- Interpreting lying on bed all the time as the same as a corpse
- Interpreting that one is no longer the same as before
- Interpreting that it is not easy to live with the changes
- Interpreting that the reminder of being sick is always there
- Interpreting that one is depending on others for everything
- Interpreting that one is burdening others
- Interpreting accepting help from others as a form of stress
- Interpreting depending on others as a sign of uselessness
- Interpreting that the children are not independent enough
- Interpreting that the waiting time to see doctors is very long
- Interpreting that the services of nurses are slow

- Interpreting that receiving chemotherapy is suffering
- Interpreting that medical students are inconsiderate
- Interpreting that the hospital food is not nutritious
- Interpreting that being sick is full of pain and suffering
- Interpreting the pain experience as a terrible experience
- Interpreting a life full of pain as a life of suffering
- Interpreting feelings as the most difficult thing about being sick
- Interpreting that God has abandoned oneself
- Interpreting that life is unfair
- Interpreting that life is not worth living

Comparing

- Comparing current disability with past ability
- Comparing current disability with past enjoyment
- Comparing current suffering with past happiness
- Comparing current quality of life with past quality of life
- Comparing the impact of bad news as the stab of a knife

Imagining

- Imagining oneself as a living corpse
- Imagining oneself like being trapped in the hospital
- Imagining oneself like being treated as an experiment
- Imagining oneself like being attacked by pain one after another

Believing

- Believing that one is giving extra work to others
- Believing that the children cannot live without oneself
- Believing that one is socially out
- Believing that nobody is ready to die at a young age
- Believing that nobody can tell how long one can live
- Believing that nobody can understand the suffering
- Believing that suffering is due to actions of past life

- Believing that what other people says of retribution is true
- Believing that one has to answer to God after death
- Believing that there is no reason to live if one cannot recover
- Believing that it is impossible not to worry

Filtering

- Focusing on loss
- Focusing on loss of function
- Focusing on loss of a happy life
- Focusing on burdening of others
- Focusing on worrying about family
- Focusing on pain
- Focusing on side effects of treatment
- Focusing on dying
- Focusing intensively on fear
- Zooming in pain and suffering
- Emphasizing loss of ability to walk
- Emphasizing side effects of treatment
- Mentioning fear repetitively
- Not focusing on what one still can do
- Not focusing on how to live until death

Magnifying

- Magnifying frequent episodes of pain to a life full of suffering
- Magnifying inability to do many things to everything
- Magnifying partial mobility restriction to complete immobility

Catastrophizing

- Catastrophizing current loss to loss of everything in the future
- Catastrophizing that bad things are going to happen one by one

Generalizing

- Generalizing that all doctors are busy
- Generalizing that everybody is scared to die
- Generalizing that nobody can remain fearless at the end of life
- Generalizing that nobody can help

Blaming

- Blaming the disease for poor quality of life
- Blaming the disease for hastening death
- Blaming God for abandoning oneself
- Blaming the devil for causing the disease

Dichotomous thinking

- Either to improve or die
- Either to remain functionally independent or die
- Either to have no pain or die
- Life is either happy or suffering

'Should' thinking

- One should depend on oneself rather than others
- One should take care of family rather than the other way round
- One should work, get married and bear children before dying
- One should do many things in life before dying

Hope and the struggles with acceptance

Hope

- Hoping for cure
- Hoping for life prolongation
- Hoping to live one day at a time
- Hoping for physical independence
- Hoping to be able to take care of oneself

- Hoping to be able to walk around freely
- Hoping for quality of life
- Hoping for a normal life
- Hoping to do many normal things in life
- Hoping to try many things in life
- Hoping to see more people
- Hoping to see the world more
- Hoping that family won't feel so sad
- Hoping to face dying later
- Hoping for hastening of death
- Hoping for death if burdening others
- Wanting to do many things but breathless
- Wanting to have own family before dying
- Wanting to know the entire picture
- Wanting to see the same doctor
- Wanting empathy from the doctor
- Intending to die if not improving
- Intending to die if suffering
- Bargaining to live longer
- Bargaining to live one extra day at a time
- Bargaining to delay death
- Expecting a cure but not possible
- Expecting life prolongation with quality
- Preferring to die if suffering
- Having no hope for recovery

Hope not

- Not wanting the disease
- Not wanting to have cancer
- Not wanting to suffer
- Not wanting to suffer anymore
- Not wanting to depend on others

- Not wanting to be disturbed
- Not wanting family to get sick from caring
- Not wanting family to suffer together
- Not wanting tubes and lines
- Not wanting to lie on hospital bed
- Not wanting to take medications
- Not wanting to wait in the clinic
- Not wanting to be treated like experiment
- Not wanting to eat hospital food
- Not wanting to die with pain
- Not wanting to die by losing bit by bit
- Having to depend on others
- Having to go through side effects of chemotherapy
- Having to wake up because of pain
- Having to walk slowly because of the pain
- Having difficulty in passing time
- Not able to do anything about the pain
- Not able to forget that one is sick
- Not able to sit still for minutes
- Not able to walk for ten minutes

The struggles with acceptance

- Not accepting the disease
- Not accepting the terminality of the disease
- Not accepting pain
- Not accepting the dependence on others
- Not accepting but no choice
- Finding it hard to accept the prognosis
- Feeling unprepared to die
- Completely unprepared to die
- Not scared of dying but not ready to die
- Not believing the told prognosis

- Arguing with the doctor for disparaging one's experience
- Complaining about lack of communication
- Complaining about lack of empathy
- Complaining about lack of care continuity
- Not satisfied with slow nursing service
- Not satisfied with hospital food
- Asking family to go home to rest

Emotions

- Feeling shocked with the diagnosis
- Feeling shocked with the prognosis
- Feeling frustrated with the disease
- Feeling angry and unfair
- Feeling bored with nothing to do
- Fear of no carer
- Fear of burdening others
- Fear of getting infection from friends
- Fear of needles
- Fear of dying
- Fear of suffering
- Fear of suffering but not dying
- Feeling fearful knowing what is cancer
- Feeling scared about many things
- Feeling scared to answer God
- Feeling scared not knowing the prognosis
- Feeling anxious
- Feeling hopeless
- Feeling lonely
- Feeling lonely in the experiencing of pain
- Feeling lonely not knowing where God is
- Feeling unhappy connected to lines
- Feeling sorry to see family having stress

- Feeling sad when diagnosed with cancer
- Feeling sad because of incurability
- Feeling sad for the family
- Feeling sad when thinking about dying
- Feeling depressed
- Feeling devastated to see family sadness
- Feeling terrible because of pain
- Feeling useless

Clinging

Ruminating

- Ruminating about the disease
- Ruminating about the pain
- Ruminating about the changes
- Ruminating about troubling family
- Ruminating about the impact on children
- Ruminating about dying
- Ruminating about dying all the time
- Ruminating about not wanting to die
- Ruminating about not the right time to die
- Ruminating about unfairness of life
- Chain of fearful thoughts
- Chain of worrying thoughts

Worrying

- Worrying about the future of oneself
- Worrying about losing the ability to walk
- Worrying about coping
- Worrying about depending on others
- Worrying about the future of family
- Worrying about the well-being of family

- Worrying about small children
- Worrying about the risk of getting infection

Wondering

- Wondering why there is no forewarning
- Wondering why this is happening
- Wondering how it is possible
- Wondering why me
- Wondering what one has done wrong
- Wondering what to do if one cannot walk
- Wondering how long one has to suffer
- Wondering where God is while in pain
- Not knowing how to describe suffering
- Not knowing what to do
- Not knowing what one is doing
- Not knowing who to turn to
- Not knowing how long one can live

Diagnosing suffering

- Screening question: Are you suffering? (Cassell 1999)

General questions for suffering assessment

- Can you tell me a little about your experience?
- How has this illness affected you physically?
- What about your emotions?
- How have your family been throughout your illness?
- What about your friends?
- How do you find the doctors and nurses here?
- How is it like staying in the hospital?
- What things do you believe in that are important to you now?
- Is there anything else that you would like to share with me about your experience?

Specific questions for suffering assessment

- Existential questions
  - Loss and change
    - Can you tell me a little about the changes in your life because of the sickness?
    - How has your routine changed?
    - Are there specific things that you are planning to do?
  - Dependence on others
    - Tell me a little about your family support
    - How about the support from your friends?
    - How do you feel about their care?
  - Witnessing family suffering
    - What are your concerns for your family?
    - What are their routines now?
    - How is your family coping?
  - Facing terminal disease and death
    - What are your concerns regarding your sickness?
    - What about your treatment?
    - What are your concerns about the future?
  - Healthcare encounter
    - How do you find the communication from doctors and nurses?
    - How would you comment on the level of care you have received?
    - What are your opinions regarding the knowledge and skills of doctors and nurses?
  - Hospital stay
    - How do you find the hospital environment?
    - How do you find the hospital food?
    - What about the hospital facilities?

- Experiential questions
  - Physical experience
    - Tell me about your physical symptoms
    - How have your symptoms affected you?
    - What are your concerns about the symptoms?
  - Emotional experience
    - Tell me a little about your mood when you go through the sickness
    - How are you affected by your emotions?
    - How do you deal with your emotions?
  - Cognitive experience
    - What are your beliefs regarding the sickness?
    - What are your hopes and expectations?
    - How do you come to terms with your sickness?
  - Spiritual experience
    - Are there things that you can't make sense when you experience the sickness?
    - How has your faith affected by the sickness?
    - What support do you look for when life is difficult?

Measuring suffering

- PRISM
  - Pictorial Representation of Illness and Self Measure
  - Measurement of self-illness-separation (SIS)
  - Red disc = illness
  - Yellow disc = self
  - Place red disc on the plate in such as way that it shows which place the illness occupies in one's life
  - SIS = distance between center of "self" and "illness" in cm
  - Range: 0-27cm

- SISC
  - Structured Interview for Symptoms and Concerns
  - 13 items
    - Pain
    - Drowsiness
    - Nausea
    - Weakness
    - Dyspnoea
    - Loss of control
    - Loss of dignity
    - Sense of burden
    - Anxiety
    - Depression
    - Loss of interest
    - Hopelessness
    - Desire for death
- Distress thermometer
  - Measures distress
  - 0 = no distress
  - 10 = extreme distress
- Suffering pictogram
  - Measures overall suffering score
    - Write at center of pictogram
    - 0 = no suffering
    - 10 = worst possible suffering
  - Also measures 8 suffering experiences
    - 0 = none
    - 1 = a little bit
    - 2 = somewhat
    - 3 = quite a bit
    - 4 = a lot

Suffering pictogram

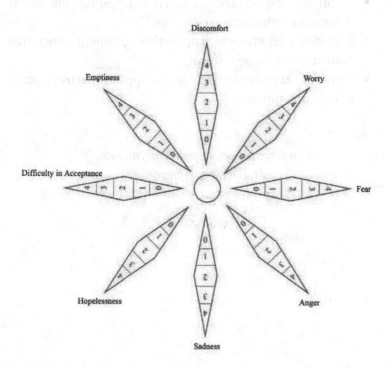

The relief of suffering

- Existential approaches (targeting events)
  - Loss and change: rehabilitation
  - Dependence on others: mobilizing support and resources
  - Witnessing family suffering: care of family caregivers
  - Terminal disease and death: disease-modifying treatment
  - Healthcare encounter: communication training
  - Hospital stay: patient-centered hospital design

- Experiential approaches (targeting experiences)
  - Physical experience: symptom control
  - Emotional experience: supportive listening, emotional processing, relaxation techniques
  - Cognitive experience: supportive listening, cognitive restructuring, hope fostering
  - Spiritual experience: spiritual support, pastoral care, nonabandonment

You treat a disease, you win, you lose.
You treat a person, I guarantee you,
you'll win, no matter what the outcome.

Patch Adams

Psychological Stages of Dying

Introduction

Elisabeth Kübler-Ross described five stages of dying in her 1969 masterpiece – On Death and Dying: What the dying have to teach doctors, nurses, clergy, and their own families.

The five stages

- Denial
- Anger
- Bargaining
- Depression
- Acceptance

Denial

- First reaction may be a temporary state of shock
- Followed by "No, not me, it cannot be true."
- A healthy way of dealing with a painful situation
- Usually a temporary defense
- Will soon be replaced by partial acceptance
- Maintained denial until the end is a rarity
- We should listen, acknowledge and allow them their defenses

Anger

- When the first stage of denial cannot be maintained any longer
- Replaced by feelings of anger, rage, envy and resentment
- The next question becomes: "Why me?"
- "Well, why couldn't it have been him?"
- The anger can be displaced in all directions
- We should not take it personally

Bargaining

- Entering into some sort of an agreement which may postpone the inevitable happening
- "If God has decided to take us from this earth and he did not respond to my angry pleas, he may be more favourable if I ask nicely."
- Wish to be rewarded for good behaviour
- Bargaining for extension of life
- Most bargains are made with God and are usually kept a secret
- The promises may be associated with quiet guilt
- We should not brush aside their remarks
- We should explore any sense of guilt and reasons behind

Depression

- Patient cannot smile it off anymore
- Numbness and stoicism, anger and rage will soon be replaced with a sense of great loss
- Reactive depression
  - A reaction to the disease and loss
  - Address the disease and symptoms
  - Address the loss
  - Encourage patient to look at the bright side
- Preparatory depression
  - A preparatory grief
  - Preparation for final separation from the world
  - Not a result of past loss but impending losses
  - Encouragements and reassurances are not meaningful
  - Allow patient to express his or her sorrow
  - Sit with patient silently
  - No or little need for words
  - Non-verbal: a touch of a hand, a stroking of the hair

Acceptance

- Patient is no longer angry nor depressed
- Has expressed feelings
- Has mourned the impending loss
- Contemplating the coming end with a certain degree of quiet expectation
- Not a happy stage
- Almost void of feelings
- It is as if the pain has gone, the struggle is over
- "The final rest before the long journey"
- Patient wishes to be left alone
- Visitors are often not desired
- Television is off
- We should focus more on non-verbal communication
- Sit in silence
- May reassure that it is alright to say nothing
- May reassure that he or she is not left alone
- Family needs more help during this stage
- A visit in the evening may lend itself best
- It is comforting for the patient to know that he or she is not forgotten

Hope

- The one thing that persists through all the stages
- Even the most accepting patients leave the possibility open for some cure, for the discovery of a new drug or the "last-minute success in a research project"
- This glimpse of hope maintains patients through their suffering
- The feeling that all this must have some meaning, will pay off eventually if they endure it for a little longer
- We should allow them to hope – realistic or unrealistic

Little sharing

My colleague said, "There is no such thing as a difficult patient or a difficult family member. They are just in a difficult situation." It is important not to judge others based on their reactions to a difficult situation because given the same situation, we may react the same too.

Hope in Palliative Care

Introduction

Many doctors think that being terminally ill means hopelessness. This is not true. Hope is present at all times.

What is hope?

> *"Hope" is the thing with feathers*
> *That perches in the soul*
> *And sings the tune without the words*
> *And never stops at all*

Emily Dickinson

- A desire for a particular thing to happen (Oxford 2010)
- A psychological function of a person that involves the desiring of a particular outcome (Tan 2014)
- A positive motivational state that is based on an interactively derived sense of successful agency [goal-directed energy] and pathways [planning to meet goals] (Snyder 1991)

The theory of hope (Snyder 2000)

- Where there is a will, there is a way
- Will power (agency thinking)
    - The will to shape the future
- Way power (pathway thinking)
    - The ability to see ways to shape the future
- Goals: provide direction and endpoint for hopeful thinking
- Barriers: things that block attainment of goals

Hope assessment

- Will power assessment (agency)
  - Could you tell me a little about your hope?
- Way power assessment (pathway)
  - What are the ways you see that can achieve your hope?

Herth Hope Index

- 12 items
  - I have a positive outlook toward life
  - I have short or long range goals
  - I feel all alone
  - I can see possibilities in the midst of difficulties
  - I have a faith that gives me comfort
  - I feel scared about my future
  - I can recall happy times
  - I have deep inner strength
  - I am able to give and receive love
  - I have a sense of direction
  - I believe that each day has potential
  - I feel my life has value and worth
- The higher the score the higher the level of hope

Types of hope of palliative care patients (Tan 2014)

- Regarding suffering
  - Hope to recover
  - Hope to live longer
  - Hope to stay independent
  - Hope to be discharged
  - Hope to be normal
  - Hope to be pain-free
  - Hope to die peacefully

- Regarding quality of life
  - Hope to do
    - Take care of family
    - Do housework
    - Go for holiday
    - Just sit and relax
    - Be a better person
    - Do charity
  - Hope to see
    - Children grow up, enter university, graduate, get married, bear children
    - Grandchildren grow up, enter university, graduate, get married, bear children
    - Harmony in the family

Hope and well-being

- Hope is a coping mechanism
- It is a positive thought that can fill the gap of a stream of negative thoughts

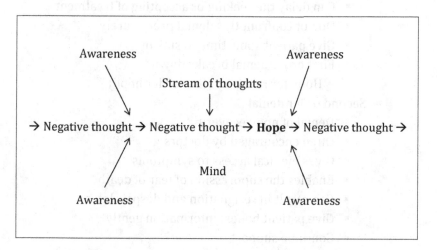

The change of hope in terminally ill patients

- Initial hope
  - Hope that the news is not true
  - Hope that there is treatment
  - Hope that treatment is effective
  - Hope that treatment is not causing any side effects
- Feeling hopeless when treatment is ineffective
- Subsequent hope
  - Hope for family
  - Hope for symptom control
  - Hope for meaningful time
  - Hope for a peaceful death
  - Hope after death
- Denial and hope (Runbold 1986)
  - First order denial
    - Denial of symptoms
    - Denying the significance of symptoms
    - Ignoring worrying symptoms
    - Enables patient to continue functioning
    - Can delay the seeking or accepting of treatment
    - Do not confront this denial prematurely
    - Give patient some time to sink in
    - First order denial breaks down
      → Hope for recovery (first order hope)
  - Second order denial
    - Denial of non-recovery
    - Often encouraged by doctors
    - Gives medical access to symptoms
    - Enables the suppression of fear of death
    - Can result in resignation and despair later
    - Give patient honest information gently
    - Continue support

422

- Second order denial breaks down
  → Despair if collusion or lack of support
  → Hope beyond recovery
  (second order hope)
    - Hope to die with dignity
    - Hope for the continuing success of children
    - Hope that partner will find the needed support
    - Hope that life's contribution will continue
- Third order denial
    - Denying the possibility that death will be the end
    - Third order denial breaks down
    → Hope that accepts the existential possibility of extinction at death, but that nevertheless finds a sense of ultimate meaning in the life that has been lived (third order hope)

Sources of hope (Herth 1990)

- Family
- Friends
- Healthcare professionals
- God or higher spiritual being

Obstacles of hope (Herth 1990)

- Abandonment and isolation
- Uncontrolled pain
- Devaluation of personhood

The Zeigarnik effect

- Nagging from the unconscious mind to fulfil a hope
- Stops when a hope is fulfilled or a plan is made
- Recommendations:fulfil patient's hope or give patient a plan

Interventions that engender hope (Herth 1990, Storey 1997)

- Adequate control of symptoms
- Fostering interpersonal connectedness and relationship
- Assistance in attaining practical goals
- Exploring spiritual beliefs
- Supporting and identifying personal attributes, such as determination, courage, and serenity
- Encouraging light-heartedness when appropriate
- Affirming worth by treating the patient as a valued individual
- Recalling uplifting memories with life review

Communicating hope

- It is important NOT to take away patient's hope by
  - Saying "there is no more hope"
  - Saying "there is nothing more can be done"
- Always give hope by saying:
  - I will never leave you in pain
  - I will never abandon you
  - I will never give up hope on you

Realistic and unrealistic hope

- Realistic hope
  - Always provide realistic hope
  - Relieve pain
  - Non-abandonment
  - Fulfil patient's wish
- Unrealistic hope
  - Never give false hope
  - Never destroy patient's hope, realistic or unrealistic
  - Communicate sensitively
  - Give patient time to sink in
  - Hope is never unrealistic from a patient's perspective

Hope from a family perspective (Catherine 2015)

- Hope is a form of strength that is always there and can be passed on from one person to another
- Giving and receiving hope can lead to a positive reaction
- It is important to realize and respect that each individual has their own perception of hope
- Communication and trust will align hopes and expectations

Hope continues to bloom

My mother, the queen of my heart,

Before... any portrait is just in that moment in time

She hopes to do her best and to give everything
So her family is happy and her kids are successful

She hopes to be healthy and active
To be able to enjoy the little things in life

She wants to live as long as possible to see my brother and I get married and have kids

I hope my 'best friend' will never leave my side
So I can always be her little girl

She was diagnosed with lung cancer stage 1
And the prognosis was grim

She hopes to be healthy and recover soon
So she gives her best and is willing to do anything

I hope my 'daughter' will be healthy again
So she can do what she loves like before

She hopes that we will not be worried or unhappy
So she continues smiling

Four months later, after radio and chemotherapy
She is already in stage 4

She hopes to be home with her loved ones
Because she does not know how long she has

I hope I can take her pain and suffering away
For I am so helpless my 'daughter' is suffering

She hopes we will be happy always and taken care of
And wish that someday she would come back as my daughter

We hope that you are happy
and having a wonderful journey wherever you are

For you have given us unconditional LOVE, JOY and HOPE

By Catherine Yee Chiew Huei

Spirituality in Palliative Care

Introduction

Spirituality is one of the most important areas in palliative care. Stricty speaking, palliative care is a form of spiritual care because treating patients as whole persons is spiritual care.

What is spirituality?

- Spirit in Latin: spiritus – breath, life, soul
- Of, or pertaining to, affecting or concerning the spirit or higher moral questions. (Oxford 1988)
- That which is deepest and most genuine in us, the ground of our being, and what we, and others, refer to as spiritual pain is the experience of alienation from this depth. (Saunders 1988)
- Whomever or whatever gives one a transcendent meaning in life. (Puchalski 1999)
- Concerned with an aspect of human nature that is rooted in our experience of relatedness to both an inner and outer world. (Cobb 2003)
- Spirituality is a fundamental element of human experience. It encompasses the individual's search for meaning and purpose in life and the experience of the transcendent. (Puchalski 2009)
- Spirituality is the aspect of humanity that refers to the way individuals seek and express meaning and purpose, and the way they experience their connectedness to the moment, to self, to others, to nature, and to the significant or sacred. (Puchalski 2009)

The meaning of life is to find your gift.
The purpose of life is to give it away.

Pablo Picasso

What is religion?

- The structured and communal aspects of belief related to one's ultimate concern (Hoffman 2008)
- Religion is a formal structure through which a person expresses spirituality within a community
- A religious community is then organized around common beliefs, attitudes, practices, traditions, and relationships

Spirituality and religion

- Not interchangeable
- The spirit is a dimension of personhood
- Religion is a construct of human making that, for some, enables conceptualization and expression of spirituality (Hill 2003)
- Spirituality explains what is important to the life of a person
- Religion is one of the many explanations
- The hand and glove analogue of Jean Radley
  - Hand
    - Spirituality
    - An integral part of human being
  - Glove
    - Religion
    - Some people find a glove that their hand can fit in
    - Some people choose to forgo the glove
- A religious person may still experience spiritual pain
- A spiritual person may have strengths even without a religion

Spiritual components

Existential component (Yalom 1980)

- 4 ultimate concerns:
- Existential freedom
    - The absence of inherent design in the universe
    - We are absolutely responsible for how we live our life
    - We are absolutely responsible for our choices
    - Causes: awareness of this terrifying responsibility, fear of this groundlessness, erecting defences to suppress the fear, passing the responsibility to others in an attempt to escape from the freedom
- Existential isolation
    - The unbridgeable gap between self and others
    - Deeper than loneliness, which is bridgeable
    - Our aloneness in the universe
    - We enter and leave the world alone
    - Causes: recognizing this basic isolation, recognizing that one's death is always solitary, recognizing the terror of feeling that there may be moments when no one in the world is thinking of us, connecting with others to buffer against the experience of existential isolation
    - A deep sense of connection does not solve the problem of existential isolation, but it provides solace
    - An important milestone in therapy is the patient's realization that, "there is a point beyond which the therapist can offer nothing more."
- Meaning
    - Finding meaning in life, although none is absolute and none is given to us
    - We create our own world and have to answer for ourselves why we live and how we shall live

- Causes: searching for meaning and purpose in life, the crisis of meaning seeking, feeling empty, passionless or pointless in life
- The big questions
  - Why me?
  - Why now?
  - Why am I living?
- If all purpose is self-authored, then one must confront the ultimate groundlessness of existence
- We create our own meaning and purpose in life
- Death
  - Existential obliteration
  - Causes: the awareness of our inevitable demise, death anxiety, fear of death, denial of death to suppress fear, projecting ourselves into the future through our children, trying to grow rich and famous, developing compulsive behaviours, or fostering an impregnable belief in an ultimate rescuer
  - Confronting death allows us to live fuller, richer, and more compassionate lives

Connectedness component (Puchalski 2009)

- The sense and experience of connectedness
  - Connectedness to the moment
  - Connectedness to self
  - Connectedness to others
  - Connectedness to nature
  - Connectedness to the significant or sacred

Religious component

- Faith
- Beliefs
- Rituals and practices
- Relationship with God
- Relationship with the ultimate

Spiritual needs (Flannelly 2005)

- Need for meaning and purpose
- Need for love and a sense of belonging
- Need for appreciation of nature and beauty
- Need for positivity, gratitude and peace
- Need for spiritual or religious practices
- Need for resolution of issues involving life and death

Spiritual assessment

- Acronym FICA (Christina Puchalski 1999)

F = Faith

- What do you believe in that gives meaning to your life?

I = Importance

- How important is your faith, religion or spirituality to you?

C = Community

- Are you part of a spiritual or religious community?

A = Address

- How would you like me to address these issues?

- Acronym SPIRIT (Maugans 1997)
    - S = spiritual belief system
    - P = personal spirituality
    - I = integration with a spiritual community
    - R = ritualized practices and restrictions
    - I = implications for medical practices
    - T = terminal events planning
- Acronym HOPE (Anandarajah 2001)
    - H = sources of hope, meaning, comfort, strength, peace, love and compassion
    - O = organized religion
    - P = personal spirituality or practices
    - E = effects on medical care and end-of-life issues
- FACIT-Sp-12 (Version 4)
    - Assess spiritual well-being
    - 12 items
    - I feel peaceful
    - I have a reason for living
    - My life has been productive
    - I have trouble feeling peace of mind
    - I feel a sense of purpose in my life
    - I am able to reach down deep into myself for comfort
    - I feel a sense of harmony within myself
    - My life lacks meaning and purpose
    - I find comfort in my faith or spiritual beliefs
    - I find strength in my faith or spiritual beliefs
    - My illness has strengthened my faith or spiritual beliefs
    - I know that whatever happens with my illness, things will be ok

Spiritual suffering

- Pain deep in your being that is not physical (Mako 2006)
  - Three domains of expression
    - An intrapsychic conflict
    - An interpersonal loss or conflict
    - In relation to the divine
- Pain caused by extinction of the being and the meaning of the self (Murata 2003)
  - Three dimensions
    - A being founded on temporality
    - A being in relationship
    - A being with autonomy
- Arises when there is a gap between a person's innermost sense of value and meaning and the external reality

Types of spiritual suffering

- Existential suffering
  - Existential groundlessness
    - The key existential dynamic is the clash between our confrontation with groundlessness and our wish for ground and structure
    - Experience (Bruce 2011)
      - Being shaken to the core
      - Recognizing life is ending
      - Profound sense of hopelessness
      - Unable to reconcile experience with their faith
      - Not understanding why God is doing this
      - Having one's belief system shattered
      - Experiencing extreme dissonance
      - Feeling of deep despair and unmalleable grief

- Existential loneliness
  - The existential conflict is the tension between the awareness of our isolation and our wish for contact, for protection, our wish to be part of a larger whole
  - Experience
    - The feeling of fundamental aloneness as human
    - Feeling "separated" from the rest of the world
    - Loneliness unrelieved by presence of others
    - Feeling nobody can understand one's feeling
    - Feeling nobody cares
- Meaninglessness
  - Conflict arising from the issue of meaning, stems from the dilemma of a meaning-seeking creature who is thrown into a universe that has no meaning
  - Experience
    - Feeling the lack of meaning and purpose in life
    - Cannot make sense of the suffering
    - Cannot make sense of what is happening
    - Feeling meaningless, hopeless and helpless
    - Feeling empty and futile: existential vacuum
    - Desire to die
- Death anxiety
  - The core existential conflict is the tension between the awareness of the inevitability of death and the wish to continue to be
  - Definitions of death anxiety
    - A negative emotional reaction provoked by the anticipation of a state in which the self does not exist (Tomer 1996)
    - Feeling of dread, apprehension and solicitude (anxiety) when one thinks of the process of dying, or ceasing to be (Farley 2010)

- Experience
  - Fear of death
  - Fear of a painful death
  - Fear of suffering
  - Fear of loss
  - Fear of separation
  - Fear of the unknown
  - Paradoxical desire to hasten death
- Connectedness-related suffering
  - Failure to live in the moment
    - Ruminating excessively about the past
    - Worrying excessively about the future
  - Disrupted self integrity
    - Hopelessness and despair
    - Grief
    - Guilt and shame
  - Impaired sense of belonging
    - Abandonment
    - Loneliness
    - Reconciliation issues
    - Dispute
  - Disconnected from nature
    - Hospital confinement
  - Disrupted spiritual practices
    - Inability to practice spirituality
- Religion-specific
  - Loss of ability to practice religion
    - Inability to pray
    - Inability to meditate
    - Inability to attend religious activities
    - Inability to observe religious ethics
    - Inability to perform rituals

- Loss of faith
  - Feeling unfair
  - Feeling being abandoned by God
  - Feeling angry at God
  - Feeling angry at religious community
  - Challenged belief system
- Religious-specific fear
  - Fear of retribution
  - Fear of punishment
  - Fear of God
- Religious-specific guilt
  - Failure to practice religion
  - Failure to progress
  - Failure to do good
  - Failure to live a moral life
- Interfaith distress
  - Lack of understanding from people of other faiths
  - Distress due to preaching from others
  - Fear of being evangelized
  - Concerns regarding different rituals and ceremonies
  - Dispute due to different faiths in the family

Spiritual care

- Spiritual care is defined as interventions, individual or communal, that facilitate the ability to express the integration of the body, mind, and spirit to achieve wholeness, health, and a sense of connection to self, others, and/or a higher power (Health Minitries Association 2005)
- Spiritual care is care that encourages and supports reflection on experience, the search for meaning and the development of inner resources for the journey

- Responding to spiritual suffering (Kearney 1997)
  - Surface-work
    - Interventions aimed at easing distress at the surface, the conscious and concrete level of an individual's experience
    - Not "superficial", but the way to the deep
    - For many, caring, effective surface-work is also depth-work and all that is needed to bring individuals into depth
  - Depth-work
    - Approach or intervention that brings individual inward and downward toward the deeper layers of the psyche
    - Helping patient to reconnect with those very simple and ordinary aspects of life that have, in the past, brought them a sense of depth or significance
    - This may involve encouraging patients
      - To share memories
      - To spend time with their loved ones
      - To visit a place of special importance to them
      - To return home from the hospital if possible
      - To bring 'home' to the hospital if cannot return
        - Photographs
        - A particular treasured object
  - Depth skills
    - Image work
    - Dream work
    - Art therapy
    - Music therapy
    - Reminiscence and biography therapy
    - Body work (including massage)
    - Meditations

- Control of physical symptoms
- Existential approaches
  - Explore fear of death
  - Explore the meaning of illness and suffering
  - Explore the sources of meaning in patient's life
  - Encourage the search for meaning and purpose
  - Fostering hope
  - Reframing goals and redefining hope
- Connectedness approaches
  - Establish a therapeutic relationship
    - Being presence
    - Supportive listening
    - Understanding suffering
    - Working with love
  - Practice non-abandonment
  - Encourage life review
  - Explore guilt, shame, remorse and regret
  - Explore the need for reconciliation
  - Encourage mindful practices to connect to the moment
  - Encourage engagement in art and music if appropriate
- Religious approaches
  - Facilitate religious expression
  - Facilitate ritual practices
  - Encourage prayers that assist healing
  - Encourage meditative practices that focus on healing
  - Involve chaplain or spiritual care workers

Specific therapy for spiritual suffering

- Existential therapy (Yalom 1980)
- Meaning-centered group therapy (Breitbart 2010)
- Dignity therapy (Chochinov 2005)
- Mindfulness-based supportive therapy (Tan 2015)

UNIPAC's acronym for spiritual care: LET GO (Storey 1997)

- Listen to the patient's story
- Encourage the search for meaning
- Tell of your concern and acknowledge the pain of loss
- Generate hope whenever possible
- Own your limitation and refer when appropriate

Life Review

Introduction

Life review is a structured evaluation of one's life with the intention to derive a sense of meaning and purpose from the recalled memories.

Life review and reminiscence (Butler 1963)

- Life review
  - Structured
  - Involves one or more life themes
  - Evaluative process
    - To derive a sense of meaning and purpose
    - To come to terms with difficult memories
- Reminiscence
  - Unstructured
  - Involves spontaneous recall of memories
  - Passive process
  - May be part of life review but not synonymous

Everybody is a story. When I was a child, people sat around kitchen tables and told their stories. We don't do that so much anymore. Sitting around the table telling stories is not just a way of passing time. It is the way the wisdom gets passed along. The stuff that helps us to live a life worth remembering.

Rachel Naomi Remen

Techniques (Butler 1963)

- Patients are asked to describe important life events
  - Time periods
    - Childhood
    - Adolescence
    - Adulthood
    - Present situation
  - Life events
    - Schooling
    - Working
    - Marriage
    - Parenting
    - Illness
- Use of mementos to enhance life review
  - Music
  - Scrapbooks
  - Photos
  - Letters
  - Cherished possessions
  - Family trees
- Create a legacy from life review
  - Audio
  - Video
  - Notebooks
  - Album with pictures
- Review the creation with patient and family
- Facilitate
  - Expression of emotions
  - Finding meaning from recalled memories
  - Coming to terms with difficult memories
  - Closure

Existential Therapy

Introduction

Existential therapy is a way of thinking about human experience. It is a philosophical approach to therapy that assumes we are free to choose and are responsible for our choices.

Basic concepts (Yalom 1980)

- Based on principles of humanistic and existential psychology
    - Humanism: emphasizes the whole person
    - Existentialism: emphasizes the four ultimate concerns of human existence
        - Existential freedom
        - Existential isolation
        - Meaninglessness
        - Death
- Assists patient
    - In confronting the ultimate concerns
        - Freedom and responsibility
        - Loneliness and loss
        - Meaninglessness and suffering
        - Death and finitude
    - To live more fully in each moment
- Focuses on
    - The person as the center of the therapeutic process
    - The subjective experience of self
    - The will and intentionality
    - The therapeutic encounter
    - The here-and-now

Existential maturity (Spira 2000)

- Hermeneutic basis of the self
  - The "self" arises from social interpretations formed from a lifetime of social conditioning
- Inauthentic assumptions of our self and our world
  - Our assumptions of our "self" and our "world" are merely mental constructions
  - We assume our "self" as fixed, stable entity
  - We assume our "world" as fixed, predictable world
  - These are inauthentic assumptions
- Breakdown of inauthentic assumptions
  - External crisis can lead to the breakdown of assumptions
  - Breakdown of our habitual assumptions leads to either covering up of the breakdown by fleeing into conveniently provided alternative social conventions and returning to inauthentic assumptions; or to existential anxiety (Angst) and feeling of a sense of dissociated depersonalization (Unheimlicheit)
- Moment of vision
  - Becoming aware of the inauthentic assumptions one has been making unconsciously in one's life
  - One may realize that they have done nothing that is truly rewarding but only things that the society or others expect of them
- Authentic commitment
  - Reevaluation of how one wants to live more fully in the remaining time
  - Choosing life acivities that will bring greatest meaning, purpose and value to one's life

- The severity of the external disruption corresponds to the extent to which assumptions breakdown (live as it has been lived), corresponds to the extent which one will recognize prior assumptions (habitual, nonchosen activities), which in turn corresponds to the extent to which new activities can be authentically chosen for greatest meaning, purpose and value in one's life

Methods of existential therapy (Spira 2000)

- Establish an authentic relationship
  - Establish rapport
    - The therapeutic stance
      - "The fellow traveller"
      - Not doctor and patient
      - Not therapist and client
      - We are all in this together
    - Sharing the essence of human conditions
    - Treat encounter as a learning experience for both
    - Active listening
    - Non-judgmental acceptance of the patient
      - Acknowledge beliefs
      - Acknowledge emotions
      - Acknowledge existential concerns
      - Acknowledge potential for existential maturity
  - Ask questions that encourage exploration of existential issues and development of existential maturity
    - What is important to you in the time you have left?
    - Are there things you would like to do for yourself that are not what others expect from you?

- Ask questions that encourage open intimacy with self and others that lead to existential process
  - Cognitive openness
    - Acceptance versus denial
    - Question: Can you give me a specific example of how that affects you personally?
  - Affective openness
    - Integrated feeling versus repression
    - Question: How does that make you feel?
  - Interpersonal
    - Open expression versus isolation
    - Question: Can you tell your family your fears about losing control?
  - Active coping
    - Explore ways to deal with what one can control and let go of what one cannot control
    - Question: What can you do to lessen your pain?
- Facilitate the breakdown
  - Acknowledge patient's suffering and explore the basis of such suffering rather than helping to cover up patient's distress
  - Assist in making unconscious assumptions conscious
    - Facilitate the development of "lateral perspective"
      - How do family members view what is going on?
      - How do friends view what is going on?
      - How do doctors view what is going on?
      - How do other patients view what is going on?
    - Facilitate appreciation of the idea that any view is personally created over a lifetime, rather than mirroring a "realistic" view of the world
    - Facilitate suspension of patient's fixed view of self and life to explore ways that allow adjustment

- Another way to facilitate the breakdown is to discuss death and dying openly

Exercise 1: Living in the face of dying

- If you have one year (month, week) to live and you want to make it the most meaningful year of your life
    - What personal characteristics (self-image, personality, assumptions about life) would you want to let go of?
    - What activities would you let go of that you find more of a burden than a joy?
    - What personal characteristics would you want to have to help you make this year a valuable one for you?
    - What activities would you want to engage in that would bring greatest meaning and value to your life?
    - What is stopping you from having these qualities and doing these activities now?
    - What can you do to overcome these barriers to live more fully?

Exercise 2: Identifying beliefs that limit ability to live fully

- When was this belief developed? Under what circumstances did you form this belief?
    - How did this belief help you at that time? How does this belief still help you now?
    - How has this belief limited you in the past? How does this belief limit you at this time?
    - What is an alternative belief that would help you at this time, and would keep the habit belief in check?
    - In what situations will the old belief influence you, and what will help you recall the alternative belief?

Exercise 3: Being in the moment

- Can you describe the present state?
- Can you discuss what you feel in your body?
- What do you see in the room?
- What sounds come to your ears?
- How do you feel in the relationship with the therapist?
- Patients can practice this each day for one minute and then use this "presencing" method to become calm whenever they start "thinking too much"

- Support a "moment of vision"
  - A moment of vision occurs when patients realize they are more than their limited view of themselves
  - They also come to appreciate that they contain all the resources they have from their entire lives, releasing their full potential for acting
  - Must allow full grieving to occur, supporting the state of despair, until such time as the patient can fully accept his or her condition without attempting to flee it
  - Must be kept in mind that different patients will have different capacities for existential maturation
  - Must be flexible enough to support patients in the way that works best for them
- Encourage the pragmatic development of commitment
  - Promote active strategies to develop meaningful actions in the patient's life
  - Assist patients in reprioritizing life activities

Exercise 4: reprioritizing life activities

- Make a list of activities you spend your time doing during a typical week

- Prioritize this list, with the activities you spend most time with at the top and those you spend less time on toward the bottom
- Prioritize these activities again, but this time list at the top the activities that bring more meaning and personal value to your life, with progressively less meaningful activities toward the bottom. To the list can also be added any activities you wish you were doing, even though you have not gotten around to them
- Examine the last two columns. If the lists are ordered differently, then it is important to ask what you can do to spend more time engaged in those activities that bring more meaning and value to your life and less in activities that you do out of habit

Principles of existential psychotherapy (Spira 2000)

- Development of an authentic relationship between therapist and patient, and between patient and others
- The valuing of patient experience, resources, and capacity for development at any point in life
- The importance of facilitating the breakdown of conditioned habitual assumptions about life
- Assisting patients to accept their suffering and potential for death without attempting to cover up
- Helping patients to trust in the present moment as the fullest experience possible in life
- Engaging in activities that bring greatest meaning, purpose, and value to one's life

Meaning-centered Therapy

Introduction

Meaning-centered therapy or logotherapy was developed by Viktor Frankl, an Austrian neurologist, psychiatrist as well as a Holocaust survivor. A short introduction to the therapy was given in his famous book, Man's Search for Meaning.

Basic concepts

- Logos = "meaning" in Greek
- Less retrospective compared to psychoanalysis
- Less introspective compared to psychoanalysis
- Focuses on the meaning to be fulfilled by patient in the future
- Primary motivational force in human
  - Freudian psychoanalysis: will to pleasure
  - Adlerian psychotherapy: will to power
  - Logotherapy: will to meaning
- Human's will to meaning can lead to existential frustration
  - Existential frustration = an existential distress
  - Not pathological
  - Not pathogenic
  - Not a mental disease
  - Can result in noögenic neurosis (vs psychogenic neurosis)
- Logotherapy assists patient to find meaning in his or her life

He who has a why to live for can bear almost any how

Nietzsche

Logodrama

- A technique based on logotherapy for discovering meaning and responding meaningfully to a life situation
- Dramatization of an imagined experience in the here-and-now
- Stages
  - Present-moment awareness
    - Awareness of bodily sensations
    - Awareness of thoughts
    - Awareness of emotions
  - Engagement
    - Counters the instinct to run away from emotions
    - Counters the instinct to run away from a person
    - Counters the instinct to run away from a situation
  - Stepping back
    - Allows one to see the situation subjectively
    - To find the choice between stimulus and response
  - Expectant presence
    - To look for meaning of what the situation is about in terms of values
    - To respond in a way that makes life worth living

Meaning-centered group psychotherapy (Breitbart 2010)

- A psychoeducational model
- Developed from logotherapy
- Designed for patients with life-threatening illness
- 6-8 weekly sessions
- 90min sessions
- Includes
  - Teachings on the philosophy of meaning
  - Discussion of topic such as "good death"
  - Engagement in experiential exercises
  - Home exercises that reinforce similar themes

- Themes
  - Summary of concepts and sources of meaning
  - Cancer and meaning
  - Meaning derived from historical context in life
  - Meaning derived from attitudinal values
  - Meaning derived from creative values and responsibility
  - Meaning derived through experiential values
  - Termination and feedback

Dignity Therapy

Introduction

Dignity therapy is a brief, individualized psychotherapeutic intervention designed to address psychosocial and existential distress among terminally ill patients.

Three major domains of dignity (Chochinov 2002)

- Illness-related concerns that influence dignity
  - Physical distress
  - Psychological distress
  - Cognitive acuity
  - Functional capacity
  - Medical uncertainty
  - Death anxiety
- Dignity conserving repertoire
  - Dignity conserving perspectives
    - Continuity of self
    - Role preservation
    - Generativity
    - Maintenance of pride
    - Hopefulness
    - Autonomy and control
    - Acceptance
    - Resilience and fighting spirit
  - Dignity conserving practices
    - Living in the moment
    - Maintaining normalcy
    - Seeking spiritual comfort

- Social dignity inventory
  - Privacy boundaries
  - Social support
  - Care tenor
  - Burden to others
  - Aftermath concerns

Dignity themes (Chochinov 2005)

- Generativity
  - The notion that, for some patients, dignity is intertwined with a sense that one's life has stood for something or has some influence transcendent of death
  - Implication: sessions are tape-recorded and transcribed, with an edited transcript or "generativity document" being returned to patient to bequeath to a friend or family member
- Continuity of self
  - Being able to maintain a feeling that one's essence is intact despite advancing illness
  - Implication: patients are invited to speak to issues that are foundational to their sense of personhood or self
- Role preservation
  - Being able to maintain a sense of identification with one or more previously held roles
  - Implication: patients are questioned about previous or currently held roles that may contribute to their core identity
- Maintenance of pride
  - An ability to sustain a sense of positive self-regard
  - Implication: providing opportunities to speak about previous accomplishments or achievements that engender a sense of pride

- Hopefulness
  - Hopefulness relates to the ability to find or maintain a sense of meaning or purpose
  - Implication: patients are invited to engage in a therapeutic process intended to instill a sense of meaning and purpose
- Aftermath concerns
  - Worries or fears concerning the burden or challenges that their death will impose on others
  - Implication: inviting the patient to speak to issues that might prepare their loved ones for a future without them
- Care tenor
  - Refers to the attitude and manner with which others interact with the patient that may or may not promote dignity
  - The tenor of dignity therapy is empathic, nonjudgmental, encouraging and respectful

Dignity psychotherapy question protocol (Chochinov 2005)

- Tell me a little about your life history; particularly the parts that you either remember most or think are the most important? When did you feel most alive?
- Are there specific things that you would want your family to know about you, and are there particular things you would want them to remember?
- What are the most important roles you have played in life (family roles, vocational roles, community-service roles, etc)? Why were they so important to you, and what do you think you accomplished in those roles?
- What are your most important accomplishments, and what do you feel most proud of?

- Are there particular things that you feel still need to be said to your loved ones or things that you would want to take your time to say once again?
- What are your hopes and dreams for your loved ones?
- What have you learned about life that you would want to pass along to others? What advices or words of guidance would you wish to pass along to your (son, daughter, husband, wife, parents, others)?
- Are there words or perhaps even instructions that you would like to offer your family to help prepare them for the future?
- In creating this permanent record, are there other things that you woud like to include?

Well-being of Palliative Care Patients

Introduction

Relieving suffering and increasing well-being are interrelated but not equal. We may be very good in relieving suffering of patients but not very good in making them happy.

Types of well-being

- Hedonic well-being
    - Advocates maximizing pleasure and minimizing pain
    - Model of subjective well-being (Diener 1984)
        - Subjective well-being (SWB) = high level of positive affect (maximizing pleasure) + low level of negative affect (minimizing pain) + high degree of life satisfaction
- Eudaimonic well-being
    - Single-minded pursuit of sensory pleasure and avoidance of pain does not lead to a lasting form of well-being
    - True well-being is found by living a virtuous life
    - Multiple models
        - Psychological well-being (Ryff 1995)
            - Self-acceptance
            - Personal growth
            - Positive relationships
            - Autonomy
            - Purpose in life
            - Environmental mastery
        - Self-determination theory (Deci 2000)
            - Competence
            - Relatedness

- Autonomy
- The theory of flow (Csikszentmihalyi 1975)
    - Flow denotes the holistis sensation present when we act with total involvement
    - Characteristics of flow (Nakamura 2002)
        - Intense and focused concentration
        - Merging of action and awareness
        - Loss of self-consciousness
        - A sense of control
        - Distortion of temporal experience
        - Experience of the activity as intrinsically rewarding (autotelic experience)
    - The authentic happiness model (Seligman 2011)
        - Positive emotions
        - Engagement
        - Meaningful life
        - Positive relationships
        - Positive accomplishments

Types of well-being of palliative care patients (Tan 2014)

- Attitudinal well-being
    - Positive attitude: the psychological tendency of a person to think, feel, or act in a particular way that is conducive to his or her own well-being
        - Acceptance: an attitude that allows things to happen as it is without any denial or resistance
        - Kindness: an attitude characterized by the concern for others
        - Resilience: the universal capacity which allows a person to overcome the damaging effects of adversity (Newman 2004)

- Volitional well-being
  - Positive volitional activities
    - Positive cognitions: thoughts that contribute to one's own well-being
      - Hope: a psychological function of a person that involves the desiring of a specific outcome
      - Optimism: the positive view of a person that enables him or her to interpret events with the best possible explanation that is conducive to his or her own well-being
      - Faith: the confident belief in something that gives the person energy to move forward irrespective of the direness of the situations
      - Wisdom: the awareness of a person regarding the truth of a situation or an experience and the ways to deal with it
    - Positive emotions: emotions that contribute to one's own well-being
      - Happiness: a pleasant emotion that occurs when one is involved in a relationship, activity, or thought that is perceived by him or her as pleasurable or meaningful
      - Calmness: an emotion that occurs when one is completely or partially free from negative thoughts or emotions
    - Positive engagement: the active participation of a person in activities that promote well-being
      - Routine activities: customary activities
      - Leisure activities: enjoyable activities
    - Positive relationships: supportive relationships
      - Practical support
      - Psychological support

- Perceptual well-being
    - Positive circumstances: situations that contribute to the well-being of a person
        - Symptom-free
        - Functional

Six approaches to enhance well-being (Tan 2014)

- Attitudinal interventions
    - Facilitate acceptance
    - Foster kindness
    - Promote resilience
- Cognitive interventions
    - Foster hope
    - Support optimism
    - Strengthen faith
    - Acknowledge wisdom
- Emotional interventions
    - Conduct practices that promote happiness
    - Conduct practices that promote calmness
- Behavioural interventions
    - Encourage engagement in meaningful routines
    - Encourage engagement in enjoyable activities
- Interpersonal interventions
    - Mobilize practical support
    - Mobilize psychological support
- Circumstantial interventions
    - Symptom control
    - Support making full use of remaining functions

Caregiver Suffering

Introduction

Suffering affects both patients and family caregivers reciprocally. However, family caregivers are often left out by healthcare professionals, to the degree that we can label their suffering as "disenfranchised suffering". Family caregivers are "second-order patients" with their own care needs requiring medical attention.

The model of compassion suffering (Tan 2013)

- Compassion is the perception of another's suffering, coupled with the intention and action to relieve it
- Compassion suffering is a state of severe distress associated with caring of another person
  - Perception component
  - Intention component
  - Action component
- Perception component
  - Empathic suffering
    - Empathic suffering from seeing
      - Seeing suffering of patient
        - Physical suffering
        - Functional decline
        - Emotional suffering
        - Treatment-related suffering
        - Death and dying
      - Seeing family stress
        - Tiredness in the family
        - Sadness in the family
        - Denial in the family

- Seeing suffering of other patients
  - Abandonment by family
- Empathic suffering from hearing
  - Hearing bad news from doctors
    - Terminal diagnosis
    - Abnormal blood results
    - Disease progression
    - Additional chemotherapy
    - Coma
    - Short prognosis
  - Hearing expression of suffering from patient
    - Expression of unbearable suffering
    - Expression of the desire to give up
    - Expression of death and dying
- Empathic suffering from worrying
  - Worrying about patient
    - Pain and suffering
    - Nutritional status
    - Complications
    - Side effects of treatment
    - Prognosis
  - Worrying about other family members
    - Grief in the family
- Anticipatory grief
  - Perceived impending death of patient
    - Perceptions
      - Recognizing dying
        - Knowing the incurability of sickness
        - Hearing treatment discontinuation
      - Witnessing dying
        - Seeing patient deteriorate
        - Seeing patient eat less

- - Seeing patient talk less
  - Seeing patient sleep most of the time
  - Seeing patient unresponsive
- Cognitions
  - Hopes for patient
    - Hope for cure
    - Hope for survival
    - Hope for function
    - Hope for quality of life
    - Hope for a good after-life
    - Hopelessness
  - Hopes for oneself
    - Hope to return to a normal life
    - Hope to be with patient
  - Beliefs
    - Belief in staying positive
    - Belief in decision of God
  - Denial
    - Complete denial
    - Partial denial
- Emotions
  - Shock
  - Fear
  - Anxiety
  - Sadness
  - Frustration
  - A mixture of emotions
- Perceived impending absence of patient
  - Current absence
    - Absence of company for daily activities
    - Absence of company at home
    - Absence of company for talking

- Absence of company for support
- Role substitution
- Perceived absence when patient can't talk
- Future absence
  - Anticipated loneliness
  - Anticipated quietness
  - Anticipated sadness
  - Anticipated aimlessness
  - Anticipated supportlessness
  - Anticipated life changes
  - Concerns about new life without patient
- Intention component
  - Obsessive-compulsive suffering
    - Compassion obsession
      - Obsession with giving the best care
      - Obsession with giving 24-hour company
      - Obsession with pleasing patient
      - Obsession with motivating patient
      - Ignoring career
      - Ignoring job and income
      - Ignoring own social life
      - Ignoring own health
      - Concealing own grief
      - Concealing own exhaustion
      - Avoidance of discussing sickness with patient
      - Avoidance of discussing death with patient
    - Existential obsession
      - Obsession with keeping patient alive
        - Seeking multiple medical opinions
        - Seeking alternative medicine
        - Seeking various nutritional supplements
        - Pressurizing medical team to treat

- Promising to do good
- Performing life-prolonging rituals
- Praying for miracle
- Willingness to sacrifice own life
- Doing compulsion
  - Compulsion to do something for patient
    - Not comfortable in doing nothing
    - Not comfortable in sitting down and cry
    - Doing something without knowing benefit
    - Doing something despite own exhaustion
- Helpless-powerless suffering
  - Lack of information
    - Not knowing what to do
      - When patient is getting weaker
      - When patient is dying
      - When patient is not eating
      - When patient is not talking
      - When patient is restless
      - When patient is in pain
      - When patient insists to go home
    - Not knowing what to say
      - When patient expresses
        - Unberable suffering
        - Burdening of family
        - Knowledge about impending death
        - Desire to give up
        - Desire to die
        - Unwillingness to die
    - Not knowing what to expect
    - Not knowing how long patient can live

- Lack of support
  - Lack of support
    - Assisting patient functionally
    - Temporary relief
    - Overnight relief
    - Home medical support
    - Home nursing support
  - Difficulty to get support
    - Everyone has own commitment
    - Lack of leave during year end
    - Dispute in scheduling care
    - Fear of troubling others
    - Belief that help should be voluntary
  - Dissatisfaction with support
    - Nonsupportive family
    - Family is not doing enough
      - Not talking to patient
      - Not motivating patient
      - Not cheering patient up
  - Criticism from family and friends
    - Criticism in the way of caring
    - Criticism in sacrificing own job for caring
- Action component
  - Obligatory suffering
    - Companionship burden
      - 24-hour company
      - Overnight company
      - Final days company
      - Final moments presence
    - Functional burden
      - Functional assistance
        - Activities of daily living

- - - Instrumental activities
  - Unfinished business
  - Decision input
- Financial burden
  - Expenses
    - Treatment
    - Hospitalization
    - Medical equipment
    - Traditional medicine
    - Daily necessities like milk and diapers
- Cheer-making burden
  - Making patient happy
    - Family gatherings
    - Outdoor activities
- Impedimental suffering
  - Patient-related obstacles
    - Difficult circumstances
      - Excessive dependence
      - Bad temper
      - Conflict in opinion
      - Desire to die
      - Confusion state
      - Withdrawal from external world
    - Lack of appreciation from patient
    - Complaints from patient
  - Family-related obstacles
    - Family conflict
      - Continuation vs stopping treatment
      - Conventional vs alternative treatment
      - Different alternative medicine options
      - Different levels of acceptance in the family
      - Different levels of involvement

- .Different ways of caring
- Healthcare-related obstacles
  - Information issues
    - Lack of medical information
      - Disease
      - Complications
      - Side effects of treatment
      - Updates on progress of patient
    - Lack of opportunity to meet doctors
  - Interaction issues
    - Poor communication
      - Lack of listening
      - Lack of sensitivity
      - Lack of hope-giving
      - Lack of nonabandonment statement
      - Told "nothing much can be done"
      - Paternalistic communication
    - Lack of empathy
    - Lack of compassion
    - Poor attitude
  - Institution issues
    - Long waiting time
    - Noisy hospital environment
    - Witnessing suffering of other patients
    - Witnessing death of other patients
- Repercussion suffering
  - Personal life repercussion
    - Physical exhaustion
    - Psychological exhaustion
      - Sadness
      - Worry
      - Rumination

- Guilt
- Regret
- Fear
- Countertransferences
  - Fear of getting cancer
  - Fear of dying
  - Fear of burdening family in the future
- Sleep disturbances
- Loss of freedom
- Loss of personal time
- Spiritual suffering
  - Questioning "Why me?"
  - Questioning God
- Social life repercussion
  - Loss of family life
  - Loss of socialization with friends
  - Loss of recreational activities
  - Loss of promotion
  - Loss of job

The relief of caregiver suffering

- Perception approaches
  - Empathic suffering
    - Palliation of patient's suffering
  - Anticipatory grief
    - Supportive listening
- Intention approaches
  - Obsessive-compulsive suffering
    - Self-care emphasis
    - Supportive listening
    - Shift of curing to caring duties

- Helpless-powerless suffering
  - Information giving
  - Mobilizing support
- Action approaches
  - Obligatory suffering
    - Mobilizing support
    - Respite care
  - Impedimental suffering
    - Conflict resolution
    - Family meeting
    - Communication training of healthcare providers
  - Repercussion suffering
    - Self-care emphasis
    - Social connection encouragement

Little advices

- Pay attention to family caregivers
- Explore caregiver suffering
- Remind caregivers to take care of themselves too
- Remind caregivers to **EAT**, **SLEEP** and **RELAX**
- Teach caregivers to practice mindful caregiving as opposed to automatic caregiving

Mindful caregiving:

   Paying attention to caregiving on purpose
   Paying attention in the present moment
   Paying attention nonjudgmentally

Grief and Bereavement

Introduction

Most bereaved family members require no specific intervention. They recover with the support of family and friends, and time. Only 10-20% of family members who remain stuck in their grief require further assistance.

Terms

- Grief: the distressing emotional response to any loss, including related feelings, cognitions and behaviours (Genevro 2004)
- Bereavement: the state of having experienced a loss resulting from death (Genevro 2004)
- Mourning: the process of adaptation to a loss, which includes expression of grief and behaviours influenced by culture, religion, and social evens, such as grieving rituals (Raphael 1983)
- Anticipated grief: the distress and related emotions, cognitions, and behaviours that occur before an expected loss (Raphael 1983)
- Pathological grief: a severely distressing and disabling abnormal emotional response to loss that involves mental and physical dysfunction (Jacobs 1993)
- Disenfranchised grief: grief that occurs with losses that are not recognized by society, resulting in less social permission to express one's grief (Doka 1989)

Theories of grief and bereavement

- The four phases of grief (Bowlby 1973, Parkes 1998)
  - Phase 1: shock and numbness
    - Feeling that the loss is not real
    - Feeling impossible to accept
    - Somatic symptoms
    - Emotional shut-down if stuck
  - Phase 2: yearning and searching
    - Acutely aware of the void left from the loss
    - The imagined future is no longer possible
    - Searching for comfort one used to have together
    - Trying to fill the void
    - Preoccupied with the person
    - Looking for reminders of the person
    - Looking for ways to be close to the person
    - Remain preoccupied with the person if stuck
  - Phase 3: despair and disorganization
    - Accepted the irreversible loss
    - Hopelessness and despair
    - Anger and questioning
    - Feeling meaningless without the person
    - Remain negative and hopeless if stuck
  - Phase 4: reorganization and recovery
    - Faith in life restored
    - New goals and patterns of day-to-day life established
    - Realizing that life can still be positive
    - Grief continues to influence oneself but no longer at the forefront of the mind

- The five phases of grief (Lindemann 1994)
  - Somatic disturbances
  - Preoccupation with the image of the deceased
  - Guilt, reviewing behaviour that occurred before the death for evidence of negligence or failure
  - Feeling of hostility or anger
  - Difficulty in carrying out everyday routines
- The five stages of grief (Kübler-Ross 1969)
  - Denial
  - Anger
  - Bargaining
  - Depression
  - Acceptance
- The four tasks of mourning (Worden 1991)
  - Task 1: to accept the reality of loss
  - Task 2: to work through and experience the pain of grief
  - Task 3: to adjust to an environment without the deceased
  - Task 4: to withdraw emotionally from or relocate the deceased and move on
- The dual process model of coping with bereavement (Stroebe and Schut 1999)
  - Loss-orientated processes
    - Grief work
    - Intrusion of grief
    - Denial or avoidance of restoration changes
    - Breaking bonds or ties
  - Restoration-orientated processes
    - Attending to life changes
    - Distraction from grief
    - Doing new things
    - Establishing new roles/identities/relationships

Prolonged grief disorder (Prigerson 2009)

- Bereavement: loss of a significant other
- Separation distress: yearning daily or to a disabling degree
- ≥ 5 symptoms
  - Confusion about one's role in life or diminished sense of self (feeling that a part of oneself has died)
  - Difficulty accepting the loss
  - Avoidance of reminders of the reality of the loss
  - Inability to trust others since the loss
  - Bitterness or anger related to the loss
  - Difficulty moving on with life
  - Numbness
  - Feeling that life is unfulfilling, empty, and meaningless
  - Feeling stunned, dazed, or shocked by the loss
- > 6 months since the death
- Social impairment
- No Major Depressive Disorder, Generalized Anxiety Disorder or Posttraumatic Stress Disorder

Addressing grief and bereavement

- Before death
  - Communicate prognosis timely and sensitively
  - Prepare family
  - Allow family to grieve
  - Facilitate expression of grief if suppressed
- At the time of death
  - Allow family to see the deceased before last office
  - Allow family time to grieve before last office
  - Give practical information on procedures after death
- After death
  - Follow up contact
    - Condolences phone call

- Sympathy card
- Home visits
- Attending funeral if appropriate
- Annual commemoration services
- Grief and bereavement counseling
  - Bereaved individuals who request help
  - High risk bereaved individuals
  - Prolonged grief disorders

Self-care

Introduction

Caring of oneself and caring of others are inseparable. If we cannot take good care of ourselves, we cannot take good care of others. If we ourselves are unhappy, it will be hard for us to make others happy, more so in terminally ill patients.

Stress

- Definitions of stress
  - The non-specific response of the body to any demand for change (Selye 1956)
  - Non-specific: different noxious stimuli → similar response
  - A constellation of physiological, cognitive, emotional and behavioural reactions as a person is confronted with perceived threat and challenges (Harrington 2013)
- Stressor: an event that provokes stress
- Acute stress reaction: fight-or-flight response (Cannon 1932)
- Chronic stress reaction (Selye 1956)
  - General adaptation syndrome
    - Alarm stage
    - Resistance stage
    - Exhaustion stage
- Types of stress
  - Eustress: positive stress
  - Distress: negative stress
- Sources of stress
  - Major life events or daily hassles
  - Internal or self-generated

The transactional model of stress and coping

- By Lazarus and Folkman 1984
- Stress is a transaction (two-way process) between a person and the situation in the form of cognitive appraisals
- Primary appraisal
    - The relevant significance of the situation as a threat
        - Motivational relevance: relevance of the situation to the person own well-being
        - Motivation congruence: congruence of the situation with the person's goals
    - Stress is the perceived discrepancy between what one has in a given situation and what one wants in that situation
- Secondary appraisal: the capacity of the person to cope
    - Problem-focused coping: the capacity to improve the situation so that it is more congruent with one's goals
    - Emotion-focused coping: the capacity to adapt to the situation when the situation remains incongruent with one's goals

Types of stressors in palliative care (Vachon 1995)

- Personal factors
    - Age
    - Sex
    - Ethnicity
    - Family status
    - Financial status
    - Work experiences
    - Qualifications
    - Personal values
    - Coping styles
    - Social support

- Work factors
  - Work environment problems
    - Communication problems within the organization
    - Inadequate resources
    - Unrealistic expectations of the system
  - Role problems
    - Role strain
    - Role ambiguity
    - Role conflict
  - Patient-family problems
    - Dealing and communicating with dying patients
    - Dealing and communicating with young patients
    - Dealing and communicating with non-coping family

Cognitive appraisals of palliative care providers

- Primary appraisals
  - Perceived mismatch between the person and the working environment
  - Perceived imbalance between job demands, job resources and workplace support
- Secondary appraisals
  - Problem-focused coping
    - Good communication with patients
    - Good communication with family members
    - Good communication with colleagues
    - Being connected with patients
    - Practice of exquisite empathy
    - Optimism
    - Self-efficacy
    - Receiving social support
  - Emotion-focused coping
    - Positive reinterpretation

- Meaning making
- Humour
- Practice of mindfulness
- Healthy lifestyle engagement
- Turning to religion
- Praying
- Taking a break

The Total Care Model of Palliative Care Stress (Tan 2013)

- Stress of palliative care providers
    - Problems in caring for others (healthcare)
    - Problems in interacting with others (interpersonal care)
    - Problems in caring for oneself (self-care)
- Healthcare
    - Organizational challenges
        - Team dysfunction
            - Lack of shared team philosophy
            - Lack of caring attitude in team members
            - Lack of team cooperation
            - Lack of competence in team members
            - Lack of team communication
            - Lack of team support
            - Inter-team dispute
        - Resources, staffing and working environment
            - Lack of hospital resources
            - Lack of staffing
            - Lack of understanding of the complex system
    - Care overload
        - Heavy workloads
            - Incapacity to attend to all distressed patients
            - Multiple calls from patients and family
            - Time-consuming nature of the work of caring

- Too many orders from the superior
- Difficult encounters
  - Uncontrolled pain
  - Repetitive requests for more analgesia
  - Difficult branula insertions
  - Unrealistic expectations from patients or family
  - Request for hastening of death
  - Pressure from family to monitor closely
  - Pressure from family to do everything possible
  - Pressure from family to give futile treatment
  - Family interfering with treatment decisions
  - Family giving instructions for doctors to follow
  - Family's impatience
  - Family's inability to accept patient's death
  - Family's begging to hasten patient's death
  - Too many visiting family members
- Interpersonal care
  - Communication challenges
    - With patients
      - Communicating prognosis
      - Dealing with strong emotions
      - Dealing with strong denial
      - Dealing with difficult questions
      - Lack of time to build rapport
      - Repetitive listening to patient's suffering
      - Language barrier
      - Attending to non-communicative patients
    - With family members
      - Being asked too many questions
      - Different relatives asking same questions
      - Dealing with big family
      - Difficult to please all family members

479

- Dealing with fussy family members
- Dealing with non-disclosure
- Dealing with intense grief
  - With colleagues
    - Lack of communication
    - Lack of consideration
    - Lack of listening
    - Lack of empathy
- Differences in opinion
  - With patients and family members
    - Disagreement in prognosis
    - Disagreement in treatment option
    - Disagreement in treatment futility
    - Disagreement in goals of care
    - Disagreement in end-of-life discussion
    - Conflicting views among different relatives
  - With colleagues
    - Disagreement in prognosis
    - Disagreement in treatment option
    - Disagreement in treatment futility
    - Disagreement in goals of care
    - Disagreement among different specialists
- Misperceptions and misconceptions
  - From patients and family members
    - Regarding palliative care referral
      - A sign of giving up
      - A sign of nothing more can be done
      - A sign of not doing anything
    - Regarding morphine and sedatives
      - Rejecting use of morphine
      - Rejecting dose titration
      - Requesting for discontinuation of sedative

- Regarding cancer
  - Cancer means suffering
  - Cancer means death
- Regarding disclosure of cancer diagnosis
  - Disclosure generates depression
  - Disclosure causes giving up
  - Disclosure expedites death
- Self-care
  - Personal expectations
    - Perception of having not done enough
      - Lack of time to see patients
      - Lack fo time to see patients regularly
      - Lack of time to attend to patients immediately
      - Feeling upset for the incapacity to fulfil request
      - Feeling guilty for not doing enough
      - Being criticized for not doing anything
    - Perceived failure
      - Failure to prevent young deaths
      - Failure to extend life of patients
      - Failure to relieve suffering
      - Failure to fulfil patient's wish
      - Failure to change misperceptions
      - Failure to help patients in strong denial
    - Perceived helplessness
      - Feeling helpless when young patients die
      - Feeling helpless when patients die alone
      - Feeling helpless when nothing can be done
      - Feeling helpless when patients gasp for breath
      - Feeling powerless when patients desire death

- Emotional involvement
  - Emotional vulnerability
    - In seeing pain and suffering
      - Patient devastated by bad news
      - Patient develops multiple problems
      - Patient confused by different information
      - Patient stuck at emergency
      - Patient has unnecessary investigations
      - Patient asked to fast for investigations
      - Patient cries
      - Patient gives up
      - Relative grieves
    - In seeing death and dying
      - Seeing patient deteriorates
      - Seeing patient dies
      - Harder to see certain patients die
        - Close patients
        - Children
        - Young patients
        - Young patients with children
        - Patients who are breadwinners
        - Elderly patients for some
      - Circumstantial vulnerability
        - Sudden death
        - Sudden absences in ward
        - Multiple deaths in short time
  - Emotional reactivity
    - Feeling sad when patient dies
    - Feeling angry with demanding family
    - Feeling frustrated when patient presents late
    - Feeling guilty when patient dies post-treatment
    - Feeling helpless when not knowing what to do

- Feeling puzzled why patient has to die
- Difficulty controlling emotions before patient
- Grieving after patient's death
- Death and dying thoughts
  - Worrying about own death
  - Worrying about how one will die in the future
  - Worrying about getting cancer
  - Worrying about dying with pain and suffering
  - Fear of death
  - Fear of suffering
  - Fear of separation with family
  - Fear of death of other family members
  - Fear of suffering of family members

Countertransference

- A result of the patient's influence on the physician's unconscious feelings (Freud 1910)
- The reactions that arise in the therapist as a result of the patient's influence on the therapist's unconscious feelings and have their origins in the therapist's identification and projection (Noyes 1963)
- The totality of feelings experienced by the clinician towards the patient – whether conscious or unconscious or whether prompted by the client's dynamics or by issues or events in the clinician's own life (Katz 2006)

Vicarious traumatization

- The negative transformation in the therapist's inner experience resulting from empathic engagement with clients' trauma material (Pearlman 1995)

Compassion fatigue

- The natural consequent behaviors and emotions resulting from knowing about a traumatizing event experienced by a significant other – the stress resulting from helping or wanting to help a traumatized or suffering person (Figley 1995)

Moral distress

- Moral distress occurs when one knows the right thing to do, but institutional constraints make it nearly impossible to pursue the right course of action (Jameton 1984)
- Moral distress is the painful psychological disequilibrium that results from recognizing the ethically appropriate action, yet not taking it, because of such obstacles as lack of time, supervisory reluctance, an inhibiting medical power structure, institution policy, or legal considerations (Corley 2001)
- Moral distress is the physical or emotional suffering that is experienced when constraints (internal or external) prevent one from following the course of action that one believes is right

Burnout

- A psychological syndrome in response to chronic interpersonal stressors on the job (Maslach 1982)
- A state of mental and physical exhaustion caused by excessive and prolonged stress (Girdin 1996)
- Dimensions of burnout
  - Emotional exhaustion
    - The basic individual stress dimension of burnout
    - The feelings of being overextended and depleted of one's emotional and physical resources
  - Depersonalization (cynicism)
    - The interpersonal context dimension of burnout

- A negative, callous, or excessively detached response to various aspects of the job
  - Personal accomplishment
    - The self-evaluation dimension of burnout
    - Feelings of incompetence and lack of achievement and productivity at work
- The 12 phases of burnout cycle (Freudenberger 2006)
  - A compulsion to prove oneself
  - Working harder
  - Neglecting own needs
  - Displacement of conflicts
  - Revision of values
  - Denial of emerging problems
  - Withdrawal
  - Obvious behavioural changes
  - Depersonalization
  - Inner emptiness
  - Depression
  - Burnout syndrome

Coping

- Coping comprises both behavioral and cognitive strategies aimed at managing the internal and external demands of stressful transactions (Lazarus 1984)
- Defence mechanism: an unconscious psychological mechanism that reduces anxiety arising from unacceptable or potentially harmful stimuli (Schacter 2011)
- Defence mechanisms are not to be confused with conscious coping strategies

- Maladaptive defence mechanisms
  - Acting out: direct expression of an unconscious wish or impulse in action, without conscious awareness of the emotion that drives that expressive behaviour
  - Blocking: temporary or transiently inhibiting thinking
  - Controlling: attempting to manage or regulate events or objects in the environment to minimize anxiety and to resolve inner conflicts
  - Delusional projection: grossly frank delusions about external reality, usually of a persecutory nature
  - Denial: refusal to accept external reality because it is too threatening
  - Displacement: redirection of an intense emotion toward someone or something that is less offensive or threatening in order to avoid dealing directly with what is frightening or threatening
  - Dissociation: temporary drastic modification of one's personal identity or character to avoid emotional distress
  - Distortion: a gross reshaping of external reality to meet internal needs
  - Externalization: tending to perceive in the external world and in external objects elements of one's own personality, including instinctual impulses, conflicts, moods, attitudes, and styles of thinking
  - Fantasy: tendency to retreat into fantasy in order to resolve inner and outer conflicts
  - Hypochondriasis: an excessive preoccupation or worry about having a serious illness
  - Idealization: unconsciously choosing to perceive another individual as having more positive qualities than he or she may actually have

486

- Identification: the unconscious modelling of one's self upon another person's character and behaviour
- Inhibition: consciously limiting or renouncing some ego functions, alone or in combinations, to evade anxiety arising out of conflict with instinctual impulses, the superego, or environmental forces or figures
- Intellectualization: concentrating on the intellectual components of a situation so as to distance oneself from the associated anxiety-provoking emotions
- Introjection: identifying with some idea or object so deeply that it becomes a part of that person
- Isolation: separation of feelings from ideas and events
- Passive aggression: aggression towards others expressed indirectly or passively such as using procrastination
- Projection: shifting one's unacceptable thoughts, feelings and impulses within oneself onto someone else, such that those same thoughts, feelings, beliefs and motivations are perceived as being possessed by the other
- Projective identification: the object of projection invokes in that person precisely the thoughts, feelings or behaviours projected
- Rationalization (making excuses): offering rational explanations in an attempt to justify attitudes, beliefs or behaviour that may otherwise be unacceptable
- Reaction formation: transforming an unacceptable impulse into its opposite
- Regression: temporary reversion of the ego to an earlier stage of development rather than handling unacceptable impulses in a more adult way
- Repression: expelling or withholding from consciousness an idea or feeling

- Somatization: converting psychic derivatives into bodily symptoms and tending to react with somatic manifestations, rather than psychic manifestations
- Splitting: segregating experiences into all-good and all-bad categories, with no room for ambiguity
- Undoing: trying to 'undo' an unhealthy, destructive or threatening thought by engaging in contrary behaviour
- Upward and downward social comparisons: looking to another individual or group who is considered to be worse off in order to dissociate oneself from perceived similarities and to make oneself feel better
- Wishful thinking: making decisions according to what might be pleasing to imagine instead of by appealing to evidence, rationality or reality
- Adaptive defence mechanisms
  - Altruism: constructive service to others that brings pleasure and personal satisfaction
  - Anticipation: realistic planning for future discomfort
  - Humour: overt expression of ideas and feelings (especially those that are unpleasant to focus on or too terrible to talk about) that gives pleasure to others
  - Sublimation: transformation of negative emotions or instincts into positive actions, behaviour, or emotion
  - Thought suppression: consciously or semiconsciously postponing attention to a conscious impulse or conflict
- Cognitive distortions: irrational thinking patterns
  - All-or-none thinking, dichotomous reasoning, polarized thinking, splitting: seeing things in absolute, black-and-white categories
  - Always being right: actively trying to prove one's actions or thoughts to be correct

- Blaming: holding other people responsible for the harm they cause
- Catastrophizing: an extreme form of magnification, giving greater weight to the worst possible outcome, however unlikely
- Control fallacies: feeling oneself as a victim of fate (external control) or assuming responsibility for the well-being of others (internal control)
- Disqualifying the positive: discounting positive events
- Emotional reasoning: thinking something is true, solely based on a feeling
- Fallacy of change: expecting others to change to suit oneself if one just pressures or cajoles them enough
- Fallacy of fairness: believing that life is fair according to your definition
- Filtering: picking out a single negative detail and dwelling on it exclusively
- Heaven's reward fallacy: expecting one's sacrifice to pay off, as if someone is keeping score
- Jumping to conclusions: making a negative interpretation though there are no definite facts that convincingly support conclusion
- Labeling: attaching a negative label to oneself or others
- Magical thinking: attributing causal relationships between actions and events which seemingly cannot be justified by reason and observation
- Magnification: exaggerating the importance of things
- Mind reading: a form of jumping to conclusion, concluding arbitrarily that someone is reacting negatively to oneself
- Minimization: shrinking things inappropriately until they appear tiny

- Overgeneralization: seeing a single negative event as a never-ending pattern of defeat
- Oversimplification: looking for incorrect mental shortcuts
- Personalization: seeing oneself as the cause of some negative external event which in fact one was not primarily responsible for
- Should statements: criticizing oneself or others with "Shoulds" or "Shouldn'ts". "Musts", "Oughts" and "Have tos" are similar offenders
- The Fortune Teller Error: a form of jumping to conclusion, anticipating that things will turn out badly
- Conscious coping strategies (Lazarus and Folkman 1984)
  - Problem-focused coping
    - To change or eliminate stressors
      - Taking control
      - Information seeking
      - Evaluating the pros and cons
  - Emotion-focused coping
    - To alleviate distress triggered by stressors
      - Disclaiming
      - Escape-avoidance
      - Accepting responsibility or blame
      - Exercising self-control
      - Positive reappraisal

Coping strategies in palliative care (Tan 2013)

Healthcare

- Organizational challenges
  - Team dysfunction
    - Adopt similar team philosophy
    - Define role clearly
    - Encourage team cooperation and commitment

- Open team communication
- Regular team meeting
- Resources, staffing and working environment
  - Mobilize resources
  - Increase staffing
  - Improve working environment
- Care overload
  - Heavy workload
    - Prioritize visits based on needs
    - Help patients bit by bit
    - Practice teamworking
  - Difficult encounter
    - Try to understand patient's perspective
    - Try to understand family's perspective
    - Cognitive reappraisal of the situation
    - Facilitate shifting of expectation
    - Facilitate grieving
    - Debriefing sessions

Interpersonal care

- Communication challenges
  - Learn and practice good communication skills
  - Practice empathy
  - Explore hope and preferences
  - Give hope
- Differences in opinion
  - Learn to agree to disagree
  - Respect differences in opinion
  - Allow time for change
- Misperceptions and misconceptions
  - Give adequate information
  - Acknowledge misperceptions and misconceptions

- Respect preferences
- Allow time for change

Self-care

- Personal expectation
  - Debriefing sessions
  - Cognitive reappraisal
  - Practice mindfulness
    - Non-appraisal
    - Non-attachment to outcome
- Emotional involvement
  - Improve emotional competence
  - Debriefing sessions
  - Practice mindfulness
    - Non-reactive
    - Letting go
  - Work-life balance
    - Eat well
    - Sleep well
    - Exercise
    - Socialize
    - Hobbies
    - Relaxation
    - Meditation
    - Taking a break
- Death and dying thought
  - Spirituality
    - Having a personal philosophy of life and death
    - Finding meaning in work
    - Finding meaning in life
    - Reflection on personal mortality
    - Imagine the deceased going to a better place

- Connect with family, friends, nature, art, music
- Connect with the significance and the sacred
- Prayer
- Meditate
- Rituals

The 3 essential practices of self-care

1. Practice mindfulness
2. Practice happiness
3. Practice kindness

Mindfulness

Introduction

While science is an excellent method to study the natural world, mindfulness is a universal human capacity to study the inner world, or the mind. The former focuses on looking "outside" and the latter focuses on "looking inside". Looking inside is crucial in the pursuit of an enduring happiness.

The three stages in practicing mindfulness

- Understanding mindfulness
- Experiencing mindfulness
- Living mindfully

What is mindfulness?

- Mindfulness = sati in Pali = bare attention
- Paying attention in a particular way: on purpose, in the present moment, nonjudgmentally (Kabat-Zinn 1994)
- When you first become aware of something, there is a fleeting instant of pure awareness just before you conceptualize the thing, before you identify it. That is a state of awareness. Ordinarily, this state is short-lived. It is that flashing split second just as you focus your eyes on the thing, just as you focus your mind on the thing, just before you objectify it, clamp down on it mentally, and segregate it from the rest of existence. It takes place just before you start thinking about it – before your mind says, "Oh, it's a dog." That flowing, soft-focused moment of pure awareness is mindfulness. (Gunaratana 2011)

Characteristics of mindfulness (Gunaratana 2011)

- Mindfulness is mirror-thought: it reflects only what is happening and in exactly the way it is happening
- Mindfulness is nonjudgmental observation: it is that ability of the mind to observe without criticism
- Mindfulness accepts whatever experience we may be having
- Mindfulness is impartial watchfulness: it does not take sides
- Mindfulness is nonconceptual awareness: it does not get involved with thoughts or concepts. It just looks.
- Mindfulness is present-moment awareness: it takes place in the here and now
- Mindfulness is nonegotistic alertness: it takes place without reference to self
- Mindfulness is awareness of change: it is observing the passing flow of experience
- Mindfulness is participatory observation: the meditator is both participant and observer at one and the same time
- Mindfulness is extremely difficult to define in words: not because it is complex, but because it is too simple and open
- Mindfulness is a presymbolic function: we can never fully express what it is

Three core elements of mindfulness (Shapiro 2006)

- Intention
  - Self-regulation
  - Self-exploration
  - Self-liberation
  - Selfless service
- Attention
  - Temporal: moment-to-moment attention
  - Quality: deep attention that "sinks" into its object

- Attitude
  - Acronym COAL (Siegel 2007)
    - Curiosity
    - Openness
    - Acceptance
    - Love
  - Nonjudging
  - Nonstriving
  - Nonattachment
  - Nonreactivity
  - Gentleness
  - Patience
  - Trust
  - Letting go

Benefits of mindfulness

- Improves pain acceptance
- Improves sleep
- Reduces stress
- Reduces anxiety and depression
- Integrates emotions
- Calms the body
- Increases cortical thickness (Lazar 2005)
- Increases telomerases and decelerates aging (Lengacher 2014)
- Improves immune function (Witek-Janusek 2008)

Mechanisms of mindfulness in stress reduction

- Paying attention on purpose
  - Attention regulation
- Paying attention in the present moment
  - Reduces rumination of the past
  - Reduces worry of the future

- Paying attention nonreactively
  - Metacognitive awareness: the ability to see one's thoughts and feelings as mental events, rather than the self
  - Decentering: the ability to observe one's thoughts and feelings as temporary, objective mental events
  - Defusion: the ability to be aware of one's thoughts, feelings and memories as passing events rather than "things" that are valid or invalid
  - Reperception: the ability to disidentify from the contents of consciousness, such as one's thoughts, feelings, and judgments and view one's moment-to-moment experience with greater clarity and objectivity

Measuring mindfulness

- Freiburg Mindfulness Inventory (Buchheld 2001)
  - 30 items
  - Nonjudgmental present-moment observation
  - Openness to negative experience
  - Designed for experienced meditators
- Mindful Attention Awareness Scale (Brown 2003)
  - 15 items
  - Awareness of present-moment experience in daily life
- Kentucky Inventory of Mindfulness Skills (Baer 2004)
  - 39 items
  - Observing present-moment experience
  - Describing: applying verbal labels
  - Acting with awareness
  - Accepting present-moment experience without judgment
- The Toronto Mindfulness Scale (Lau 2006)
  - 13 items
  - Curiosity
  - Decentering

- The Five Facet Mindfulness Questionnaire (Baer 2006)
  - 39 items
  - Observing
  - Describing
  - Acting with awareness
  - Non-judging of inner experience
  - Non-reactivity to inner experience
- The Cognitive and Affective Mindfulness Scale (Feldman 2007)
  - 12 items
  - Attention
  - Awareness
  - Present-focus
  - Acceptance
  - Non-judgment of thoughts and feelings
- The Southampton Mindfulness Questionnaire (Chadwick 2008)
  - 16 items
  - Mindful observation
  - Letting go
  - Non-aversion
  - Non-judgment
- The Philadelphia Mindfulness Scale (Cardaciotto 2008)
  - 20 items
  - Awareness
  - Acceptance

Slowing down

Slowing down is a prerequisite for the practice of mindfulness. With the current pace of our modern society, we rush a lot. We seldom have time for ourselves. The first step in establishing mindfulness is to slow down and to stop rushing. Then, it is easier for us to pay full attention to whatever we are doing. Try not to multi-task. Do one thing at a time, with our full attention.

The four foundation practices to establish mindfulness

- From <u>The Discourse on the Foundations of Mindfulness</u>
- Or <u>Satipatthana Sutta</u> in Pali
  - Mindfulness of the body
  - Mindfulness of feelings
  - Mindfulness of mind
  - Mindfulness of reality

Mindfulness of the body

- The first way to establish mindfulness
- The simplest and most direct way to reduce stress
- The basis of all other practices

Mindfulness of the breath

Exercise 1: conscious breathing

- Go to a quiet place
- Sit down comfortably
- Fold or cross legs; or sit on a chair
- Sit upright
- Observe the breath at the nose area
- Breathing in, I know I am breathing in
- Breathing out, I know I am breathing out
- Do not control the breath in any way
- Breathe naturally
- Do not be distracted by other thoughts
- Come back to the breath once we are distracted
- Practice for our own welfare , others and even the whole world
- Just be aware of the breath
- Breathe with full awareness of each breath

Exercise 2: following the breath

- Follow the breath closely
- Follow the entire length of the breath: "the breath body"
- Do not allow any distracting thought to enter
- Breathing in a long breath,
  I know I am breathing in a long breath
- Breathing out a long breath,
  I know I am breathing out a long breath
- Breathing in a short breath,
  I know I am breathing in a short breath
- Breathing out a short breath,
  I know I am breathing out a short breath
- Do not force ourselves to take long or short breath
- Breathe naturally
- Just be aware of the entire length of the breath
- Breathe with full awareness of the entire length of the breath
- As we follow the breath, the breath will calm naturally
- The breath will become smooth, regular and harmonious
- The flow of air will change from turbulent to laminar

Exercise 3: bringing our mind home to the body

- Use our breathing to bring our mind home to our body
- Stop ruminating about the past
- Stop worrying about the future
- Bring our mind back to the present moment
- Bring our mind and body together as one
- Breathing in, I am aware of my whole body
- Breathing out, I am aware of my whole body
- Feel the different parts of our body, from the top to the bottom
- Feel the body as a whole, fully united with the mind
- Feel the wholeness of ourselves with each breath

Exercise 4: calming the body

- Once our breath is harmonious, it will calm our body naturally
- Breathing in, I calm my body
- Breathing out, I calm my body
- Notice whether there is any tension in any part of our body
- Breathe and relax the tension one by one, from top to bottom
- Then relax the whole body all at once
- Feel the breath entering our body and calming all parts of body
- Feel the breath leaving our body and taking away our tiredness
- Feel the breath and the body calm down together

Mindfulness of postures

Exercise 5: awareness of postures

- Be aware of our bodily postures
- When sitting, I know I am sitting
- When sitting, just sit
- When standing, I know I am standing
- When standing, just stand
- When walking, I know I am walking
- When walking, just walk
- When lying down, I know I am lying down
- When lying down, just lie down
- The benefits of mindfulness of postures
  - It helps to maintain the continuity of mindfulness
  - It reveals our states of mind
  - It reveals the three universal characteristics of reality
    - The reality of impermanence (time)
    - The reality of selflessness (space)
    - The reality of suffering (mind)

- The reality of impermanence (anicca in Pali)
  - Notice the big changes from one posture to another
  - Notice the minute changes of sensation during movement
  - Slow down to notice the minute sensations
- The reality of selflessness (anatta in Pali)
  - Notice the different body parts during different postures
  - Notice the contact between the body and any support
  - Observe "who" is sitting, standing, walking or lying down
  - Observe the intention that initiates each action
  - Find out what and where is the "I" during each posture
- The reality of suffering (dukkha in Pali)
  - Notice the discomfort that causes us to change posture
  - Notice the temporary relief of discomfort with movement

Mindfulness of activities

Exercise 6: awareness of activities

- Practice full awareness of every activity
  - Waking up and falling asleep
  - Eating and drinking
  - Urinating and defecating
  - Sitting, standing and walking
  - Talking and keeping silent
- Full awareness (sampajanna)
  - Awareness of the purpose of an activity
    - Notice the purpose of an activity
    - Is the purpose wholesome or unwholesome?
    - Is the activity beneficial to us and others?
    - Notice the possibility to choose
    - Choose a wholesome activity
  - Awareness of the appropriateness of an activity
    - Notice the appropriateness of a wholesome activity
    - Is it the right time and place to perform the activity?

- Awareness of the four fields of practice
    - Knowing which field we are practicing
        - Mindfulness of the body
        - Mindfulness of feelings
        - Mindfulness of mind
        - Mindfulness of reality
    - Knowing when we are distracted
- Awareness of the three universal characteristics of reality
    - Notice the impermanent nature of each activity
        - The big change of an activity
        - The small change of an activity
    - Notice the selfless nature of each activity
        - The "self" is just a mental construction
        - The "self" is just a combination of:
            - The physical body
            - Sensations
            - Perceptions
            - Mental activities: cognitions and emotions
            - Consciousness
        - The "doing" without a "doer"
    - Notice the unsatisfactory nature of each activity

Mindfulness of the physical body

Exercise 7: bodily awareness

- Scan our body bottom-up from the soles of our feet
- Scan our body top-down from the top of the hair
- Scan the different parts of the body
    - Superficial somatic: head hair, body hair, nails, teeth, skin
    - Deep somatic: fat, muscles, tendon, ligament, bones, bone marrow, diaphragm
    - Solid visceral: brain, heart, lungs, liver, kidneys, spleen
    - Hollow visceral: stomach, small bowel, large bowel, feces

- Excretion fluid: tears, saliva, phlegm, mucus, sweat, urine
- Body fluid: bile, blood, lymph, pus, synovial fluid
- Notice the attractive and unattractive aspects of the body parts
- The benefits of mindfulness of the physical body
  - To decondition our strong identification with the body
    - Liking the superficial parts
    - Disliking the deeper parts
  - To lessen suffering that results from that identification
  - To deepen understanding of the three characteristics
    - Notice the impermanent nature of the body
      - The changes of the body
    - Notice the selfless nature of the body
      - The interdependent nature of the body
    - Notice the unsatisfactory nature of the body
      - The changes that we cannot accept

Exercise 8: awareness of body composition

- Be aware of the presence of earth elements in our body
  - Earth element: the solid nature of matter
- Be aware of the presence of water elements in our body
  - Water element: the liquid nature of matter
- Be aware of the presence of fire elements in our body
  - Fire element: the heat nature of matter
- Be aware of the presence of air elements in our body
  - Air element: the movement nature of matter
- Notice similar elements that constitute the earth and universe
- Notice the interrelated nature of our body and the earth
- Notice the interrelated nature of our body and the universe
- See our lives outside our bodies
- Transcend the boundary between self and nature
- Go beyond the limiting concepts of life and death

Exercise 9: contemplation of decomposition of a corpse

- The benefits of this exercise
  - Helps us to understand the decaying nature of our body
  - Helps us to become less attached to our body
  - Helps us to use and care for the body without attachment
  - Helps us to see the preciousness of life
  - Helps us to see the preciousness of time
- Visualize a corpse in various stages of decay
  - The body is bloated, discolored, festered and stinky
  - The body is crawling with insects and worms
  - The body is eaten by animals
  - The body is left with skeleton with little flesh and blood
  - The body is left with skeleton with no flesh but little blood
  - The body is left with skeleton with no more blood
  - The body is left with scattered bones
  - The body is left with bleached bones
  - The body is left with dried bones
  - The bones are reduced to a pile of dust
  - The dust disappears with a gust of wind
- It is not a pleasant exercise
- It is meant for someone with good physical and mental health
- The effect of this exercise can be liberating

Mindfulness of feelings

- Feeling is the English translation of the Pali word *vedana*
- Feeling in English can be a sensation, an emotion or an opinion
- Vedana carries a more specific meaning
  - It refers to the feeling tone
  - The quality of pleasantness, unpleasantness or neutrality
  - Key factor to free us from our deepest conditioning
  - Key factor to eliminate stress permanently

- The conditioning of reaction and action by *vedana*
  - Pleasant feeling
    - Reaction: craving, attachment
    - Action: addictive behaviour
  - Unpleasant feeling
    - Reaction: hate, aversion
    - Action: avoidance behaviour
  - Neutral feeling
    - Reaction: indifference, delusion
    - Action: couldn't-care-less behaviour
- The benefits of mindfulness of feelings
  - To recognize the transitory nature of feelings
  - To recognize our ingrained habitual reactions to feelings
  - To recognize our reactions to feelings, and not the object
  - To become less identified with feelings
    - Less attached to pleasant feeling
    - Less resistant to unpleasant feeling
    - Less unaware of neutral feeling
  - To become less judgmental and reactive
  - To foster calmness and equanimity

Exercise 10: identifying the feeling tone

- When a feeling arises, notice its feeling tone
- Watch the arising, maintaining and disappearing of the tone
- Do not attempt to control or change the feeling tone
- Just observe and return our attention to the breath
- Feeling a pleasant feeling,
  I know I am feeling a pleasant feeling
- Feeling an unpleasant feeling,
  I know I am feeling an unpleasant feeling
- Feeling a neutral feeling,
  I know I am feeling a neutral feeling

- Abandon the tendency to crave for pleasant feeling
- Abandon the tendency to hate unpleasant feeling
- Abandon the tendency to ignore neutral feeling
- Practice nonreactivity towards feeling
- Notice the moment-to-moment changes of feelings
- Notice the suffering that arises from resisting painful feeling
- Notice the suffering that arises from craving pleasant feeling
- Whether the feeling is pleasant, unpleasant or neutral
    - Contemplate impermanence in those feelings
    - Watch the feelings come, stay and fade away
    - Let the feelings come when they come
    - Let the feelings stay when they stay
    - Let the feelings fade away when they fade away
    - Do not cling to any feeling
- When we do not cling to anything, we are not agitated
- When we are not agitated, we experience stresslessness

Exercise 11: identifying the source of the feeling tone

- Notice the source of the feeling tone
- Is it from the body or from the mind?
- Feeling a pleasant feeling from the body,
  I know I am feeling a pleasant feeling from the body
- Feeling a pleasant feeling from the mind,
  I know I am feeling a pleasant feeling from the mind
- Feeling an unpleasant feeling from the body,
  I know I am feeling an unpleasant feeling from the body
- Feeling an unpleasant feeling from the mind,
  I know I am feeling an unpleasant feeling from the mind
- Feeling a neutral feeling from the body,
  I know I am feeling a neutral feeling from the body
- Feeling a neutral feeling from the mind,
  I know I am feeling a neutral feeling from the mind

- Notice the source of the feeling tone
  - From sight?
  - From hearing?
  - From smell?
  - From taste?
  - From touch?
  - From thoughts?
- Notice the source of the feeling tone
  - Is it a physical sensation?
  - Is it an internally generated emotion?
- Notice how the sensation or emotion changes

Exercise 12: identifying worldly and unworldly feelings

- Notice whether it is a worldly or unworldly feeling
  - Worldly pleasant feeling
    - Sensory pleasure
    - Psychological pleasure
  - Worldly unpleasant feeling
    - Sensory pain
    - Psychological pain
  - Worldly neutral feeling
    - Sensory indifference
    - Psychological indifference
  - Unworldly pleasant and unpleasant feeling
    - Spiritual pleasure and pain
      - Practicing generosity without expectation
      - Practicing love without attachment
      - Practicing compassion without attachment
      - Practicing renunciation
      - Practicing mindfulness and meditation
  - Unworldly neutral feeling
    - Equanimity in mindfulness and meditation

- Both kinds of feelings will arise naturally in our lives
- Recognize the tendencies of the worldly feelings
  - Chasing worldly pleasant feeling
  - Running away from worldly painful feeling
  - Ignoring worldly neutral feeling
- Abandon these tendencies
- Appreciate and cultivate the unworldly feelings

Mindfulness of mind

- Two mental states
  - Unwholesome mental states
    - The mental state of craving (attachment)
    - The mental state of hating (aversion)
    - The mental state of indifference (delusion)
  - Wholesome mental states
    - The mental state of non-craving (non-attachment)
    - The mental state of non-hating (non-aversion)
    - The mental state of awareness (non-delusion)

Exercise 13: identifying unwholesome/wholesome mental states

- Notice our mental state
- The mental state of craving
  - Notice the arising of craving thoughts
  - Observe the craving thoughts without following them
  - Observe until the craving thoughts fade away
  - Recognize that the craving thoughts have gone
  - Reflect on the nature of a craving-free mind
  - It is free, happy, generous, loving and compassionate
- The mental state of hating
  - Notice the arising of hateful thoughts
  - Observe the hateful thoughts without following them
  - Observe until the hateful thoughts fade away

- Recognize that the hateful thoughts have gone
- Reflect on the nature of a hate-free mind
- It is free, happy, relaxed, peaceful and friendly
- The mental state of awareness
  - The mind is clear and aware before delusion arises
  - Notice the arising of delusion
  - Once we pay attention, the clouds of delusion fade away
  - Recognize the re-appearance of the clear mind
  - Recognize the nature of a delusion-free mind
  - It is clear, aware, sky-like and luminous
- Delusion
  - A false belief based on incorrect inference about external reality that is firmly sustained despite what almost everyone else believes and despite what constitutes the inconvertible and obvious proof or evidence to the contrary (DSM IV)
  - Delusion in the context of mindfulness
    - Is not similar to DSM IV definition
    - Is *moha* in Pali
    - Is the unawareness of the reality
      - The reality of impermanence (time)
        - That things change from time to time
      - The reality of selflessness (space)
        - That things are conditioned
      - The reality of suffering (mind)
        - That suffering arises when we cannot accept things as they are
  - Delusion of permanence: the false belief that things remain unchanged all the time (reality: nothing lasts)
  - Delusion of self: the false belief that the self is an independent entity (reality: the self is just a mental construction)

- Delusion of happiness: the false belief that true happiness is achieved through avoiding pain and the pursuit of sensory pleasure (reality: pain is inevitable in life, pleasure is transient, true happiness is achieved through abandoning the root causes of suffering and practicing the eight noble paths – please refer to mindfulness of reality)

Exercise 14: the removal of distracting thoughts

- This exercise combines mindfulness of thoughts and cognitive methods to remove distracting thoughts
- From <u>The Discourse on The Removal of Distracting Thoughts</u>
- Or <u>Vitakkasanthana Sutta</u> in Pali
- 5 cognitive methods in the removal of distracting thoughts
  - Replacing the thoughts
    - Identify unwholesome thoughts
    - Notice the arising of craving, hate or delusion
    - Replace the thoughts with wholesome thoughts
    - Metaphor: like a carpenter striking hard at, pushing out, and getting rid of a coarse peg to replace it with a fine one
  - Reflecting on the negative effects of the thoughts
    - When unwholesome thoughts remain
    - Examine the danger of the unwholesome thoughts
    - Reflect on the negative effects of the thoughts
    - Metaphor: like a well-dressed young man or woman feeling disgusted with the carcass of a snake hung around his or her neck
  - Ignoring the thoughts
    - When unwholesome thoughts remain
    - Pay no attention to the unwholesome thoughts
    - Metaphor: like a man shutting his eyes or looking away from a visible object

- Removing the source of the negative thoughts
  - When unwholesome thoughts remain
  - Reflect on the removal of the source
  - Metaphor: like a man slowing down because he found no reason to walk fast
- Suppressing unwholesome thoughts
  - When unwholesome thoughts remain
  - Use all our energy to suppress the thoughts
  - With teeth clenched and tongue pressed on palate
  - Metaphor: like a strong man holding a weaker man by the head or shoulders, restraining, subduing and beating him down

Exercise 15: identifying the eight pairs of mental states

- Pause and look at our mind
- Recognize whether the mind is:
  - Greedy or not greedy
    - Greedy: burning with the fire of craving
    - Not greedy: calm, cool, peaceful and relaxed
  - Angry or not angry
    - Angry: gripped by anger or hate
    - Not angry: calm, cool, peaceful and relaxed
  - Deluded or not deluded
    - Deluded: being trapped in the net of cognitive errors
    - Not deluded: calm, cool, peaceful, clear and free
  - Contracted/distracted or not contracted/distracted
    - Contracted: dull and heavy, collapsing inward
    - Distracted: agitated and restless, expanding outward
  - Narrow or wide
    - Narrow: our day-to-day ordinary consciousness
    - Wide: altered consciousness in meditation, the mind is calm, peaceful, tranquil, harmonious, relaxed

- Not supreme or supreme
  - Not supreme: not in the highest state of meditation
  - Supreme: in the highest state of meditation
- Not concentrated or concentrated
  - Not concentrated: not in meditative states
  - Concentrated: in meditative states
- Not liberated or liberated
  - Not liberated: bound by problems; greedy, angry or deluded; narrow, not supreme or not concentrated
  - Liberated: free of all problems; not greedy, not angry and not deluded; wide, supreme, concentrated

Mindfulness of reality

- The three universal characteristics of reality
  - Temporal reality: the reality of impermanence
  - Spatial reality: the reality of selflessness
  - Psychological reality: the reality of suffering

Exercise 16: recognizing impermanence

- Be mindful of impermanence
- Watch the arising, maintaining, dissolving and disappearing of:
  - The breath and other bodily experiences
  - Feelings: pleasantness, unpleasantness, neutrality
  - The ordinary mind: mental states, thoughts and emotions
  - The meditative mind: altered mental states
- Recognize the impermanence of impermanence awareness
  - Drifting of mind from unawareness of impermanence to awareness of impermanence
  - Drifting of mind from awareness of impermanence back to unawareness of impermanence again
- Recognize the freedom when we reduce our clinging to the idea of permanence (the wish for pleasant things to stay the same)

Exercise 17: recognizing selflessness

- Recognize that the sense of "self":
  - Is a faulty mental construction
  - Is not an independent entity
  - Is dependent on various causes and conditions
  - Arises as we think about our body, feelings, perceptions, mental formations and consciousness
  - Is impermanent
- Recognizing selflessness (conditionality)
  - That conditioned things change
  - That things arise, maintain, dissolve and disappear based on causes and conditions
  - The body: birth, aging, sickness and death
  - Feelings: come and go based on causes and conditions
  - Mental states: change from time to time based on causes and conditions
- Recognize the freedom when we reduce our clinging to the idea of self (the wish for things the way "I" want, not as they are)

Time Magazine 2002

After more than a century looking for it, brain researchers have long since concluded that there is no conceivable place for a self to be located in the physical brain, and that it simply does not exist.

Exercise 18: recognizing suffering

- Suffering is not inherent in the phenomena of the world
- It exists only in the way the ordinary mind experiences it
- It arises when we are unable to accept changes
- It arises when we cannot accept the reality of impermanence and conditionality
- The 4 noble truths
  - The truth of suffering
  - The truth of causes of suffering
  - The truth of cessation of suffering
  - The truth of paths leading to cessation of suffering
- The truth of suffering (dukkha in Pali)
  - Notice the arising of suffering when it arises
  - Notice the suffering as it is
  - Notice the unsatisfactory nature of suffering
  - Contemplate on the 8 types of suffering associated with:
    - Birth
    - Aging
    - Sickness
    - Death
    - Separating from what or who we love
    - Not getting what we want
    - Getting what we do not want
    - Clinging to our body and mind
  - Contemplate on the 3 types of suffering
    - Suffering due to unpleasant experiences
      - The obvious biopsychosocial-spiritual suffering
    - Suffering due to impermanence
      - The potential suffering hidden in all changes
    - Suffering due to conditionality
      - The potential suffering hidden in conditioned things

- The truth of causes of suffering (samudaya in Pali)
  - Notice the arising of the causes of suffering
    - Delusion: the mistaken belief of the reality
      - The belief that things are permanent
      - The belief that things are independent
      - The belief that long-lasting happiness can be achieved by indulging in things we crave
      - The belief that suffering can be removed totally by resisting or avoiding things we hate
    - Attachment: the craving of things that one likes
    - Aversion: the hating of things that one dislikes
  - When delusion arises, I know this is delusion
  - Notice delusion as it is without sustaining it
  - When attachment arises, I know this is attachment
  - Notice attachment as it is without sustaining it
  - When aversion arises, I know this is aversion
  - Notice aversion as it is without sustaining it
  - Watch how suffering arises based on causes & conditions
    - Notice the arising of feeling tone
      - Pleasant
      - Unpleasant
      - Neutral
    - Notice the conditioned reactions to feeling tones
      - Pleasant feeling → attachment
      - Unpleasant feeling → aversion
      - Neutral feeling → delusion
    - Notice the reaction to attachment/aversion
      - Clinging
        - Holding on to attachment
        - Holding on to aversion
        - Holding on to delusion

- Notice the arising of suffering
    - From feelings to attachment/aversion
    - From attachment/aversion to clinging
- The truth of cessation of suffering (nirodha in Pali)
    - Suffering arises, maintains, dissolves and disappears due to impermanence and conditionality
    - Observe the mind when it is free of suffering
    - Delusion, craving and hate arise, maintain, dissolve and disappear due to impermanence and conditionality
    - Observe the mind when it is free of the causes of suffering
        - Free of delusion
        - Free of craving
        - Free of hate
    - Observe the mind when it is free of clinging
    - Feel the radical freedom that is independent of favourable or unfavourable conditions
    - Feel the extinction of negative mental states
- The truth of paths (magga in Pali)
    - Notice the paths/factors leading to cessation of suffering
    - The 8 noble paths
        - Right understanding
            - Understanding the reality as it is
            - Understanding the 4 noble truths
        - Right intention
            - The intention to do no harm
            - The intention to do good
        - Right speech
            - Communicating truthfully
            - Communicating meaningfully
            - Communicating sensitively
            - Communicating timely

- Right action
  - To protect life
  - To give
  - To preserve dignity
  - To listen deeply and speak with love
  - To promote health
- Right livelihood
  - Not engaging in profession that may do harm
  - Engaging in profession that may do good
- Right progress
  - Prevent negative thoughts from arising
  - Abandon negative thoughts that have arisen
  - Invite positive thoughts that have not arisen
  - Sustain positive thoughts that have arisen
- Right mindfulness
  - Mindfulness of the body
  - Mindfulness of feelings
  - Mindfulness of mind
  - Mindfulness of reality
- Right meditation
  - Meditation to calm down our mind
  - Meditation to look inside our mind
    - Insight into reality of impermanence
    - Insight into reality of selflessness
    - Insight into reality of suffering
- Notice the arising of these factors from time to time
- Notice the cessation of suffering with these factors
- Practice the 8 noble paths continuously

Mindfulness in Palliative Care

Introduction

Although mindfulness has great potential in reducing suffering, the practice of mindfulness in palliative care has many challenges.

Challenges of practicing mindfulness in palliative care

- Patients/families may not have the intention to practice
- Patients/families may be too tired to pay attention
- Patients/families may be too overwhelmed with suffering
- Patients may experience rapid change in suffering
- Patients may experience rapid change in physical strength
- Patients may experience rapid change in conscious level
- Healthcare staff may be too busy with work

Mini-mindfulness meditation (MMM)

- Designed for palliative care patients since most patients do not have the time or energy to attend formal mindfulness practices
- Recommended duration: at least 5 minutes a day
- Flexibility
  - Can choose from any of the following practices
  - Can practice for 5min, 15min, 30min, or more
  - Can practice for any number of sessions
  - Can practice at any setting
  - Can stop at any time
  - Can be a practice for family members
  - Can be a practice for healthcare providers
  - Can be a guided practice except mindful bathing
  - Can be a self-practice

Two breaths to relieve stress

Breathing in, I calm down.
Breathing out, I smile.
Breathing in, present moment.
Breathing out, wonderful moment.

by Thich Nhat Hanh
(Vietnamese Zen Master)

Instructions for mindful breathing

- Make yourself comfortable
- Relax your body
- Close your eyes gently
- Take two deep breaths slowly
- Then, breathe naturally
- Notice the flow of air through your nose
- Rest your attention gently on your breath
- If you are distracted by any sounds, body sensations, thoughts or feelings, gently come back to your breath
- Be aware of the breath for the next five minutes

Instructions for mindful eating

- Enjoy your breathing while waiting for the food
- Feel grateful when the food arrives
- Be there fully for the food
- Put your food gently into your mouth
- Chew slowly
- Feel the taste, texture and temperature of the food
- Feel every nook and corner of the food
- Feel the movement of the food as you chew and swallow

- Follow the food down to the foodpipe and stomach
- Take the next portion or sip a drink when you are ready
- If you are lost in thinking, gently come back to your meal

Instructions for mindful movement

- Breathe in and out to center yourself
- Stop rushing
- Move slowly
- It can be any exercise or walking
- Feel the joint movement
- Feel the muscles contraction and relaxation
- Feel the skin and the gentle wind caused by the movement
- Synchronize you breathing with your movement
- As you stop moving, rest your attention on your posture
- If you are distracted, gently come back to yourself
- Rest your attention on movement for the next five minutes

Instructions for mindful bathing

- Breathe in and out
- Lock the door
- Take off your clothes slowly
- Turn on the shower
- Bathe slowly
- Feel the contact and flow of the running water
- Feel the temperature of the water
- Wipe your body with soap
- Feel the soap and the foam
- Focus on the skin sensation
- Do not get lost in thoughts
- If your mind wanders, come back to your skin sensation
- Wash away all your worries and stress
- Rest your attention on the water showering all over your body

Instructions for mindful smiling

- Breathe in and out to center yourself
- Imagine your face as a flower bud
- Choose your favourite flower
- Visualize the flower blooming as you start to smile
- Smile very slowly until your smile is blooming fully
- Rest your mind in the feeling of happiness
- Let the feeling spread to your whole body as you breathe
- Do not let other feelings, thoughts or sensations distract you
- Stay with this feeling of happiness for the next five minutes

Instructions for mindful chanting

- Breathe in and out to center yourself
- Choose a positive phrase
- Phrases: may I be happy, may I be calm, may I be peaceful
- Rest your mind on this phrase
- Chant it slowly and silently in your mind
- Use it as an anchor to stabilize your mind
- If you are distracted, come back to it again and again
- Rest your mind on it for the next five minutes

Instructions for mindfulness of love

- Love is an intention to bring happiness to someone
- Breathe in and out naturally
- Imagine your loved one in front of you
- Imagine sending love to the person
- Visualize him or her getting happier and happier
- Let go of any distraction
- Rest your attention on your love to the person
- Then, imagine receiving love from the person too
- See yourself getting happier and happier with the love
- Stay with the feeling of love for the next five minutes

Instructions for mindfulness of nature

- Choose a leaf, a flower, a tree, the sky or a picture of nature
- Breathe in and out naturally
- If you have chosen a leaf, look at it deeply
- Appreciate the general characteristics of the leaf
- Then, appreciate its details
- See the beauty of the leaf
- See until you can picture the leaf completely in your mind
- Let go of any distraction
- Rest your attention on the leaf and be one with it

Instructions for mindfulness of pain

- Seek help from your doctor for analgesia
- Breathe in and out to center yourself
- Breathe until you feel you are calmer
- Bring your attention to the pain
- Try to keep a curious mind to see what pain is
- Notice the sensations, emotions and thoughts of pain
- Pay particular attention to the unpleasantness of pain
- Notice how the mind resists pain
- Relax the resistance
- Smile to your pain

Instructions for mindful suffering

- Relax your body
- Take two deep breaths slowly
- Then, breathe naturally
- Allow your mind to settle down
- When you feel calmer, bring your attention to your suffering
- Observe the sensations, emotions and thoughts of suffering
- Watch suffering like an observer rather than an experiencer
- Notice how your suffering arises and disappears naturally

- Do not increase your suffering by overthinking about it
- Do not reject your suffering
- Embrace your suffering with kindness
- Imagine breathing in kindness to dissolve your suffering
- Imagine breathing out the remnants of suffering
- Continue breathing in and out for the next five minutes

Instructions for mindfulness of death

- Recommended for advanced mindfulness practitioners
- May cause considerable distress for those who are not
- Death is a natural process in life
- It can happen to us at anytime and anywhere
- Breathe in and out to center yourself
- Openly acknowledge that death can happen to you at anytime
- Imagine you are dying and lying on a bed surrounded by family
- Imagine the sensations caused by failure of many organs
- Imagine the negative thoughts and emotions that can arise
- Watch them and let them be as they are without rejecting them
- If fear arises, just breathe and let go
- If anger arises, just breathe and let go
- If worry arises, just breathe and let go
- If sadness arises, just breathe and let go
- Breathing in, I see dying as falling leaves
- Breathing out, I smile in peace
- Breathing in, I embrace my journey of living and dying
- Breathing out, mindfulness is my lead
- Rest your mind on the imagined scene for the next 5 minutes

Mindfulness-based supportive therapy (MBST)(Tan 2015)

- Designed for healthcare providers (HCP)
- Allow HCP to practice mindfulness during patient care
- Recommended duration: limited by available time of HCP
- Flexibility
  - No restriction in time
  - No restriction in number of sessions
  - Can be delivered by any HCP
  - Can be delivered to patients, family members or both
  - Can be delivered at hospital, home or hospice
  - Can be terminated at any time
  - Can be a bridge to other psychotherapies
- Reciprocity
  - May alleviate suffering of patients and family members
  - May reduce stress of HCP
- Simultaneity
  - Allow HCP to practice mindfulness at work
  - No need to change any schedule

The foundations of MBST (refer to chapter of suffering)

- Based on the theory of suffering in palliative care
  - Patients: the existential-experiential model of suffering
  - Families: the model of compassion suffering
- Open-ended questions for assessment of suffering
  - General questions
  - Specific questions
- Types of suffering as a guide in the diagnosis of suffering
  - Suffering of patients
  - Suffering of family caregivers

The framework of MBST

- Mindful presence
- Mindful listening
- Mindful empathy
- Mindful compassion
- Mindfulness of boundaries

The application techniques of MBST

- Directing attention (paying attention on purpose)
- Sustaining attention (paying attention on purpose)
- Distraction monitoring
    - Temporal distraction
      (paying attention in the present moment)
    - Reactive distraction
      (paying attention nonreactively)

Instructions for mindful presence

- Practice mindful breathing
    - Breathe consciously
    - Follow the entire length of the breath
    - Feel your whole body while you are breathing
    - Calm your body
- Give patient 100% of your attention
- Treat patient as if he or she is the only person in the world
- Maintain good eye contact from moment to moment
- See patient as a whole
- Observe his or her facial expression and body movement
- If you find yourself judging patient, feeling anxious or rushing, breathe and relax your body and mind again
- Be there fully for the patient during the entire encounter

Instructions for mindful listening

- Continue with mindful breathing
- Listen to patient with 100% of your attention
- Do not interrupt unnecessarily
- Do not judge patient
- Do not give your opinion prematurely
- Listen to the speech
- Listen to the rate, rhythm, pitch and volume
- Be comfortable with the speech and the silence in between
- Listen with an open and curious heart to understand patient
- Create a safe space for patient to express his or her suffering
- Try to understand what is being expressed
- Try to understand what is behind the expression
- If you are distracted by your judgment, just breathe and relax
- Let the barrier between you and patient dissolves
- Listen with all of yourself during the entire encounter

Instructions for mindful empathy

- Continue with mindful breathing
- Imagine "entering into" the feelings and perspectives of patient
- Imagine experiencing the emotions and thoughts of patient
- Imagine yourself going through the same experience
- If you notice any overimagination, just breathe and relax
- Try to understand what are the hopes, expectations and wishes
- Allow patient to express everything, thoughts and emotions
- Allow silence
- Abandon your impulse to block any form of expression
- Acknowledge, validate or normalize the expression if necessary
- Continue to put yourself in patient's shoes from time to time

Instructions for mindful compassion

- Continue with mindful breathing to anchor your attention
- Compassion is the motivation to relieve suffering
- Cultivate the sincere motivation to alleviate patient's suffering
- Repeat silently: May you be free from suffering
- Focus on the thoughts and feelings of compassion
- Let compassion manifest in your speech and action
- Speak consciously in consistent with the hopes, expectations, wishes and preferences of patient
- Act consciously in consistent with the hopes, expectations, wishes and preferences of patient
- Be mindful not to speak or act unwisely
- If you are excessively concerned in fixing the suffering, breathe
- If you are excessively attached to any expectation, breathe
- Breathe, relax and come back to compassion

Instructions for mindfulness of boundaries

- Mindfulness of boundaries is a practice of self-awareness
- Continue to practice mindful breathing
- Consciously monitor boundary issues that arise during your practices of presence, listening, empathy and compassion
- Be aware when boundaries are approached
- Cross boundaries consciously only if you are convinced that crossing boundary in that particular situation is beneficial to patient and the therapeutic relationship, without violating your professional conduct or compromising the equity of care
- Mindfulness of boundaries protects you from burnout due to:
    - Time constraint (presence)
    - Countertransferences (listening)
    - Vicarious traumatization (empathy)
    - Compassion fatigue (compassion)
- Maintain self-awareness throughout the encounter

The Neuroscience of Mindfulness

Introduction

With regular practice, mindfulness can change the brain areas involved in attention regulation, emotional regulation and self-awareness.

Default mode network (DMN)

- The wandering mind
- Active when we are not engaged in performing a task
- Active when we are not processing external events
  - Daydreaming or mind wandering
  - Thinking about ourselves or others
  - Thinking about the past or future
- Comprises 3 midline regions and inferior parietal lobule
  - Ventromedial prefrontal cortex (vmPFC)
    - Emotion processing
  - Dorsomedial prefrontal cortex (dmPFC)
    - Self-referential processing
  - Posterior cingulate cortex (PCC) + adjacent precuneus
    - Recollection of prior experiences
  - Inferior parietal lobule (IPL)
    - Perspective taking
- Mindfulness practices
  - Reduce activation of DMN (mPFC and PCC)
    - Less mind wandering
  - Increase connectivity between PCC, dACC and dlPFC
    - More self-monitoring and cognitive control
  - Increase DMN functional connectivity
    - More communication within DMN

The habit loop

- 3Rs
    - Reminder: cue, stimulus
    - Routine: triggered behaviour
    - Reward: the benefit that makes us repeat the loop
- Habit learning
    - Basal ganglia (the habit center)
        - Dorsal striatum: caudate, putamen
        - Ventral striatum: nucleus accumbens
        - Globus pallidus
    - Basal-ganglia-thalamocortical loops
        - Cortex → striatum
            - Caudate nucleus and vmPFC
                - Initial learning
                - Flexible goal-directed behaviour
            - Putamen
                - Later
                - Stimulus-driven habitual behaviour
        - Striatum → globus pallidus
        - Globus pallidus → thalamus
        - Thalamus → cortex
- Neurotransmitter
    - Dopamine: released in response to reward
        - Food
        - Sex
        - Money
        - Praise
- Mindfulness practices
    - Increase functional connectivity
        - Caudate nucleus
        - Basal-ganglia-thalamocortical loops
            - Mindfulness becomes more spontaneous

Shifting from DMN to mindfulness

- Mind wandering
  - Activation of vmPFC, dmPFC, PCC
- Awareness of mind wandering
  - Activation of dorsal anterior cingulate cortex (dACC)
    - Salience network
    - Conflict monitoring and error detection
- Shifting and sustaining attention to the breath
  - Activation of dorsolateral prefrontal cortex (dlPFC)
    - Central executive network
    - Cognitive and emotional regulation

Summary of brain regions involved in mindfulness

- Anterior cingulate cortex (ACC)
  - Salience network
    - Attention regulation
    - Cognitive regulation
    - Emotional regulation
    - Self-regulation
- Dorsolateral prefrontal cortex (dlPFC)
  - Central executive network
    - Cognitive regulation
    - Emotional regulation
    - Meta-awareness: consciously aware of awareness
- Insular cortex
  - Body awareness
- Striatum
  - Habit formation
- Amygdala
  - Shrinks after 8 weeks of mindfulness practices
  - Fight-or-flight center
    - Emotional learning

Happiness

Introduction

If we are not happy, it is difficult for us to make patients happy. To be happy, we have to study and practice happiness.

Terms

- Positive psychology: the study of happiness
- Hedonism
  - Living a pleasant life
  - Pursuing pleasure and avoiding pain
    - Sensory pleasures are short-lived
    - Constant pursuit is needed
    - Tendency to adapt: hedonic treadmill or adaptation
    - May not lead to personal growth
    - Pain is inevitable in life
  - Model of subjective well-being (Diener 1984)
    - Subjective well-being
      - High level of positive affect
      - Low level of negative affect
      - High degree of life satisfaction
  - The happiness pie chart (Lyubomirsky 2005)
    - Happiness set point 50%
    - Intentional activities 40%
    - Life circumstances 10%
  - Happiness set point
    - An average level of happiness after temporary highs and lows in emotionality
    - Attributed to genetic predeterminism
    - Assumed to be fixed and stable over time

- Eudaimonia
  - Living a good life
  - Pursuing virtues and strengths
    - Happiness from living a virtuous life is more stable
    - Promotes personal growth
  - The authentic happiness model (Seligman 2011)
    - Positive emotions
    - Engagement
    - Meaningful life
    - Positive relationships
    - Positive accomplishments
  - Flourishing (Fredrickson 2005)
    - Living within an optimal range of human functioning
    - One that connotes goodness, generativity, growth and resilience
  - Mental health functioning (Keyes 2002)
    - Flourishing: high well-being, low mental illness
    - Struggling: high well-being, high mental illness
    - Floundering: low well-being, high mental illness
    - Languishing: low well-being, low mental illness
  - Resilience (Newman 2004)
    - A universal capacity which allows a person, group or community, to prevent, minimize or overcome damaging effects of adversity
  - Flow (Csikszentmihalyi 1975)
    - The holistic sensation present when we act with total involvement

Savouring: the pursuit of pleasure

- Noticing and appreciating the positive aspects of life
- Positive counterpart of coping
- Involves mindfulness and conscious attention to pleasure

- Types of savouring (Bryant 2005, 2007)
    - Anticipation: enjoying future pleasure
    - Being in the moment: enjoying present pleasure
        - Luxuriating: indulging in sensory pleasure
        - Marveling: feeling wonderful
        - Basking: receiving praise
        - Thanksgiving: expressing gratitude
    - Reminiscing: enjoying past pleasure

Flow: the pursuit of optimal experience

- The psychology of optimal experience
- The process of total involvement in life
- The elements of enjoyment
    - Involved in a challenging activity that requires skills
    - The merging of action and awareness
    - Clear goals, immediate feedback and sense of reward
    - Concentration on the task at hand
    - The paradox of control
    - The loss of self-consciousness
    - The transformation of time

The pursuit of love (Sternberg 1986)

- Passion: an intense emotional response to another person
- Intimacy: warmth, closeness, sharing of self in a relationship
- Commitment: decision to maintain the relationship
- Infatuation: passion alone
- Liking: intimacy alone
- Empty love: commitment alone
- Romantic love: passion + intimacy
- Fatuous love: passion + commitment
- Companionate love: intimacy + commitment
- Consummate love: passion + intimacy + commitment

The pursuit of excellence

- Excellence: the acquisition of extraordinary skill in a specific area of expertise (Ericsson 1994)
- Elements of excellence
  - Cognitive: large knowledge base in one's specific domain
  - Motivational: passion and commitment
  - Action: consistent deliberate practice, persistence
- Grit (Duckworth 2007)
  - Passion + persistence
- Ten-year rule
  - It takes at least a decade of dedicated, consistent practice before one can attain a high level of excellence

Aesthetics: the pursuit of beauty

- Aesthetics: an appreciation of the beautiful and the sublime
- Four attributes of the aesthetic experience
  - Pleasure
  - Absorption
  - Intrinsic interest
  - Challenge

The pursuit of creativity

- Creativity: adaptive originality (Simonton 2009)
  - Adaptive: provides a useful solution to a real-life problem
  - Originality: original, novel, surprising or unexpected
- The creative process
  - Preparation: gathering information
  - Incubation: subconscious processing of information
  - Illumination: rapid emerging of a creative solution
  - Verification: turning an insight into real-world solution

The pursuit of virtues and strengths (Martin Seligman 2002)

- Virtue: good character or moral excellence
- Strength: route in achieving virtue
- The six virtues and twenty four strengths
  - Wisdom
    - Curiosity
    - Love of learning
    - Open-mindedness
    - Creativity
    - Emotional intelligence
    - Perspective
  - Courage
    - Bravery
    - Perseverance
    - Integrity
  - Love
    - Kindness
    - Loving and loved
  - Justice
    - Responsibility
    - Fairness
    - Leadership
  - Temperance
    - Self-control
    - Prudence
    - Humility
  - Spirituality
    - Appreciation of beauty
    - Gratitude
    - Hope and optimism
    - Sense of purpose
    - Forgiveness

- Humour
- Passion

The reward system

- Reward: the attractive and motivational property of a stimulus that induces approach behaviour (Schultz 2015)
- Reward system: a group of neural structures responsible for:
    - Liking or pleasure
    - Wanting or desire (incentive salience)
    - Learning or positive reinforcement
- Intrinsic rewards
    - Unconditioned rewards that are attractive and motivate behaviour because they are inherently pleasurable
- Extrinsic rewards
    - Conditioned rewards that are attractive and motivate behaviour, but are not pleasurable
- Neuroscience of the reward system
    - Primarily within cortico-basal ganglia-thalamic loop
    - Pleasure centers or hedonic hotspots
        - Mediate pleasure or "liking"
            - Subcortical
                - Nucleus accumbens shell
                - Ventral pallidum
                - Parabrachial nucleus of pons
            - Cortical:
                - Orbitofrontal cortex
                - Insular cortex
                - Medial prefrontal cortex
                - Anterior cingulate cortex
    - Mesolimbic dopamine pathway
        - Ventral tegmental area (VTA) to nucleus accumbens
        - Mediates motivational processes or "wanting"

- Medial forebrain bundle (MFB)
  - Fibers from basal olfactory regions
  - Fibers from periamygdaloid region
  - Fibers from the septal nuclei
  - Fibers from ventral tegmentum area (VTA)
  - Integration of reward and pleasure
- Basal ganglia
  - Mediates learning and drives activities
    - Dorsal striatum: caudate and putamen
    - Substantia nigra
    - Globus pallidus
- Possible neural correlates of eudaimonic happiness
  - Link between cortical and hedonic brain circuits
  - Cortical regions
    - Orbitofrontal cortex
    - Medial prefrontal cortex
    - Anterior cingulate cortex
    - Dorsolateral prefrontal cortex
    - Insular cortex

Happiness activities (Sonja Lyubomirsky 2008)

- Expressing gratitude
- Cultivating optimism
- Avoiding overthinking
- Practicing acts of kindness
- Nurturing social relationships
- Develop strategies for coping with stress
- Learning to forgive
- Increasing flow experiences
- Savouring life's joys
- Committing to our goals
- Practicing spirituality or religion

- Practicing mindfulness or meditation
- Exercise
- Smile

Little quote

If you want others to be happy, practice compassion.
If you want to be happy, practice compassion.

Dalai Lama

Kindness

Introduction

Kindness is the most important quality of a human being. If we cultivate kindness every day, it will grow every day and embrace everyone. We will become happier. Everyone around us will become happier.

Kindness

- The quality of being friendly, generous and considerate
- Synonyms of kindness
    - Altruism
    - Benevolence
    - Big-heartedness
    - Care
    - Compassion
    - Concern
    - Charitableness
    - Friendliness
    - Generosity
    - Gentleness
    - Goodwill
    - Helpfulness
    - Humaneness
    - Kind-heartedness
    - Love
    - Selflessness
    - Thoughtfulness
    - Understanding
    - Warm-heartedness

The four mental states of kindness

Love

- The intention and capacity to bring happiness
- Requires
    - Attentive looking and listening
    - Empathy and understanding
        - Knowing what to think and what not to think
        - Knowing what to say and what not to say
        - Knowing what to do and what not to do
- Love with understanding brings happiness
- Love without understanding causes suffering
- Love starts with ourselves
- If we cannot love ourselves, it can be hard to love others

Compassion

- The intention and capacity to relieve suffering
- Roots: passion (suffer) and com (with)
- We do not need to 'suffer with' to relieve another's suffering
- Requires
    - Attentive looking and listening
    - Empathy and understanding
    - Deep concern
    - Calmness, clarity and strength
- Calmness, clarity and strength are needed in relieving suffering
- Otherwise we will be overwhelmed by suffering

If your compassion does not include yourself, it is incomplete.

Jack Kornfield

Joy

- The intention and capacity to abide in a state of joy
- Requires
    - Feeling blessed for many things in life
    - Feeling grateful to many persons in life
    - Rejoicing in our own happiness
    - Rejoicing in others' happiness
- A joy that is filled with peace and contentment

Equanimity

- The intention and capacity to abide in a state of freedom
- The state of freedom
    - Freedom from judgment and conditions
    - Freedom from attachment to outcome
    - Freedom from discrimination
- The practices of love, compassion and joy are incomplete without the practice of freedom
    - Practice love without judgment and conditions
    - Practice compassion without attachment to outcome
    - Practice joy without discrimination
- Associated with the cognition of clarity
- Associated with the emotion of calmness

Guided meditations on the four mental states of kindness

Love meditation (metta meditation)

- Sit comfortably and relax your body
- Breathe in and breathe out naturally
- Make a wish from the depth of your heart: I am going to train myself in developing love for the sake of all beings
- Imagine someone you love in front of you
- Imagine receiving unconditional love from the person

- Feel the love from the bottom of your heart
- Rest in this love for a few moments
- Make a sincere wish for this person to be happy
- "May he or she be happy"
- Imagine sending unconditional love toward the person
- Rest in this love for the next few moments
- Now imagine extending unconditional love to:
  - All family members
  - All friends
  - All strangers
  - All enemeies
  - All beings
- Take time to deepen your unconditional love to each group
- End by imagining the whole universe filled with boundless love

Compassion meditation (karuna meditation)

- Sit comfortably and relax your body
- Breathe in and breathe out naturally
- Make a wish from the depth of your heart: I am going to train myself in developing compassion for the sake of all beings
- Imagine someone you love suffering in front of you
- Open your heart to feel the suffering of the person
- Feel the suffering from the bottom of your heart
- Rest in this suffering for a few moments
- Make a sincere wish for this person to be free from suffering
- "May he or she be free from all suffering"
- Imagine directing your compassion toward the person
- Rest in this compassion for the next few moments
- Now imagine extending compassion to:
  - All family members
  - All friends
  - All strangers

- All enemies
- All beings
- Take time to deepen your compassion to each group
- Imagine the whole universe filled with boundless compassion

Joy meditation (mudita meditation)

- Sit comfortably and relax your body
- Breathe in and out naturally
- Make a wish from the depth of your heart: I am going to train myself in developing joy for the sake of all beings
- Imagine you are with a very joyful person
- Feel the lightness and joy that this person brings to others
- Rejoice in his or her joy
- Feel his or her joy flowing into every part of your body
- Rest in this joy for a few moments
- Make a sincere wish for everyone to be full of joy
- "May everyone be full of joy"
- Imagine radiating this joy to:
    - Everyone in the northern direction
    - Everyone in the southern direction
    - Everyone in the eastern direction
    - Everyone in the western direction
    - All living beings above
    - All living beings below
- Take time to radiate joy to each direction
- Imagine the whole universe filled with boundless joy

Equanimity meditation (upekkha meditation)

- Sit comfortably and relax your body
- Breathe in and out naturally
- Make a wish from the depth of your heart: I am going to train myself in developing equanimity for the sake of all beings

- Imagine you are with a very calm and peaceful person
- Feel the calmness and peace of this person
- Imagine the peace of this person entering your body
- Feel the peace flowing into every part of your body
- Rest in this feeling of peace for a few moments
- Let go of everything in your mind
    - Your body
    - Your feelings
    - Your perceptions
    - Your thoughts and emotions
    - Your consciousness
- Just let them be as they are
- Do not try to change or manipulate any of them
- Just let them be as they are
- Feel the freedom and peace when you have let go of everything
- Rest in this freedom of your mind for the next few moments
- Make a sincere wish for everyone to be full of peace
- "May everyone be calm and peaceful"
- Imagine radiating this peace to:
    - Everyone in the northern direction
    - Everyone in the southern direction
    - Everyone in the eastern direction
    - Everyone in the western direction
    - All living beings above
    - All living beings below
- Take time to radiate peace to each direction
- Imagine the whole universe filled with boundless peace

18 qualities of kindness (Piero Ferrucci 2006)

- Honesty: everything becomes easier
- Warmth: the temperature of happiness
- Forgiveness: live in the present

- Contact: to touch and be touched
- Sense of belonging: I belong, therefore I am
- Trust: are you willing to risk?
- Mindfulness: the only time is now
- Empathy: expansion of consciousness
- Humility: you are not the only one around
- Patience: have you left your soul behind?
- Generosity: redefining boundaries
- Respect: look and listen
- Flexibility: adapt or perish
- Memory: have you forgotten anyone?
- Loyalty: don't lose your thread
- Gratitude: the easiest way to be happy
- Service: a wonderful opportunity
- Joy: our natural state

Cultivating the qualities of kindness

Generosity

- Sit down and listen to a patient
- Help a patient to pour water
- Help a patient to eat or drink
- Help a patient to adjust the bed linen
- Help a patient to comb hair
- Help a patient to adjust shoes or slippers
- Give a hand for a patient to sit up
- Bring flowers to a patient
- Buy a handheld fan for a patient with breathlessness
- Arrange a hairstylist to cut hair for a long-staying patient
- Arrange a musician to play music for a patient
- Hand out balloons for paediatric patients
- Make a patient smile
- Call and visit a dying patient

- Sit beside a dying patient
- Ask a family member "How are you doing?"
- Give a lazy chair to a family member
- Serve a drink to a family member
- Say something nice to a family member
- Bring a colleague out for lunch
- Write a small note of appreciation to a colleague
- Bring a small gift for a colleague
- Be a friend to a new colleague
- Buy a copy of book on kindness and give to a colleague
- Give a compliment to a colleague
- Allow staff to go home a bit earlier
- Write a thank you note to boss
- Take a picture with staff
- Offer to help the nurses during bed-making
- Give some cookies to a medical attendant
- Create a kindness board for daily kindness quote
- Plant some indoor flowers in the hospital
- Give our loved ones 100% of our attention
- Give our loved ones little surprises
- Listen with our heart
- Give a big hug to a friend
- Make a new friend
- Smile to a stranger
- Say something nice to everyone we meet
- Crack a joke
- Press the lift button for a stranger
- Say hello to a stranger
- Make some kindness bookmark and distribute it
- Play with a children
- Pick up a rubbish
- Plant a tree

Patience

- Slow down
- Stop rushing
- Listen to a patient without interrupting
- Give a patient time to come to terms with illness
- Give a patient time to come to terms with dying
- Allow a talkative patient to talk a bit more
- Allow an angry patient to express anger
- Allow an anxious patient to ask question
- Continue to review an unappreciative patient
- Continue to review a withdrawn patient
- Acknowledge differences in opinion with family member
- Acknowledge request for futile treatment from family member
- Respect the mistaken belief of family member
- Agree to disagree with a colleague
- Accept criticism of a colleague and respond thoughtfully
- Respect the impatience of a colleague
- Give a colleague time to change
- Listen attentively to a nagging spouse
- Keep calm and respond thoughtfully to a negative remark
- Keep calm and respond thoughtfully to a noisy neighbour
- Remain mindful during a queue
- Let someone cut in front of us in line
- Be a courteous driver
- Let someone merge into our lane in traffic
- Enjoy a traffic jam
- Leave nice comments on social media
- Complain less
- Say a timely apology
- Respect politicians
- Clean the toilet
- Keep calm and smile

Humility

- Avoid seeing a patient with a huge team
- See a patient in small group if necessary
- See a patient one-to-one if possible
- Sit down at the same level as patient
- Remove our sense of superiority over patient
- Spend more time listening than talking
- Learn from the experiences of a patient
- Speak without medical jargon
- Speak at the same level as patient
- Accept our limitations
- Accept credit when credit is due
- Give other people credit when it is due
- Avoid showing off
- Ask for help when appropriate
- Work as a team
- Recognize the contribution of each team member
- Acknowledge the importance of each team member
- Stop identifying ourselves as the center of the universe
- Stop identifying ourselves as someone very important
- Stop identifying ourselves as someone special
- Stop identifying our stress as something very overwhelming
- Stop identifying our contributions as highly important
- Learn to develop concern for others
- Learn to see others as very important person
- Learn to see others as very special person
- Learn to understand others' pain and suffering
- Learn to appreciate the contribution of others
- Adopt the beginner mind
- Keep an open mind
- Accept kindness from others
- Show gratitude to others

Forgiveness

- Forgive ourselves
- Write down our past mistake
- Feel the burden we are carrying: pain, guilt, fear, regret
- Make a confession
- Say sorry for any wrongs
- Ask for forgiveness
- Let go of our past misconduct
- Do not repeat similar mistake
- Begin anew
- Make a wish to act in a more caring way
- Dedicate our lives to others
- Do something to redeem the past if necessary
- Forgive ourselves if we are not ready to forgive completely
- Practice forgiving ourselves regularly
- Practice empathy for ourselves
- Open our heart to ourselves fully
- Forgive others
- Forgive the person, not the misdeeds
- Look deeply into the reasons causing the misdeeds
- Look deeply into the life of the person
- Practice empathy for the person
- Release our heart from the grip of anger or hatred
- Free ourselves from the past
- Let go of our judgment
- Do not force forgiveness
- Forgive little by little if necessary
- Open our heart to the person fully
- Do something to change the person skilfully
- Do something to change the world little by little
- Make peace with the past
- Live in the present moment

Gratitude

- Do not take things for granted
- Complain less
- Criticize less
- Judge less
- Gossip less
- Appreciate everyone and everything
- Express our gratitude to our family and friends
- Express our gratitude to our colleagues
- Express our gratitude to patients and their family members
- Express our gratitude to strangers
- Express our gratitude to enemies: they teach us patience
- Keep a gratitude journal
- Write down things you are grateful for daily
- Express thank you daily
- Appreciate and learn from adverse situations
- Praise a colleague
- Give a thank you card to a colleague
- Slow down our pace of life
- Breathe in and out to calm ourselves
- Count our blessing daily
- Start our day with lovely words

Waking up in the morning, I smile,
twenty-four brand new hours are before me,
I vow to live fully in each moment
and to look at all beings with eyes of compassion.

Thich Nhat Hanh

- Appreciate life and all its beauty from moment-to-moment
    - The sleeping faces of our loved ones
    - The first step out of bed
    - The smell of toothpaste
    - The cold running tap water
    - The mentally constructed "me" in the mirror
    - The breakfast
    - The flowers in our garden
    - The morning sun
    - The clouds
    - The swaying trees
    - The road full of cars
    - The rushing pedestrians
    - The ground that we walk as we arrive at work
    - The smile of our colleagues
    - The smile of patients or their family members
    - The tears
    - The silent grief
    - The faces of pain relief
    - The lunch
    - The wind and the falling leafs
    - The dinner
    - The time with our own family
    - The laughters and tears of our own children
    - The television
    - The book
    - The cozy sofa
    - The bed waiting for us for a whole day
- End our day with gratitude
    - Be thankful for every person that we meet that day
    - Be thankful for every little things in our life
    - Realize how blessed we are

Humour

- Practice light-heartedness
- Practice laughing without reasons when nobody is watching
- Learn to laugh at ourselves
- Learn to laugh at our adversities
- Watch a comedy
- Do some research on humour
- Memorize a few jokes every week
- Pay attention when others are joking
- Think three times before joking while breaking bad news
- Tell a patient our pulse is weaker while feeling their pulses
- Prescribe food in the medication chart
- Prescribe smiles from nurses three times a day in the care plan
- Request KY jelly from a nurse during PR, not the edible jelly
- Tell your colleague a correct PR examination can be enjoyable
- Put some jokes on the notice board
- Do not share dirty jokes openly unless boss is not around
- Laugh when others are laughing
- Avoid sarcastic jokes
- Avoid laughing at others unless they are not paying attention
- Avoid laughing when others are grieving
- Stand close to a door to escape when our joke is not funny
- Imagine the joke if it is inappropriate to share
- Look for opportunity to laugh in everyday life
- Learn from children how they laugh
- Hang around more with friends who can understand our jokes
- Type more LOLs in social media, appropriately
- Exaggerate our stories a bit while joking
- Use funny comparisons
- Treat our life as a joke
- Laugh at death, but not in front of patients
- Laugh five seconds before sleeping if we are sleeping alone

The social brain

- Neural networks that synchronize around relating to others
- Sensory stimuli: humans
- Key regions of the social circuitry
  - Amygdala
  - Fusiform gyrus
  - Superior temporal sulcus
  - Prefrontal cortex
- Amygdala
  - Two almond-shaped nuclei within the temporal lobe
  - Part of the limbic system: the emotional brain
  - Functions
    - Attaches emotional significance to sensory stimuli
    - Forms and stores emotional memories
    - Detects threat
    - Shapes social life
      - How we interact with people
      - How we react to people
  - Amygdala volume correlates with social network size
- Fusiform gyrus
  - Spindle-shaped
  - Also called occipitotemporal gyrus
  - Part of occipital lobe and temporal lobe
  - Function: facial recognition
- Superior temporal sulcus (STS)
  - Separates superior temporal from middle temporal gyrus
  - Function: social perception
    - Recognizes voices as opposed to sounds
    - Recognizes stories as opposed to nonsense speech
    - Recognizes moving faces as opposed to objects
    - Detects biological motion

- Prefrontal cortex
  - Orbitofrontal cortex (OFC)
    - Medial OFC: stimulus-reward association
    - Lateral OFC: stimulus-outcome association
    - Functions
      - Judges facial attractiveness
      - Supports the "reward" feelings
- The resonance circuit of empathy
  - Components
    - Mirror-neuron system for reflexive empathy
      - Broca's area
      - Premotor cortex
      - Motor cortex
      - Posterior superior temporal sulcus (STS)
      - Inferior parietal lobule
    - Emotional empathy
      - Amygdala
      - Fusiform gyrus
      - Superior temporal sulcus
    - Cognitive empathy
      - Middle prefrontal cortex
        - Orbitomedial prefrontal cortex
          - Orbitofrontal cortex
          - Medial prefrontal cortex
        - Anterior cingulate cortex
        - Ventrolateral prefrontal cortex
    - Insular cortex
      - Connects mirror neurons to limbic system for the development of emotional empathy
      - Connects limbic system and bodily information to middle prefrontal cortex for the empathic imagination of cognitive empathy

Index

Printed in the United States
By Bookmasters

Beginning Mathematica and Wolfram for Data Science

Applications in Data Analysis, Machine Learning, and Neural Networks

Second Edition

Jalil Villalobos Alva

Apress®

Beginning Mathematica and Wolfram for Data Science: Applications in Data Analysis, Machine Learning, and Neural Networks

Jalil Villalobos Alva
Mexico City, Mexico

ISBN-13 (pbk): 979-8-8688-0347-5
https://doi.org/10.1007/979-8-8688-0348-2

ISBN-13 (electronic): 979-8-8688-0348-2

Managing Director, Apress Media LLC: Welmoed Spahr
Acquisitions Editor: Melissa Duffy
Development Editor: James Markham
Editorial Project Manager: Gryffin Winkler
Copyeditor: Kim Burton

Cover designed by eStudioCalamar

Cover image designed by Mathew Schwartz on Unsplash (www.unsplash.com)

Distributed to the book trade worldwide by Springer Science+Business Media New York, 1 New York Plaza, Suite 4600, New York, NY 10004-1562, USA. Phone 1-800-SPRINGER, fax (201) 348-4505, e-mail orders-ny@springer-sbm.com, or visit www.springeronline.com. Apress Media, LLC is a California LLC and the sole member (owner) is Springer Science + Business Media Finance Inc (SSBM Finance Inc). SSBM Finance Inc is a **Delaware** corporation.

For information on translations, please e-mail booktranslations@springernature.com; for reprint, paperback, or audio rights, please e-mail bookpermissions@springernature.com.

Apress titles may be purchased in bulk for academic, corporate, or promotional use. eBook versions and licenses are also available for most titles. For more information, reference our Print and eBook Bulk Sales web page at http://www.apress.com/bulk-sales.

Any source code or other supplementary material referenced by the author in this book is available to readers on GitHub. For more detailed information, please visit https://www.apress.com/gp/services/source-code.

If disposing of this product, please recycle the paper

To my family, who supported me in all aspects

Table of Contents

About the Author

Jalil Villalobos Alva is a Wolfram Language programmer and Mathematica user. He graduated with a degree in engineering physics from the Universidad Iberoamericana in Mexico City. His research background comprises quantum physics, bioinformatics, proteomics, and protein design. His academic interests cover the topics of quantum technology, bioinformatics, machine learning, artificial intelligence, stochastic processes, and space engineering. During his idle hours, he likes playing soccer, swimming, and listening to music.

About the Technical Reviewer

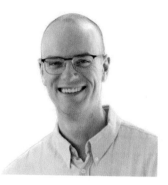

Andrew Yule is a co-founder and managing partner of Pontem Analytics, a global consulting company in the energy industry specializing in combining domain expertise with data-driven solutions. Andrew has over 13 years of professional experience leveraging the Wolfram Language and was the recipient of the Wolfram Innovator Award in 2017. He is an editor for the Society of Petroleum Engineers, The Way Ahead magazine, and is also currently a member of the Young Entrepreneurial Council. His technical background includes a bachelor's degree in chemical engineering from the Colorado School of Mines and a master's degree in data science from Southern Methodist University.

Acknowledgments

I want to thank the collective support and guidance received throughout the development of this project's second edition. The contributions of numerous past and present individuals have played an integral role in shaping this work. Their assistance, feedback, and mentorship have been invaluable, enriching the content and presentation of this edition. I also want to thank the technical and staff reviewers for their valuable comments and feedback during this manuscript. They both helped me improve the material's presentation and theoretical work. And finally, I would like to thank Las Des Nestor and "Los Betos" for teaching me great mastery.

Introduction

Welcome to *Beginning Mathematica and Wolfram for Data Science.*

Why is data science important nowadays? Data science is an active topic that is evolving daily; new methods, techniques, and data are created daily. Data science is an interdisciplinary field involving scientific methods, algorithms, and systematic procedures to extract data sets and thus better understand the data in its different structures. It is a continuation of some theoretical data analysis fields such as statistics, data mining, machine learning, and pattern analysis. With a unique objective, to extract quantitative and qualitative information of value from the data being recollected from various sources, and thus be able to objectively count an event for decision-making, product development, pattern detection, or identification of new business areas.

Data Science Roadmap

Data science carries out a series of processes to solve a problem, which includes data acquisition, data processing, model construction, communication of results, and data monitoring or model improvement. The first step is to formalize an objective in the investigation. From the object of the investigation, you can proceed to the data acquisition sources. This step focuses on finding the right data sources. The product of this path is usually raw data, which must be processed before it can be handled. Data processing includes transforming the data from a raw form to a state in which it can be reproduced to construct a mathematical model. Proceeding to the construction of the model, a stage that intends to obtain the information by making predictions in accordance with the conditions established in the early stages. Here, the appropriate techniques and tools, which consist of different disciplines, are used. The objective is to obtain a model that provides the best results. The next step is to present the outcome of the study. Which consists of reporting the results obtained and whether they are congruent with the established research objective. Finally, it comes to data monitoring, with the intention of keeping the data updated because data can change constantly and in different ways.

Data Science Techniques

Data science includes analysis techniques from different disciplines, such as mathematics, statistics, computer science, and numerical analysis. The following are some disciplines and techniques used.

- Statistics (linear, multiple regressions, least squares method, hypothesis testing, analysis of variance (ANOVA), cross-validation, resampling methods)

- Graph theory (network analysis, social network analysis)

- Artificial intelligence

- Machine learning

- Supervised learning (natural language processing, decision trees, naive bayes, nearest neighbors. support vector machine)

- Unsupervised learning (cluster analysis, anomaly detection, K-means cluster)

- Deep learning (artificial neural networks, deep neural networks)

- Stochastic processes (Monte Carlo methods, Markov chains, time series analysis, nonlinear models)

Even though many techniques exist, this list only shows a part of it since research on data science, machine learning, and artificial neural networks is constantly increasing.

Prerequisites

This book is intended for readers who want to learn about Mathematica / Wolfram Language and implement it in data science; it focuses on the basic principles of data science as well as for programmers outside of software development, that is, people who write code for their academic and research projects, including students, researchers, teachers, and many others. The general audience is not expected to be familiar with Wolfram Language or with the front-end program Mathematica, but little or any experience is welcome. Previous knowledge of the syntax would be an advantage in understanding how the commands work in Mathematica. If this is not the case, the book provides the basic concepts of the Wolfram Language syntax. The fundamental structure of expressions in the Wolfram Language. Basic handling and understanding of Mathematica notebooks.

Prior knowledge or some experience with programming, mathematical concepts such as numbers, trigonometric functions, and basic statistics are useful, along with some understanding of mathematical modeling, which is also helpful but not compulsory.

Wolfram Language is different from many other languages but very intuitive and user-friendly to learn.

The book aims to teach the general structure of the Wolfram Language, data structures, objects, and rules for writing efficient code, and at the same time, teach data management techniques that allow them to solve problems in a simple and effective way. Provide the reader with the basic tools of the Wolfram Language, such as creating structured data, to support the construction of future practical projects.

For this new version, all the programming was carried out on a MacBook Air M1 with Sonoma 14 environment with the installation of version 13.3.1.0 and 14 of Wolfram Mathematica. Wolfram Mathematica is currently supported in other environments such as Linux, Windows, and macOS. The code found in the book works with both the Pro and Student versions.

Book Conventions

Throughout the book, you may come across different words written distinctly from others. Throughout the book, the words command, built-in functions, and functions may be used as synonyms that mean Wolfram Language commands written in Mathematica. So, a function will be written in the form of the real name; for example, RandomInteger.

The evaluation of expressions appears in the Mathematica In/Out format; the same applies to blocks of code.

```
In[#]:= "Hello World!"
Out[#]= "Hello World!"
```

The Layout

The book is written in a compact and focused way to cover the basic ideas behind the Wolfram Language and cover details on more complex topics. Some chapters have been revised and redesigned in this new version to focus on novice and advanced topics.

Chapter 1 discusses the starting topics of the Wolfram Language, basic syntax, and basic concepts with some example application areas, followed by an overview of the basic operations and debugging techniques, and concludes by discussing security measures within a Mathematica session.

Chapter 2 provides the key concepts and commands for data manipulation, sampling, types of objects, and some concepts of linear algebra—the introduction to lists, an important concept to understand in the Wolfram Language.

Chapter 3 discusses how to work properly with data and the initiation of the core structures for creating a dataset object, introducing concepts like associations and association rules are discussed with a conclusion remarking how associations and dataset constructions can be interpreted as a generalization of a hash table aiming to expose a better understanding of internal structures inside the Wolfram Language, including an overview of performing operations on a list and between lists and then discussing various techniques applied to dataset objects.

Chapter 4 exposes the main ideas behind importing and exporting data with examples throughout the chapter with common and newly added file formats. It also presents a very powerful command known as SemanticImport, which can import data elements that are natural language.

Chapter 5 covers the topic areas for new data visualization, common data plots, data colors, data markers, and how to customize a plot. Basic commands for 2D plots and 3D plots are presented, too.

Chapter 6 introduces the statistical data analysis. Starting with random data generation begins by introducing some standard statistical measures, followed by a discussion on creating statistical charts and performing an ordinary least square method.

Chapter 7 exposes the basis for data exploration and reviews a central discussion on the Wolfram Data Repository. Performing descriptive statistics and data visualization inside Fisher's Irises dataset objects is also covered.

Chapter 8 starts with machine learning concepts and techniques, such as gradient descent, linear regression, logistic regression, and cluster analysis, including examples from various datasets like the Boston and Titanic datasets and newly implemented features.

Chapter 9 introduces the key ideas and the basic theory to understand the construction of neural networks in the Wolfram Language, such as layers, containers, and graphs. The MXNet framework in the Wolfram Language scheme is also discussed.

Chapter 10 concludes the book by discussing training neural networks in the Wolfram Language. In addition, the Wolfram Neural Net Repository is discussed with an example application, examining how to access data inside Mathematica and the retrieval of information, such as credit risk modeling fraud detection, and concluding with the example of the LeNet neural network, reviewing the idea behind this neural network and exposing the main points on the architecture with the help of the MXNet graph operations and a final road map on the creation, evaluation, and deployment of predictive models with the Wolfram Language. In this new version, LLM (large language model) features are introduced with the connection to GPT services, use of chat cells, and presentation of the GPT-1 and GPT-2 models.

CHAPTER 1

Introduction to Mathematica

The chapter begins with a preliminary introduction to why Mathematica is a useful and practical tool. It explores the core concepts of the Wolfram Language and its syntax. It starts by explaining the internal structure of Mathematica and how to add code effectively. The concept of a notebook is introduced, which is important to understand the type of format that Mathematica handles. The chapter examines this interface class and demonstrates how notebooks simultaneously support code and text. In this way, a notebook is a computable text file. Next, you inspect various add-ons that can be employed within a notebook to help the user maximize their code's capabilities.

The next section demonstrates how to write expressions in Mathematica, examining topics such as arithmetic, algebra, symbols, global and local variables, built-in functions, date and time formats, plotting functions, logical operators, performance measures, delayed expressions, and accessing Wolfram Alpha. You then look at how Mathematica performs code computations, including its accepted varieties of inputs and the evaluation of these inputs. This chapter concludes with tips for seeking support within Mathematica, managing and handling errors, searching for solutions, and safely dealing with security concerns in notebooks that incorporate dynamic content.

Why Mathematica?

Mathematica is a mathematical software package created by Stephen Wolfram more than 35 years ago. Its first official version (Mathematica 1.0) emerged in 1988 and was created as an algebraic computational system capable of handling symbolic computations. However, Mathematica has established itself as a tool capable of performing complex tasks efficiently, automatically, and intuitively. Mathematica is

© Jalil Villalobos Alva 2024
J. Villalobos Alva, *Beginning Mathematica and Wolfram for Data Science*,
https://doi.org/10.1007/979-8-8688-0348-2_1

widely used in many disciplines like engineering, optics, physics, graph theory, financial engineering, game development, and software development.

Mathematica provides a complete, integrated platform to import, analyze, and visualize data. Mathematica does not require plug-ins. It also has a mixed syntax, performing both symbolic and numerical calculations. It provides an accessible way to read the code with the implementation of notebooks as a standard format, which also serves to create detailed reports of the processes carried out. Mathematica can be characterized as a powerful platform enabling efficient and concise forms of work. Among computer languages, the Wolfram Language falls into the group of programming languages classified as a high-level, multi-paradigm interpreted language. Unlike conventional programming languages, the Wolfram Language adheres to unique rules, facilitating order and clear, compact code composition.

The Wolfram Language

Mathematica is powered by the Wolfram Language, an interpreted high-level programming language that covers both symbolic and numeric capabilities. To understand the Wolfram Language, it is necessary to remember that the language's core nature resembles a normal mathematical text, as opposed to other programming languages' syntax. The following describes some remarkable features of the Wolfram Language.

- The first letter of a built-in function word is uppercase and is also human-readable.

- Any element introduced in the language is taken as an expression.

- Expressions take values consisting of the Wolfram Language atomic expressions.

  - A symbol made up of letters, numbers, or alphanumeric contents

  - Four types of numbers: integers, rational, real, and complex

  - The default character string is written within the quotation marks (" ")

- In Mathematica, there are three ways to group expressions.

  - Parentheses group terms within an expression (expr1 + expr2) + (expr3).

  - Command entries are enclosed by brackets [ ]. Also, square brackets enclose the arguments of a built-in function, F[x].

  - Mathematica uses curly braces {} (e.g., {a, b, c}) to represent lists, arrays, matrixes, and other collections.

Structure of Mathematica

Before entering code, you need to get the layout of Mathematica. To launch Mathematica, go to your Applications folder and select the Mathematica icon. This action brings up the new welcome screen, illustrated in Figure 1-1.

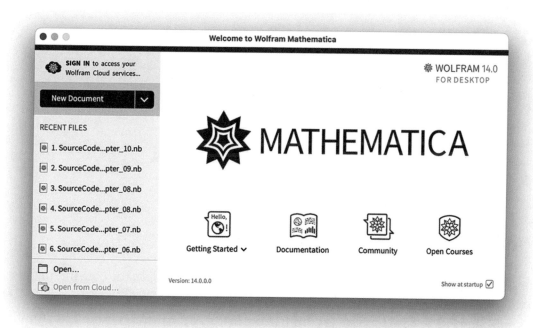

Figure 1-1. *The default welcome screen for Mathematica's latest version*

Tip   The startup window offers valuable information for new and adept users, including the Mathematica version, access to documentation, resources, and the Wolfram community, among other things.

After the startup screen appears, you can create a new notebook by selecting the New Document button, and a blank page should appear like the one shown in Figure 1-2. New documents can also be created by selecting File ➤ New ➤ Notebook or with the ⌘+N (macOS) or Ctrl+N (Win) keyboard shortcut command.

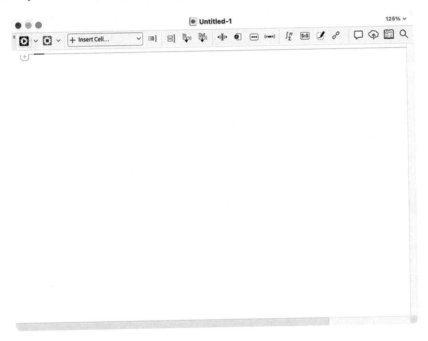

Figure 1-2. A blank notebook ready to receive input

The blank document that appears is called a notebook, and it's the core interaction between the user and Mathematica. Notebooks can be saved locally from the menu bar by selecting File ➤ Save (or Save as). Initializing Mathematica always exhibits an untitled notebook. Notebooks serve as the standard document format. They can be customized to display text alongside computations. However, the key feature of Mathematica lies in its capacity to perform computations, extending beyond numerical calculations, regardless of the notebook's purpose.

> **Note**   Mathematica version 13.1 introduced a new default assistant toolbar.

Mathematica's notebooks are separated into input spaces called cells. Cells are represented by the square brackets on the notebook's right side. Each input and output cell has its bracket. Brackets enclosed by larger brackets are related computations, whether input or output. Grouped cells are represented by nested brackets that contain the whole evaluation cell. Other cells can be grouped by selecting and grouping them with the right-click option. Cells can also have the capability to show or hide input by simply double-clicking the cells. To add a new cell, move the text cursor down, and a flat line should appear, marking the new cell ready to receive input expressions. The plus tab in the line is the assistant input tab, showing the various types of input supported by Mathematica. Figure 1-3 displays grouped input (In[-]) and output (Out[-]) cells.

$$In[\circ]:=\ \texttt{"Hello World"}$$
$$Out[\circ]=\ \texttt{Hello World}$$

Figure 1-3. *Expression cells are grouped by input and output*

There are four main input types. The default input is the Wolfram Language code input. Free-form input is involved with Wolfram knowledge-base servers, and the results are shown in Wolfram Language syntax. Wolfram Alpha query is associated with results explicitly shown on the Wolfram Alpha website. External Language Input is built-in support for common external programming supported by Mathematica.

There are four main input types.

- Default input: Wolfram Language code input

- Free-form input: involved with Wolfram knowledge-base servers and the results are shown in Wolfram Language syntax

- Wolfram Alpha query: associated with results explicitly shown on the Wolfram Alpha website

- External language input: built-in support for common external programming supported by Mathematica

These are illustrated in Figure 1-4.

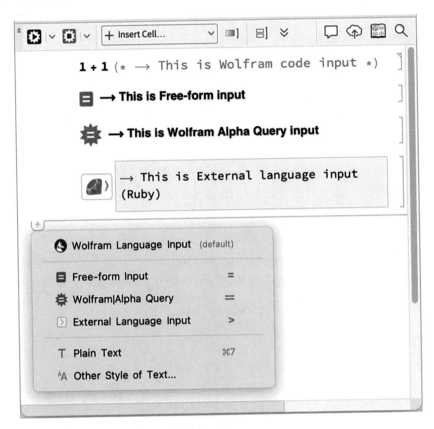

Figure 1-4. *Main input types in Mathematica*

Tip   Keyboard shortcuts for front-end instruction commands are shown on the right or left side of each panel.

Design of Mathematica

Now that you have the lay of the land of Mathematica's basic format, you can learn the internal structure of how Mathematica works. Inside Mathematica, there are two fundamental processes: the Mathematica kernel and the graphical interface. The Mathematica kernel is the one that takes care of performing the programming computations; it is where the Wolfram Language is interpreted and is associated with each Mathematica session. The Mathematica interface allows the user to interact with the Wolfram Language functions and, at the same time, document your progress.

Each notebook contains cells, where the commands that the Mathematica kernel receives are written and then evaluated. Each cell has an associated number. There are two types of cells: the Input cell and the Output cell. These are associated with each other and have the following expressions: In[n]:= Expression and Out [n]: = Result or ("new expr"). The evaluations are listed according to which cell is evaluated first and continue in ascending order. When quitting the kernel session, all the information, computations made, and stored variables are relinquished, and the kernel is restarted, including the cell expressions. To quit a kernel session, select Evaluation ➤ Quit Kernel ➤ Local.

Tip   To start a new kernel session, click Evaluation ➤ Start Kernel ➤ Local.

To begin, try typing the following computation.

```
In[1] := (11*17) + (4/2)
Out[1] = 189
```

The computation shows that In and Out have a number enclosed. This number is the number associated with the evaluated expression.

A suggestion bar appears after every expression is evaluated (see Figure 1-5). The suggestion bar in Mathematica is always visible unless the user hides it. But the suggestion bar offers suggestions for possible new commands or functions to be applied to the generated output. The suggestion bar can sometimes be helpful if you are unsure what to code next; if used wisely, it might be helpful.

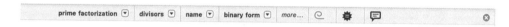

Figure 1-5. *Suggestion bar for more possible evaluations*

The input form of Mathematica is intuitive; to write in a Mathematica notebook, you just have to put the cursor in a blank space, and the cursor indicates that you are inside a cell that has not been evaluated. To evaluate a cell, click the keys [Shift + Enter], instructing Mathematica kernel to evaluate the expression written. The next chapter looks at the new form to evaluate expressions using the new toolbar.

To evaluate the whole notebook, go to the Evaluation tab on the toolbar and select Evaluate Notebook. If the execution of calculations takes more time than expected, you make a wrong execution of code, or if you want to seize a computation, Mathematica provides several ways to stop calculations. To abort a computation, go to

Evaluation ➤ Abort Evaluation. Alternatively, use the keyboard shortcut in Windows [Alt + .] or macOS [⌘ + .].

When a new notebook is created, the default settings are applied to every cell (input style). Nevertheless, preferences can be edited in Mathematica with various options. To access them, go to Edit ➤ Preferences. On macOS, the Preferences (settings) menu is located in the application menu, go to Mathematica ➤ Settings.

Once opened, a pop-up window appears (see Figure 1-6) with multiple tabs (Interface, Appearance, AI Settings, etc.). Basic customizations involve magnification, language settings, and other general instructions. The Appearance tab is related to code syntax color (i.e., symbols, strings, comments, errors, etc.). The AI Settings tab is the new tab associated with the LLM (large language model) evaluator. Other options belong to advanced settings that are not used in this book. Feel free to navigate each option.

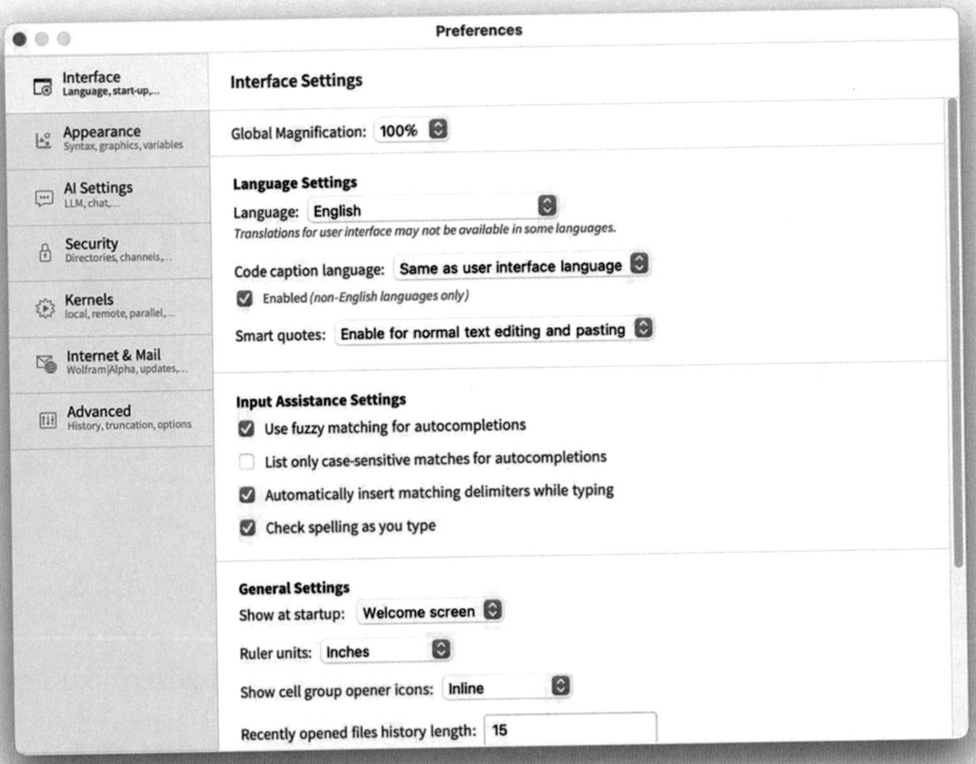

Figure 1-6. *Preferences window*

Later, you learn about in-depth settings and customization options for the notebook interface that allow you to tailor preferences.

Mathematica Environment

This section explores the user interface of Mathematica, with a focus on the notebook interface, as well as the other user experience functionalities.

Notebook Interface

Mathematica is always on the quest to improve user experience and boost productivity. In version 13.1, a big enhancement has been introduced—the seamless integration of a default toolbar (see Figure 1-7) across all standard notebook user interfaces (UIs).

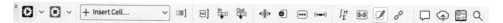

Figure 1-7. *The new UI default toolbar showcases essential tools and functionalities for efficient code development. Toolbar icons may vary by Mathematica version*

This new toolbar (described left to right) includes several new features to enhance user experience. Evaluate allows users basic and costume code evaluation. Abort lets users cancel queued cells and remove chosen ones; both options are shown in Figure 1-8. These features can also be accessed via the keyboard, as previously mentioned.

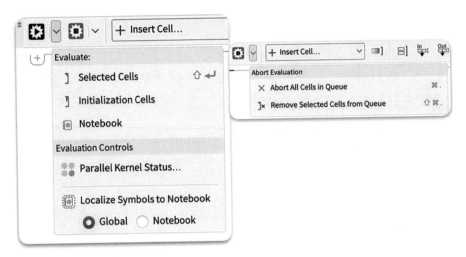

Figure 1-8. *Extensive options for code evaluation and abort options in a notebook interface; the double arrow-like shape hides the toolbar*

The other options integrate text cell formatting, offering styling options like cell style (title, subtitle, etc.) and cell color background. Users also benefit from the convenient cell management functions, such as grouping, dividing, merging cells, and inserting input/output of cells, all reduced to simple buttons. Continuing to options like extend selection, convert natural language into Wolfram Language code, collapse cells, insert comment, math form input, and LATEX rendering, users also have access to drawing canvas and hyperlink features. Finally, the rightmost section of the toolbar includes buttons for chat notebooks (utilizing LLM features), saving or publishing to the Wolfram Cloud, accessing documentation (local or web-based), and searching within the notebook.

Note   Different buttons may appear based on the selected cell type where the cursor resides, ranging from text to code formatting. Figure 1-7 shows for Wolfram Language code input cell. Figure 1-9 shows for text display cell.

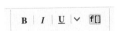

Figure 1-9. *Text cell options for bold, italic, and underline and insert code text evaluation and abort options in a notebook interface*

This essential addition provides a coherent user experience and fosters a more streamlined, productive programming environment within Mathematica. For example, Figure 1-10 shows a code input cell with a colored background.

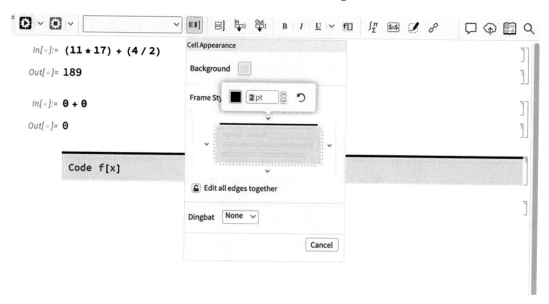

Figure 1-10. *Light-green code input cell, with a 2pt black top margin*

Besides the default toolbar, more improvements were made to the other toolbars, Ruler, Formatting, Templating, and Testing, as Figure 1-11 shows. The last two are not shown since they are more associated with a specific type of programmatic notebook, which is beyond the scope of this book.

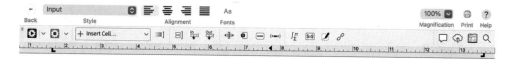

Figure 1-11. *Notebook application toolbar menu showcasing three distinct toolbars: formatting (upper), default (central), and ruler (lower)*

Note   To show or hide any toolbar, go to Window ➤ Toolbar. Toolbar availability varies by version.

The prominent toolbar Ruler indicates and adjusts the text margins of specified cells using draggable marks, offering control over the text format. The Formatting toolbar brings advanced textual design options, while the Templating and Testing toolbars (not shown in the image) facilitate the efficient creation of new templates and testing programmatic notebooks.

Text Processing

Notebooks can include explanatory text, titles, sections, and subsections. The Mathematica notebook resembles a computable document rather than a programming command line. Text is useful for describing code and can be inserted into cells as text cells, which often relate to the corresponding computations. Mathematica allows you to work with multiple forms of text cells, including lines of text, chapters, formulas, items, bullets, and more. Like a word-processing tool, notebooks can have titles, chapters, sections, and subsections. By selecting Format ➤ Style, additional options become available. For more control over style cells, use the formatting toolbar (see Figure 1-12) found by navigating to Window ➤ Toolbar Formatting in the menu bar. The formatting toolbar streamlines cell styling, allowing users to justify text left, center, right, or fully.

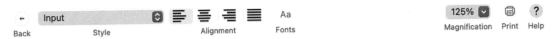

Figure 1-12. *The Style Format toolbar has a user-friendly interface for customizing text appearance*

The cell types can be arranged in different forms, depending on the notebook's format. There are numerous forms to add text in a cell; the most straightforward is to type the text in the input cell, and the Assistant tab input automatically suggests converting it to text. Another alternative is to choose the cell type from the toolbars, with the input chooser or the shortcut (⌘+7 or Ctrl+7).

Styled text can be created with the formatting toolbar or by selecting the desired style in Format ➤ Style ➤ (title, chapter, text, code, input, etc.). In the Style menu, note the keyboard shortcuts for all the available text styles. It can be used instead of going into the menu bar every time. Plain text can also be converted into input text by formatting the cell in the Input style. There is no restriction in converting text; text can be converted into whatever style is supported in the format menu.

Note   To convert text, highlight the text or select the cell that contains the text.

As shown in Figure 1-13, styled cells look different from others. Each style has a unique order by which a notebook is organized into cell groups. A title cell has a higher order in a notebook, so the other cells are anchored to the title cell, as shown in Figure 1-13, but it does not mean that if another title cell is added, both titles are grouped. If the title cell is collapsed, the title is the only displayed text.

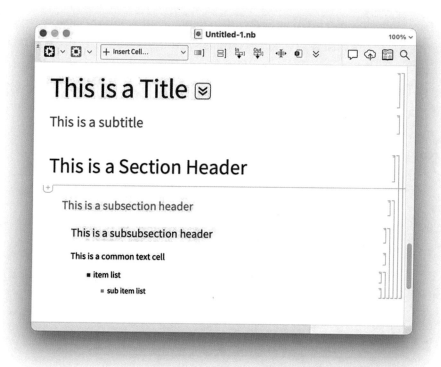

Figure 1-13. *A notebook with different format styles; this includes title, subtitle, section, subsections, plain text, item list, and subitem list*

Text can be given a particular style, changed, and different formats applied throughout the notebook. By selecting Font or Show Fonts (macOS users) from the Format menu, a pop-up window appears, allowing you to change the font, font style, size, and other characteristics.

Tip   To clear the format style of a cell, select the cell and then the right-click button and choose Clear Formatting.

Palettes

Palettes show different ways to enter various commands into Mathematica. A diverse quantity of special characters and typesetting symbols are used in the Wolfram Language, which can be typed within expressions to more closely resemble mathematical text. The best way to access these symbols is by using the pallets built into Mathematica. To select a simple pallet, go to Pallets ➤ Basic Math Assistant. Each pallet has different tabs that stand for different categories with distinct commands and a variety of characters or placeholders that can be inserted using the pallets. To enter the symbol, type **ESC** followed by the name of the symbol, then ESC again. Try typing (**ESC a ESC**) to type the lowercase alpha Greek letter. Figure 1-14 shows the basic math assistant pallet in Mathematica.

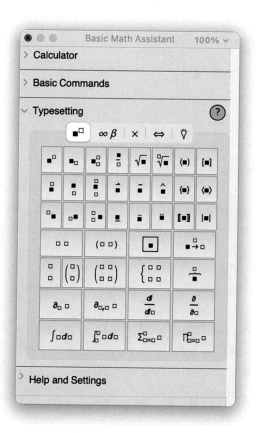

Figure 1-14. *The Basic Math Assistant palette*

Note   Hovering the mouse cursor over a symbol or character, an information tip pops up, showing the keyboard shortcut. This also applies to placeholders.

Notebook Style and Features

In the new versions comprising version 13.0 and beyond, Mathematica has been refining and polishing its notebook interface by adding new features for a smoother user experience. One considerable enhancement involves the handling of extensive outputs within the user interface. Users can efficiently manage and interpret sizable outputs without overwhelming the notebook display or causing memory issues. The following example generates a large amount of data, which can be suppressed, displayed, or even stored in the notebook (see Figure 1-15).

```
In[2]:= Table[i^12,{i,1,10^4}]
Out[2]=
```

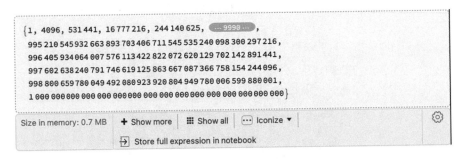

Figure 1-15. *Large output menu displaying additional user control*

Figure 1-15 shows that the input code returns a responsive output. Users can expand, show, iconize, or select to store the whole data expression. Additionally, the data can be fully stored in the notebook, preserving the entire output for future manipulation and consuming 0.7MB of memory. If you iconize large outputs, a summary of the data structure, length, and size is displayed. See Figure 1-16.

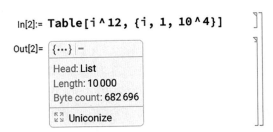

Figure 1-16. *List structure with 10,000 items and a byte count of 682,696*

Another aspect that has been renewed is the preference settings. The whole settings display has undergone notable refreshment in terms of customization options, as illustrated in Figure 1-6. Specifically, regarding the notebook front end, by selecting the Appearance tab (see Figure 1-17), users can tailor their choices to optimize their notebook code style, resulting in a more personalized experience.

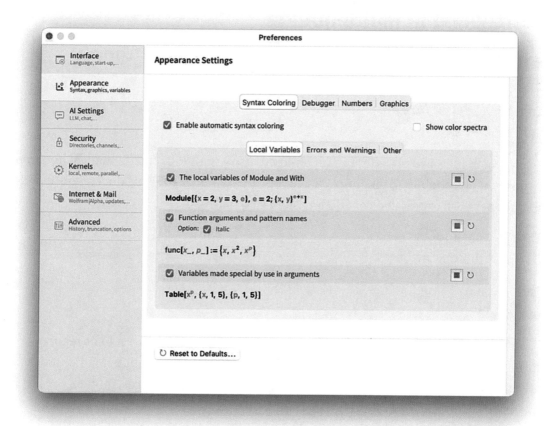

Figure 1-17. *Notebook settings customization*

Figure 1-17 shows Appearance Settings window. The Syntax Coloring tab is related to the visual representation of code elements (variables, errors, automatic coloring, highlighting, etc.). The Debugger tab includes coloring options about debugger highlights, breakpoints, and evaluation points. The Numbers tab offers multiple choices based on formatting and configuration choices, a few mentions are digits control numerical notation, among others. The Graphics tab allows you to choose the render of 2D and 3D graphics, from lowest to highest quality.

Note   To change the colors of the code syntax options in the Appearance windows. Select the variables checkbox and click the green square. A color wheel pops up, allowing you to change the color. This process is the same for the three code setting options. Also, as you can see, there are different tabs.

Expression in Mathematica

Basic arithmetic operations can be performed in Mathematica with a common, intuitive form.

```
In[3]:= (3*3) + (4/2)
Out[3] = 11
```

Mathematica also provides the capability to use a traditional mathematical notation. To insert a placeholder in the form, click [Ctrl + 6]. To indicate the product operation, use a space between expressions or add an asterisk (*) between.

```
In[4]:= 100² * 10
Out[4]= 100000
```

```
In[5]:= 2 1
Out[5]= 2
```

The standard Mathematica format aims to deliver the value closest to its regular form, so when dealing with decimal numbers or general math notation, Mathematica always gives you the best precision (involving, in some circumstances, infinite precision). However, it allows you to manipulate expressions numerically, to display numeric values, you use the N function. To insert the square root, type [Ctrl + 2].

```
In[6]:= 1/2 +√2
Out[6]= 1/2 + √2
```

```
In[7]:= N[1/2+√2]
Out[7]= 1.91421
```

You can manage the number precision of a numeric expression. In this case, you establish 10 decimal places.

```
In[8]:= N[77/13,10]
Out[8]= 5.923076923
```

For a shortcut to work with the decimal point, just type a dot (.) anywhere in the expression, and with this, you are telling Mathematica to calculate the value with machine precision.

$$In[9]:=\frac{4.}{2}+\frac{2}{13}$$

Out[9]= 2.15385

Mathematica performs the sequence of operations from left to right, in line with the written expression, while adhering to the standard order of mathematical operations. To evaluate an expression without showing the result, you add a semicolon (;) after the end of the first term. In the following example, the 11/7 is evaluated but not shown, and the other term is displayed.

```
In[10]:= 11/7; Sqrt[4]
Out[10]= 2
```

The last form of code is called a compound expression. Expressions can be written in a single line of code, and with compound expressions, they are evaluated in the intended sequence. If you write the semicolon in each expression, Mathematica does not return the values, but they are evaluated.

```
In[11]:= 3*4; 100*100; Sqrt[4];Power[2,2];
Out[11]=
```

There is no output, but all the expressions have been evaluated. Later, you use compound expressions to understand the concept of delayed expressions. This basic feature of the Wolfram Language makes it possible for expressions to be evaluated but not displayed to save memory.

Assigning Values

In the Wolfram Language, each variable requires a unique identifier that distinguishes it from the others. A variable in the Wolfram Language can be a union of more than one letter and digits; it must also not coincide with protected words—reserved words that refer to commands or built-in functions. Keep in mind that the Wolfram Language is case-sensitive. User variables are advised to be lowercase to avoid confusion with built-in symbols.

Note   Mathematica supports assigning values to variables, which enables the effective handling of algebraic variables.

Undefined variables or symbols appear in blue font, while defined or recognized built-in functions appear in black. It is also true that the previously mentioned characteristics can be changed in the preferences window.

Use the keyboard shortcut Esc pi Esc (pi number) to write special constants and Greek letters. A symbol of a vertical ellipsis (:) should appear every time Esc is typed. Another choice is to write the first letter of the name, and a sub-menu showing a list of options should appear.

```
In[12]:= a=Pi
x=11
z+y
Out[12]= π
Out[13]= 11
Out[14]= y+z
```

In the previous example, Mathematica expresses each output with its cell, even though the input cell is just one. That is because Mathematica gives each cell a unique identifier. To access previous evaluations, the symbol (%) is used. Additionally, Mathematica lets you retrieve previous values using the cell input/output information by the % # command and the number of the cell or by explicitly writing the command with In [# of cell] or Out [# of cell]. As demonstrated in the next example, Mathematica gives the same value for each expression.

```
In[15]:=
%12
In[12]
Out[12]

Out[15]= π
Out[16]= π
Out[17]= π
```

To determine whether a word is reserved within the Wolfram Language, use the Attributes command; this displays the attributes to the associated command. Attributes are general aspects that define functions in the Wolfram Language. When the word "Protected" appears in the attributes, it means that the word of the function is reserved. The next example shows whether the word "Power" is reserved.

```
In[18]:= Attributes[Power]
Out[18]= {Listable,NumericFunction,OneIdentity,Protected}
```

As seen in the attributes, "Power" is a protected word. Importantly, most of the built-in functions in Mathematica are listable—that is, the function is interleaved to the lists that appear as arguments to the function.

Variables can be presented in a notebook in the following ways: (1) global variables, or those that are defined and can be used throughout the notebook, like the ones in the earlier examples; and (2) local variables, which are defined in only one block that corresponds to what is known as a module, in which they are only defined within a module. A module has the following form: Module [symbol1, symbol 2... body of module].

```
In[19]:= Module[{l=1,k=2,h=3},h Sqrt[k+1] + k + 1]
Out[19]= 3 + 3 √3
```

Variables inside a module turn green by default; this is a handy feature for seeing the code inside a module block. A local variable only exists inside the module, so if you try to access them outside their module, the symbol is unassigned, as shown in the following example.

```
In[20]:= {l,k,h}
Out[20]= {l,k,h}
```

Variables can be cleared with multiple commands, but the most suitable command is the Clear[symbol], which removes assigned values from the specified variable or variables. So, if you evaluate the variable after Clear, Mathematica treats it as a symbol, and you can check it with the command Head; Head always gives you the head of the expression, which is the type of object in the Wolfram Language.

```
In[21]:= Clear[a,x]
```

And if you check the head a, you see that "a" is a symbol.

```
In[22]:= Head[a]
Out[22]= Symbol
```

Symbols or variables assigned during a session remain in the memory unless they are removed or the kernel session ends.

Note   Remove is an alternative to Clear.

Built-in Functions

Built-in commands or functions are written in common English with the first letter capitalized. Some functions have abbreviations, while others employ PascalCase notation with two capital letters. Here, different examples of functions are presented. Built-in functions and group expressions often require arguments, which are values that the function needs to execute the correct operation. Functions may or may not accept arguments; they are separated by commas.

```
In[23]:= RandomInteger[]
Out[23]= 0
```

Note   RandomInteger, with no arguments, returns a random integer from the interval of 0 to 1, so do not panic if the result is not the same.

```
In[24]:= Sin[90 Degree] + Cos[0 Degree]
Out[24]= 2

In[25]:= Power[2,2]
Out[25]= 4
```

Built-in functions can also be assigned symbols.

```
In[26]:= d=Power[2,2]
  F=Sin[π] + Cos[π]
Out[26]= 4
Out[27]= -1

In[28]:= Clear[d,F]
```

Some commands or built-in functions in Mathematica have options that can be specified in a particular expression. To see whether a built-in function has available options, use Option. In the next example, the RandomReal function creates a pseudo-random real number between an established interval.

```
In[29]:= Options[RandomReal]
Out[29]= {WorkingPrecision → MachinePrecision}
```

RandomReal has only one option for specifying specific instructions within the WorkingPrecision command. The default value for this option is MachinePrecision. WorkingPrecision defines the number of digits of precision for internal computations, while MachinePrecision is the symbol used to approximate real numbers, denoted by $MachinePrecision. To see the value of MachinePrecision, type $MachinePrecision. The next example observes the difference between using default values for an option and employing custom values.

```
In[30]:= RandomReal[{0,1},WorkingPrecision->MachinePrecision]
RandomReal[{0,1},WorkingPrecision->30]
Out[30]= 0.19858
Out[31]= 0.451259323577871140781571594337
```

Tip   In the Wolfram Language, global constants, which can be considered environmental variables, always start with a dollar sign (e.g., $MachinePrecision).

The first one returns a value with six digits after the decimal point, and the other returns a value with 30 digits after the decimal point. However, some built-in functions, such as Power, do not have any options associated with them.

```
In[32]:= Options[Power]
Out[32]= {}
```

Dates and Time

The DateObject command provides results for concretely manipulating dates and times (see Figure 1-18). Date and time input and basic words are supported.

```
In[33]:=DateObject[]
Out[33]=
```

> Wed 13 Sep 2023 12:44:31 GMT−6

Figure 1-18. *The date of Wed 13 Sept 2023 and time zone*

DateObjects with no arguments give the current date, as shown in Figure 1-19. Natural language is supported in Mathematica—for instance, getting the date after Wed 13 Sept 2023.

```
In[34]:= Tomorrow
Out[34]=
```

> Thu 14 Sep 2023

Figure 1-19. *The date of Thu 14 Sep 2023*

The date format is entered as year, month, and day. It also supports string date formats and different calendars, as the next code dates show.

```
In[35]:= DateString[DateObject[{2020,6,10}]]
Out[35]= Wed 10 Jun 2020
```

```
In[36]:= DateString[DateObject[Today,CalendarType->"Julian"]]
DateString[DateObject[Today,CalendarType->"Jewish"]]
Out[36]= Wed 31 Aug 2023
Out[37]= Yom Revi'i 27 Elul 5783
```

The command also supports options that are related to a time zone.

```
In[38]:= DateString[DateObject[{2010,3,4},TimeZone->"America/Belize"]]
Out[38]= Thu 4 Mar 2010
```

Your current location's sunrise and sunset times can be calculated (support data is downloaded).

```
In[39]:= DateString[Sunset[Here,Now]]
DateString[Sunrise[Here,Yesterday]]

Out[39]= Wed 13 Sep 2023 18:41:27
Out[40]= Tue 12 Sep 2023 06:23:34
```

To get the current time, use TimeObject with zero arguments (see Figure 1-20). It can be entered in the format of 24h or 12h. To introduce the time, enter the hour, minute, and second.

```
In[41]:= TimeObject[]
Out[41]=
```

```
13:22:37
```

Figure 1-20. *Wed 13 Sep GMT-6 time*

Time zone conversion is supported; convert 5 p.m. from GMT-5 Cancun time to Pacific Time Los Angeles. You can also use DatesString to use pure string objects.

```
In[42]:=
DateString[TimeZoneConvert[TimeObject[{17,0,0},TimeZone-> "America/
Cancun"],"America/Los_Angeles"]]
Out[42]= 15:00:00
```

Strings

Text can be useful when a description of the code is needed. Mathematica allows you to input text into cells and create a text cell related to your computations. Mathematica has different forms to work with text cells. Text cells can have lines of text, and depending on the purpose of the text, you can work with different text formats, like creating chapters, sections, or just general text. In contrast, to text cells, you can introduce comments to expressions that need an explanation of their purpose or just a description. For that, you simply write the comment within the symbols (* *). And the comments are shown with different colors; comments also always remain as unevaluated expressions. Comments can be single-line or multiline.

Mathematica can work with strings. To input a string, enclose the text in quotation marks "text"; Mathematica knows that it is dealing with text. Characters can be whatever you type or enter into the cells.

```
In[43]:= "Hello World" (*This is a comment*)
Out[43]= Hello World
```

Mathematica assumes that what you enter is text by being enclosed in quotation marks, although you can always impel it to explicitly treat it as text using the ToString command. You can check the head of the expression to make sure you are dealing with strings.

```
In[44]:= ToString[23.423563]
Out[44]= 23.4236
```

```
In[45]:= % // Head(*We use Head to know what type of object is*)
Out[45]= String
```

Strings appear without apostrophes when entered because it is the default format.

```
In[46]:= "Welcome to Mathematica"
Out[46]= Welcome to Mathematica
```

Whenever you put the type cursor over a string in Mathematica and enter input, it automatically appears surrounded by apostrophes. In this way, you can know you are working with strings.

Later, you learn about the functionality of AtomQ. The following demonstrates that strings cannot have subexpressions in the Wolfram Language. The output, true, indicates that the string input is a single, indivisible unit.

```
In[47]:= AtomQ["The sky is blue and tomorrow is expected to rain"]
Out[47]= True
```

You can also separate a string by characters.

```
In[48]:= Characters["Hello World"] (*Function that breaks the string into
its characters*)
Out[48]= {H,e,l,l,o, ,W,o,r,l,d}
```

Replace particular characters in a string with a rule operator ($\rightarrow$ or ->, in plain text).

```
In[49]:= StringReplace["Hello this is a string ",{"h","H"}->"4"] (*This
function replaces the string each time it appears for rule of the
pattern,that is 4*)
Out[49]= 4ello t4is is a string
```

Convert a text string to uppercase or lowercase.

```
In[50]:= ToUpperCase["hello my name is"]
Out[50]= HELLO MY NAME IS
```

```
In[51]:= ToLowerCase["HELLO MY NAME IS"]
Out[51]= hello my name is
```

Join a text string.

```
In[52]:= StringJoin["Nice","to","have","you","back"]
Out[52]= Nicetohaveyouback
```

Or with the string join symbol (<>).

```
In[53]:= "Nice"<>"to"<>"have"<>"you"<>"back"
Out[53]= Nicetohaveyouback
```

Basic Plotting

The Wolfram Language offers a basic description to easily create two-dimensional and three-dimensional graphics. It has a wide variety of graphics, such as histograms, contour, density, and time series. To graph a simple mathematical function, use the Plot command, accompanied by the variable symbol and the interval where you want to graph (see Figure 1-21).

```
In[54]:= Plot[x^3,{x,-20,20}]
Out[54]=
```

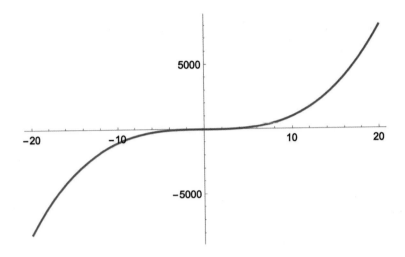

Figure 1-21. *A cubic plot*

The plot function also supports handling more than one function; simply gather the functions inside curly braces. Figure 1-22 shows the two functions in the same graph; each with a unique color.

```
In[55]:= Plot[{Tan[x],x},{x,0,10}]
Out[55]=
```

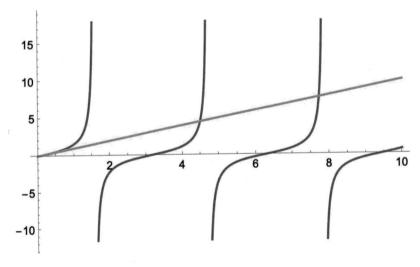

Figure 1-22. *Multiple functions plotted*

You can also customize graphics in color if the curve is thick or dashed; this is done with the PlotStyle option (see Figure 1-23).

```
In[56]:= Plot[Tan[x],{x,0,10},PlotStyle->{Dashed,Purple}]
Out[56]=
```

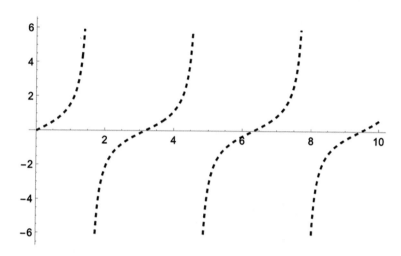

Figure 1-23. *Dashed tangent function*

The PlotLabel option allows you to add basic descriptions to your graphics by adding a title. On the other hand, the AxesLabel option lets you add names to axes, both x and y, as depicted in Figure 1-24.

```
In[57]:= Plot[E^x,{x,0,10},PlotStyle->{Blue}, PlotLabel -> "eˣ" ,AxesLabel->
{"x-axis","y-axis"}]
Out[57]=
```

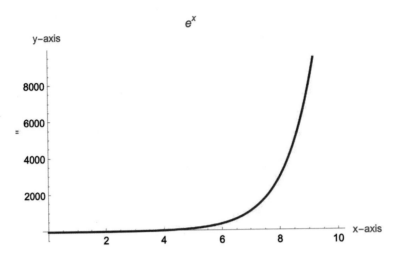

Figure 1-24. *A plot with title and labeled axes*

Logical Operators and Infix Notation

Infix notation and logical operators are commonly used in logical statements or comparisons of expressions, and the result values are either true or false. Table 1-1 shows the relation operators of the Wolfram Language.

Table 1-1. *Operators and Their Definitions*

Definition	Operator Form
Greater than	>
Less than	<
Greater than or equal	≥
Less than or equal	≤
Equal	=
Unequal	!= or ≠
Structural Equality	===

Relational operators, also called *comparison operators* and *logical binary operators*, check the veracity or falsity of certain relationship proposals. The expressions that contain them are called relational expressions. They accept various types of arguments, and the result can be true or false—that is, they are Boolean results. As you can see, they are all binary operators, of which two are of equality condition == and !=. These serve to verify the equality or inequality of expressions.

```
In[58]:= 6*1>2
Out[58]= True
```

```
In[59]:= 6*1<2
Out[59]= False
```

$$In[60]:= \frac{1}{2} >= 1/2$$
```
Out[60]= True
```

$$In[61]:= 1/4 <= \frac{1}{2}$$
```
Out[61]= True
```

```
In[62]:= 3.12 == 2.72
Out[62]= False
```

$$In[63]:= \pi \; != \sqrt{-1}$$
```
Out[63]= True
```

```
In[64]:= 2===2.
Out[64]= False
```

Boolean operands produce a true or false result or test whether a condition is satisfied. Table 1-2 shows Boolean operators of the Wolfram Language.

Table 1-2. *Boolean Operators and Their Definitions*

Definition	Operator Form
AND	&& or ∧
OR	‖ or ∨
XOR	⊻
Equivalent	⇔
Negation	¬

The AND operator returns a true value if both expressions are true. Otherwise, the result is false.

```
In[65]:= 2==1 && 3.12==2
Out[65]= False
```

The OR operator returns true if any of the expressions is true. Otherwise, it returns false. This operator has an analogous operation to the previous one.

```
In[66]:= 2*2==3||23*2==1
Out[66]= False
```

The XOR operator is an exclusive "or" operator that returns true when both expressions differ. Otherwise, it returns false when the expressions have the same value.

```
In[67]:= 2==1 \[Xor] 2==2
Out[67]= True
```

The equivalent operator returns true if expressions are powered from each other. Otherwise, it returns false.

```
In[68]:= Power[1,2] \[Equivalent] 1^2
Out[68]= True
```

The negation operator, also called logical negation, returns a value that can be an expression that evaluates to a result. The result of this operator is always a Boolean type.

```
In[69]:= \[Not]2==1
Out[69]= True
```

Another approach, instead of using Boolean operators, is to use different functions with postfix (Q), which consists of testing whether an object meets the condition of the built-in function. A few honorable mentions are SameQ, UnsameQ, AtomQ, IntegerQ, and NumberQ. The next example tests whether a number is a float expression or an integer.

```
In[70]:=
IntegerQ[1]
IntegerQ[1.]
Out[70]= True
Out[71]= False
```

The valuable application of the AtomQ function can tell you whether an expression is subdivided into subexpressions. Later, you are shown how to deal with subexpressions with lists. If the result is true, then the expression cannot be subdivided into subterms, and if it is false, then the expression has subterms.

```
In[72]:= AtomQ[12]
Out[72]= True
```

As shown, numbers cannot be subdivided because a number is a canonic expression; the same applies to strings, as seen before.

Algebraic Expressions

The Wolfram Language can work with algebraic expressions. For instance, perform symbolic computations, algebraic expansions, and simplifications. Many words used in common language in algebra are preserved in Mathematica. To expand an algebraic expression, use Expand.

```
In[73]:= Expand[((x^2)+y^2)*(x+y)]
Out[73]= x^3+x^2 y+x y^2+y^3
```

Adding a space between variables is the same as adding the multiplication operator. This can be checked by a*x==a x.

```
In[74]:= Expand[a x^2*(a x)^3]
Out[74]= a^4 x^5
```

But be careful when writing algebraic expressions because the ax symbol is not the same as an x. This also is checked using the SameQ[ax, a x] or the short notation a x === ax.

To simplify an expanded expression, use Simplify or FullSimplify.

```
In[75]:= Simplify[x^3+x^2 y+x y^2+y^3]
FullSimplify[x^3+x^2 y+x y^2+y^3]
Out[75]= x^3+x^2 y+x y^2+y^3
Out[76]= (x+y) (x^2+y^2)
```

The difference is that the latter tries transformations to simplify the expression more broadly. To unite terms over a repeated denominator, use Together. To expand into partial fraction decomposition, use Apart.

In[77]:=
Together$[\frac{1}{z}+\frac{1}{z+1}-\frac{1}{z+2}]$

Apart$[\frac{2+4z+z^2}{z(1+z)(2+z)}]$
Out[77]= (2+4 z+z^2)/(z (1+z) (2+z))
Out[78]= 1/z+1/(1+z)-1/(2+z)

Solving Algebraic Equations

Various functions are accessible for finding solutions to algebraic equations. The most common is the Solve function. The first argument is the equation or expression to be solved, and the second is for the variable to be solved.

In[79]:= Solve[z^2+1==2,z]
Out[79]= {{z → -1},{z → 1}}

Note   As you might remember, equal is expressed as double equal (==); do not use one equal (=) because that means assigning a value to a symbol or variable.

The result means that z has two solutions: one is –1, and the other is 1. Each result is expressed in the form of a rule. A rule expression changes the assignment of the left side to the one on the right side (left → right) whenever it applies. For example, z → 1 is the same as Rule [z, 1].

To verify the solution, the values of z (–1, 1) must be replaced in the original equation. For this, you can use the ReplaceAll operator (/.) along with the rule command → or Rule, which is used to apply a transformation to a variable or a pattern with other expressions.

In[80]:= z^2+1 /.Rule[z,{1,-1}]
Out[80]= {2,2}

The other option is to type the solutions explicitly in the equation.

```
In[81]:= {1^2+1==2, (-1)^2+1==2}
Out[81]= {True,True}
```

Multiple equations can be solved, too, given a system of equations and a list of interested variables. To solve the equations, place the system of equations in one list and the variables in another.

For example, solve the next system of equations.

$$x + y + z == 2$$
$$6x - 4y + 5z == 3$$
$$5x + 2y + 2z == 1$$

The solution is

```
In[82]:= Solve[{x+y+z == 2, 6x-4y+5z == 3, x+2y+2z == 1},{x,y,z}]
```
$$Out[82] = \left\{ \left\{ x \to 3, y \to \frac{10}{9}, z \to -\frac{19}{9} \right\} \right\}$$

Note   The results are listed. Lists are essential structures in the Wolfram Language and are discussed in the next chapter.

The latter process is also applicable to equations assigned to variables. You can write this with the use of compound expressions.

```
In[83]:=
EQ1=x+y+z==2;
EQ2=6 x-4 y+5 z==3;
EQ3=x+2 y+2 z==1;
Solve[{EQ1,EQ2,EQ3},{x,y,z}]
```
$$Out[83] = \left\{ \left\{ x \to 3, y \to \frac{10}{9}, z \to -\frac{19}{9} \right\} \right\}$$

The Solve function also works with pure algebraic equations.

```
In[84]:= Solve[{x + y + z == a, 6 x - 4 y + 5 z == b, x + 2 y + 2 z == c},
{x, y, z}]
```
$$Out[84] = \left\{ \left\{ x \to 2a - c, y \to \frac{1}{9}(7a - b - c), z \to \frac{1}{9}(-16a + b + 10c) \right\} \right\}$$

35

The Solve function supports expressions with a mixture of logical operators, expressing y and x in terms of z.

In[85]:= Solve[EQ1 && EQ2, {x, y}]

$$Out[85]=\left\{\left\{x\rightarrow\frac{1}{10}(11-9z), y\rightarrow\frac{9-z}{10}\right\}\right\}$$

It also uses the OR operator.

In[86]:= Solve[x^2 + y^2 == 0 || x - 2 y == 1, x]
Out[86]= {{x → − iy}, {x → iy}, {x → 1 + 2y}}

The Solve function returns the solution for each of the equations entered.

Establishing a condition with the AND operator lets you return solutions that satisfy a condition; for example, the following equation has two solutions 1 and –1, but you can solve the equation with the condition that z must be different from 1.

In[87]:= Solve[z^-2 + 1 == 2 && z != 1, z]
Out[87]= {{z → -1}}

To obtain more general results, Reduce is used, as shown in the following example.

In[88]:= Reduce[Cos[x]==-1,x]
Out[88]= $c_1 \in Z$ & & $(x = = -\pi + 2\pi c_1 \,\|\, x = = \pi + 2\pi c_1)$

Here, the alternative solutions are separated by the OR operator, and the condition is established by the AND. So this means that there are two possible solutions $-\pi + 2\pi c1$ or $\pi + 2\pi c1$ and that the constant $c1$ must be a number that belongs to the integers (Z). In addition, Reduce can also solve inequalities.

In[89]:= Reduce[h^2+k2<11,{h,k}]

$$Out[89]= -\sqrt{11} < h < \sqrt{11} \text{ \& \& } -\sqrt{11-h^2} < k < \sqrt{11-h^2}$$

Here, the simultaneous equations are for h and k. Furthermore, Reduce can show the combination of equations with certain conditions.

In[90]:= Reduce $[\alpha + \beta * \alpha \wedge 2 = = E, \alpha]$

$$Out[90]= (\beta == 0 \text{ \& \& } \alpha == e) \,\Big\|\, \left(\beta \neq 0 \text{ \& \& } \left(\alpha == \frac{-1-\sqrt{1+4e\beta}}{2\beta} \,\Big\|\, \alpha == \frac{-1+\sqrt{1+4e\beta}}{2\beta}\right)\right)$$

The first solution is that α and β must be the number e and zero. The second solution is in terms of α and the condition that β must differ from zero.

Using Wolfram Alpha Inside Mathematica

A really good application inside Mathematica uses the Wolfram Alpha computable knowledge base. Wolfram Alpha can be called from Mathematica with the Wolfram Alpha query. To enter the Wolfram Alpha query, type the double equal sign before typing any expression; an orange asterisk with a white equal sign should appear, meaning that the input typed is a query with natural language. To execute the cell, click the Enter key.

So, for example, algebraic equations can be solved using the Wolfram Alpha query. Type the double equal sign (==) in an input cell, and the Wolfram Alpha query symbol should appear (see Figure 1-25). Alternatively, select Wolfram Alpha query as a new input from the + menu (left of the horizontal line) for a new cell.

In[91]:=

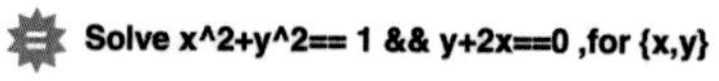

> ⚙ **Solve x^2+y^2== 1 && y+2x==0 ,for {x,y}**

Figure 1-25. *Wolfram Alpha query input*

Out[91]=

Figures 1-25 and 1-26 show the input and output of the Wolfram Alpha query.

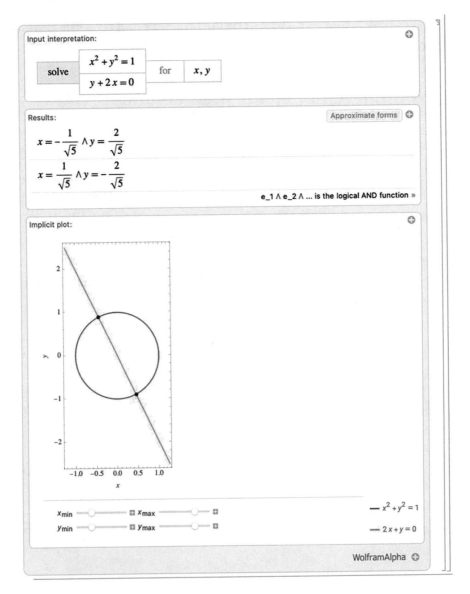

Figure 1-26. *Wolfram Alpha query output*

As shown, the system returns the solutions for x and other calculations. The cell represents the calculations in the Wolfram Alpha form. Clicking the plus icon shows a list of different forms of input. To see the equivalent in the Wolfram Language, select the Input option. The other related way to use Wolfram Alpha is with free-form input. It is worth mentioning that words associated with Mathematica commands, like Reduce, can be used too. Figure 1-27 shows the input cell in the free-form input. Clicking the plus icon shows more calculations, like in the Wolfram Alpha query. The following code is the equivalent in the Wolfram Language of input typed. Clicking the code, replace it with the Wolfram Language syntax.

> Reduce x^2+y^2== 1 && y+2x==0 ,for {x,y}
>
> Reduce[{x^2 + y^2 == 1, y + 2*x == 0}, {x, y}]

Figure 1-27. *Input code in the free-form input*

In[91]:=

Out[91]= $\left(x == -\dfrac{1}{\sqrt{5}} \;||\; x == \dfrac{1}{\sqrt{5}} \right) \&\& y == -2x$

A clarification here, not just calculations can be made. With Wolfram Alpha, access to curated data for various topics is available; for example, getting the financial data for a particular stock in March (see Figure 1-28) or the population of Australia, as depicted in Figure 1-29.

In[93]:=
Out[93]=

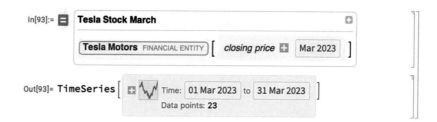

Figure 1-28. *Input and output of the Tesla stock in March 2023. Identified by the financial entity and returns a TimeSeries object, made possible by the latest version of Mathematica*

In[94]:=
Out[94]=

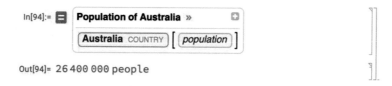

Figure 1-29. *Input for the population of Australia*

Both free-form input and Wolfram Alpha queries can be useful and practical tools. For example, if you do not know the appropriate syntax of a function or command, try using the free-form input in natural language so that, when evaluated, you can get the equivalent Wolfram Language syntax of that function. Nevertheless, a downside of the Wolfram Alpha query is that the computations are done outside Mathematica, meaning that the computations are made on the Wolfram Alpha servers. In contrast, calculations with free-form input can be reproduced inside Mathematica. Sometimes it is preferable to work directly with the Wolfram Language to better manage the results, as extracting results from Wolfram Alpha can be tedious. It should be noted that to access these two features from Mathematica, it is necessary to have access to Wolfram servers via an online network.

Delayed and Immediate Expressions

The Wolfram Language has two important features. First, let's look at how the Set mechanism works. The symbol = is the script for Set, and := is for SetDelayed. The Set mechanism is represented by W = expr. W is the variable you are assigning a value to, and expr is the expression or value you are assigning to W. This means that Mathematica evaluates the expression straightaway, then each time the variable or defined function is called, the value of W is written, and the result is shown. On the contrary, using W:= expr means that the expression is not evaluated until called, so each time the W is called, it evaluates the stored expression every time.

```
In[95]:= W=RandomReal[]
Out[95]= 0.536369
```

Test whether W equals W.

```
In[96]:= W==W
Out[96]= True
```

The condition is true in this case because Set is used for declaring the W variable with the RandomReal function, which returns a pseudo-random choice from 0 to 1. The same approach is used for SetDelayed, and the result is false because every time W appears, the function is called for a new evaluation. You can write the code as a compound expression.

```
In[97]:= Clear[W];W:=RandomReal[];W
Out[97]= 0.550058
```

Let's check.

```
In[98]:= W==W
Out[98]= False
```

The result is false since the RandomReal function is evaluated again each time W is called. So, the first W evaluates RandomReal, and the second W again evaluates RandomReal, even though they are the same symbol.

The same approach applies to Rule ($\rightarrow$) for immediate evaluation and RuleDelayed ($:\rightarrow$) for evaluation only when used. Consider the following example.

```
In[99]:=
z=2; (*Assigning 2 to z*)
R=z->z^3; (*Rule example*)
RD=z:>z^3; (*RuleDelayed example*)
R
RD
Out[102]= 2 → 8
Out[103]= 2 :→ z³
```

The expression returns $2 \rightarrow 8$ since z is evaluated immediately, while the expression $z :\rightarrow z^\wedge 3$ delays the evaluation of z^3 until it is applied. These operators can be used with the ReplaceAll operator (/.) as previously seen with algebraic equations.

Improving Code

Code efficiency is essential to achieve performance and decrease resource consumption, leading to faster execution times and improved maintenance. One specific context where these matters are improving code for increased efficiency and reliability in Mathematica and Wolfram Language. As a developer, you can achieve greater readability and facilitate easier troubleshooting by using the built-in functions. Also, built-in symbols are optimized for efficiency, making them preferable to defining your own.

Code Performance

In Mathematica, there are many ways to write an expression in the same form. However, when you carry out long code operations, there may be a better notation to improve the performance of the code and thus not consume too many computational resources. This can be achieved by the relative performance of different functions for the development of the same result. The Wolfram Language provides a measure of this. The timing function shows the performance in units of seconds to each process in relation to the value of $TimeUnit, which is the CPU time it takes for the Wolfram Language kernel to carry out the process. $TimeUnit varies from system to system, so you might get something different—such as 1/1000.

Note   A lower value of $TimeUnit would be considered more precise than using it, as it provides a higher granularity or resolution in the time measurements.

The following example shows how long it takes to calculate the expression with a built-in function and a common power expression. Timing returns two values: the unit time and the calculation result, but the output is suppressed because it is a very big value.

```
In[104]:= Timing[Power[10,10^8];]
Out[104]= {1.1401,Null}
```

```
In[105]:= Timing[10^10^8;]
Out[105]= {1.54863,Null}
```

As you see, there is a difference between each; this has to do with how the Wolfram Language processes each computation and your computer specs. To look at the absolute

```
In[106]:= AbsoluteTiming[10^10^8;];]
Out[106]= {1.13833,Null}
```

```
In[107]:= AbsoluteTiming[Power[10,10^8];]
Out[107]= {1.13189,Null}
```

There is a difference, too, as in the case with Timing. To restrain a computation by time, use TimeConstrained. With this command, time constraints can be added to a calculation. The evaluation is aborted if the code is still running and the time limit has been reached. For example, abort the evaluation after 1 second has passed.

```
In[108]:= TimeConstrained[10^10^8,1]
Out[108]= $Aborted
```

The EchoTiming function has been improved and can display the timing information of an evaluated expression. EchoTiming supports the latter methods of Timing and AbsoluteTiming.

```
In[109]:=
EchoTiming[Power[10,10^8];,"Time in seconds:",Method->Timing]
EchoTiming[Power[10,10^8];,"Time in seconds:",Method->AbsoluteTiming]
Out[109]= Time in seconds:   1.13813
Out[110]= Time in seconds:   1.12619
```

Handling Errors

Mistakes may be commonplace, as you most commonly develop code as you continue to learn. When a function fails, Mathematica displays a message below the written function. The message form provides the name of the function associated with the error, along with a possible description of the cause of the error.

Next, let's look at how this works (see Figure 1-30).

```
In[111]:= StringJoin["hello","I am ",Jeff]
Out[111]= helloI am <>Jeff
```

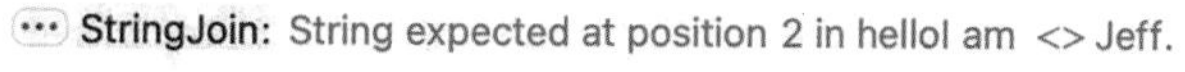

··· **StringJoin:** String expected at position 2 in helloI am <> Jeff.

Figure 1-30. *Error message for the code entered*

The associated function in the message appears in red (see Figure 1-20). What happens here is that the StringJoin function works only for strings, and you are writing a Jeff variable, not a string, hence the error.

To learn more about the error, click the red ellipsis icon. A menu appears, listing the different options available to handle the error. To review the error in the documentation, you must click the error option, which is the option that has an open book icon. This option takes you to the documentation of the associated function.

Another option from the pop-up menu that appears is Show Stack Trace. This option shows you graphically and in blocks how the function and its expressions are being evaluated. This option is analogous to the Trace command. Let's look at the next example error and Figure 1-31.

```
In[112]:= Power[x/0,2]
Out[112]= ComplexInfinity
```

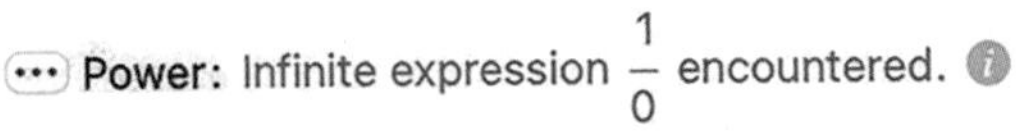

Figure 1-31. *Error message for infinite expression*

Here, the error is that Mathematica encounters a division by zero, which is undefined, and you can see the trace of the function with Stack Trace in Figure 1-32.

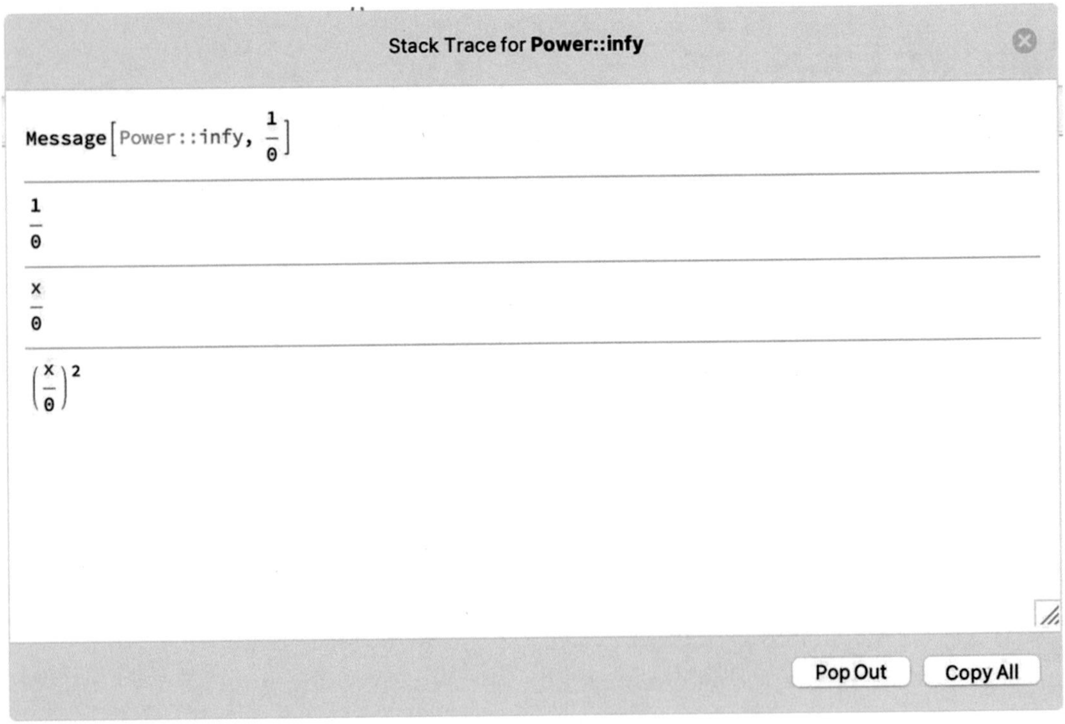

Figure 1-32. *Show Trace Stack pop-up window*

Debugging Techniques

In Mathematica, debugging practices help programmers identify, diagnose, and fix errors or unusual behavior in their written segments of code. Traditional code operations using the Wolfram Language built-in functions like Trace, Echo, and Print, among others, let you follow each step of your code as it runs. This makes it easier to focus on the specific implementation details and not the whole abstract operations that the code does, providing a flexible and robust sense of what the code or code block should do.

Since version 13, a few improved built-in functions, like EchoLabel and EchoEvaluation, have been added to the repertoire, as seen in the following example.

```
In[113]:=
x=2;
Echo[x];x=x^2+1;
Echo[x];x=x^2+1;
Echo[x];

Out[114]=
>> 2
>> 5
>> 26
```

Let's go over what happened here. Initially, the value 2 is assigned to x. The first Echo prints the value of x, which is 2. Then, in the 2nd operation, x is updated based on its original form. Subsequently, the second Echo prints the new value, 5, which continues until the final value of 26 is reached (5^2 + 1).

The same can be achieved using EchoLabel and EchoEvaluation but tagging costume messages.

```
In[117]:=
x=2;
Echo[x,"Initial Value: "];
x=x^2+1;
EchoLabel["First Iteration: "][x];
x=x^2+1;
EchoEvaluation[x=x^2+1,"Second Iteration: "->"Output :"];
```

```
Out[118]=
>> Initial Value:    2
>> First Iteration:    5
<< Second Iteration:    x=x^2+1
<< Output :   677
```

The previous example performs three iterations of the same operation on the same initial value. The first Echo prints the value of x. The second EchoLabel prints the output of the first iteration with a costume label and finalizes with the last evaluation and label association. Before evaluation, the initial label is printed, followed by the second label being printed once the evaluation is complete. Throughout the process, it displays results next to symbols with different colors: orange (>>) and blue (<<). The first symbol represents output, and the second symbol represents input.

Now, by utilizing operations to measure the time, as seen before, you can combine them to pinpoint which stages demand more time to compute, as exemplified in the following example.

```
In[123]:=
x=2;
EchoTiming[Echo[x,"Initial Value: "]];
x=x^2+1;
EchoTiming[EchoLabel["First Iteration: "][x]];
x=x^2+1;
EchoTiming[EchoEvaluation[x=x^2+1,"Second Iteration: "->"Output :"]];
Clear[x];

Out[124]=
>> Initial Value:    2
⊘ 0.013603
>> First Iteration:    5
⊘ 0.018695
<< Second Iteration:    x=x^2+1
>> Output :   677
⊘ 0.031909
```

As seen, the last evaluation took the longest time (0.031909 seconds), while the initial value estimation was the fastest (0.013603 seconds). These techniques are useful when program flow is broken into small chunks of digestible code, like visualizing variable values at key points and gauging computation time for performance breakdown.

How Mathematica Works

This section explores the internal workings of computations and discovers ways to visualize data using multiple basic yet powerful commands.

How Computations are Made (Form of Input)

Each time Mathematica receives a computation in the input cell, it uses the StandardForm, which is the output representation of expressions in the Wolfram Language and has many aspects of common mathematical notation. Input can be written in various forms, but to know how the expression is written in the Wolfram Language, StandardForm is used.

```
In[130]:= StandardForm[1/x+x^2]
Out[130]//StandardForm=
```

$$\frac{1}{x} + x^2$$

InputForm works similarly but produces the output acceptable to be entered as Wolfram Language input.

```
In[131]:= {InputForm[1/x+x²], InputForm[aˣ], InputForm[aₓ], InputForm[√2]}
Out[131]= {x^(-1) + x^2,a^x, Subscript[a, x], Sqrt[2]}
```

Every type of format has its equivalent in one line of code text, like the square root symbol ($\sqrt{\ }$), which means the same as Sqrt[ ]. To convert input into StandardForm, InputForm, and other forms, select the cell block and head to Cell ➤ Convert To ➤ StandardFrom, and InputForm, among others. StandardForm and InputForm apply to every expression in the Wolfram Language. Try using InputForm on the previous plots to see how the expression is written completely. To understand better how Mathematica works, you want to know how symbolic or numeric computations are performed or written. The FullForm and TreeForm commands can be applied to view how expressions are represented symbolically. TreeForm represents the command in a graphical format, while FullForm represents the form of the expression managed internally by the Wolfram Language.

```
In[132]:= FullForm[t/2+2^2]
Out[132]//FullForm= Plus[4,Times[Rational[1,2],t]]
```

FullForm also represents the input as a one-line output code, like InputForm. But even if InputForm also returns a one-line output code, why not use InputForm? The reason is that FullForm represents what Mathematica understands as input. With this in mind, FullForm is useful because it lets you know what Mathematica interprets about the written input. In Mathematica, the mathematical order of operations is preserved. So the previous output is as follows: first, Mathematica detects the rational number 1/2 (Rational[1,2]) and the symbol t, followed by the multiplication of these two elements (Times[Rational[1,2],t]) followed by the addition of 22 (Plus[4, Times[Rational[1,2],t]]).

Another type of command that helps in creating a visualization of how Mathematica manipulates expressions is TreeForm. TreeForm returns the expression as a tree plot (see Figure 1-33). Alternatively, you can apply commands using the postfix form 'expr // function', rather than writing in the canonical form 'F[expression]'.

```
In[133]:= t/2+2^2//TreeForm

Out[133]//TreeForm=
```

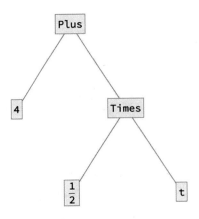

Figure 1-33. *Tree plot representation*

In short terms, Mathematica detects the multiplication of 1/2 times t and then proceeds to add the result of the product with the result of two squared. The tree graph is read from bottom to top until you reach the top of the tree.

One more helpful command is Trace. Trace returns individual forms corresponding to the evaluation line, which contains the sequence of forms of the evaluated expression.

In[134]:= Trace[Plus[4,Times[Rational[1,2],t]]]

Out[134]= {{{Rational[1,2], $\frac{1}{2}$}, $\frac{t}{2}$}, 4+$\frac{t}{2}$}

So here, the sequence of operations is as follows: first use the term Rational [1, 2], followed by 1/2, then 1/2 is multiplied by t, and the result is added to 4. Using FullForm in Trace lets you see how the internal structure changes.

In[135]:= FullForm[Trace[Plus[4,Times[Rational[1,2],t]]]]
Out[135]//FullForm= List[List[List[HoldForm[Rational[1,2]],HoldForm[Rationa
l[1,2]]],HoldForm[Times[Rational[1,2],t]]],HoldForm[Plus[4,Times[Rational[
1,2],t]]]]

It can be seen that the terms change each step. The HoldForm command is used to see the output in an unevaluated form. As a complement to Trace, FullForm and TreeForm can be combined to see the hierarchy of operations in an expression internally, as seen in Figure 1-34.

In[136]:= Trace[$\frac{t}{2}$+2^2]//TreeForm

Out[136]//TreeForm=

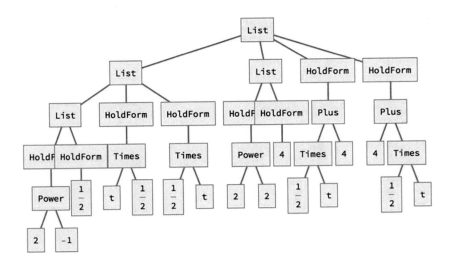

Figure 1-34. *TreeForm and Trace combined*

Here, the tree shows how changes are made and read from left to right. Reading the tree, you see that Mathematica recognizes that 1/2 is 2^-1; this is followed by t times 1/2, followed by 2^2, which is 4, and so on until the end. Moving the cursor over each block displays a representation of the operation being held. There may be occasions when you encounter operations or expressions you do not understand. A solution to this would be using the previous commands, which allow you to see the expression's inner structure and thus understand how the operation is performed.

Searching for Assistance

The Wolfram Documentation Center contains the registry of all built-in functions. Documentation of functions can be accessed through the front end by opening a new window, clicking the Help tab on the toolbar, or entering expressions. Since version 13.1, the documentation can also be accessed through the toolbar's rightmost icon, which is an open book icon. The Input Assistant is displayed as an autocomplete or suggestion bar when a command or related sensible options are written. When writing a built-in function or command, Mathematica tries to automatically complete the phrase.

Like in Figure 1-35, type the word **Random**, and different associated commands appear as suggestions. If the desired command is listed, you can select it with the cursor pointer.

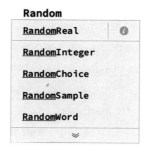

Figure 1-35. *Autocomplete pop-up menu*

To access the documentation for a particular command, click the "i" document icon next to the command name, and the documentation windows should appear.

Note   Autocomplete also works for assigned symbols.

When writing the built-in function or command followed by the left square bracket, the completion menu appears; if you click the double-down arrow, it displays the input forms supported by that command, as shown in Figure 1-36.

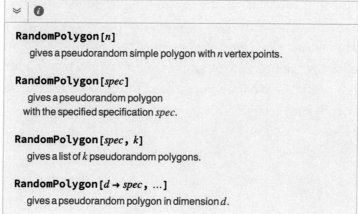

Figure 1-36. *Built-in function RandomPolygon with different input forms*

As seen in the example, the RandomPolygon function has four types of input forms; also, in the menu, you can see text related to the different forms of the input.

To learn how a function works or how built-in functions are written, the best resource is to consult the Wolfram Documentation Center. You can also check if an alternative input expression can be used. So, if you need help understanding how the Head function works, you input a question mark (?) before the function's name, giving you a simple understanding of how the command works (see Figure 1-37). If you want additional information related to the attributes of the function, a double question mark (??) can be employed. As a piece of advice, the Wolfram Documentation Center can be used for more in-depth options. Use the F1 shortcut, which opens the Documentation Center. If you highlight the symbol name and press F1, you are taken directly to the documentation page for that symbol.

```
In[137]:= ?Head
Out[137]=
```

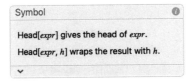

Figure 1-37. *Output information for the Head command*

The previous command showed how to show information related to a specific function. But if you don't recall the exact spelling, you can write the first letters of the name followed by an asterisk (*), and Mathematica provides a list that matches your query. In the following example, the output is the functions whose names start with "Hea" (see Figure 1-38). The Wolfram documentation can be used in a scenario that needs more in-depth knowledge.

```
In[138]:= ?Hea*
Out[138]=
```

? Hea∗

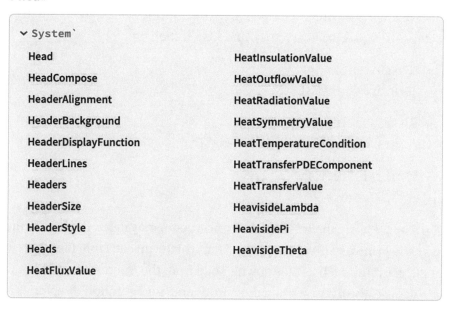

Figure 1-38. *Output information for the commands starting with the letters Head*

Notebook Security

The Wolfram Language provides creation and the ability to run dynamic content. These contents allow the user to create programs that can perform useful and complex tasks; on certain occasions, unwanted content may be executed or code misused. A notebook may or may not contain dynamic content as part of its code. Notebooks containing dynamic content can be instantly downloaded without any user action. Sometimes, Mathematica alerts the user when a notebook contains dynamic content, displaying a message like that shown in Figure 1-39.

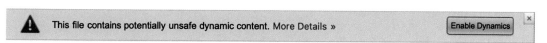

Figure 1-39. *Warning message of dynamic content*

If the notebook is not found in a trusted directory, a message warns the user that the notebook contains unreliable dynamic content. The dynamic content is executed without displaying a previous message to the user if the notebook is located in a reliable directory. To find out if a notebook is located in a trusted directory with the name TrustedPath, check out the trusted math directories, which are found in (1) $ BaseDirectory, (2) $ UserBaseDirectory, and (3) $ InitialDirectory.

```
In[139]:= $BaseDirectory
Out[139]= /Library/Mathematica
```

```
In[140]:= $UserBaseDirectory
Out[140]= /Users/macosx/Library/Mathematica
```

```
In[141]:= $InitialDirectory
Out[141]= /Users/macosx
```

In this case, these are the trusted directories; yours may defer. By default, the directories called UntrustedPath are those from which you can store files that can be potentially harmful, such as files downloaded from the Internet. For this, in the Wolfram Language, the user's writing directories and configuration directories are called UntrustedPath. To add, change, or remove the trusted and untrusted directories, go to the Preferences menu and then to the Security tab. There are options to edit unreliable and trusted directories.

Summary

This chapter served as an introduction to Mathematica, a comprehensive software used for mathematical computation and analysis. The chapter also introduced the unique Wolfram Language used within the software, focusing on its notebook interface, text processing, palettes, and various styles and features. It also delved into expressions in Mathematica and concluded with topics related to code performance, error and debugging management, and ensuring security.

CHAPTER 2

Data Manipulation

This chapter reviews the basics of data creation and data handling in the Wolfram Language. The chapter begins with the concept of lists and structures within the language. Numbers, digits, and simple ways to use them with common math functions are discussed. Next, you are introduced to lists of objects, representing, and generating lists, delving into data arrays and examining nested lists, vectors, matrixes, and relevant operations for various purposes. The chapter ends with study list manipulation techniques—retrieving, assigning, or removing data—and structuring lists to offer a general guide to understanding list manipulation in the Wolfram Language.

Lists

Lists are the core of data construction in the Wolfram Language. Lists can gather objects, construct data structures, create tables, store values or variables, make elementary to complex computations, and characterize data. A list can represent any expression in the Wolfram Language (numbers, text, data, images, graphics, etc.)—that is, any set of whichever data.

If you access the information structure of a list, as demonstrated in Figure 2-1, you can see the typical format to form a list. Lists are represented by curly braces or the List command. In the Wolfram Language, almost every data object result can be listable; in other words, lists allow you to group data that maintain some type of relationship, even if they are of a different type, by manipulating all together (using the same identifier) or each separately.

```
In[1]:= ??List
Out[1]=
```

J. Villalobos Alva, *Beginning Mathematica and Wolfram for Data Science*, https://doi.org/10.1007/979-8-8688-0348-2_2

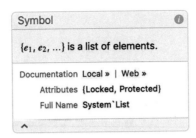

Figure 2-1. *List definition in the Wolfram Language*

As seen in the evaluation, commas separate elements, and the whole list is between curly braces. Also, List is a protected variable, meaning you cannot assign values to the name List.

Types of Numbers

The fundamental number types in the Wolfram Language are represented by integers, rational, real, and complex numbers.

First, the integers have an exact result since they are numbers that cannot be represented by a decimal point.

```
In[2]:= {10, InputForm[10]}
Out[2]= {10,10}
```

Therefore, integers in the Wolfram Language are handled with infinite precision and infinite accuracy.

```
In[3]:= {10//Accuracy, InputForm[10]//Precision}
Out[3]= {∞, ∞}
```

Second, rational numbers can be represented as a quotient of two integers.

```
In[4]:= {5/10,InputForm[10/12]}
Out[4]= {1/2, 5/6}
```

Mathematica treats rational numbers exactly as with integers, so whenever Mathematica deals with rational numbers, it returns the minimum expression in which that number is represented.

```
In[5]:= {5/10 //Accuracy,InputForm[10/12] //Precision}
Out[5]= {∞, ∞}
```

Third, real numbers—typically known as floating-point numbers—are represented in the Wolfram Language by any number with a decimal point.

```
In[6]:= {2.72 //Precision, InputForm[2.72]}
Out[6]= {MachinePrecision,2.72}
```

Since real numbers are approximate, they do not have an exact precision. These numbers are considered machine numbers, which have the precision of the $MachinePrecision variable. It should be noted that in the Wolfram Language, numbers 1 and 1.0 are treated differently. Although Mathematica recognizes that they are equivalent expressions, it must be taken into account that they are not the same object within the Wolfram Language.

To corroborate this, let's look at the following example, where you use SameQ to test if the expressions are the same for 1 and 1.0.

```
In[7]:= SameQ[1,1.0]
Out[7]= False
```

The heads of the expressions are different because one is an integer and the other a real number.

```
In[8]:= {Head[1],Head[1.0]}
Out[8]= {Integer, Real}
```

Complex numbers are numbers that contain a real part and an imaginary part. The form of a complex number is a + bi, where "a" is the real part and "b" is the imaginary part. The symbol "i" represents the square root of the negative number –1.

```
In[9]:= 10+19I
Out[9]= 10+19I
```

The type of precision in these numbers can be exact or approximate since these numbers can be built from the numbers described previously.

```
In[10]:= {Precision[I], Precision[1 + 0.3I], FullForm[11+1I]}
Out[10]=  {∞, Machineprecision, Complex[11, 1]}
```

Though complex numbers appear as a single atomic expression, these numbers can be subdivided into different expressions, such as when extracting the real or imaginary parts.

```
In[11]:= 1+I //AtomQ
Out[11]= True
```

```
In[12]:= {ReIm[1+3I],Re[1+0.3I],Im[Complex[1,0.2]]}
Out[12]= {{1,3},1.,0.2}
```

When you deal with transcendental numbers like pi and the golden ratio, these numbers are treated as symbols—that is, Mathematica has reserved these symbols since they are important numerical constants. Therefore, they have an exact precision despite being real numbers.

```
In[13]:= {Accuracy[\[Pi]],Precision[E],Accuracy[I],Precision[GoldenRatio]}
//NumberQ
Out[13]= False
```

To determine whether a given value is considered a number within the Wolfram Language, use the NumberQ command. It returns "True" if the expression is a number and "False" if not. This can be observed in the previous command (for transcendental numbers) and the following examples.

```
In[14]:= {NumberQ[1/2],NumberQ[1],NumberQ[E]}
Out[14]= {True,True,False}
```

As a result, you can see how a rational number and an integer are numbers, but the number E is not. In fact, E is a type of symbol.

```
In[15]:= {Head[E],FullForm[E]}
Out[15]= {Symbol,E}
```

Generally speaking, there is no restriction on combining the different types of numbers within the Wolfram Language. You can perform operations between different types.

```
In[16]:= {1+0.2+1/2+1+11+1I}
Out[16]= {13.7 +1. I}
```

Conversion between approximate numbers to exact numbers is carried out with Rationalize.

```
In[17]:= Rationalize[2.72]
Out[17]= 68/25
```

Also, alternative number notations like scientific notation are supported. Scientific notation is a useful tool to represent large numbers in powers of ten.

```
In[18]:= {ScientificForm[N@E/1000000],2.71828*^-6}
Out[18]={2.71828 × 10⁻⁶, 2.71828 × 10⁻⁶}
```

You know that the N function is used to calculate approximate numbers. It converts an exact expression to an approximate one, keeping in mind that the desired precision can also be specified.

Different forms can generally be extrapolated to all the built-in function notations of the Wolfram Language.

- Employing the direct application of the N function [ ] to the expression

  ```
  In[19]:= N[13/7]
  Out[19]= 1.85714
  ```

- Utilizing the infix notation, ~N~

  ```
  In[20]:= E~N~E
  Out[20]= 2.72
  ```

- Through the postfix notation, // N

  ```
  In[21]:= E//N
  Out[21]= 2.71828
  ```

- Using the prefix notation, N@

  ```
  In[22]:= N@E
  Out[22]= 2.71828
  ```

When the precision is not defined, Mathematica uses the value of $MachinePrecision to determine the standard precision of the approximate number. The value of $MachinePrecision varies since it is a float number established by Mathematica according to the characteristics of each computer.

```
In[23]:= $MachinePrecision
Out[23]= 15.9546
```

Setting arbitrary precision with SetPrecision or using machine precision.

```
In[24]:= SetPrecision[E, 17]
Out[24]= 2.7182818284590452
```

The following uses machine precision.

```
In[25]:= SetPrecision[E,MachinePrecision]
Out[25]= 2.71828
```

When precision is not introduced, Mathematica uses MachinePrecision numbers.

```
In[26]:= SetPrecision[e,MachinePrecision] == N@e
Out[26]= True
```

Another way to enter approximate numbers with some precision is by adding the grave accent symbol (') after the real number, followed by the precision. For example, use it for six-digit precision.

```
In[27]:= 77/3`6
Out[27]= 25.6667
```

Working with Digits

To extract digits that make up an exact number, use the IntegerDigits function.

```
In[28]:= IntegerDigits[234544553]
Out[28]= {2,3,4,5,4,4,5,5,3}
```

RealDigits for approximate numbers.

```
In[29]:= {RealDigits[321.4546554],RealDigits[N@E]}
Out[29]={{{3,2,1,4,5,4,6,5,5,4,0,0,0,0,0,0},3},{{2,7,1,8,2,8,1,8,2,8,4,5,9,
0,4,5},1}}
```

In the case of a complex number, it would consist of extracting its real and imaginary parts and then extracting the digits of each part, as the case may be.

```
In[30]:= RealDigits[ReIm[113+2.7213I]]
Out[30]= {{{1,1,3,0,0,0,0,0,0,0,0,0,0,0,0,0,0,0},3},{{2,7,2,1,3,0,0,0,0,0,0,0,
0,0,0,0},1}}
```

By default, the two previous functions give results in the decimal base. To define a base, enter the base you want as the function's second argument; for example, using base 2.

```
In[31]:= RealDigits[321.4546,2]
Out[31]= {{1,0,1,0,0,0,0,0,1,0,1,1,1,0,1,0,0,0,1,1,0,0,0,0,0,1,0,1,0,1,0,1,
0,0,1,1,0,0,1,0,0,1,1,0,0,0,0,0,1,1,0,0,0,0,0},9}
```

Specifying the three digits of the number e in base-10 notation.

```
In[32]:= RealDigits[N@E, 10, 3]
Out[32]= {{2,7,1},1}
```

Reconstructing a number from the representation of their integers is possible with the FromDigits function.

```
In[33]:= FromDigits[{2,7,1,1}]
Out[33]= 2711
```

Also, it is possible to form a float point number.

```
In[34]:= N@FromDigits[{{2,7,1,1},1}]
Out[34]= 2.711
```

and to measure the length of an integer number.

```
In[35]:= IntegerLength[2711]
Out[35]= 4
```

A Few Mathematical Functions

The Wolfram Language offers a wide repertoire of mathematical functions, ranging from the most basic to the most specialized. These functions can be managed numerically or symbolically, facilitating pure analytical manipulation.

Trigonometric functions are available either in radians or in degrees. Typing a number alone calculates and returns the value in radians.

```
In[36]:= Cos[Pi]
Out[36]= -1
```

Entering the number followed by the Degree unit or the symbol of degrees (°) calculates and returns the value in degrees.

```
In[37]:= Sin[90 Degree]==Sin[90\[Degree]]
Out[37]= True
In[38]:= Sin[90\[Degree]]
Out[38]= 1
```

The same applies to hyperbolic trigonometric functions and inverse trigonometric functions.

```
In[39]:= N[Cosh[Pi]]
N[Tanh[45 Degree]]
Out[39]= 11.592
Out[40]= 0.655794
```

```
In[41]:= N[ArcTan[Pi]]
N[ArcSinh[45 Degree]]
Out[41]= 1.26263
Out[42]= 0.721225
```

Logarithmic functions and exponential functions are written like common math notation. Logarithms with only a number compute the natural logarithm.

```
In[43]:= Log[E]
Out[43]= 1
```

To specify a base, type the number as the first argument and the base as the second argument.

```
In[44]:= Log[10,10]
Out[44]= 1
```

Exponentials can be written with Exp or with the constant E.

```
In[45]:= Exp[2]==E^2
Out[45]= True
```

The factorial is represented by either typing the exclamation mark after the number or by using Factorial.

```
In[46]:= 12!
Out[46]= 479001600
```

```
In[47]:= Factorial[12]
Out[47]= 479001600
```

Numeric Function

In the Wolfram Language, functions are available for manipulating numerical data, these functions can work with any types of numbers, including real, integer, rational, and complex. Users can handle precision either exactly or using floating-point precision.

To truncate a number, z, to its closest integer (z), use the Round function with no arguments. By adding a second argument, the Round function rounds z to the nearest multiple of the second provided number.

```
In[48]:=Round[8.9](*Rounds to 9 because it is the closest number*)
Out[48]= 9
```

```
In[49]:=Round[8.9,2](*Rounds to 8 because it is the closest multiple of
2, 2^3*)
Out[49]= 8
```

Other similar functions that can truncate numbers given a number z are Floor and Ceiling. The Floor function rounds to the largest integer less than or equal to the number typed. The Ceiling function rounds to the smallest integer larger than or equal to the typed number.

```
In[50]:= Floor[Pi]
Out[50]= 3
```

```
In[51]:= Ceiling[Pi]
Out[51]= 4
```

The Floor and Ceiling functions can be written in their mathematical notation, $\lfloor z \rfloor$ for Floor and $\lceil z \rceil$ for Ceiling, by typing the key **ESC lf ESC** for the left Floor and **ESC rf ESC** for the right Floor. The same applies to Ceiling—just change **lf** for **lc** (left Ceiling) and **rf** for **rc** (right Ceiling).

```
In[52]:= ⌊Pi⌋
Out[52]= 3
```

```
In[53]:= ⌈Pi⌉
Out[53]= 4
```

Converting a float point number to a rational approximation can be done with Rationalize. However, adding the number 0 as the second argument can force the calculation to find the most exact form of a float point number; for example, a rational approximation to the number E.

```
In[54]:= Rationalize[N[E],0]
Out[54]= 325368125/119696244
```

The Max and Min functions return the maximum and minimum number of a list of numbers.

```
In[55]:= Max[{9,8,7,0,3,12}]
Out[55]= 12
```

```
In[56]:= Min[{0987,32,9871}]
Out[56]= 32
```

Lists of Objects

This section extends the concept of lists in the Wolfram Language, focusing on techniques for creating and managing lists, nesting them through specialized functions, and effectively storing data in a variable. The topic covers how to create datasets and how they can be derived from various functions, as the composition of a list can include a wide range of elements, such as sets of numbers, text strings, equations, arithmetic operations, or any expression in Mathematica. Despite this, you explore concepts like arrays and sparse arrays and their respective object types. Additionally, this section discusses the nested lists and multiple ways to create data in a nested form.

List Representation

The curly braces denote a list of general objects, with each member separated by a comma. The simplest form to create a list is to enclose data in curly braces, or by using the List function. The following examples demonstrate how to assign lists to variables and gather objects in a list.

```
In[57]:= {x2+1, "Dog", π}
List[1,P,Power[3,2]] (* Power[3,2] represents 3 raised to the power of 2 *)
Out[57]= {x2+1, "Dog", π}
Out[58]= {1,P,9}
```

The list identifier or symbol is an optional name to create the structure.

```
In[59]:= List["23.22","Dog", π,2,4,6,456.,56,2==3 && 3==2]
Out[59] = {23.22,Dog, π,2,4,6,456.,56,False}
```

Inside a list, between the braces, you can define all the elements that you consider suitable to be listed.

```
In[60]:= {1+I, π + π,"number 4",Sin[23 Degree],425+I-413-3I,24,4456., "dog"
+ "cat"}
Out[60]= {1+I, 2π,number 4,Sin[23°],12-2 I,24,4456.,cat+dog}
```

In Mathematica, there are different types of objects. To identify an object type, you have to use the Head function. The returning value is the head of the expression, known as the data type. If you apply Head to a list, you get that the head of the expression is a list.

```
In[61]:= % //Head
Out[61]= List
```

This means that the object you have created is a List object.

Generating Lists

Lists can be created with costume values, but Mathematica has a variety of functions to create automated lists, such as Range and Table. Both Range and Table functions create an equally spaced list of numbers. However, the Table generates a list with specified intervals, like when "i" goes from 1 to 10. Wolfram Language also lets you incorporate built-in functions inside a list.

```
In[62]:= Range[10]
Table[i,{i,1,10}]
Table["Soccer",{i,1,15}]
Out[62]= {1,2,3,4,5,6,7,8,9,10}
Out[63]= {1,2,3,4,5,6,7,8,9,10}
Out[64]= {Soccer,Soccer,Soccer,Soccer,Soccer,Soccer,Soccer,Soccer,Soccer,
Soccer,Soccer,Soccer,Soccer,Soccer,Soccer}
```

The Table function can also be used to create indexed lists. Each interval is specified within the curly braces { }, as shown in the previous and following examples.

```
In[65]:= Table["Red and Blue",5]
Range[-5,5]
Out[65]= {Red and Blue,Red and Blue,Red and Blue,Red and Blue,Red and Blue}
Out[66]= {-5,-4,-3,-2,-1,0,1,2,3,4,5}
```

The Table function can work with or without an inner iterator, but to create structured lists, using an iterator is recommended.

```
In[67]:= Table[i^i,{i,1,5}]
Out[67]= {1,4,27,256,3125}
```

This shows the function without an iterator.

```
In[68]:= Table[10^3,{5}]
Out[68]= {1000,1000,1000,1000,1000}
```

Note   When using the iterator, make sure to properly write the expression to avoid errors. When the table recognizes the iterator, it changes colors because the letter is no longer a symbol.

You can create a list of lists. This type of structure is considered a nested list.

```
In[69]:= {Range[5], Table[h, {h, -6, 2}]}
Out[69]= {{1, 2, 3, 4, 5}, {-6, -5, -4, -3, -2, -1, 0, 1, 2}}
```

The iterator can also be an alphanumeric variable.

```
In[70]:= Table[data2, {data2, 0, 6}]
Out[70]= {0, 1, 2, 3, 4, 5, 6}
```

Structures of arrays with the same data can also be created, such as an array of 2×2.

```
In[71]:= Table[11,{2},{2}]
Out[71]= {{11,11},{11,11}}
```

The Table function supports multiple iterators, which is useful when constructing tabular data.

```
In[72]:= Table[i+j+k,{i,1,4},{j,1,4},{k,1,4}]
Out[72]={{{3,4,5,6},{4,5,6,7},{5,6,7,8},{6,7,8,9}},{{4,5,6,7},{5,6,7,8},
{6,7,8,9},{7,8,9,10}},{{5,6,7,8},{6,7,8,9},{7,8,9,10},{8,9,10,11}},
{{6,7,8,9},{7,8,9,10},{8,9,10,11},{9,10,11,12}}}
```

To display a list in a more structured way using the Grid command.

```
In[73]:= Table[i-j,{i,1,2},{j,1,2}]//Grid
Out[73]= 0     -1
         1      0
```

An alternative to the Grid command is the TableForm command, which lets you display the list created as a table. This command is explained in detail later.

```
In[74]:= Table[i+j,{i,1,2},{j,4,6}]//TableForm
Out[74]//TableForm= 5    6    7
                    6    7    8
```

There is no limitation on the intervals of the iterators. You can choose that "i" goes from 0 to 3 and "j" from "i" to 3 and use TableForm to view it.

```
In[75]:= Table[{i,j},{i,3},{j,i,3}]//TableForm
Out[75]//TableForm= 1 1 1
                    1 2 3
                    2 2
                    2 3
                    3
                    3
```

You can even use other syntax notations like the increment (++) or decrement (--) in the interval iterator.

```
In[76]:= Table[{i,j},{i,2},{j,i++,2}]
Out[76]= {{{2,1},{2,2}},{{3,2}}}
```

The increment (++) and decrement (--) operators can also be used in assigned variables; this operator can have precedence or posteriority. When written before the variable, they are called PreIncrement or PreDecrement.

```
In[77]:= x=0;x++;x (*applied on the current value and shown next time x is
called*)
Out[77]= 1
```

```
In[78]:= Clear[x];x=0;--x (*applied on the current value and shown when x
is called*)
Out[78]= -1
```

Alternatively, you can apply replacement rules with the symbol (/.). For example, you create a list of random integers consisting of 0s or 1s, then replace the 1s with 2s whenever they appear. Add a space between the condition expressions to avoid a typo error and the correct right arrow (\[Rule]). Another form of Table can also be used with explicit values for the iterator.

```
In[79]:= Table[RandomInteger[],{i,1,10}]/. 1->2
Out[79]= {2,0,2,0,2,2,0,0,2,2}
```

```
In[80]:= Table[i^2,{i,{1,2,3,4,5}}]
Out[80]= {1,4,9,16,25}
```

Arrays of Data

There are different forms to create an array. The most used form is a list, as you saw in the previous section. But as an alternative to the Table command or Range command, arrays can be created with the Array command, which generates a list with a specific function applied to the elements created. The Array, ConstantArray, and SparseArray functions can also be used to build lists. The form of these functions is analogous to the previous ones.

```
In[81]:= Array[Cos[90 Degree],{3,3}]//Grid
Out[81]= 0[1,1]    0[1,2]    0[1,3]
         0[2,1]    0[2,2]    0[2,3]
         0[3,1]    0[3,2]    0[3,3]
```

What happens with Array is that it constructs an array from a function. In the previous example, you generated an array from the numerical value of the cosine of 90 degrees, followed by the structure of the array, which is 3×3. The indices on the right side of the array values are the positions of each element in the array.

If you generalize to any function, you can better see how Array works.

```
In[82]:= Array[F,{2,2}]//Grid
Out[82]= F[1,1]    F[1,2]
         F[2,1]    F[2,2]
```

As you can observe, the F function is applied and is respective to each element of the arrangement.

To create an array of constant values the ConstantArray function is used. To write the function, first write the value you want to repeat, followed by the times you want it to repeat.

```
In[83]:= ConstantArray[\[Pi],5]
Out[83]= {π,π,π,π,π}
```

You can also create arrangements with defined dimensions.

```
In[84]:= ConstantArray[\[Pi],{4,4}]
Out[84]= {{π,π,π,π},{π,π,π,π},{π,π,π,π},{π,π,π,π}}
```

To display a data array, there is the MatrixForm command, which, as its name suggests, shows the array in matrix form.

```
In[85]:= ConstantArray[\[Pi],{4,4}]//MatrixForm
```

$$
Out[85]//MatrixForm=
\begin{pmatrix}
\pi & \pi & \pi & \pi \\
\pi & \pi & \pi & \pi \\
\pi & \pi & \pi & \pi \\
\pi & \pi & \pi & \pi
\end{pmatrix}
$$

A sparse arrangement is one in which the elements generally have the same value. The SparseArray command lets you define the values of the array positions. By standard, if any position is not defined, the value is 0.

The SparseArray command generates an object of type SparseArray, shown in Figure 2-2, with the name of the command and a gray box that appears.

```
In[86]:= SparseArray[{{1,1},{2,2}}->{1,2}]
Out[86]=
```

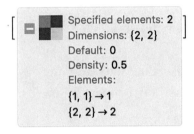

Figure 2-2. *SparseArray object*

If you click the + icon, you see the array's characteristics and its rules; this is shown in Figure 2-3.

[
Specified elements: 2
Dimensions: {2, 2}
Default: 0
Density: 0.5
Elements:
{1, 1} → 1
{2, 2} → 2
]

Figure 2-3. *Specifications of the array*

In the Wolfram Language, there is no limitation on the content of a SparseArray. Furthermore, you can create an array with the same values on its diagonal.

Figure 2-4 illustrates elements of the same values in the array appear in one color, and different values appear in another.

```
In[87]:= SpArray=SparseArray[{{1,1}->"A",{2,2}->"A",{3,3}->"A",{4,4}->
"A"},{4,4}]
Out[87]=
```

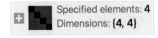

Figure 2-4. *Sparse Array with more elements*

With the help of MatrixForm, you can visualize the arrangement as a matrix.

```
In[88]:= MatrixForm[%]
Out[88]//MatrixForm=
```

$$\begin{pmatrix} A & 0 & 0 & 0 \\ 0 & A & 0 & 0 \\ 0 & 0 & A & 0 \\ 0 & 0 & 0 & A \end{pmatrix}$$

To convert the sparse array object to a list object, use Normal to normalize into expression form.

```
In[89]:= Normal[SpArray]
Out[89]= {{A,0,0,0},{0,A,0,0},{0,0,A,0},{0,0,0,A}}
```

And now you deal with a list.

```
In[90]:= Head[%]
Out[90]= List
```

Nested Lists

A nested list is a list of lists where the elements of the lists correspond to another list, and so on. Nested lists can be used for ordered or unordered data structures. To create a nested list, you can use curly braces within curly braces or built-in functions.

```
In[91]:= {{"This","is","A"},{"Nested","List","."}}
Out[91]= {{This,is,A},{Nested,List,.}}
```

You can also use the Table function.

```
In[92]:= Table[Prime[i]+Prime[j],{i,1,3},{j,2,4}]
Out[92]= {{5,7,9},{6,8,10},{8,10,12}}
```

To measure a list, you must use the Length command.

```
In[93]:= NestL=Table[Prime[i]+RandomReal[j],{i,1,3},{j,1,3}];
Length[NestL]
Out[93]= 3
```

The length of the list is 3 because Length is properly used with flattened lists. To properly measure the depth of a nested list, Dimensions is more suited for the task.

```
In[94]:= Dimensions[NestL]
Out[94]= {3,3}
```

Dimensions provide a general aspect of the dimensions of the nested list, meaning that a list of three sublists constitutes your list and that the sublists each have three elements. Mathematica constructs a list with three elements, in which those three elements are also a list, and those lists have three elements, and each element corresponds to a specific value form.

Note   You might want to use TreeForm to explore how Mathematica deals with nested list expressions; for instance, (*TreeForm[NestL]*).

The ArrayDepth command measures the depth of a nested list or an array.

```
In[95]:= ArrayDepth[NestL]
Out[95]= 2
```

Now you know programmatically that NestL has a depth of 2.

Vectors

Mathematica handles vectors the same way as with lists. Usual calculations of linear algebra can be symbolic or numeric.

```
In[96]:= V={6,3,2}
Out[96]= {6,3,2}
```

A vector is always shown as a list. To see a vector in regular notation, the MatrixForm command is used.

```
In[97]:= MatrixForm[V]
Out[97]//MatrixForm=
```

$$\begin{pmatrix} 6 \\ 3 \\ 2 \end{pmatrix}$$

The VectorQ command can tell you if the list you are dealing with is a vector.

```
In[98]:= VectorQ[V]
Out[98]= True
```

To see the rank of the vector, use either ArrayDepth or TensorRank.

```
In[99]:= {TensorRank[V],ArrayDepth[V]}
Out[99]= {1,1}
```

Vectors are created with the same commands that create a list: Table, Array, Range, curly braces, SparseArray, ConstantArray, and so forth. Also, common operations of vectors are performed like normal lists.

```
In[100]:=
Print["Addition: "<>ToString[V+V]]
Print["Subtraction: "<>ToString[V-V]]
Print["Scalar product: "<>ToString[2*V]]
Print["Cross product: "<>ToString[Cross[V,{1,3,2}]]]
Print["Norm: "<>ToString[Norm[V]]]
Addition: {12, 6, 4}
Subtraction: {0, 0, 0}
Scalar product: {12, 6, 4}
Cross product: {0, -10, 15}
Norm: 7
```

Matrixes

A matrix is a square list or list of lists arranged in n-rows and m-columns, where n and m are the dimensions of the matrix.

$$A_{m \times n} = \begin{pmatrix} a_{11} & a_{12} & \cdots & a_{1n} \\ a_{21} & a_{22} & \cdots & a_{2n} \\ \vdots & \vdots & \ddots & \vdots \\ a_{m1} & a_{m2} & \cdots & a_{mn} \end{pmatrix}$$

The easiest form is to create a list of lists.

```
In[105]:= {{3,3,1},{7,8,7}}//MatrixForm
Out[105]//MatrixForm=
```

$$\begin{pmatrix} 3 & 3 & 1 \\ 7 & 8 & 7 \end{pmatrix}$$

Another way is to go to Insert ➤ Table/Matrix ➤ New. A pop-up menu appears; select Matrix and specify the rows and columns within this menu. With this option, you can also specify to fill contents and the diagonal and add a grid or frames, such as in the next example that has drawn lines between columns.

$$In[106]:= A = \begin{pmatrix} 1 & 0 & 0 \\ 0 & 1 & 0 \\ 0 & 0 & 1 \end{pmatrix}$$

```
Out[106]:= {{1,0,0},{0,1,0},{0,0,1}}
```

To test whether a list of lists is a matrix, use MatrixQ.

```
In[107]:= MatrixQ[A]
Out[107]= True
```

Transpose returns the transpose of a matrix—that is, changing its rows by columns. For matrix **A**, the transpose is denoted by A^T.

```
In[108]:= Transpose[{{0,1,0},{0,1,0},{0,1,0}}]//MatrixForm
Out[108]//MatrixForm=
```

$$\begin{pmatrix} 0 & 0 & 0 \\ 1 & 1 & 1 \\ 0 & 0 & 0 \end{pmatrix}$$

Matrix Operations

Common operations between matrixes are performed by the rules of linear algebra: addition, subtraction, and multiplication. Remember that when multiplying two matrixes, **A** and **B,** the number of columns in **A** must match the number of rows in **B**. In mathematical terms: $A_{m \times n} \times B_{n \times l} = C_{m \times l}$.

```
In[109]:= B={{0,1,0},{0,1,0},{0,1,0}};
Print["Addition: "<>ToString[A+B]]
Print["Subtraction: "<>ToString[A-B]]
Print["Product: "<>ToString[Dot[B,V]]]
Addition: {{1, 1, 0}, {0, 2, 0}, {0, 1, 1}}
Subtraction: {{1, -1, 0}, {0, 0, 0}, {0, -1, 1}}
Product: {3, 3, 3}
```

To calculate the determinant, use Det.

```
In[113]:= {Det[A],Det[B]}
Out[113]= {1,0}
```

To construct a diagonal matrix, use the DiagonalMatrix command; for the identify matrix, use the IdentityMatrix command. DiagonalMatrix is for costume values, and IdentityMatrix returns a matrix with a diagonal with the same elements.

```
In[114]:= DiagonalMatrix[{X,Y,Z}]//MatrixForm
IdentityMatrix[{2,2}]//MatrixForm(*Identity matrix of 2 by 2*)
Out[114]//MatrixForm=
```

$$\begin{pmatrix} X & 0 & 0 \\ 0 & Y & 0 \\ 0 & 0 & Z \end{pmatrix}$$

```
Out[115]//MatrixForm=
```

$$\begin{pmatrix} 1 & 0 \\ 0 & 1 \end{pmatrix}$$

Restructuring a Matrix

Matrix restructuring is done with the same commands to restructure a list, like replacing an element with a new value.

```
In[116]:= ReplacePart[A,{{1,1},{2,2}}-> 3]//MatrixForm
Out[116]//MatrixForm=
```

$$\begin{pmatrix} 3 & 0 & 0 \\ 0 & 3 & 0 \\ 0 & 0 & 1 \end{pmatrix}$$

Also, it can be done by assigning the value. To access the elements of a matrix, enter the symbol followed by the subscript of the element of interest with the double bracket notation ([[ ]]). Later, you see the proper functionality of this short notation. In this case, you change the value of the element in position 1,1 of the matrix.

```
In[117]:= A[[1,1]] = 2;
MatrixForm[A]
Out[118]//MatrixForm=
```

$$\begin{pmatrix} 2 & 0 & 0 \\ 0 & 1 & 0 \\ 0 & 0 & 1 \end{pmatrix}$$

If matrix A is called again, the new value is preserved. To invert a square matrix, use Inverse.

```
In[119]:= Inverse[A]//MatrixForm
Out[119]//MatrixForm=
```

$$\begin{pmatrix} 1/2 & 0 & 0 \\ 0 & 1 & 0 \\ 0 & 0 & 1 \end{pmatrix}$$

Measuring the dimensions of a matrix is done by using Dimensions.

```
In[120]:= Dimensions[A]
Out[120]= {3,3}
```

Manipulating Lists

The previous section demonstrated different ways to create lists, including arrays, nested lists, and tables. This section describes how to manipulate these lists through referenced names, functions, and compact notation. You learn how to access the data of a list depending on its position. You learn how to add and delete elements in a list, replace single parts, and change the value of a specific element. You also examine restructuring lists once it has been built, ordering them, and converting nested lists to linear lists based on their depth. Finally, the section investigates how to see data from a list through patterns and examine pattern behavior in the Wolfram Language.

Retrieving Data

Several functions exist for handling elements of a list. The Part ["list", i] function allows you to select index parts of a list with index i.

Note   The index in a list starts at 1. Index 0 is for the head of the list.

For example, let you define a list called list1 and use Part to access the elements inside the list. The Part function works by defining the position of the element you want.

```
In[121]:= list1={1,2};
Part[{1,2},1]
Out[122]= 1
```

It also works with index notation.

```
In[123]:= {1,2}[[1]]
Out[123]= 1
```

Lists can be fully referenced by using their assigned names. Elements inside the structure can be accessed using the notation of double square brackets [[i]] or with the special character notation of double brackets, ⟦ ⟧.

Tip   To introduce the double square bracket character, type Esc [[Esc and Esc]] Esc.

```
In[124]:= list1[[1]] (*[[i]] gives you access to the element of the list in
the position i.*)
Out[124]= 1
```

Note   Square brackets ([[ ]]) are the short notation for part Esc.

To access the elements of the list by specifying the positions, you can use the span notation, which is with a double semicolon (;;).

```
In[125]:= list2=List[34,6,77,4,5,6];
Part[list2,1;;4] (*from items 1 to 4*)
Out[126]= {34,6,77,4}
```

You can also use backward indices, where the counts start from right to left, which is from the last element to the first. Let you now select from position –6 to –4.

```
In[127]:= list2[[-6;;-4]]
Out[127]= {34,6,77}
```

For the nested list, the same process is applied. The concept can be extended into a more general aspect. The next example creates a nested list with three levels and select a unique element.

```
In[128]:= list3=List[2^3,2.72,{\[Beta],ex,{Total[1+2],"Plane"}}];
list3[[3,3,2]]
Out[129]= Plane
```

In the previous example, you created a nested list of depth three. Next, you select the third element of the list {8, 2.72, {β, ex, { Total[1 + 2], "Plane"}}, then from that list, select the third element of the previous list, which is {Total[1 + 2], "Plane"}. Finally, you select the element in the second position of the last list, which is "Plane".

If you are dealing with a nested list, use the same concept you saw with the span notation. The next example selects the third element of the list3 and then display from position 1 to 2.

```
In[130]:= list3[[3,1;;2]]
Out[130]= {β, ex}
```

The same is done to a more in-depth list; you use the list's third element, then display from position 3 to 3 and select part 1.

```
In[131]:= list3[[3,3;;3,1]]
Out[131]= {3}
```

Segments of data can be displayed based on what parts of the data you are interested in. For example, the Rest function shows the data elements, except for the first. Most display the whole list except for the last element(s), depending on the type of list.

```
In[132]:= Rest[list3]
Out[132]= {2.72,{ β,ex,{3,Plane}}}
```

```
In[133]:= Most[list3]
Out[133]= {8,2.72}
```

An alternative to the previous functions is the Take function, which lets you select more broadly the data in a list. There are three possible ways to accomplish this.

- By specifying the first i elements

  ```
  In[134]:= Take[list3,2]
  Out[134]= {8,2.72}
  ```

- By specifying the last -i elements

  ```
  In[135]:= Take[list3,-1]
  Out[135]= {{ β,ex,{3,Plane}}}
  ```

- By selecting the elements from i to j

  ```
  In[136]:= Take[list3,{1,3}]
  Out[136]= {8,2.72,{ β,ex,{3,Plane}}}
  ```

Assigning or Removing Values

Once a list is established—if you have defined a name for it—it can be used just like any other type. This means that elements can be replaced by others. To change a value or values, select the position of the item, and then set the new value.

```
In[137]:= list4={"Soccer","Basketball",0,9};
list4[[2]]=1 (*position 2 corresponds to the string Basketball and we
change it for the number 1*)
Out[138]= 1
```

You can check that the new values have been added.

```
In[139]:= list4
Out[139]= {Soccer,1,0,9}
```

In addition to using the abbreviated abbreviation notation, you can use the Replace function part of specific values and choose the list, the new element, and the position.

```
In[140]:= ReplacePart[list4,Exp[X],4]
Out[140]= Soccer, 1, 0, e^X
```

To add new values, use PrependTo and AppendTo; the first adds the value on the left side of the list, whereas the second adds it by the right side of the list. Append and Prepend operate the same but with storing the new value in the original variable.

```
In[141]:= PrependTo[list4,"Blue"]
Out[141]= {Blue,Soccer,1,0,9}
```

```
In[142]:= AppendTo[list4,4]
Out[142]= {Blue,Soccer,1,0,9,4}
```

```
In[143]:= list4(*we can check the addition of new values.*)
Out[143]= {Blue,Soccer,1,0,9,4}
```

To remove the values of the list, you use Drop. Drop can work with the level of the specification or the number of elements to be erased.

```
In[144]:= Drop[list4,3];(*first 3 elements,Delete[list3,3]*)
Drop[list4,{5}](*or by position,position, number 5*)
Out[145]:= {Blue,Soccer,1,0,4}
```

The Delete command can also do the job by defining the particular positions on the list—for example, deleting the contents in positions 1 and 5.

```
In[146]:= Delete[list4,{{1},{5}}]
Out[146]= {Soccer,1,0,4}
```

As an alternative to Append and Prepend, there is the Insert function, with which you can add elements indicating the position where you want the new data. Given the expression (list4), insert the new element (2/43.23) at the third position. Consequently, the number 2/43.23 now occupies the list's third slot.

```
In[147]:= Insert[list4,2/43.23,3]
Out[147]= {Blue,Soccer,0.0462642,1,0,9,4}
```

The Insert function allows the use of several positions at the same time; for example, inserting the number 0.023 at positions –6 (second) and 7 (the last position).

```
In[148]:= Insert[list4,0.023,{{-6},{7}}]
Out[148]= {Blue,0.023,Soccer,1,0,9,4,0.023}
```

If you want to add repetitive terms or remove terms to a list or an array, you can use the ArrayPad function. The standard value is zeros if the term to be added is not defined.

```
In[149]:= ArrayPad[list4,1](*number 1 means one zero each side*)
Out[149]= {0,Blue,Soccer,1,0,9,4,0}
```

If you want to add one-sided terms, it is written as follows.

```
In[150]:= ArrayPad[list4,{1,2}](*1 zero to the left and 2 zeros to
the right*)
Out[150]= {0,Blue,Soccer,1,0,9,4,0,0}
```

To add values other than zero, you must write the value to the right of the number of times the value is repeated.

```
In[151]:= ArrayPad[list4,{0,3},"z"](*Adding the letter z three times only
the right side*)
Out[151]= {Blue,Soccer,1,0,9,4,z,z,z}
```

With ArrayPad you can add reference lists; for example, add a new list of values either left or right.

```
In[152]:= newVal={0,1,4,9}; (*Here we add them on the left side*)
ArrayPad[list4,{4,0},newVal]
Out[153]= {4,9,0,1,Blue,Soccer,1,0,9,4}
```

ArrayPad also can remove elements from a list symmetrically using negative indices.

```
In[154]:= ArrayPad[list4,-1](*it deletes the first and last elements*)
Out[154]= {Soccer,1,0,9}
```

Note   With ArrayPad, addition and deletion are symmetric unless otherwise specified.

Structuring List

When you work with lists, in addition to the different forms of access and removing its content, you might encounter cases where a list needs to be accommodated, sectioned, or restricted. The following explores several forms to achieve these tasks.

To sort a list into a specific order, use Sort followed by the sorting function.

```
In[155]:= Sort[{1,12,2,43,24,553,65,3},Greater]
Out[155]= {553,65,43,24,12,3,2,1}
```

Sort by default sorts values from less to greater, either numbers or text.

```
In[156]:= Sort[{"b","c","zz","sa","t","p"}]
Out[156]= {b,c,p,sa,t,zz}
```

To reverse a list, use the Reverse command.

```
In[157]:= Reverse[{1,12,2,43,24,553,65,3}]
Out[157]= {3,65,553,24,43,2,12,1}
```

To create a nested list in addition to that previously seen, you can generate partitions to a flat list by rearranging the elements of the list. For example, you create partitions of a list to subdivide the list into pairs.

```
In[158]:= Partition[{1,12,2,43,24,553,65,3},2]
Out[158]= {{1,12},{2,43},{24,553},{65,3}}
```

You can choose a partition with successive elements included.

```
In[159]:= Partition[{1,12,2,43,24,553},3,1]
Out[159]= {{1,12,2},{12,2,43},{2,43,24},{43,24,553}}
```

Depending on how you want a nested list, you can add an offset to the partition; for example, a partition in two with an offset of four.

```
In[160]:= Partition[{"b","c","zz","sa","t","p"},2,4]
Out[160]= {{b,c},{t,p}}
```

To return to a flat list, the Flatten function is used.

```
In[161]:= Flatten[{{1,12},{2,43},{24,553},{65,3}}]
Out[161]= {1,12,2,43,24,553,65,3}
```

Depending on the depth of the list, you can decide how deep the Flatten should be.

```
In[162]:= Flatten[{{{{1},1},1},1},1] (*here we flatten a list with a level
1 depth.*)
Out[162]= {{{1},1},1,1}
```

The ArrayReshape function lets you reshape data into a specific rectangular array with; for example, create an array of 3×3.

```
In[163]:= ArrayReshape[{1,12,2,43,24,553,65,3},{3,3}]
Out[163]= {{1,12,2},{43,24,553},{65,3,0}}
```

Elements that complete the array form are zeros. This is shown in the next example using ArrayShape to create an array of 2×2 from one element in the list.

```
In[164]:= ArrayReshape[{6},{2,2}]
Out[164]= {{6,0},{0,0}}
```

When dealing with a nested list, SortBy is also used, but instead of a sorting function, a built-in function is used. For example, order a list by the result of their approximate value.

```
In[165]:= SortBy[{1,4,553,12.52,4.3,24,7/11},N]
Out[165]= {7/11,1,4,4.3,12.52,24,553}
```

Criteria Selection

Particular values of a list can be selected with certain conditions; conditions can be applied to lists by using the Select command. The function selects the elements of the list that are true to the criteria established; the functions used for criteria can be order functions.

```
In[166]:= nmbrList=List[12,5,6,345,7,3,1,5];
Select[nmbrList,EvenQ] (*only the values that return True are selected, in
this case values that are even*)
Out[167]= {12,6}
```

Pick is also an alternative to Select.

```
In[168]:= Pick[nmbrList,PrimeQ @ nmbrList]
Out[168]= {5,7,3,5}
```

Pattern matching is used in the Wolfram Language to decree whether a given criterion should be associated with an expression. In the context of the Wolfram Language, three distinct types of patterns exist.

- The underscore symbol (_) represents any expression within the Wolfram Language.

- The double underscore symbol (__) represents a sequence containing one or more expressions.

- The triple underscore symbol (___) represents a sequence containing zero or more expressions.

Every pattern has its built-in function name. One underscore is Blank, two underscores are BlankSequence, and three underscores are BlankNullSequence.

To better understand the following examples in the channels, you use the Cases function, which allows you to select data that corresponds to the pattern.

The following is a list of data pairs where you write the selection pattern (_).

```
In[169]:= Cases[{{1,1},{1,2},{2,1},{2,2}},{_}]
Out[169]={}
```

It does not choose any element because it does not have the form of the list pattern; for example, the form {a, b}. Now if you change this shape, you see that it selects all the elements that match the shape of the pattern.

```
In[170]:= Cases[{{1,1},{1,2},{2,1},{2,2}},{_,_}]
Out[170]= {{1,1},{1,2},{2,1},{2,2}}
```

The same result can be obtained if you use the double underscore.

```
In[171]:= Cases[{{1,1},{1,2},{2,1},{2,2}},{__}]
Out[171]= {{1,1},{1,2},{2,1},{2,2}}
```

The following example shows how to select data from a list that contains numerical and categorical data. You use the RandomChoice function, which gives you a random selection from a list. In this case, it is a random selection between the words Red or Blue. The next chapter explains how this random function works in the Wolfram Language.

```
In[172]:= SeedRandom[1234]; (*Employ SeedRandom[s] to ensure the same
sequence of pseudorandom in the following examples.*)
tbl=Table[{i,j,k,RandomChoice[{"Red","Blue"}]},{i,1,3},{j,1,3},{k,1,3}]//
TableForm
Out[173]//TableForm=
1 1 1 Blue        1 2 1 Red         1 3 1 Red
1 1 2 Blue        1 2 2 Red         1 3 2 Red
1 1 3 Blue        1 2 3 Red         1 3 3 Red

2 1 1 Blue        2 2 1 Blue        2 3 1 Blue
2 1 2 Blue        2 2 2 Red         2 3 2 Red
2 1 3 Red         2 2 3 Red         2 3 3 Blue

3 1 1 Blue        3 2 1 Red         3 3 1 Red
3 1 2 Red         3 2 2 Blue        3 3 2 Red
3 1 3 Blue        3 2 3 Red         3 3 3 Red
```

The numbers on the right side are named Red or Blue. For example, you can use Cases to choose the values in the Blue or Red category. Since this is a nested list of depth four, you must specify the level ({4}) at which Cases should search for patterns.

```
In[174]:= Cases[tbl,{_,_,_,"Blue"},{4}]
Out[174]=
{{1,1,1,Blue},{1,1,2,Blue},
{1,1,3,Blue},{2,1,1,Blue},{2,1,2,Blue},
{2,2,1,Blue},{2,3,1,Blue},{2,3,3,Blue},
{3,1,1,Blue},{3,1,3,Blue},{3,2,2,Blue}}
```

Furthermore, the same result can be obtained using the double underscore. Using only the number 4, search in levels from 1 through 4.

```
In[175]:= Cases[tbl,{__,"Blue"},{4}]
Out[175]=
{{1,1,1,Blue},{1,1,2,Blue},
{1,1,3,Blue},{2,1,1,Blue},{2,1,2,Blue},
{2,2,1,Blue},{2,3,1,Blue},{2,3,3,Blue},
{3,1,1,Blue},{3,1,3,Blue},{3,2,2,Blue}}
```

You can even count how much of the Blue category you have.

```
In[176]:= Count[Tbl,{__,"Blue"},{4}]
Out[176]= 11
```

Count works in the next form, Count["list", pattern, level of spec].

Now that you understand the underscore function, you can use the Cases function to check conditions and filter values. To attach a condition, use the form (/; "condition"), where the symbol /; followed by a rule or pattern indicates that the subsequent expression is a condition or pattern in Mathematica. In the next example, the x_ represents an arbitrary element x, which represents the list's elements in this case. The condition that x is greater than 5 is then applied.

```
In[177]:= Cases[nmbrList,x_ /;x>5]
(*only the values greater than 5 are selected.*)
(*x can be replaced by any arbitrary symbol try using z_ and z > 5, the
result should be the same *)
Out[177]= {12,6,345,7}
```

As you saw in the previous example, what happens when you use _ means that the expression x_ must be applied to the condition > 5 since _ means any expression, which is the list.

Cases can also select data where the condition is true for the established pattern or set of rules. The next example selects data that are integers. The pattern objects are represented by an underscore or a rule of expression.

```
In[178]:=mixList={1.,1.2,"4",\[Pi],{"5.2","Dog"}, 3,66,{Orange,Red}};
Cases[mixList,_Integer]
(*We now select the numbers that are integers*)
Out[179]= {3,66}
```

The underscore can be applied to patterns that check the head of an expression, which is an integer. Cases compare each element to see if they are integers.

As for conditional matching, if the blanks of a pattern are accompanied by a question mark (?) and then the function test, the output is a Boolean value.

```
In[180]:= MatchQ[mixList,_?ListQ](*we test if mixlist has a head of List*)
Out[180]= True
```

You can select the level of specification with Cases. The next example selects the cases that are a string; you write two as a level of specification because mixList is a nested list with two sublists.

```
In[181]:= Cases[mixList,_?StringQ,2]
Out[181]= {4,5.2,Dog}
```

You can include several patterns with alternatives. To test different alternatives, place a (|) between patterns, so it resembles the form "pattern1" | "pattern2" |"pattern3 "| ...

```
In[182]:= Cases[mixList, _?NumberQ| _?String] (*We select the numbers and
the strings*)
Out[182]= {1.,1.2,3,66}
```

Summary

This chapter serves as an opening to the concept of lists, which are a core structure employed in Mathematica. It emphasizes the utility of lists and presents the unique Wolfram Language syntax. The chapter covers diverse types of objects that can be represented as lists. It concludes with basic functionalities for manipulating lists based on data requirements.

CHAPTER 3

Working with Data and Datasets

This chapter reviews the basics of working with data and datasets in the Wolfram Language. It starts by reviewing how to apply functions to a list, followed by how to define user functions that can be used throughout a notebook. Next, you are introduced to how to write code in one of the powerful syntaxes used in the Wolfram Language, called pure functions. Naturally, you then delve into associations, explaining how to associate keys with values and why they are fundamental for proper dataset construction in the Wolfram Language. The chapter concludes with an overview of how associations are abstract constructions of hierarchical data representations.

Operations with Lists

Let's look at how to perform operations on and between lists. This is important since, for the most part, results in Mathematica can be treated as lists. This section explains how to perform arithmetic operations, addition, subtraction, multiplication, division, and scalar multiplication. You also learn how to apply functions to a list using Map and Apply. These tools are helpful when dealing with linear and nested lists because they allow you to specify a function's depth level of application. This section also discusses how to make user-defined functions, their syntax, term grouping, receive groups, and apply the function like any other. It reviews an important concept of the Wolfram Language, which is pure functions, since these are very important for carrying out powerful tasks and activities and compactly writing code.

© Jalil Villalobos Alva 2024
J. Villalobos Alva, *Beginning Mathematica and Wolfram for Data Science*,
https://doi.org/10.1007/979-8-8688-0348-2_3

Arithmetic Operations to a List

This section discusses how lists support different arithmetic operations between numbers and between lists. You can perform basic arithmetic operations like addition, subtraction, multiplication, and division with lists.

Addition and Subtraction

The following are examples of addition and subtraction operations.

```
In[1]:= List[1,2,3,4,5,6]+1
Out[1]= {2,3,4,5,6,7}
In[2]:= List[1,2,3,4,5,6]-5
Out[2]= {-4,-3,-2,-1,0,1}
```

Division and Multiplication

The following are examples of division and multiplication operations.

```
In[3]:= List[1,2,3,4,5,6]/ π
```

$$Out[3]= \left\{ \frac{1}{\pi}, \frac{2}{\pi}, \frac{3}{\pi}, \frac{4}{\pi}, \frac{5}{\pi}, \frac{6}{\pi} \right\}$$

Scalar multiplication operations can also be performed.

```
In[4]:= List[1,2,3,4,5,6]*2
Out[4]= {2,4,6,8,10,12}
```

Exponentiation

The following is an example using exponentiation.

```
In[5]:= List[1,2,3,4,5,6]^3
Out[5]= {1,8,27,64,125,216}
```

Lists can also support basic arithmetic operations between lists.

```
In[6]:= List[1,2,4,5]-List[2,3,5,6]
Out[6]= {-1,-1,-1,-1}
```

You can also use mathematical notation to perform operations.

$$In[7]:= \frac{\{"Dog",2\}}{\{2,1\}}$$

$$Out[7]= \left\{\frac{Dog}{2},2\right\}$$

To perform computations between lists, the length of the lists must be the same; otherwise, Mathematica returns an error specifying that lists do not have the same dimensions, like in the following example.

```
In[8]:= {1,3,-1}+{-1}
During evaluation of In[8]:= Thread::tdlen: Objects of unequal length in
{1,3,-1}+{-1} cannot be combined.
Out[8]= {-1}+{1,3,-1}
```

Joining a List

To join one list with another—that is, to join the two lists—there is the Union command, which joins the elements of the lists and shows it as a new list.

```
In[9]:= Union[List["1","v","c"],{13,4,32},List["adfs",3,1,"no"]]
Out[9]= {1,3,4,13,32,1,adfs,c,no,v}
```

In addition to the Union command, there is the Intersection command, which has a function analogous to what it represents in set theory. This command lets you observe the common elements in the list or lists.

```
In[10]:= Intersection[{7,4,6,8,4,7,32,2},{123,34,6,8,5445,8}]
Out[10]= {6,8}
```

As seen the lists only have in common the numbers 6 and 8.

Applying Functions to a List

Functions can be concisely applied and automated to a list. The most used functions are Map and Apply. A short notation is to use the symbol @ instead of the square brackets [ ]; f@ "expr" is equivalent to f[expr].

```
In[11]:= Max@{1,245.2,2,5,3,5,6.0,35.3}
Out[11]= 245.2
```

Map has the following form, Map[f, "expr"]; another way of showing it is with the shorthand notation using the symbol @. f /@ "expr" and Map[f, "expr"] are equivalent. This function also supports nested lists.

```
In[12]:= Factorial/@List[1,2,3,4,5,6]
Out[12]= {1,2,6,24,120,720}
```

Map can be applied to nested lists.

```
In[13]:= Map[Sqrt,{{1,2},{3,4}}]
Out[13]= {{1,Sqrt[2]},{Sqrt[3],2}}
```

The Map function is applied to each element of the list. Map can also work with nested lists, as in the previous example. The next example creates a list of 10 elements with Table. Those elements are random numbers between 0 and 1, and then you map a function to convert them to string expressions.

```
In[14]:= data=Range[RandomReal[{0,1}],10];(*List*)
ToString/@data (*mapping a to convert to string*)
Head/@% (*Checking the data type of every element*)
Out[15]= {0.526418,1.52642,2.52642,3.52642,4.52642,5.52642,6.52642,7.52642,
8.52642,9.52642}
Out[16]= {String,String,String,String,String,String,String,String,String,
String}
```

Let's look at how to apply a function to a list with additional functions. Apply has the form Apply [f, "expr"] and the shorthand notation is f @@ "expr".

```
In[17]:= Apply[Plus,data](*It gives the sum of the elements of Data*)
Out[17]= 50.2642
```

```
In[18]:= Plus@@data
Out[18]= 50.2642
```

Also, commands can be applied to a list in the same line of code, which is helpful when dealing with large lists. For example, if you want to know whether an element satisfies a condition, instead of going through each value, the element can be gathered into a list and tested for the specified condition.

```
In[19]:= primelist=Range[100];Map[PrimeQ,primelist]
Out[19]= {False,True,True,False,True,False,True,False,False,False,True,False,
True,False,False,False,True,False,True,False,False,False,True,False,False,
False,False,False,True,False,True,False,False,False,False,False,True,False,
False,False,True,False,True,False,False,False,True,False,False,False,False,
False,True,False,False,False,False,False,True,False,True,False,False,False,
False,False,True,False,False,False,True,False,True,False,False,False,False,
False,True,False,False,False,True,False,False,False,False,False,True,False,
False,False,False,False,False,False,True,False,False,False}
```

The previous example created a list from 1 to 100 and then tested which of the numbers satisfies the condition of being a prime number with the PrimeQ function. Other functions can be used to test different conditions with numbers and strings. Also, a more specific function for testing logical relations in a list can be used (MemberQ, SubsetQ).

Defining Own Functions

User functions can be written to perform repetitive tasks and reduce the size of a program. Segmenting the code into functions allows you to create pieces of code that perform a certain task. Functions can receive data from outside when called through parameters and return a fixed result.

A function can be defined with the set or set delayed symbol, but remember, using the set symbol assigns the result to the definition. To define a function, first write the name or symbol, followed by the reference variable and an underscore. As with cases, the underscore tells Mathematica that you are dealing with a dummy variable. As a warning, defined functions cannot have space between letters. Functions can also receive more than one argument.

```
In[20]:= MyF[z_]:=12+2+z;MyF2[x_,z_]:=z/x
```

Now, you can call the function with different z values.

```
In[21]:= List[MyF[1],MyF[324],MyF[5432],MyF2[154,1],MyF2[14,4],MyF2[6,9]]
```
$$Out[21]= \left\{ 15, 338, 5446, \frac{1}{154}, \frac{2}{7}, \frac{3}{2} \right\}$$

Also, another way to write functions is to write compound functions. This concept is similar to compound expressions; expressions of different classes are written within the definition. Each computation can or cannot be ended with a semicolon. The following example shows the concept.

```
In[22]:= StatsFun[myList_]:={Max@myList,Min@myList,Mean@myList,Median
@myList,Quantile@@{myList,1}(*25 percent*)(*to write a function with
multiple arguments with shorthand notation use curly braces*)}
```

You can also send a list as an argument.

```
In[23]:= myList=Table[m-2,{m,-2,10}];
StatsFun[myList]
Out[24]= {8,-4,2,2,8}
```

You can have multiple operations within a function, with the option to create conditions for the arguments to meet. To write a condition, use the dash and semicolon (/;) symbols. When the condition is true, the function is evaluated; otherwise, if the condition is not true, the function is not evaluated. Compound functions need to be grouped; otherwise, Mathematica treats them as though they are outside the body of the whole function.

The next example creates a function that tells you if an arbitrary string is a palindrome, which is when the word is the same when written backward.

```
In[25]:= PalindromeWord[string_/;StringQ@string==True]:=(*we can check if
the input is really a string*)
(ReverseWord=StringJoin[Reverse[Characters[string]]];
(*here we separate the characters,reverse the list and join them into a
string*)
ReverseWord==string (*then we test if the word is a palindrome,the output
of the whole function will be True or False*))
```

Let's test the new function.

```
In[26]:= PalindromeWord/@{"hello","room","jhon","kayak","civic","radar"}
Out[26]= {False,False,False,True,True,True}
```

When you have a local assignment on a compound function or functions, the symbols used are still assigned, so if the symbol(s) are called outside the function, it can cause coding errors. One thing to consider is that you can clear the function and local symbols when the function is no longer used. Clearing only the function name does not remove local assignments. Another solution is to declare variables inside a module since the variables are only locally treated, as shown in the following form.

```
In[27]:= MyFunction[a0_,b0_]:=Module[{m=a0,n=b0},(*local variables*)m+n
(*body of the module*)](*end of module*)
In[28]:= Clear[MyF,MyF2,StatsFun,PalindromeWord,ReverseWord] (*To remove
tag names of the functions and local symbols *)
```

Pure Functions

Pure functions, also known as anonymous functions, are a powerful feature of the Wolfram Language. They allow the execution of a function without referencing a name and can be explicitly assigned to an operation. Arguments within pure functions are denoted with a hashtag (#). To refer to a specific argument, append a number to the hashtag (e.g., #1, #2, (#3, ... for the first, second, third, ... argument). An ampersand (&) is used at the end of the definition to signify the use of the hashtag references. Pure functions can be constructed with the Function keyword or using the shorthand notation of hashtag and ampersand.

```
In[29]:= Function[#^-1][z]==#^-1&[z]
#^-1&[z] (*both expression mean 1/z*)
Out[29]= True
Out[30]= 1/z
```

Some examples of pure functions.

```
In[31]:= {#^-1&[77],#1+#2-#3&[x,y,z] (*we can imagine that #1,#2,#3 are the
1st,2nd and 3rd variables*),Power[E,#]&[3]}
Out[31]= {1/77,x+y-z,E^3}
```

You can use pure functions along with Map and Apply to pass each argument of a list to a specific function. The # represents each element of the list, and the & represents that # is filled and tested for the elements of the list.

```
In[32]:= N[#]&/@ {1,1,1,12,3,1}
Sqrt[#]&/@{-1,2,4,16}
Out[32]= {1.,1.,1.,12.,3.,1.}
Out[33]= {I,Sqrt[2],2,4}
```

Code can be written more compactly using Apply and pure functions, as shown in the next example. You can select the numbers bigger than 10.

```
In[34]:= Select@@{{1,22,41,7,62,21},#>10&}
Out[34]= {22,41,62,21}
```

Indexed Tables

You can create and display results in tables to provide a quick way to observe and manage a group of related data, which leads to how to create tables in the Wolfram Language, such as giving titles to columns and names to rows. A series of examples to help you learn the essentials of using the tables so that you can present your data properly are featured in this section.

Tables with the Wolfram Language

Tables are created with nested lists, and those lists are shown with TableForm.

```
In[35]:= table1={{"Dog","Wolf"},{"Cat","Leopard"},{"Pigeon","Shark"}};
TableForm[table1]
Out[36]//TableForm=
Dog     Wolf
Cat     Leopard
Pigeon  Shark
```

The format of TableForm is ["list", options]. Formatting options let you justify the columns of tables in three ways: left, center, and right. In the next example, the contents of the table are centered.

```
In[37]:= TableForm[table1,TableAlignments\[RightArrow]Right]
Out[37]//TableForm=
Dog      Wolf
Cat      Leopard
Pigeon  Shark
```

Titles can be added with the TableHeadings option command and by specifying whether the rows and column labels are exposed or just one of them. Choosing the Automatic option gives index labels to the rows and columns. Remember to write strings between the apostrophes or to use ToString.

```
In[38]:= TableForm[table1,TableHeadings->{{"Row 1","Row 2","Row
3"},{"Column 1","Column 2"}}]
Out[38]//TableForm=
        | Column 1  Column 2
_____|_____
Row 1  | Dog        Wolf
Row 2  | Cat        Leopard
Row 3  | Pigeon     Shark
```

Labeled rows and columns can be customized with desired names.

```
In[39]:= colname={"Domestic Animals","Wild Animals"};
rowname={"Animal 1","Animal 2","Animal 3"};
TableForm[table1,TableHeadings->{rowname,colname}]
Out[41]//TableForm=
        | Domestic Animals   Wild Animals
_____|_____
Row 1  | Dog                Wolf
Row 2  | Cat                Leopard
Row 3  | Pigeon             Shark
```

The same concept applies to labeling just columns or rows by typing None on the rows or columns option.

```
In[42]:= TableForm[table1,TableHeadings->{None,{"Domestic Animals","Wild
Animals"}}]
Out[42]//TableForm=
```

Domestic Animals	Wild Animals
Dog	Wolf
Cat	Leopard
Pigeon	Shark

Automated forms of tables can be created with the use of Table and Range. By applying the Automatic option in the TableHeadings, you can create indexed labels for the data.

```
In[43]:=tabData={Table[i,{i,7}],Table[5^i,{i,7}]};TableForm[tabData,TableHe
adings->Automatic]
Out[43]//TableForm=
```

	1	2	3	4	5	6	7
1	1	2	3	4	5	6	7
2	5	25	125	625	3125	15625	78125

For exhibit reasons, a table can be transposed too.

```
In[44]:= TableForm[Transpose[tabData],TableHeadings->Automatic]
Out[44]//TableForm=
```

	1	2
1	1	2
2	2	25
3	3	125
4	4	625
5	5	3125
6	6	15625
7	7	78125

Another useful tool is Grid, which displays a list or a nested list in tabular format. Like TableForm, Grid can also be customized to exhibit data more properly.

Note   Grid works with any expression.

```
In[45]:= tabData2=Table[{i,Exp[i],N@Exp[i]},{i,7}];
Grid[tabData2]
Out[46]=
```

i	Exp^i	Numeric approx.
1	e	2.71828
2	e^2	7.38906
3	e^3	20.0855
4	e^4	54.5982
5	e^5	148.413
6	e^6	403.429
7	e^7	1096.63

To add headers, insert them in the original list as strings and in position 1.

```
In[47]:= Grid[Insert[tabData2,{"i","Exp^i","Numeric approx."},1]]
Out[47]=
```

i	Exp^i	Numeric approx.
1	e	2.71828
2	e^2	7.38906
3	e^3	20.0855
4	e^4	54.5982
5	e^5	148.413
6	e^6	403.429
7	e^7	1096.63

You can add dividers and spacers too. With Dividers and Spacing, you can divide or space the y and x axes.

```
In[48]:= Grid[Insert[tabData2,{"i","Expⁱ","Numeric approx."},1],
Dividers->{All,False},Spacings->{1,1}]
Out[48]=
| i | Expⁱ | Numeric approx.
| 1 | e    | 2.71828
| 2 | e²   | 7.38906
| 3 | e³   | 20.0855
| 4 | e⁴   | 54.5982
| 5 | e⁵   | 148.413
| 6 | e⁶   | 403.429
| 7 | e⁷   | 1096.63
```

Background can be added with the Background option. This option allows specific parts of the table or column table to be colored.

```
In[49]:= Grid[Insert[tabData2,{"i","Exp i","Numeric approx."},1],Dividers ->
{All,False},Spacings -> {Automatic,0},Background -> {{LightYellow,None,LightBlue}}]
Out[49]=
```

i	Exp^i	Numeric approx.
1	e	2.71828
2	e²	7.38906
3	e³	20.0855
4	e⁴	54.5982
5	e⁵	148.413
6	e⁶	403.429
7	e⁷	1096.63

Associations

Associations are fundamental in developing the Wolfram Language; associations are used to index lists or other expressions and create more complex data structures. Associations, much like dictionaries in many other programming languages, are a more structured construct that allows you to provide a process for creating pairs of keys and values. Later, you see that they are important for handling datasets in the Wolfram Language.

Associations are of the form Association["key_1" → val_1, key_2 →val_2 ...] or <| "key_1"→ "val_1", "key_2" → "val_2" ... | >; they associate a key to a value. Keys and values can be any expression. The Association command is used to construct an association, or you can use the symbolic entry <| --- |>.

```
In[50]:= Associt=<|1->"a",2->"b",3->"c"|> (*is the same as Association
[a\[RightArrow]"a",b\[RightArrow]"b",c\[RightArrow]"c"]*)
Associt2=Association[dog->"23","score"->\[Pi]*\[Pi],2*2->Sin[23 Degree]]
Out[50]= <| 1 → a, 2 → b, 3 → c | >
Out[51]= <| dog → 23, score → π², 4 → Sin[23°] | >
```

Entries in an association are ordered, so data can be accessed based on the key of the value or by the position of the entries in the association, like with lists. The position is associated with the values (position of the entries), not the keys, as the order of the keys is not always preserved.

```
In[52]:= Associt[1](*this is key 1 *)
Associt2[[2]] (*this is position of key 2, which is π² *)
Out[52]= a
Out[53]= π²
```

As seen in the latter example, the position is associated with the values, not the key. So, if you want to show parts of the association, use the semicolon.

```
In[54]:= Associt[[1;;2]]
 Associt2[[2;;2]]
Out[54]= <|1→a,2→b|>
Out[55]= <|score→ π² |>
```

Values and keys can be extracted with the Keys and Values commands.

```
In[56]:= Keys@Associt2
Values@Associt2
Out[56]= {dog, score, 4}
Out[57]= {23, π², Sin[23 °]}
```

You get an error if you ask for a key without a proper reference.

```
In[58]:= Associt["a"](*there is no "a" key in the association, thus
the error*)
Out[58]= Missing[KeyAbsent,a]
```

Associations can also be associations. The next example shows how to associate associations, thus producing an association of associations. This concept is basic for understanding how a dataset works in the Wolfram Language.

```
In[59]:= Association[Associt,Associt2]
Out[59]= <| 1 → a, 2 → b, 3 → c, dog → 23, score → π², 4 → Sin[23°] |>
```

You can also make different associations with lists using AssociationThread. The keys correspond to the first argument and the values to the second. AssociationThread threads a list of keys to a list of values like the next form: < | {"key_1", "key_2", "key_3" ...} → {"val_1", "val_2", "val_3" ... } | >. The latter form can be seen as a list of keys marking a list of values. When you have defined the lists of keys and values, the command can associate a list with another list. You can also create a list of associations to read keys as a row and a column.

```
In[60]:=AssociationThread[{"class","age","gender","survived"},{"Economy",
29,"female",True}]
Out[60]= <| class → Economy, age → 29, gender → female, survived → True |>
```

You can construct the list of keys and values.

```
In[61]:= keys={"class","age","gender","boarded"};
values={"Economy",29,"female",True};
AssociationThread@@{keys,values}
Out[63]= <| class → Economy, age → 29, gender → female,
boarded → True |>
```

More complex structures can be created with associations. For example, the next association creates a data structure based on the information about a sports car, with the model name, engine, power, torque, acceleration, and top speed.

```
In[64]:= Association@{"Model name" -> "Koenigsegg CCX",
"Engine" -> "Twin supercharged V8",
"Power" -> "806 hp",
 "Torque" -> "5550 rpm",
"Acceleration 0-100 km/h" -> "3.2 sec",
"Top speed" -> "395 Km/h"}
Out[64]= <|Model name→Koenigsegg CCX, Engine→Twin supercharged V8,
Power→806 hp, Torque→5550 rpm, Acceleration 0-100 km/h→3.2 sec, Top
speed→395 Km/h|>
```

You can see how labels and their elements are created in a grouped way. In addition to that, it is shown how the curly braces mark how each row can arrange the key/value pair.

Dataset Format

Associations are an essential part of making structured forms of data. Datasets in the Wolfram Language offer a way to organize and exhibit hierarchical data by providing a method for accessing data inside a dataset. This section features examples of how to convert lists, nested lists, and associations to a dataset. It also covers how to add values, access values in a dataset, drop and delete values, map functions over a dataset, deal with duplicate data, and apply functions by row or column.

Constructing Datasets

Datasets are for constructing hierarchical data frameworks, where lists, associations, and nested lists have an order. Datasets are useful for exhibiting large data in an accessible, structured format. Datasets can show enclosed structures in a sharp format with row headers, column headers, and numbered elements. Having the data as a dataset allows you to look at the data in multiple ways.

Datasets can be constructed in four forms.

- A list of lists; a table with no denomination in rows and columns

- A list of associations, a table with labeled columns; a table with repeated keys and different or same values

- An association of lists, a table with labeled rows; a table with different keys and different or same values

- Association of associations; a table with labeled rows and columns

The most common form to create a new dataset is from a list of lists. Create a list within the curly braces {} using the Dataset function. Each brace represents the parts of the table. Figure 3-1 shows the output of the Dataset function.

```
In[65]:= Dataset@{{"Jhon",23,"male","Portugal"},{"Mary",30,"female","USA"},
{"Peter",33,"male","France"},{"Julia",53,"female","Netherlands"},{"Andrea",
45,"female","Brazil"},{"Jeff",24,"male","Mexico"}}
Out[65]=
```

Jhon	23	male	Portugal
Mary	30	female	USA
Peter	33	male	France
Julia	53	female	Netherlands
Andrea	45	female	Brazil
Jeff	24	male	Mexico

Figure 3-1. *Dataset object created from the input code*

By hovering the mouse cursor over the elements of the dataset, you can see their position in the lower-left corner. The name France corresponds to row 3 and column 4. The notation of a dataset is first rows, then columns. If you have labeled columns, rows, or both, you see the column name and row name instead of the numbers.

Constructing a dataset with a list of associations is performed by creating associations first with repeated keys and then enclosing them in a list. First, create the associations; the repeated keys specify each column header. The values represent the contents of the columns. Datasets have a head expression of Dataset.

```
In[66]:=
Dataset@{
<|"Name"->"Jhon","Age"->23,"Gender"->"male","Country"->"Portugal"|>,
<|"Name"->"Mary","Age"->30,"Gender"->"female","Country"->"USA"|>,
<|"Name"->"Peter","Age"->33,"Gender"->"male","Country"->"France"|>,
<|"Name"->"Julia","Age"->53,"Gender"->"female","Country"->"Netherlands"|>,
<|"Name"->"Andrea","Age"->45,"Gender"->"female","Country"->"Brazil" |>,
<|"Name" -> "Jeff", "Age" -> 24, "Gender" -> "male", "Country" -> "Mexico"
|>}(*Head @ % *)
Out[66]=
```

As seen in Figure 3-2, Mathematica recognizes that Name, Age, Gender, and Country are column headers, which is why the color of the box is different.

Name	Age	Gender	Country
Jhon	23	male	Portugal
Mary	30	female	USA
Peter	33	male	France
Julia	53	female	Netherlands
Andrea	45	female	Brazil
Jeff	24	male	Mexico

Figure 3-2. *Dataset with column headers*

When passing the cursor over the column labels, they are highlighted in blue, thus making it possible to click the name of the label, and then it produces only the selected label and not the whole dataset, as seen in Figure 3-3.

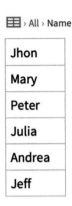

> All > Name

Figure 3-3. *Column name selected in the dataset*

When this happens, the name of the column also appears. To return to the whole dataset, hit the spreadsheet icon ▦ in the upper-left corner or the name All. This type of layout is practical when dealing with a big set of rows and columns, and you want to focus only on a few sections of the dataset.

In an association of lists, the keys represent the label of the rows, and the values are the list of the elements of the rows; then, you associate the whole block. The next block of code generates an association of a list.

Note   The same is true here. Whenever you click a row's name, it only displays that row.

```
In[67]:=  Dataset@
<|"Subject A"->{"Jhon",23,"male","Portugal"},
"Subject B"->{"Mary",30,"female","USA"},
"Subject C"->{"Peter",33,"male","France"},
"Subject D"->{"Julia",53,"female","Netherlands"},
"Subject E"->{"Andrea",45,"female","Brazil"},
"Subject F"->{"Jeff",24,"male","Mexico"}|>
Out[67]=
```

As seen in Figure 3-4, the rows are now labeled.

Subject A	Jhon	23	male	Portugal
Subject B	Mary	30	female	USA
Subject C	Peter	33	male	France
Subject D	Julia	53	female	Netherlands
Subject E	Andrea	45	female	Brazil
Subject F	Jeff	24	male	Mexico

Figure 3-4. *Dataset with labeled rows*

Row labels are recognized and displayed in the color box. When selecting the row's label, it display only that row, as shown in Figure 3-5.

⊞ › Subject E

Andrea	45	female	Brazil

Figure 3-5. *Subject E row selected*

In an association of associations, the repeated keys of the association of associations are the column labels and the values of the dataset. In the second association, the keys are the labels of the rows, and the first associations are the values of the second association. The next example clarifies this.

```
In[68]:= Dataset@
<|"Subject A"-><|"Name"->"Jhon","Age"->23,"Gender"->"male","Country"->
"Portugal"|>,"Subject B"-><|"Name"->"Mary","Age"->30,"Gender"->
"female","Country"->"USA"|>,"Subject C"-><|"Name"->"Peter","Age"->33,
"Gender"->"male","Country"->"France"|>,
"Subject D"-><|"Name"->"Julia","Age"->53,"Gender"->"female","Country"->
"Netherlands"|>,"Subject E"-><|"Name"->"Andrea","Age"->45,"Gender"->
"female","Country"->"Brazil"|>,"Subject F"-><|"Name"->"Jeff","Age"->
24,"Gender"->"male","Country"->"Mexico"|>|>
Out[68]=
```

	Name	Age	Gender	Country
Subject A	Jhon	23	male	Portugal
Subject B	Mary	30	female	USA
Subject C	Peter	33	male	France
Subject D	Julia	53	female	Netherlands
Subject E	Andrea	45	female	Brazil
Subject F	Jeff	24	male	Mexico

Figure 3-6. *Dataset with names in rows and columns*

As can be seen in Figure 3-6, the rows and columns are now labeled. Like the previous examples, the column and row labels are recognized and displayed in the color box. When selecting the label of the row or a column, it displays only that row or column, as seen in Figure 3-7.

⊞ › Subject F

Name	Age	Gender	Country
Jeff	24	male	Mexico

Figure 3-7. *Only a row selected*

If you select only a particular value, then that value is solely displayed. Figure 3-8 shows its form.

⊞ › Subject F › Name

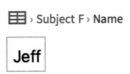

Figure 3-8. *Name for subject F*

Creating a dataset from associations of associations is best for compact datasets because sometimes it can get messy to extract values and keys. However, the best approach is the one that works best for you.

Accessing Data in a Dataset

Mathematica gives each element a unique index; so if you are interested in selecting data from a dataset, assign a symbol to the dataset and proceed to specify each output in the next form. The first and second positions of the arguments represent row and column [nth row, mth column]. So, to extract data based on a column name or a set of columns, enclose the columns in brackets. You can also use double-bracket notation. If only one argument is received, it is only the rows. First, let's create the dataset.

```
In[69]:=Dst=Dataset@{
<|"Name"->"Jhon","Age"->23,"Gender"->"male","Country"->"Portugal"|>,
<|"Name"->"Mary","Age"->30,"Gender"->"female","Country"->"USA"|>,
<|"Name"->"Peter","Age"->33,"Gender"->"male","Country"->"France"|>,
<|"Name"->"Julia","Age"->53,"Gender"->"female","Country"->"Netherlands"|>,
<|"Name"->"Andrea","Age"->45,"Gender"->"female","Country"->"Brazil"|>,
<|"Name"->"Jeff","Age"->24,"Gender"->"male","Country"->"Mexico"|>};
```

The notation [[ ]] works the same as the special character for double brackets (⟦ ⟧). Also, you can select data using the specific keys of the value, as shown in Figure 3-9.

```
In[70]:= Dst[[1,2]](*This is for row 1,column 2*)
Dst[1](*row 1*)
Out[70]= 23
Out[71]=
```

Name	Jhon
Age	23
Gender	male
Country	Portugal

Figure 3-9. *Row 1 for Dst*

Let's look at the following and Figure 3-10.

```
In[72]:= Dst[1;;3](*to manipulate data of the column try Dst[1;;3,1;;3]*)
Out[72]=
```

Name	Age	Gender	Country
Jhon	23	male	Portugal
Mary	30	female	USA
Peter	33	male	France

Figure 3-10. *Values from rows 1 to 3 and columns 1 to 3*

This case selected data from positions 1 to 3, from John to Peter. The same is applied to columns.

You can also show specific columns and maintain all the fixed rows with their keys. The same process is applied when having a label in each row. Typing All means all the elements in the column or the row. The output is shown in Figure 3-11.

```
In[73]:= Dst[All,{"Name","Age"}] (*If more than 1 column label is added
then enclosed the labels by curly braces.*)
Out[73]=
```

Name	Age
Jhon	23
Mary	30
Peter	33
Julia	53
Andrea	45
Jeff	24

Figure 3-11. *Values for column name and age*

Alternatively, you can extract a column or a row as a list to better manipulate them in the Wolfram Language. To do that you need to use the Normal function and the Values command. Remember that you are dealing with associations, so if you want the values, you use the Values command and then Normal to convert it to a normal expression.

```
In[74]:= Normal@Values@Dst[All,{"Name","Age"}](*values of the name and age
columns*)
Out[74]= {{Jhon,23},{Mary,30},{Peter,33},{Julia,53},{Andrea,45},{Jeff,24}}
```

It is the same idea for the rows: if they have a label, you can use them.

```
In[75]:= Normal@Values@Dst[[1,All]]
Out[75]= {Jhon,23,male,Portugal}
```

The result is the same if you first do Normal and then Values.

```
In[76]:= Values@Normal@Dst[[1,All]]
Out[76]= {Jhon,23,male,Portugal}
```

Another function that can be used is Query, a specialized function that works with datasets. Queries must be applied to the symbol of the dataset or directly to the dataset. Queries are helpful because they allow easy selectivity of the values; you can extract rows or columns and get individual records.

```
In[77]:= Query[All,"Country"]@Dst
Query[3]@%
Out[77]=
```

Figure 3-12 shows that you can extract columns and values with Query.

Portugal
USA
France
Netherlands
Brazil
Mexico

Figure 3-12. *Country values*

Out[78]= France

Another function that works more intuitively is Take, in which you can specify the symbol of the dataset and then how many rows and columns to display. Take comes in handy when dealing with large datasets, and you want to only view a specific part of the data.

```
In[79]:= Take[Dst,2] (*First 2 rows*)
(*Take[Dst,3,3] First 3 rows and columns*)
Out[79]=
```

Figure 3-13 shows you can use Take as an alternative.

Name	Age	Gender	Country
Jhon	23	male	Portugal
Mary	30	female	USA

Figure 3-13. *First two rows of a dataset*

Adding Values

Now that you have examined how to access the elements of a dataset, you can add new
values to the dataset. You can add rows with Append or Prepend, but remember that
AppendTo and PrependTo can be used too. However, they assign the new result to the
assigned variable. Append adds at the last and Prepend at the first.

To add a row, you would need to write the new row like you write the associations
with repeated keys, calling the dataset and then the function, followed by the new row,
as shown in Figure 3-14.

```
In[80]:= Dst[Append[<|"Name"->"Anya","Age"->19,"Gender"->
"female","Country"->"Russia"|>]]
Out[80]=
```

Name	Age	Gender	Country
Jhon	23	male	Portugal
Mary	30	female	USA
Peter	33	male	France
Julia	53	female	Netherlands
Andrea	45	female	Brazil
Jeff	24	male	Mexico
Anya	19	female	Russia

Figure 3-14. *New row added at the end of the dataset*

The operator form of the Append function was used in this case. Operator forms
in the Wolfram Language allows for a more concise and readable code syntax. They
essentially allow function to be used directly without square brackets. This form
can be used with other function, like Apply, to make expression with a more natural
representation. For example, to add a new row at the top of the dataset, try using the
code, Dst@Prepend[<|"Name"->"Anya", "Age"->19, "Gender"->"female", "Country"->
"Russia"|>], which is the same as Dst[Prepend[<|"Name"->"Anya","Age"->19,
"Gender"->"female", "Country"->"Russia"|>]].

Adding a new column of only single values can be done by simply assigning a value to the side of the columns of the dataset with the key name, which is the column name. Figure 3-15 shows the new column added.

```
In[81]:= Dst[All,Prepend["ID number"->1]]
Out[81]=
```

ID number	Name	Age	Gender	Country
1	Jhon	23	male	Portugal
1	Mary	30	female	USA
1	Peter	33	male	France
1	Julia	53	female	Netherlands
1	Andrea	45	female	Brazil
1	Jeff	24	male	Mexico

Figure 3-15. *ID column added*

To add a list of values as a column, first create a list of values. Next, use AssociationThread to associate each value with the same key, creating an association of values for the repeated key. Then you create a dataset of the new association and combine it with the original dataset with the Join function. This merges expressions of the same head.

```
In[82]:= Id={1,2,3,4,5,6};(*our list of values*)
ID=AssociationThread["ID"->#]&/@Id (*the process is threaded in the list*)
Out[82]= {<|ID->1|>,<|ID->2|>,<|ID->3|>,<|ID->4|>,<|ID->5|>,<|ID->6|>}
```

Each element needs to be associated one by one for the later block because AssociationThread suppresses repeated keys, so you would only have one association, and you need to have a repeated key marking different values.

Next, create the new dataset with the same key shown in Figure 3-16.

```
In[83]:= Dataset[ID]
Out[83]=
```

ID
1
2
3
4
5
6

Figure 3-16. *ID column dataset*

Finally, join the same objects; here, Join is used with a level of specification of 2 because the new dataset is a sublist of depth 2. If you want to add the column on the left side, the new column goes first, followed by the dataset; for the right side, it is the opposite. Figure 3-17 shows the output dataset.

```
In[84]:= Join[%,Dst,2]
Out[84]=
```

ID	Name	Age	Gender	Country
1	Jhon	23	male	Portugal
2	Mary	30	female	USA
3	Peter	33	male	France
4	Julia	53	female	Netherlands
5	Andrea	45	female	Brazil
6	Jeff	24	male	Mexico

Figure 3-17. *ID column added*

The previous cases worked with a dataset from a list of associations; since you are working with tagged rows only or tagged rows and columns, adding a row or column is preserved by adding the same structure to the dataset. So, adding a new row to an association of lists would take the form < | "key" → {elem, ... } |>; for columns, this would be the process of creating a dataset and joining them. In the case of a list of lists, adding a row would be the same approach but without a key. For the case of association of associations, to add a row would be <| "key" → < |"key 1" → "val 1", ... | > |>, and for columns, it would be the same as before, a key associated with a value. Nevertheless, there is no restriction on how data can be accommodated.

Finally, to change unique values, select the item and give it the new content. In the case that you have labels on rows and columns, the original form is still preserved: "rows", "columns"}. So, if you want to replace Jhon's age, use the ReplacePart function by calling the symbol of the dataset and specifying the column tag and then with the new value, which is 50. If you were working with only a row label or a column label, the process would be the same, but using the row or column label and then the number position of the element. Figure 3-18 shows the new value is 50.

```
In[85]:= ReplacePart[Dst,{1,"Age"}->50](*Also using the index will produce
the same output,that would be {1,2} -> 50*)
Out[85]=
```

Name	Age	Gender	Country
Jhon	50	male	Portugal
Mary	30	female	USA
Peter	33	male	France
Julia	53	female	Netherlands
Andrea	45	female	Brazil
Jeff	24	male	Mexico

Figure 3-18. Jhon age value changed to 50

Dropping Values

You can eliminate the contents of a row or column without deleting the entire table structure. To accomplish this, use the Drop function or the Delete function. When using Drop, you enclose the number of the row or column with { } to delete a unique row or column (see Figure 3-19).

```
In[86]:= Drop[Dst,{1}](*in the instance we want to delete more than one
then we write m through n dropped {m,n}*)
Out[86]=
```

Name	Age	Gender	Country
Mary	30	female	USA
Peter	33	male	France
Julia	53	female	Netherlands
Andrea	45	female	Brazil
Jeff	24	male	Mexico

Figure 3-19. *Drop row 1*

Figure 3-19 shows that the first row has been dropped. You can also drop rows and columns at the same time. Figure 3-20 shows the second row and last column dropped.

```
In[87]:= Drop[Dst,{2},{4}]
Out[87]=
```

Name	Age	Gender
Jhon	23	male
Peter	33	male
Julia	53	female
Andrea	45	female
Jeff	24	male

Figure 3-20. *New dataset after dropping row 2 and column 4*

Another way is to use Delete on a row or column label, as shown in Figure 3-21.

```
In[88]:= Dst[All,Delete["Age"]] (*to delete a row use["label of row",All]*)
Out[88]=
```

Name	Gender	Country
Jhon	male	Portugal
Mary	female	USA
Peter	male	France
Julia	female	Netherlands
Andrea	female	Brazil
Jeff	male	Mexico

Figure 3-21. *Age column deleted*

Filtering Values

Having the data as a dataset allows you to look at the data in multiple ways. Let's now work with the tagged dataset to better expose how filtering values work. For starters, you use the labeled dataset shown in Figure 3-22.

```
In[89]:= Clear[Dst];(*Let's clear the symbol "Dst" of previous
assignments*)
Dst=Dataset@
<|"Subject A"-><|"Name"->"Jhon","Age"->23,"Gender"->"male","Country"->
"Portugal"|>,"Subject B"-><|"Name"->"Mary","Age"->30,"Gender"->
"female","Country"->"USA"|>,"Subject C"-><|"Name"->"Peter","Age"->33,
"Gender"->"male","Country"->"France"|>,
"Subject D"-><|"Name"->"Julia","Age"->53,"Gender"->"female","Country"->
"Netherlands"|>,"Subject E"-><|"Name"->"Andrea","Age"->45,"Gender"->
"female","Country"->"Brazil"|>,"Subject F"-><|"Name"->"Jeff","Age"->24,
"Gender"->"male","Country"->"Mexico"|>
|>
Out[90]=
```

	Name	Age	Gender	Country
Subject A	Jhon	23	male	Portugal
Subject B	Mary	30	female	USA
Subject C	Peter	33	male	France
Subject D	Julia	53	female	Netherlands
Subject E	Andrea	45	female	Brazil
Subject F	Jeff	24	male	Mexico

Figure 3-22. *Tagged dataset*

As with lists, you can create one or more filter conditions; for example, you can select an age greater than 30 and get a dataset object (see Figure 3-23).

```
In[91]:= Cases[Dst[All,"Age"],x_/;x>30](*also we can select data that
matches exactly 30 with the==sign*)
Out[91]=
```

33
53
45

Figure 3-23. *Filtered data from the age column*

Figure 3-23 shows the filtered data. Data can be selected based on True or False results. For that, you can use the Select function. Figure 3-24 shows the selected subjects.

```
In[92]:= Select[Dst[All,"Age"],EvenQ]
Out[92]=
```

Subject B	30
Subject F	24

Figure 3-24. *Selected subjects*

The use of pure functions can be applied too. Remember that the #Age resembles the elements in the Age column, as shown in Figure 3-25.

```
In[93]:= Dst[Select[#Age>30&]]
Out[93]=
```

	Name	Age	Gender	Country
Subject C	Peter	33	male	France
Subject D	Julia	53	female	Netherlands
Subject E	Andrea	45	female	Brazil

Figure 3-25. *Selected values using pure function syntax*

Also, you can count categorical data values, as shown in Figure 3-26. This is helpful when you want to identify how many types of a class you have in the data. For example, you can count how many females and males are in the dataset.

```
In[94]:= Counts[Dst[All,"Gender"]] (*alternative
form:Dst[Counts,"Gender"]*)
Out[94]=
```

male	3
female	3

Figure 3-26. *Count data for class male and female*

More complex groups can be made based on a class; for instance, you can group the dataset by gender, as shown in Figure 3-27.

```
In[95]:= Dst[GroupBy["Gender"],Counts,"Age"]
Out[95]=
```

male	23	1
	33	1
	24	1
female	30	1
	53	1
	45	1

Figure 3-27. *Data arranged by class and age*

As a good practice, clear symbols when they are no longer used.

In[96]:= Clear[Dst]

Applying Functions

Functions can be applied to the dataset to get statistics, determine dimensions, or transform the data. Functions can be applied to single columns or a unique element in the data structure. First, let's create a dataset comprising 10 items, whose columns are the factorial of 1 to 10, a random real number from 1 to 0, and the natural logarithm from 1 to 10. Figure 3-28 shows the new dataset.

In[97]:= DataNumbr=Dataset@Table[<|"Factorial"->Factorial[i],"Random
number"->RandomReal[{0,1}],"Natural Logarithm"->Log[E,i]|>,{i,1,10}]
Out[97]=

Factorial	Random number	Natural Logarithm
1	0.556204	0
2	0.747067	0.693147
6	0.986582	1.09861
24	0.905028	1.38629
120	0.395201	1.60944
720	0.507363	1.79176
5040	0.5893	1.94591
40 320	0.168404	2.07944
362 880	0.904704	2.19722
3 628 800	0.211938	2.30259

Figure 3-28. *Numeric dataset*

And now you can compute basic operations on the data, like getting the mean of the factorials and random numbers, as shown in Figure 3-29.

```
In[98]:= DataNumbr[Mean,{"Factorial","Random number"}]//N
Out[98]=
```

Factorial	403 791.
Random number	0.597179

Figure 3-29. *Mean for values in Factorial and Random number columns*

Parenthesis and the composition of functions can also be used to relate operations applied to the data by using the @ *(composition) symbol. Figure 3-30 shows the data for random numbers sorted from less to greater.

```
In[99]:= DataNumbr[All,"Random number"]@(Sort@*N)
Out[99]=
```

0.168404	0.211938	0.395201	0.507363	0.556204
0.5893	0.747067	0.904704	0.905028	0.986582

Figure 3-30. Sorted data in canonical order

You can apply different functions to the data. As shown in Figure 3-31, the dataset shows numbers in decimal form; otherwise, it would not fit in the square box.

```
In[100]:= DataNumbr[{Total,Max,Min},"Natural Logarithm"]
Out[100]=
```

15.1044	2.30259	0

Figure 3-31. Total, Max, and Min value for Natural Logarithm column

You can also apply your own functions; let's use a previously constructed function. Figure 3-32 shows the function you created previously applied to a dataset column.

```
In[101]:= DataNumbr[{StatsFun},"Natural Logarithm"]
Out[101]=
```

2.30259	0	1.51044	1.7006	2.30259

Figure 3-32. StatsFun applied to the Natural Logarithm column

Functions to restructure the dataset can be applied too, like Reverse, as shown in Figure 3-33.

```
In[102]:= DataNumbr[Reverse,All]
Out[102]=
```

Factorial	Random number	Natural Logarithm
3 628 800	0.211938	2.30259
362 880	0.904704	2.19722
40 320	0.168404	2.07944
5040	0.5893	1.94591
720	0.507363	1.79176
120	0.395201	1.60944
24	0.905028	1.38629
6	0.986582	1.09861
2	0.747067	0.693147
1	0.556204	0

Figure 3-33. *Reversed elements of the dataset*

Map can also apply functions, as you saw with lists in the previous sections. The next example maps a function directly into the dataset, as shown in Figure 3-34.

```
In[103]:= Map[Sqrt,DataNumbr]
Out[103]=
```

Factorial	Random number	Natural Logarithm
1	0.745791	0
1.41421	0.86433	0.832555
2.44949	0.993268	1.04815
4.89898	0.95133	1.17741
10.9545	0.62865	1.26864
26.8328	0.712294	1.33857
70.993	0.767659	1.39496
200.798	0.410371	1.44203
602.395	0.951159	1.4823
1904.94	0.460367	1.51743

Figure 3-34. *The square root function mapped in the dataset*

Transposition is an operation that consists of converting columns to rows and rows to columns and can sometimes help you observe data differently. To obtain the transposition of the dataset, use the Transpose function applied to the dataset. Figure 3-35 shows all columns are now rows and displayed compactly because it is a large row.

```
In[104]:= DataNumbr//Transpose
Out[104]=
```

Factorial	$\{\cdots_{10}\}$
Random number	$\{\cdots_{10}\}$
Natural Logarithm	$\{\cdots_{10}\}$

Figure 3-35. *Dataset values by Mathematica due to large contents*

If you click a row, you should get the values for the corresponding row.

Functions by Column or Row

Another approach is to directly apply a function to the values of a column, and you can specify a rule of transformation. For example, you can round to the smallest integer greater than or equal to all the values in the Natural Logarithm column. Figure 3-36 shows the output.

```
In[105]:= DataNumbr[All,{"Natural Logarithm"->Ceiling}](*The same can be
done using the index number of the columns,DataNumbr*)
Out[105]=
```

Factorial	Random number	Natural Logarithm
1	0.54158	0
2	0.223704	1
6	0.473125	2
24	0.726243	2
120	0.371648	2
720	0.37111	2
5040	0.581207	2
40 320	0.316827	3
362 880	0.254744	3
3 628 800	0.463658	3

Figure 3-36. *Ceiling function applied as a rule*

You can apply the square root to the first row. Map can also be used to apply functions to rows. Figure 3-37 shows the output generated

```
In[106]:= DataNumbr[1,Sqrt] (*Map[Sqrt,DataNumbr[1;;2,All]] can also do the
work for the first 2 rows*)
Out[106]=
```

Factorial	1
Random number	0.735921
Natural Logarithm	0

Figure 3-37. *Output generated from the earlier code*

When you want to apply a function to a defined level, you can use MapAt. MapAt has the form MapAt[f, "expr", {i, j, ...}], where {i, j} means the level of the position, as shown in Figure 3-38.

```
In[107]:= MapAt[Exp,DataNumbr,{1}](*for first position of row 1 only*)
(*Double semi-colon can be used to define from row to row,try using 4;;6.
Caution you might get big numbers*)
Out[107]=
```

Factorial	Random number	Natural Logarithm
2.71828	1.71872	1
2	0.223704	0.693147
6	0.473125	1.09861
24	0.726243	1.38629
120	0.371648	1.60944
720	0.37111	1.79176
5040	0.581207	1.94591
40 320	0.316827	2.07944
362 880	0.254744	2.19722
3 628 800	0.463658	2.30259

Figure 3-38. *Exponentiation for the first row only with MapAt*

Occasionally, you might encounter duplicate data, making it hard to understand the data, especially if something goes wrong. One approach can be to remove an entire row or column, as you saw in previous sections; but as an alternative, you can use built-in functions that can do the job. The DeleteDuplicates function is the most common. DeleteCases can be used, too, but it removes data that matches a pattern, in contrast to DeleteDuplicates. Let's create a dataset for the example.

```
In[108]:= Sales = Dataset@{
<|"Id" -> 1, "Product" -> "PC", "Price" -> "800 €",  "Sale Month" ->
"January"|>,
<|"Id" -> 2, "Product" -> "Smart phone", "Price" -> "255 €", "Sale Month"
-> "January"|>,
<|"Id" -> 3, "Product" -> "Anti-Virus", "Price" -> "100 €",  "Sale Month"
-> "March"|>,
<|"Id" -> 4, "Product" -> "Earphones", "Price" -> "78 €", "Sale Month" ->
"February"|>,
<|"Id" -> 5, "Product" -> "PC", "Price" -> "809 €",  "Sale Month" ->
"March"|>,
<|"Id" -> 5, "Product" -> "PC", "Price" -> "809 €", "Sale Month" ->
"March"|>,
 <|"Id" -> 6, "Product" -> "Radio", "Price" -> "60 €", "Sale Month" ->
"January"|>,
 <|"Id" -> 7, "Product" -> "PC", "Price" -> "700 €", "Sale Month" ->
"February"|>,
 <|"Id" -> 8, "Product" -> "Mouse", "Price" -> "100 €", "Sale Month" ->
"March"|>,
 <|"Id" -> 9, "Product" -> "Keyboard", "Price" -> "125 €", "Sale Month" ->
"January"|>,
 <|"Id" -> 10, "Product" -> "USB 64gb", "Price" -> "90 €", "Sale Month" ->
"March"|>,
 <|"Id" -> 11, "Product" -> "LED Screen", "Price" -> "900 €", "Sale Month"
-> "February"|>,
 <|"Id" -> 11, "Product" -> "LED Screen", "Price" -> "900 €", "Sale Month"
-> "February"|>}
Out[108]=
```

Figure 3-39 reveals two duplicated rows in the dataset: ID numbers 5 and 11. The DuplicateFreeQ function can detect whether the dataset appears to have duplicates. The function returns False when there is duplicate data and True when there is not. It can be applied straight to the dataset, or you can detect the rows that appear to be duplicated.

Id	Product	Price	Sale Month
1	PC	800 €	January
2	Smart phone	255 €	January
3	Anti–Virus	100 €	March
4	Earphones	78 €	February
5	PC	809 €	March
5	PC	809 €	March
6	Radio	60 €	January
7	PC	700 €	February
8	Mouse	100 €	March
9	Keyboard	125 €	January
10	USB 64gb	90 €	March
11	LED Screen	900 €	February
11	LED Screen	900 €	February

Figure 3-39. *Dataset example for duplicate data*

Let's check if there are duplicates in rows 1 through 7.

```
In[109]:= DuplicateFreeQ[Sales[1;;7,All]]
Out[109]= False
```

Duplicate data was programmatically found in the dataset. You can also check for duplicates by column.

```
In[110]:= Sales[All,{"Id"}]@DuplicateFreeQ
Out[110]= False
```

To delete duplicates, the DeletDuplicates function is used. It can be applied to the dataset, column, or row as a function. The output generated is shown in Figure 3-40.

```
In[111]:= DeleteDuplicates[Sales] (*Datas[All,{"ID"}]@DuplicateFreeQ*)
Out[111]=
```

Id	Product	Price	Sale Month
1	PC	800 €	January
2	Smart phone	255 €	January
3	Anti–Virus	100 €	March
4	Earphones	78 €	February
5	PC	809 €	March
6	Radio	60 €	January
7	PC	700 €	February
8	Mouse	100 €	March
9	Keyboard	125 €	January
10	USB 64gb	90 €	March
11	LED Screen	900 €	February

Figure 3-40. *Dataset without duplicates*

An alternative is to use GroupBy to identify which data is duplicated in the dataset. Notice in Figure 3-41 that the repeated data is stacked together.

```
In[112]:= GroupBy[Sales,"Id"]
Out[112]=
```

	Id	Product	Price	Sale Month
1	1	PC	800 €	January
2	2	Smart phone	255 €	January
3	3	Anti–Virus	100 €	March
4	4	Earphones	78 €	February
5	5	PC	809 €	March
	2 total ›			
6	6	Radio	60 €	January
7	7	PC	700 €	February
8	8	Mouse	100 €	March
9	9	Keyboard	125 €	January
10	10	USB 64gb	90 €	March
11	11	LED Screen	900 €	February
	2 total ›			

Figure 3-41. *Dataset grouped by duplicates*

Joining and Merging Datasets

Combining multiple datasets into one based on shared attributes is a frequent task. This process can be achieved depending on how a dataset should be joined. The three different functions that operate on datasets are Join, JoinAcross, and Merge.

The first function combines two datasets end-to-end, effectively concatenating them into a single dataset (see Figure 3-42).

```
In[113]:= dataset1={<|"a"->1,"b"->2|>,<|"a"->3,"b"->4|>};
dataset2={<|"a"->5,"b"->6|>};
Join[dataset1,dataset2]//Dataset
Out[116]=
```

a	b
1	2
3	4
5	6

Figure 3-42. *Dataset grouped by the Join function*

The second function combines datasets on a specified key or keys, similar to how relational databases join tables based on common keys (see Figure 3-43). Similar to operations from relational databases like join, left join, right join, inner join, outer join, and more.

```
In[117]:= dataset3={<|"ID"->1,"Value"->"A"|>,<|"ID"->2,"Value"->"B"|>};
dataset4={<|"ID"->1,"Score"->95|>,<|"ID"->2,"Score"->90|>};
JoinAcross[dataset3,dataset4,"ID"]//Dataset
Out[119]=
```

ID	Value	Score
1	A	95
2	B	90

Figure 3-43. *Dataset combined by the JoinAcross function*

The third function combines datasets, using a function f to combine values with the same key, returning a single value (see Figure 3-44).

```
In[120]:= Merge[Dataset[JoinAcross[dataset3,dataset4,"ID"]],Total]
Out[120]=
```

ID	3
Value	"A" + "B"
Score	185

Figure 3-44. *Dataset combined by the Merge and Total functions of each key*

Customizing a Dataset

Datasets can be customized depending on how you want to show the data. Working with datasets can be personalized based on preferences. To explore this, the next block loads example data from the Wolfram reference servers to discover how to personalize data for your needs. When loading data from the server, depending on your Internet connection, it might pop up a loading frame trying to access the Wolfram servers.

Let's load the data by using ExampleData and then choosing statistics of animal weights and converting the list into a dataset. By using the MaxItem option, you can display how many rows or columns to exhibit from the dataset. The first four rows and the first three columns are shown in this example. When viewing the dataset, scroll bars appear on the left and top sides; use them to move over the dataset. Alternatively, you can align the contents on the left, center, or right sides. In Figure 3-45, only the left scrollbars appear.

```
In[121]:= AnimalData=ExampleData[{"Statistics","AnimalWeights"}];
Dataset[AnimalData,MaxItems->{4,3},Alignment->Center] (*To align a
sole column,Alignment-> "Col_name" -> Left}*)
Out[121]=
```

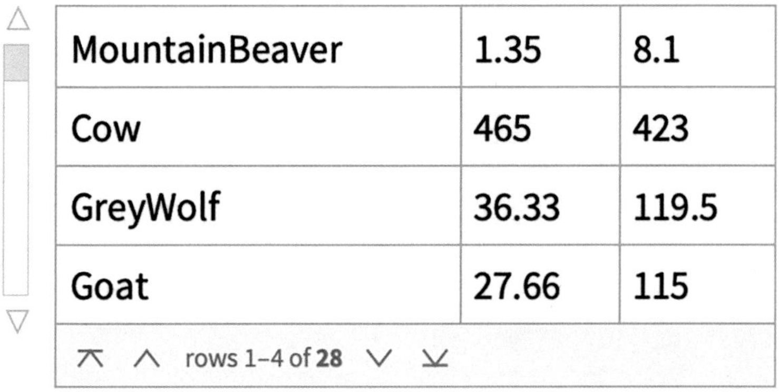

MountainBeaver	1.35	8.1
Cow	465	423
GreyWolf	36.33	119.5
Goat	27.66	115

rows 1–4 of **28**

Figure 3-45. *Animal dataset*

The Background option is used to color the dataset's contents; the colors of the notation {row, col} are preserved. To paint the whole data, enter only the color. To paint by row or column, enter the colors as a nested list—that is, {{"color_row1", "color_row2", ... }, {"color_col1", "color_col2", ... } }. Mixing colors can also be done by nesting the nested colors. For specific values, the position of the values would need to be entered. The next example colors the first two columns, as shown in Figure 3-46.

```
In[122]:= Dataset[AnimalData,MaxItems->{4,3},Background-> {{None},{LightBlue,
LightYellow}},ItemSize->{12}]
Out[122]=
```

MountainBeaver	1.35	8.1
Cow	465	423
GreyWolf	36.33	119.5
Goat	27.66	115

△ ∧ rows 1–4 of **28** ∨ ∨

Figure 3-46. *Columns 1 and 2 colored*

For particular values, the position of the values would need to be entered. Another option is the size of the items, which is controlled with the ItemSize option. If you want to edit the same options but with headers, you would use HeaderAlignment for placing the text left, center, or right; HeaderSize for the size of the titles; and ItemStyle for the style of the font of the items. Figure 3-47 shows the dataset in bold style.

```
In[123]:= Dataset[AnimalData,MaxItems->{4,3},Background->{{4,3}->
Yellow},ItemSize->{12},ItemStyle->Bold]
Out[123]=
```

MountainBeaver	**1.35**	**8.1**
Cow	**465**	**423**
GreyWolf	**36.33**	**119.5**
Goat	**27.66**	**115**

△ ∧ rows 1–4 of **28** ∨ ∨

Figure 3-47. *Dataset with bold style*

Another useful option is HiddenItems, which hides items that should not be displayed. Therefore, to hide row 1 and column 1, use HiddenItems → {"row #", "col #"}. Columns can be hidden with their associated labels. Figure 3-48 illustrates the form of suppressed rows and columns in the dataset. For specific values, nest the value's position and try HiddenItems → {{2,3}}.

```
In[124]:= Dataset[AnimalData,MaxItems->{4,3},HiddenItems->{1,1}]
Out[124]=
```

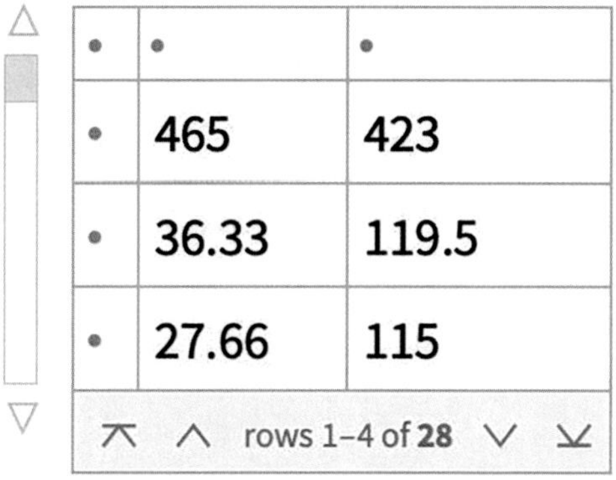

Figure 3-48. *Column 1 and row 1 suppressed*

You can add headers to each column in the new dataset with the Query command. To rename the columns, the same procedure is applied; the new names would be ruled to the old names—that is, "New name" → "Animal Name," as shown in Figure 3-49.

```
In[125]:= Query[All,<|"Animal Name"->1,"Body Weight"->2,"Brain
Weight"->3|>]@Dataset[AnimalData]
(*for display motives we put row 7 to 9,use All for the whole data set*)
(*or "symbol_of_the_dataset"[All,<|"Animal Name"-> 1,"Body Weight"->2,
"Brain Weight"->3|>]*)
Out[125]=
```

Animal Name	Body Weight	Brain Weight
MountainBeaver	1.35	8.1
Cow	465	423
GreyWolf	36.33	119.5
Goat	27.66	115
GuineaPig	1.04	5.5
Diplodocus	11 700	50
AsianElephant	2547	4603
Donkey	187.1	419
Horse	521	655
PotarMonkey	10	115
Cat	3.3	25.6
Giraffe	529	680
Gorilla	207	406
Human	62	1320
AfricanElephant	6654	5712
Triceratops	9400	70
RhesusMonkey	6.8	179
Kangaroo	35	56
GoldenHamster	0.12	1
Mouse	0.023	0.4

⎏ ⋀ rows 1–20 of 28 ⋁ ⌄

Figure 3-49. *Animal dataset with added column headers*

Generalization of Hash Tables

A hash table is an associative data structure that allows data storage and, in turn, the rapid retrieval of elements (values) from objects called keys. Hash tables can be implemented inside arrays, where the main components are the key and the value. The way to search for an element in the array is by using a hash function, which maps the keys to the pairs of values and gives you the place where it is in the array (index).

In other words, the hash function searches for a certain key, evaluates that key, and returns an index. This process is known as hashing. Figure 3-50 shows a representative schema of a hash table.

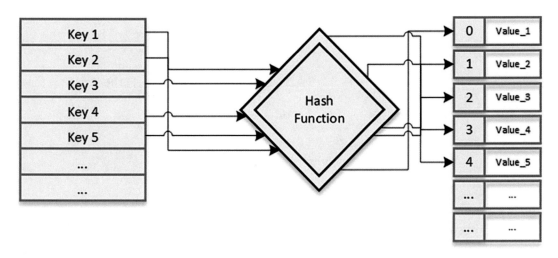

Figure 3-50. *Graphic representation of a hash table*

Inside the hash table, the number of keys and values can go on and on, which is one of the reasons hash tables are very useful; they can store large amounts of information. Inside the Wolfram Language, associations can represent hash tables. Primarily, this is because associations are an abstract data structure with fundamental components such as keys and values, just like a hash table. This combines the structure of an associative array and an indexed list, more like a nest of hash arrays. With the crucial property that associations are immutable, each association-type object is unique and the reference to one association has no link to another, even though they are referenced to the same symbol.

Other special commands are available. Let's first create an association. Nested associations are defined as associations that have associations within them—in other words, a key that points to a bucket of values that correspond to keys that have other values inside (see Figure 3-51).

```
In[126]:= Asc=<|"User"->
<|"Edgar"-> <|"id"->01, "Parameters"-><|"Active"->True,"Region"->
"LA","Internet Traffic"->"1 GB"|>|>,
<|"Anya"-><|"id"->02,"Parameters"-><|"Active"->False,"Region"->
"MX","Internet Traffic"->"3 GB"|>|>
```

```
|>|>|>;
Dataset[%]
Out[127]=
```

		id	Parameters		
			Active	Region	Internet Traffic
User	Edgar	1	True	LA	1 GB
	Anya	2	False	MX	3 GB

Figure 3-51. *Nested associations in the dataset format*

Executing operations like accessing items, updating values, and deleting is supported by the commands associated with keys and values. Remember that Keys returns the keys of the association and Values the values. Keys only work at the surface level inside a nested association, as seen in the following code.

```
In[128]:= Keys[Asc]
Out[128]= {User}
```

Applying the Keys command returns only the key user. The Keys command needs to be applied to deeper levels to see the keys inside a nested association, which is achieved with Map by specifying the sublevel only.

```
In[129]:= Map[Keys,Asc,#]&/@{{0},{1},{2}}//Column
Out[129]= {User}
<|User->{Edgar,Anya}|>
<|User-><|Edgar->{id,Parameters},Anya->{id,Parameters}|>|>
```

As seen on the surface level (0), the key is User. The next sublevel has the keys Edgar and Anya, and the last level has the keys ID and parameters for each of the keys Edgar and Anya. MapIndexed lets you look inside the whole association and apply Keys to sublevels to show the predecessors of the keys.

```
In[130]:=
Print["Level 0: "<>ToString@MapIndexed[Keys,Asc,{0}]]
Print["Level 1: "<>ToString@MapIndexed[Keys,Asc,{1}]]
Print["Level 2: "<>ToString@MapIndexed[Keys,Asc,{2}]]
Out[130]=
Level 0: {{}[User]}
Level 1: <|User -> {{Key[User]}[Edgar], {Key[User]}[Anya]}|>
Level 2: <|User -> <|Edgar -> {{Key[User], Key[Edgar]}[id], {Key[User],
Key[Edgar]}[Parameters]}, Anya -> {{Key[User], Key[Anya]}[id], {Key[User],
Key[Anya]}[Parameters]}|>|>
```

At level 0, only the User key exists, and the predecessor is {}. At level 1, the User predecessor and the Edgar and Anya keys are values of the User key. At level 2, the predecessor keys are Edgar/Anya and User for the ID and Parameters keys. In other words, the expression {Key[User], Key[Anya]}[id] means that ID corresponds to the Anya key and Anya to the User key, and so on. This is also useful because it means that access to a value or values of a key is done with the operator form applied to the association specifying the keys.

```
In[133]:= Asc["User"]["Edgar"]["id"](*{Key[User],Key[Anya]}[id],*)
Out[133]= 1
```

As shown, you get the value that corresponds to the ID inside Edgar inside User key. To see a graphical representation of the previous expression, you can use MapIndexed to label the positions of the keys and dataset applied, for example, in sublevel 4 (see Figure 3-52).

```
In[134]:= Dataset@MapIndexed[Framed[Labeled[#2,#1],FrameMargins->0,
RoundingRadius->5]&,Asc,{4}] (*Try changin the number to see how the
expression changes*)
Out[134]=
```

		id		Parameters
User	Edgar	1	Active	{Key[User], Key[Edgar], Key[Parameters], Key[Active]} True
			Region	{Key[User], Key[Edgar], Key[Parameters], Key[Region]} "LA"
			Internet Traffic	{Key[User], Key[Edgar], Key[Parameters], Key[Internet Traffic]} "1 GB"
	Anya	2	Active	{Key[User], Key[Anya], Key[Parameters], Key[Active]} False
			Region	{Key[User], Key[Anya], Key[Parameters], Key[Region]} "MX"
			Internet Traffic	{Key[User], Key[Anya], Key[Parameters], Key[Internet Traffic]} "3 GB"

Figure 3-52. *Dataset representation marking the keys inside the nested association*

Each box contains the values of the predecessor key. This is why 1 GB corresponds to {Key[User],Key[Edgar],Key[Parameters],Key[Internet Traffic]}. To see the whole expression, the level of specification is Infinity (see Figure 3-53).

```
In[135]:=MapIndexed[Framed[Labeled[#2,#1,ImageMargins->0,Spacings->0],
FrameMargins->0,RoundingRadius->5]&,Asc,Infinity]
Out[135]=
```

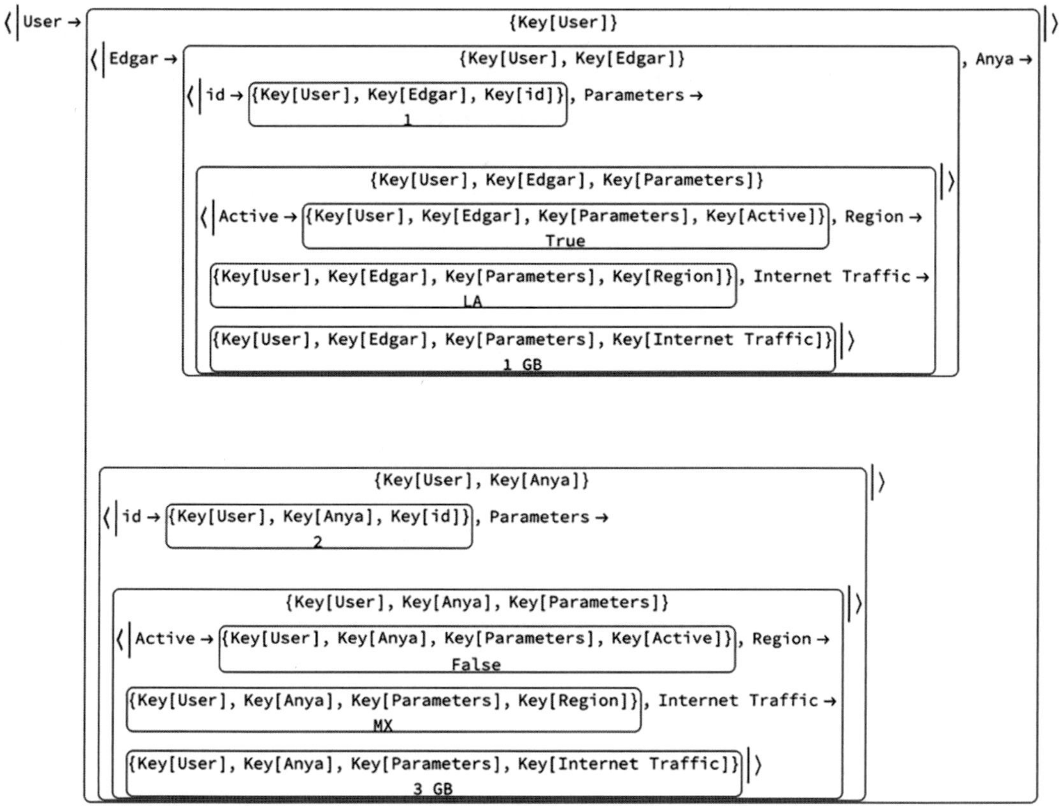

Figure 3-53. *Framed levels of the keys in a nested association*

Values use the same approach as with Keys. To test if a key exists, use KeyExistQ; this returns true if the key exists. Otherwise, it is false. To test inside deeper levels, use Map.

```
In[136]:={KeyExistsQ[Asc,"User"],Map[KeyExistsQ["Anya"],Asc,{1}],Map
[KeyExistsQ["Anya"],Asc,{2}]}
Out[136]= {True,<|User->True|>,<|User-><|Edgar->False,Anya->False|>|>}
```

Another way to test whether a key in a particular form exists inside an association, use KeyMemberQ—for example, if there is a string pattern key.

```
In[137]:= KeyMemberQ[Asc["User"]["Anya"],_String]
Out[137]= True
```

To test if a value exists given a key, use Lookup.

```
In[138]:= Lookup[Asc["User"]["Anya"],"Parameters"]
Out[138]= <|Active->False,Region->MX,Internet Traffic->3 GB|>
```

143

To select a key based on criteria, use KeySelect.

```
In[139]:= KeySelect[Asc["User"]["Anya"],StringQ]
Out[139]= <|id->2,Parameters-><|Active->False,Region->MX,Internet
Traffic->3 GB|>|>
```

Or use KeyTake to grab a particular key.

```
In[140]:= KeyTake[Asc["User"]["Anya"]["Parameters"],{"Region","Internet
Traffic"}]
Out[140]= <|Region->MX,Internet Traffic->3 GB|>
```

To remove a key, use KeyDrop.

```
In[141]:= KeyDrop[Asc["User"],"Edgar"]
Out[141]= <|Anya-><|id->2,Parameters-><|Active->False,Region->MX,Internet
Traffic->3 GB|>|>|>
```

To assign a new value, the value associated with the key is assigned with the new value

```
In[142]:= Asc["User"]["Edgar"]["Parameters"]["Region"]="CZ"
Out[142]= CZ
```

Passing this into a dataset, you can look for the new assigned value (see Figure 3-54).

```
In[143]:= Dataset[Asc]
Out[143]=
```

		id	Parameters		
			Active	Region	Internet Traffic
User	Edgar	1	True	CZ	1 GB
	Anya	2	False	MX	3 GB

Figure 3-54. *Dataset with the region value changed to CZ*

To add a key and a value to the association, you can insert the new expression by specifying the position to insert it with the key (see Figure 3-55).

```
In[144]:= Insert[Asc["User"],"Alexandra"-><|"id"->0,"Parameters"-
><|"Active"->False,"Region"->"RS","Internet Traffic"->"12
GB"|>|>,Key["Edgar"]]//Dataset
Out[144]=
```

	id	Parameters		
		Active	Region	Internet Traffic
Alexandra	0	False	RS	12 GB
Edgar	1	True	CZ	1 GB
Anya	2	False	MX	3 GB

Figure 3-55. *New row added by the key position*

Summary

This chapter continued to build upon the list operations introduced in Chapter 2. You explored the unique syntax of pure functions in the Wolfram Language and delved into several methods for creating indexed tables and associations. Additionally, you transitioned to the powerful capabilities of datasets, which provide a structured and organized way to handle and analyze data. The chapter wrapped up by providing insights into the essential components of associations and key-value management.

CHAPTER 4

Import and Export

This chapter reviews the import and export of data, including the relevant Wolfram Language commands and the import and export formats that Mathematica supports. Experimental data can come from different sources; the way to process this external data is to import it through Wolfram Language. Data that has been calculated or obtained externally can be transferred to Mathematica and exported for use on other platforms. However, Mathematica has tools to handle different data types (numbers, text, audio, graphics, and images). This chapter focuses on working with numerical and categorical data, the most frequently used data types for analysis.

Importing data from multiple sources into Mathematica allows you to load data into a notebook for analysis. The Wolfram Language supports numerous import formats; to see which are supported, type the dollar symbol ($) accompanied by the ImportFormats command. Currently, Mathematica supports 256 file formats. As shown in the following code, new formats have been added and updated since the last version of this book.

```
In[1]:= Short[$ImportFormats,4](* Length[$ImportFormats] --> 256 formats*)
Out[1]//Short= {3DS,7z,AC,ACO,Affymetrix,AgilentMicroarray,AIFF,ApacheLog,
ArcGRID,ASC,ASE,AU,AVI,Base64,BDF,Binary,BioImageFormat,Bit,BLEND,BMP,
<<216>>,WAV,Wave64,WDX,WebP,WL,WLNet,WMLF,WXF,X3D,XBM,XGL,XHTML,XHTMLMathML,
XLS,XLSX,XML,XPORT,XYZ,ZIP,ZSTD}
```

There are a lot of formats in the list, including audio, image, and text. But let's focus on the text-based formats. To import any file, the Import command is used. Import receives two arguments: the file's path and options. Options can vary between file format, elements, and other types of objects in Mathematica, like cloud and local. To select a file path, head to the toolbar and then to Insert ➤ File Path. A file explorer should appear; search the file you would like to import and select it. The path is enclosed in apostrophes like a string.

© Jalil Villalobos Alva 2024
J. Villalobos Alva, *Beginning Mathematica and Wolfram for Data Science*,
https://doi.org/10.1007/979-8-8688-0348-2_4

Another option is the named file in the Insert menu. In contrast to File Path, the File option introduces the file's contents directly without receiving prior formatting from Mathematica. File is better suited for importing notebooks or other Wolfram formats.

Note   The next series of imported files are included in the source code. The files are located in the host Desktop folder for ease of use.

Let's look at transferring a simple text file. First, select the HelloWorld.txt file path using the Import command.

```
In[2]:= Import["/Users/macosx/Desktop/Hello_World.txt"]
Out[2]= Hello world!
```

Note   Based on your operating system, the file path shows forward slashes (Linux, macOS) or back slashes (Windows file system delimiter).

You have imported your first file. Mathematica recognizes it based on the file extension and then imports it automatically. If you import a file with no file extension but you know the type of format used in the file, you can choose the proper format as an option.

```
In[3]:= Import["/Users/macosx/Desktop/Hello_World.txt","Text"]
Out[3]= Hello world!
```

Importing Files

Importing simple text files is easy and intuitive. However, based on the type of file you want to import, the options and format to display the data inside Mathematica can vary.

CSV and TSV Files

This section focuses on how to import files into Mathematica. The examples work with comma-separated value (CSV) files, tab-separated value (TSV) files, and Excel spreadsheet-style files. CSV and TSV files are files that include text and numeric values. In CSV files, fields are separated by a comma; each row is one line record. Meanwhile, in TSV files, each record is separated with a tab space.

With Import, you can import TSV or CSV files with the .tsv or .csv file extension, respectively. Let's first import a regular CSV file by introducing the file path and then the CSV option.

```
In[4]:= Import["/Users/macosx/Desktop/Grocery_List.csv","CSV"]
Out[4]= {{id,grocery item,price,sold items,sales per day},{1,milk,4$,4,4
Jun 2019},{2,butter,3$,2,6 Jun 2019},{3,garlic,2$,1,7 Jun
2019},{4,apple,2$,4,1 Jun 2019},{5,orange,3$,5,8 Jun 2019},{6,orange
juice,5$,2,8 Jun 2019},{7,cheese,5$,2,6 Jun 2019},{8,cookies,2$,5,9 Jun
2019},{9,grapes,4$,3,21 Jun 2019},{10,potatoe,2$,5,26 Jun 2019}}
```

Now that the contents of the file are imported, depending on the format of the contents, the data is presented as a nested list or not. The elements of the nested list represent rows, and the elements of the whole list represent columns.

When importing data, parts of the data can be imported—that is, if you only need a row or a column.

```
In[5]:=Import["/Users/macosx/Desktop/Grocery_List.csv",{"Data",5;;10}]
Out[5]= {{4,apple,2$,4,1 Jun 2019},{5,orange,3$,5,8 Jun 2019},{6,orange
juice,5$,2,8 Jun 2019},{7,cheese,5$,2,6 Jun 2019},{8,cookies,2$,5,9 Jun
2019},{9,grapes,4$,3,21 Jun 2019}}
```

The previous example imported data from row 5 to row 10.

You can use the following form when you are only interested in single values.

```
In[6]:=Import["/Users/macosx/Desktop/Grocery_List.csv",{"Data",6,2}]
Out[6]= orange
```

Depending on the maximum bytes of the expression, Mathematica truncates the imported data and shows you a suggestion box of a simplified version of the whole data. To see the maximum byte size, go to Edit ➤ Advanced tab, and in "Maximum output size before truncation," enter the new number of bytes before truncation. This preference applies to every output expression in Mathematica.

Let's use the same approach to import TSV files. With the short command, you can show a part of the data, just in case the data is extensive.

```
In[7]:= Short[Import["/Users/macosx/Desktop/Color_table.tsv","TSV"]]
(*Rest,to view the remain*)
Out[7]//Short= {{number,color},{1,red},<<7>>,{9,magenta},{10,brown}}
```

149

Consequently, in the result, a seven appears among the elements of the imported file. This result happens because the file contains seven elements that are not visible. Now that you have learned how to import CSV and TSV files, you can display the imported data in table format using Grid or TableForm.

```
In[8]:= Import["/Users/macosx/Desktop/Grocery_List.csv","CSV"];
Grid[%]
Out[9]=
```

id	grocery item	price	sold items	sales per day
1	milk	4$	4	4 Jun 2019
2	butter	3$	2	6 Jun 2019
3	garlic	2$	1	7 Jun 2019
4	apple	2$	4	1 Jun 2019
5	orange	3$	5	8 Jun 2019
6	orange juice	5$	2	8 Jun 2019
7	cheese	5$	2	6 Jun 2019
8	cookies	2$	5	9 Jun 2019
9	grapes	4$	3	21 Jun 2019
10	potato	2$	5	26 Jun 2019

Once you have imported the file, data can be treated as a list or any other structure inside the notebook. Parts of the data are named after the imported data, and the contents can now be extracted, as discussed in later chapters.

XLSX Files

The following example shows how to import data, display data as a spreadsheet, and transform it into a dataset. Let's use the XLSX grocery list file rather than the CSV file for exemplification purposes. To start, you need first to import the data. To start, you need first to import the data.

```
In[10]:= path="/Users/macosx/Desktop/Grocery_List.xlsx";
Import[path,"Data"]
Out[11]= {{{id,grocery item, price, sold items,sales per day},{1.,milk,4
$,4.,4-Jun-2019},{2.,butter,3$,2.,6-Jun-2020},{3.,garlic,2
$,1.,7-Jun-2021},{4.,apple,2 $,4.,1-Jun-2022},{5.,orange,3
```

```
$,5.,8-Jun-2023},{6.,orange juice,5 $,2.,8-Jun-2024},{7.,cheese,5
$,2.,6-Jun-2025},{8.,cookies,2 $,5.,9-Jun-2026},{9.,grapes,4 $,3.,21-Jun-20
27},{10.,potatoe,2 $,5.,26-Jun-2028}}}
```

As can be seen, the imported data appears as a nested list because Excel files can have multiple sheets inside a file. For this case, you have only one sheet. To see the number of sheets and the name of the sheets, use SheetCount and Sheets, respectively.

```
In[12]:= Import[path,#]&/@{"SheetCount","Sheets"}
Out[12]= {1,{Grocery_List}}
```

To show data as a spreadsheet, you use the TableView command (see Figure 4-1). The following format is used as an option to select a sheet: {"Data," # of sheet}. To select a character encoding, use the CharacterEncoding option. Also, custom rows or columns can be imported, preserving the format: {"Data," # of the sheet, # row, # column}.

```
In[13]:= TableView[Import[path,{"Data",1},CharacterEncoding->"UTF-8"]]
Out[13]=
```

	1	2	3	4	5
1	id	grocery	price	sold	sales per day
2		1. milk	4 $		4. 4 – Jun – 2019
3		2. butter	3 $		2. 6 – Jun – 2020
4		3. garlic	2 $		1. 7 – Jun – 2021
5		4. apple	2 $		4. 1 – Jun – 2022
6		5. orange	3 $		5. 8 – Jun – 2023
7		6. orange	5 $		2. 8 – Jun – 2024
8		7. cheese	5 $		2. 6 – Jun – 2025
9		8. cookies	2 $		5. 9 – Jun – 2026
10		9. grapes	4 $		3. 21 – Jun – 2027
11		10. potatoe	2 $		5. 26 – Jun – 2028

Figure 4-1. *Spreadsheet view with TableView command*

Note   With "Data", import the data as a nested list.

You can now see the data in spreadsheet format. Now, with TableView, you can view the data like in spreadsheet software, with selection tools, scrollbars, and text editing of the contents. However, one of the downsides is that with TableView, you cannot directly access the file's contents; neither can calculations be performed. To do the latter, you can transform it into a dataset.

You can convert data into a dataset for better handling in Mathematica. By typing the "Dataset" as the option instead of "Data", the imported file becomes a dataset but without headers (see Figure 4-2). To add the headers, use the HeaderLines option and choose the specification of the header by row or column type HeadLines → {# row, # column}. The file used is Grocery List 2.xlxs.

```
In[14]:=file="/Users/macosx/Desktop/Grocery_List_2.xlsx";Import[file,
{"Dataset",1},HeaderLines->1]
Out[14]=
```

id	grocery item	price	sold items
1.0	milk	4$	4.0
2.0	butter	3$	
3.0	garlic	2$	1.0
4.0	apple	2$	4.0
5.0	orange		5.0
6.0	orange juice	5$	2.0
7.0	cheese	5$	2.0
8.0	cookies		5.0
9.0	grapes	4$	
10.0	potato	2$	5.0

Figure 4-2. *Incomplete Grocery List dataset*

You have imported incomplete data. EmptyField is implemented as a rule of transformation to treat empty spaces. If the data has empty spaces and no rule is expressed, the spaces are treated as empty strings. Figure 4-3 shows the output.

```
In[15]:= Import[file,{"Dataset",1},"EmptyField"->"NaN",HeaderLines->1]
Out[15]=
```

id	grocery item	price	sold items
1.0	milk	4$	4.0
2.0	butter	3$	NaN
3.0	garlic	2$	1.0
4.0	apple	2$	4.0
5.0	orange	NaN	5.0
6.0	orange juice	5$	2.0
7.0	cheese	5$	2.0
8.0	cookies	NaN	5.0
9.0	grapes	4$	NaN
10.0	potato	2$	5.0

Figure 4-3. *NaN-filled dataset*

JSON Files

The JavaScript Object Notation (JSON) file extension is a data representation file. JSON files store data as an ordered list of values, and a collection of value pairs constitutes each list. To import a JSON file, specify the two options: JSON or RawJSON.

```
In[16]:=json=Import["/Users/macosx/Desktop/Sports_cars.json","JSON"]
Out[16]=
{{Model->Enzo Ferrari,Year->2002,Cylinders->12,Horsepower HP->660,Weight
Kg->1255},{Model->Koenigsegg CCX,Year->2000,Cylinders->8,Horsepower HP->
806,Weight Kg->1180},{Model->Pagani Zonda,Year->2002,Cylinders->12,
Horsepower HP->558,Weight Kg->1250},{Model->McLaren Senna,Year->2019,
Cylinders->8,Horsepower HP->800,Weight Kg->1309},{Model->McLaren 675 LT,
Year->2015,Cylinders->8,Horsepower HP->675,Weight Kg->1230},{Model->
Bugatti Veyron,Year->2006,Cylinders->16,Horsepower HP->1001,Weight Kg->
1881},{Model->Audi R8 Spyder,Year->2010,Cylinders->10,Horsepower HP->525,
Weight Kg->1795},{Model->Aston Martin Vantage,Year->2009,Cylinders->8,
Horsepower HP->926,Weight Kg->1705},{Model->Maserati Gran Turismo,Year->
2010,Cylinders->8,Horsepower HP->405,Weight Kg->1955},{Model->Lamborghini
Aventador S,Year->2017,Cylinders->12,Horsepower HP->740,Weight Kg->1740}}
```

Given the nature of the JSON file structure, Mathematica recognizes each structure and interprets each key to its values when importing them. As you saw in the previous output, keys correspond to Model, Year, Cylinders, Horsepower, and Weight, and each key has its values. Everything said so far explains that all records are in a nested list. This outcome leads you to conclude that if you want to present it in a dataset, you cannot directly apply Association, and Association suppresses repeated keys. You must create an association for each record since it is a nested list, which you achieve with Map, specifying the depth level of the Association command. This is shown in the following code.

```
In[17]:= Map[Association,Json,1]
Out[17]= {<|Model->Enzo Ferrari,Year->2002,Cylinders->12,Horsepower HP->
660,Weight Kg->1255|>,<|Model->Koenigsegg CCX,Year->2000,Cylinders->8,
Horsepower HP->806,Weight Kg->1180|>,<|Model->Pagani Zonda,Year->2002,
Cylinders->12,Horsepower HP->558,Weight Kg->1250|>,<|Model->
McLaren Senna,Year->2019,Cylinders->8,Horsepower HP->800,Weight Kg->
1309|>,<|Model->McLaren 675 LT,Year->2015,Cylinders->8,Horsepower HP->675,
Weight Kg->1230|>,<|Model->Bugatti Veyron,Year->2006,Cylinders->16,
Horsepower HP->1001,Weight Kg->1881|>,<|Model->Audi R8 Spyder ,Year->2010,
Cylinders->10,Horsepower HP->525,Weight Kg->1795|>,<|Model->Aston Martin
Vantage,Year->2009,Cylinders->8,Horsepower HP->926,Weight Kg->1705|>,
<|Model->Maserati Gran Turismo,Year->2010,Cylinders->8,Horsepower HP-
>405,Weight Kg->1955|>,<|Model->Lamborghini Aventador S,Year->2017,
Cylinders->12,Horsepower HP->740,Weight Kg->1740|>}
```

You already have each record as an association, and now you can convert it to a dataset, as shown in Figure 4-4.

```
In[18]:= Dataset[%]
Out[18]=
```

Model	Year	Cylinders	Horsepower HP	Weight Kg
Enzo Ferrari	2002	12	660	1255
Koenigsegg CCX	2000	8	806	1180
Pagani Zonda	2002	12	558	1250
McLaren Senna	2019	8	800	1309
McLaren 675 LT	2015	8	675	1230
Bugatti Veyron	2006	16	1001	1881
Audi R8 Spyder	2010	10	525	1795
Aston Martin Vantage	2009	8	926	1705
Maserati Gran Turismo	2010	8	405	1955
Lamborghini Aventador S	2017	12	740	1740

Figure 4-4. *Cars dataset*

You can now handle a JSON file as a dataset. However, there is another way to do it without requiring as much calculation as before. When importing the file, you must import it as RawJson because, with RawJson, the Wolfram Language identifies and imports each record as a list of associations rather than a sole nested list, as shown here. This reason is because of the nature of the key and value of the JSON file extension.

```
In[19]:= Import["/Users/macosx/Desktop/Sports_cars.json","RawJSON"]
Out[19]=
{<|Model->Enzo Ferrari,Year->2002,Cylinders->12,Horsepower HP->660,Weight
Kg->1255|>,<|Model->Koenigsegg CCX,Year->2000,Cylinders->8,Horsepower HP->
806,Weight Kg->1180|>,<|Model->Pagani Zonda,Year->2002,Cylinders->12,
Horsepower HP->558,Weight Kg->1250|>,<|Model->McLaren Senna,Year->2019,
Cylinders->8,Horsepower HP->800,Weight Kg->1309|>,<|Model->McLaren 675
LT,Year->2015,Cylinders->8,Horsepower HP->675,Weight Kg->1230|>,<|Model->
Bugatti Veyron,Year->2006,Cylinders->16, Horsepower HP->1001,Weight Kg->
1881|>,<|Model->Audi R8 Spyder ,Year->2010,Cylinders->10,Horsepower HP->
525,Weight Kg->1795|>,<|Model->Aston Martin Vantage,Year->2009,
Cylinders->8,Horsepower HP->926,Weight Kg->1705|>,<|Model->Maserati Gran
Turismo,Year->2010,Cylinders->8,Horsepower HP->405,Weight Kg->1955|>,
<|Model->Lamborghini Aventador S,Year->2017,Cylinders->12,Horsepower
HP->740,Weight Kg->1740|>}
```

The file is imported as an association in each record, and you can convert it into a dataset.

```
In[20]:=Cars=Dataset[%];
```

As a complement, once the data is imported, you can perform operations on the dataset, such as ordering the models by year from low to high.

```
In[21]:=Cars[SortBy[#Year&]];
```

Note   The previous example is also possible using the query command. (Query [SortBy[#Year &]][Cars]).

Web Data

On the other hand, web data is also supported with Import. Instead of inserting the file path, the URL site is inserted as the argument of the Import command. The next example imports a simple text file from the National Oceanic and Atmospheric Administration (NOAA). The text file contains the list of country codes used for the Integrated Global Radiosonde Archive (IGRA). The parent directory where files are located is https:// www1.ncdc.noaa.gov/pub/data/igra/, but let's only import the country list file. You need an Internet connection to make this work.

```
In[22]:=Short[Import["https://www1.ncdc.noaa.gov/pub/data/igra/igra2-
country-list.txt","HTML"]]
Out[22]//Short= AC Antigua and Barbuda AE United Arab Emirates AF ...  WS
Samoa YM Yemen ZA Zambia ZI Zimbabwe ZZ Ocean
```

The file is a plain text, but you can change how the data is imported by inserting a file format as an option. You can import it as a CSV file, for instance.

```
In[23]:=Short[Import["https://www1.ncdc.noaa.gov/pub/data/igra/igra2-
country-list.txt","CSV"]]
Out[23]//Short= {{AC Antigua and Barbuda},{AE United Arab
Emirates},<<215>>,{ZI Zimbabwe},{ZZ Ocean}}
```

This is useful when you try to make computations with the data imported. Alternatively, you can use URL commands to check the status of an online file and then download it. To check the status of the online file, use URLRead. When the file is online, you should get an HTTP response object like the one shown in Figure 4-5. You can even perform this approach before importing data, ensuring the content is available online.

```
In[24]:= URLRead["https://www1.ncdc.noaa.gov/pub/data/igra/igra2-country-
list.txt"]
Out[24]=
```

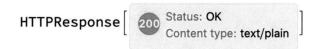

Figure 4-5. *HTTPResponse object of the URL entered*

Now that you know the status, you can download the data file with URLDownload.

```
In[25]:= URLDownload["https://www1.ncdc.noaa.gov/pub/data/igra/igra2-
country-list.txt"]
Out[25]=
```

You should get a file object with the file's location (see Figure 4-6), the name, and the extension; in this case, it is in a temporary folder.

File [/private/var/folders/zs/hxtbpjpd5xb0krb6581764xm0000gn/T/igra2–country–list–b7add4af–0a18–4cea–bbcd–3ec04b94f363.txt »]

Figure 4-6. *File object with the locations of the file downloaded*

Click the double chevron icon to open the file in an external viewer.

Semantic Import

So far, you have seen how to import files of different formats, but there is another tool called SemanticImport that allows you to import files semantically and returns a dataset as a result. Let's looks at a simple example with the CSV file.

```
In[26]:= sImprt=SemanticImport["/Users/macosx/Desktop/Grocery_List.csv"]
Out[26]=
```

Figure 4-7 shows that when you use semantic import Mathematica, it imports the data in the form of a dataset, and when it does this, it recognizes some quantities.

id	grocery item	price	sold items	sales per day
1	milk	$4	4	Tue 4 Jun 2019
2	butter	$3	2	Thu 6 Jun 2019
3	garlic	$2	1	Fri 7 Jun 2019
4	apple	$2	4	Sat 1 Jun 2019
5	orange	$3	5	Sat 8 Jun 2019
6	orange juice	$5	2	Sat 8 Jun 2019
7	cheese	$5	2	Thu 6 Jun 2019
8	cookies	$2	5	Sun 9 Jun 2019
9	grapes	$4	3	Fri 21 Jun 2019
10	potato	$2	5	Wed 26 Jun 2019

Figure 4-7. *File imported as a dataset with SemanticImport*

These quantities correspond to the magnitude and its units, such as in the case of the elements of the column of price and sales per day. When dealing with quantities, the color of the elements changes; as you see in the dataset, the elements appear differently from the other contents because a semantic-type object now represents them. Semantic objects include quantities, entities, dates, and geolocation. In other words, they are interpretations made by the freeform interpreter related to the Wolfram Knowledgebase.

Note   To check if the data is recognized as a quantity or semantic-type object, use Normal[sImprt]; you should see the entities colored differently.

In the case of imported data, there are two date-type objects, which you saw in the first chapter, and quantity type. It should be understood that to work with quantities, you must understand where they come from.

Quantities

The Quantity command converts a magnitude with units to a quantity type to convert the magnitude with their respective units; the magnitude is entered first, followed by its units in string type. When you do this, Mathematica displays the autocomplete menu as on other occasions. The following example shows it.

```
In[27]:= Quantity[2,"USDollars"]
Out[27]= $2
```

Thus, it is transformed into a quantity type. When you hover over the result, an ad is displayed, marking that a result is already a unit. In this case, it is a unit of US dollars. Now, if you check the head of the expression, it shows that it is a type of quantity.

Note   Quantities are shown in light brown color.

```
In[28]:= Quantity[2,"USDollars"]//Head
Out[28]= Quantity
```

You can also use the inline freeform input in the menu bar: Insert ➤ Inline Freeform Input. This input type is associated with the Wolfram Alpha search engine , so the inline freeform input transforms natural language into Wolfram Language input.

Inside the box, you'll find the magnitude and quantity written. One of the advantages of this type of input is that it allows for using natural language. The following example writes the amount of 77 min, which means 77 minutes. Figure 4-8 shows the input cell of the inline freeform input.

```
In[29]:=
```

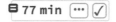

Figure 4-8. *Free inline freeform input for the quantity of 77 minutes*

```
Out[29]= 77min
```

To run the code, click ENTER since it gives you a result. Some tabs appear where you can click a submenu or a checkmark. If you click the checkmark, it is to accept the interpretation made. If you believe that the interpretation is different, you can click the other option, which is alternate interpretations, and it shows a small pop-up where it lists different interpretations. Figure 4-9 show the pop-up for the example.

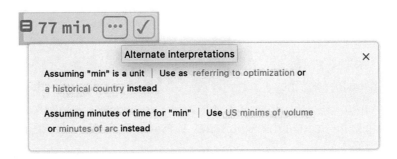

Figure 4-9. *Options for the quantity entered*

Once the interpretation is accepted, the result changes color and is a quantity-type object. And it can be used like any other quantity-type object.

When you have quantities, you cannot make operations between numbers; quantities are already different types. For these, there are two options: convert the data to quantities or extract the magnitude of a quantity. The QuantityMagnitude command is used to extract the magnitude. Make sure to copy the entity (light brown output), not the pure text 77 min.

```
In[30]:= {QuantityMagnitude[77 min],Head[%]}
Out[30]= {77,Quantity}
```

You have already extracted the magnitude, and it is already an integer. In the supposed case of wanting the units, the QuantityUnit command extracts the units.

```
In[31]:= QuantityUnit[77 min]
Out[31]= Minutes
```

Datasets with Quantities

Another aspect to emphasize: To carry out operations, the concept of performing arithmetic operations among physical quantities is maintained; otherwise, the operation is not possible, and you get an error in which the units do not agree. When you carry out an operation between quantities, the result is also of the quantity type.

```
In[32]:= {77min-77min,77min+77min,77min*77min,77min/77min,77min*3m}
Out[32]= {0min,154min,5929(min)^2,1,231m min}
```

This example shows how the results are of type quantity. Except for the division, it is already a quotient between the same units. The last one is 231 meters per minute.

Returning to the imported data, you can extract the data from the price column, as shown in Figure 4-10.

```
In[33]:= sImprt[[All,"price"]]
Out[33]=
```

$4	$3	$2	$2	$3
$5	$5	$2	$4	$2

Figure 4-10. *Price column*

If you want to have them in a list, you must use the Normal command.

```
In[34]:= Normal[%]
Out[34]= {$ 4,$ 3,$ 2,$ 2,$ 3,$ 5,$ 5,$ 2,$ 4,$ 2}
```

The result is the list but in quantity type. It is fair to say that you can do operations with quantities, but if what matters are the magnitudes, you can extract them. It's worth noting that working with magnitudes alone is generally faster and more efficient, which reduces the overhead or additional quantity processing. Unless a specific quantity is required, converting to pure numbers may be preferable.

Let's look at how.

```
In[35]:= QuantityMagnitude[#]&[%]
Out[35]= {4,3,2,2,3,5,5,2,4,2}
```

You are now working with only the magnitudes.

You can even work with dates and quantities, as shown in Figure 4-11, starting by displaying the ID of the products and the date they were sold.

```
In[36]:= sImprt[[All,{"id","sales per day"}]]
Out[36]=
```

id	sales per day
1	Tue 4 Jun 2019
2	Thu 6 Jun 2019
3	Fri 7 Jun 2019
4	Sat 1 Jun 2019
5	Sat 8 Jun 2019
6	Sat 8 Jun 2019
7	Thu 6 Jun 2019
8	Sun 9 Jun 2019
9	Fri 21 Jun 2019
10	Wed 26 Jun 2019

Figure 4-11. *ID and sales per day columns*

Having done this, you can extract the values and work directly with the date object types.

```
In[37]:= Normal[Values[%]]//InputForm
Out[37]//InputForm=
{{1, DateObject[{2019, 6, 4}, "Day"]},
 {2, DateObject[{2019, 6, 6}, "Day"]},
 {3, DateObject[{2019, 6, 7}, "Day"]},
 {4, DateObject[{2019, 6, 1}, "Day"]},
 {5, DateObject[{2019, 6, 8}, "Day"]},
 {6, DateObject[{2019, 6, 8}, "Day"]},
 {7, DateObject[{2019, 6, 6}, "Day"]},
 {8, DateObject[{2019, 6, 9}, "Day"]},
 {9, DateObject[{2019, 6, 21}, "Day"]},
 {10, DateObject[{2019, 6, 26}, "Day"]}}
```

Each value represents a date using DateObject, which is easily converted to numeric values using AbsoluteTime. It is handy for numerical operations involving dates, making the data handling more flexible and efficient.

Note   You should get the date object when testing the code instead of the pure word; here, the InputForm is used to avoid image conflicts.

Knowing this, you can make an association between the IDs of each product and when it was sold, applying the Rule command inside the nested list and creating the associations.

```
In[38]:= Association[Apply[Rule,%,1]]//InputForm
Out[38]//InputForm=
<|1 -> DateObject[{2019, 6, 4}, "Day"],
 2 -> DateObject[{2019, 6, 6}, "Day"],
 3 -> DateObject[{2019, 6, 7}, "Day"],
 4 -> DateObject[{2019, 6, 1}, "Day"],
 5 -> DateObject[{2019, 6, 8}, "Day"],
 6 -> DateObject[{2019, 6, 8}, "Day"],
 7 -> DateObject[{2019, 6, 6}, "Day"],
 8 -> DateObject[{2019, 6, 9}, "Day"],
 9 -> DateObject[{2019, 6, 21}, "Day"],
 10 -> DateObject[{2019, 6, 26}, "Day"]|>
```

To illustrate this, create a visualization in a timeline, as shown in Figure 4-12, marking the product sold and the date of its sale.

```
In[39]:= TimelinePlot[%]
Out[39]=
```

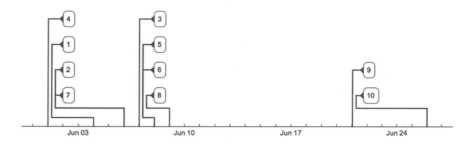

Figure 4-12. *Timeplot*

The date of each grocery item sold is shown by ID. A tooltip shows the exact date when the cursor is passed over the number in the timeline.

The idea is that when you use SemanticImport, you can integrate different forms of the Wolfram Language and how you can use this to your advantage when importing data. Semantic import makes it possible to compare data with other selected data. SemanticImport provides you with tools to work among various types of semantic objects. What is essential to observe is that instead of importing standard text, you can import currency types, dates, and any magnitude with the respective unit, as in the previous examples. This allows that data to be associated with different commands within the Wolfram Language.

Costume Import (Dealing with Large Datasets)

Having said all this about semantic import, you can import data and choose how each column in the imported file should be interpreted. However, based on the same idea that you saw earlier, with semantic import, you can also choose what data to import (e.g., if it is only one column or several), as illustrated in Figure 4-13.

```
In[40]:= SemanticImport["/Users/macosx/Desktop/Grocery_List.csv",{"Integer",
"String","Currency","Real","Date"}]
Out[40]=
```

id	grocery item	price	sold items	sales per day
1	milk	$ 4	4.0	Tue 4 Jun 2019
2	butter	$ 3	2.0	Thu 6 Jun 2019
3	garlic	$ 2	1.0	Fri 7 Jun 2019
4	apple	$ 2	4.0	Sat 1 Jun 2019
5	orange	$ 3	5.0	Sat 8 Jun 2019
6	orange juice	$ 5	2.0	Sat 8 Jun 2019
7	cheese	$ 5	2.0	Thu 6 Jun 2019
8	cookies	$ 2	5.0	Sun 9 Jun 2019
9	grapes	$ 4	3.0	Fri 21 Jun 2019
10	potato	$ 2	5.0	Wed 26 Jun 2019

id	grocery item	price	sold items	sales per day
1	milk	$4	4	Tue 4 Jun 2019
2	butter	$3	2	Thu 6 Jun 2019
3	garlic	$2	1	Fri 7 Jun 2019
4	apple	$2	4	Sat 1 Jun 2019
5	orange	$3	5	Sat 8 Jun 2019
6	orange juice	$5	2	Sat 8 Jun 2019
7	cheese	$5	2	Thu 6 Jun 2019
8	cookies	$2	5	Sun 9 Jun 2019

Figure 4-13. *Dataset with excluded rows*

With this result, observe that the first column imported contains integers, the second contains text, the third contains a currency type quantity, the fourth contains a real number, and the last contains a date object. Having done this, it is possible in the same way that with spreadsheet files, you can import certain types of information in list form, either by column or by row. The following example imports rows 1 through 5.

```
In[41]:=SemanticImport["/Users/macosx/Desktop/Grocery_List.
csv",Automatic,"Rows"][[1;;5]]//InputForm
Out[41]//InputForm= {{1, "milk", Quantity[4, "USDollars"], 4,
DateObject[{2019, 6, 4}, "Day"]}, {2, "butter", Quantity[3, "USDollars"],
2, DateObject[{2019, 6, 6}, "Day"]}, {3, "garlic", Quantity[2,
"USDollars"], 1, DateObject[{2019, 6, 7}, "Day"]}, {4, "apple", Quantity[2,
"USDollars"], 4, DateObject[{2019, 6, 1}, "Day"]}, {5, "orange",
Quantity[3, "USDollars"], 5, DateObject[{2019, 6, 8}, "Day"]}}
```

As indicated, columns can also be imported from columns 1 to 2.

```
In[42]:=SemanticImport["/Users/macosx/Desktop/Grocery_List.
csv",Automatic,"Columns"][[1;;2]]
Out[42]= {{1,2,3,4,5,6,7,8,9,10},{milk,butter,garlic,apple,orange,orange ju
ice,cheese,cookies,grapes,potato}}
```

It is necessary to emphasize that if you want to exclude data, importing with the ExcludedLines statement is recommended. For example, exclude rows 9 and 10, remembering that the titles are in row 1, as shown in Figure 4-13.

```
In[43]:=SemanticImport["/Users/macosx/Desktop/Grocery_List.csv",ExcludedLin
es->{{10},{11}}]
Out[43]=
```

When working with large datasets, it's crucial to manage memory usage. Review if your system can handle big sizes of data. If it's too large to import at once, try importing it in smaller pieces and filtering/managing the data as needed. The following example effectively selects the first ten buildings (see Figure 4-14) from the buildings.dat dataset based on the specified condition using a pure function within Select.

```
In[44]:= SemanticImport["ExampleData/buildings.dat",<|"Name"->
Automatic,"City"->Automatic,"Country"->Automatic,"Year"->
Automatic|>,HeaderLines->1];
Select[%,#[[4]]<=2000&][[1;;10]]
Out[45]=
```

Name	City	Country	Year
Petronas Tower 1	Kuala Lumpur	Malaysia	1998
Petronas Tower 2	Kuala Lumpur	Malaysia	1998
Sears Tower	Chicago	United States	1974
Jin Mao Building	Shanghai	China	1999
CITIC Plaza	Guangzhou	China	1996
Shun Hing Square	Shenzhen	China	1996
Empire State Building	New York City	United States	1931
Central Plaza	Hong Kong	China	1992
Bank of China	Hong Kong	China	1989
Emirates Tower One	Dubai	United Arab Emirates	1999

Figure 4-14. *Buildings dataset with selected rows*

To filter the data dataset based on the condition that the Year column (index 4) is less than or equal to 2000. Then, use [[1;; 10]] to select the first ten elements from the filtered dataset, which are the first ten buildings that meet the condition.

Export

Mathematica supports many formats; to view all supported formats, type $ExportFormat.

```
In[46]:= Short[$ExportFormats,5]
Out[46]//Short= {3DS,AC,ACO,AIFF,ASE,AU,AVI,Base64,Binary,Bit,BLEND,BMP,
BREP,BSON,Byte,BYU,BZIP2,C,CDF,<<167>>,WDX,WebP,WL,WLNet,WMLF,WXF,X3D,XBM,
XGL,XHTML,XHTMLMathML,XLS,XLSX,XML,XPORT,XYZ,ZIP,ZPR,ZSTD}
```

Exporting data is carried out using the Export command. Export has the form Export["directory path," expr, "format"].

First, you need to set up a working directory. If not, the file is exported to the default Mathematica working directory. To see the working default directory, use Directory.

```
In[47]:= Directory[]
Out[47]= /Users/macosx
```

In this case, the default directory is the Desktop folder.

Two commands are key; one is SetDirectory, whose argument is the path of the new working directory, and the other is NotebookDirectory, which is the file's location.

First, let's set the new working directory to export files to the notebook location. Using the notebook directory as the argument on SetDirectory, you tell Mathematica that the new working directory is the location of the notebook in which you are currently working.

```
In[48]:= SetDirectory[NotebookDirectory[]]
Out[48]= /Users/macosx/Desktop
```

Now that you have set up a new directory, you can export data created in Mathematica. The next example exports a list of prime numbers from 1 to 10 as a table in a text file and a CSV file. An option applies as well as Import, but if the file extension is added, it is not compulsory to write the format option.

Note   There is no restriction about whether to assign a name to the list of data or to create the data directly in the export.

```
In[49]:= mydata=Table[Prime[i],{i,1,10}];
{Export["New_File.txt",mydata,"Table"], Export["New_File.csv",mydata]}
Out[50]= {New_File.txt,New_File.csv}
```

The output generates the name of the new file exported. An alternative is manually entering the desired location of the file instead of setting a new working directory; in this case, Desktop was set as the new location.

```
In[51]:= Export["/Users/macosx/Desktop/New_File.TSV",mydata,"TSV"]
Out[51]= /Users/macosx/Desktop/New_File.TSV
```

Now that you have exported the data into a new location, the output is the full path of the new file. If you want to open the file from Mathematica, you can use SystemOpen. This command opens the operating system explorer.

```
In[52]:= SystemOpen["/Users/macosx/Desktop/New_File.TSV"]
```

SystemOpen lets you open the notebook directory folder to open other files inside the notebook directory.

```
In[53]:= SystemOpen[NotebookDirectory[]]
```

On the other hand, when dealing with tabular data, it can be exported as a spreadsheet. The next example export a tabular data structure and then export it into a spreadsheet format.

To create tabular data, let's use the Table command.

```
In[54]:=
tabD1=Table[i,{i,4}];
tabD2=SetPrecision[Table[i/11,{i,4}],3];
```

Now that you have a set of coordinates, you can export the data to different sheets by typing the reference name of the data into a list of options: {data_sheet 1,data_sheet 2, ...}

```
In[56]:= Export["Tabular_data.xls",{{tabD1},{tabD2}}]
Out[56]= Tabular_data.xls
```

By opening the file with a spreadsheet viewer, you should get that TabD1 is in sheet 1 and TabD2 is in sheet 2.

To customize the name of the sheets, you need to enter the names as a list of rules with the rule operator (➤).

```
In[57]:= Export["Tabular_data_2.xls",{"Page number 1"->tabD1,"Page number
2"->tabD2}]
Out[57]= Tabular_data_2.xls
```

If you open the file, now you should have two sheets with the names you have set.

In addition to this, there is the possibility to add the same data in a single spreadsheet. You only have to enclose the data you want in the same sheet in curly braces to do this.

```
In[58]:= Export["New_data.xls",Transpose[{tabD1,tabD2}]]
Out[58]= New_data.xls
```

After opening the file, you should see something like the following code.

```
In[59]:= Grid[Transpose[{tabD1,tabD2}]]
Out[59]=
1    0.0909
2    0.182
3    0.273
4    0.364
```

You can even export tables.

```
In[60]:= table1={{"Dog","Wolf"},{"Cat","Leopard"},{"Pigeon","Shark"}};
Export["Animal_table.xls",table1]
Out[61]= Animal_table.xls
```

Other Formats

By advancing the topic, it is possible to export the data to simple formats such as TXT, DAT, CSV, and CSV. To do this, you only have to put the path of the file where you want it to be exported, along with the name of the new file, followed by the extension of the desired file. The second argument writes the data to be exported or the variable that contains the data. The third argument is what designates the format you want the data to import.

Let's look at the following example, which exports new data to text and DAT formats. In this case, you only write the file's name, which indicates that you want it to be exported to the working directory established earlier, corresponding to the notebook's directory.

```
In[62]:= newD=Table[{i+j,i*j},{i,1,5},{j,1,5}];
{Export["File_text.txt",newD,"Text"],Export["File_dat.dat",newD,"Table"]}
Out[63]= {File_text.txt,File_dat.dat}
```

It is advisable to pause for a moment. As shown in the earlier code, the Table format is used for the DAT file. This is because a Table is used so that the exported data becomes an expression in the Wolfram Language. After you have exported, verify that the files have been exported. Likewise, you can choose the format for a file. For example, instead of typing text, you export it in the TSV format.

```
In[64]:= Export["File_text.txt",newD,"TSV"]
Out[64]= File_text.txt
```

Similarly, you can export CSV and TSV files.

```
In[65]:={Export["File_csv.csv",newD,"CSV"],Export["File_tsv.
tsv",newD,"TSV"]}
Out[65]= {File_csv.csv,File_tsv.tsv}
```

It is possible to add titles to the columns of the data for when they are exported, either CSV or TSV.

```
In[66]:= Export["File_csv.csv",newD,"CSV",TableHeadings->{"column
1","column 2","column 3","column 4","column 5"}]
Out[66]= File_csv.csv
```

It is also possible to define a list of names for the columns as follows.

```
In[67]:= labels={"Coordinates 1","Coordinates 2","Coordindates
3","Coordinates 4","Coordindates 5"};Export["File_csv.csv",newD,"CSV",
TableHeadings->labels]
Out[67]= File_csv.csv
```

In the same way, you can export datasets to known formats. Let's use automobile braking distance statistics based on speed. For this, the data is loaded using the ExampleData command. Inside this, search "Statistics"; within that, search "CarStoppingDistances".

```
In[68]:= spData=ExampleData[{"Statistics","CarStoppingDistances"}]
Out[68]={{4,2},{4,10},{7,4},{7,22},{8,16},{9,10},{10,18},{10,26},{10,34},
{11,17},{11,28},{12,14},{12,20},{12,24},{12,28},{13,26},{13,34},{13,34},
{13,46},{14,26},{14,36},{14,60},{14,80},{15,20},{15,26},{15,54},{16,32},
{16,40},{17,32},{17,40},{17,50},{18,42},{18,56},{18,76},{18,84},{19,36},
{19,46},{19,68},{20,32},{20,48},{20,52},{20,56},{20,64},{22,66},{23,54},
{24,70},{24,92},{24,93},{24,120},{25,85}}
```

To get the dataset's columns and a description, add Description and ColumnDescriptions.

```
In[69]:= ExampleData[{"Statistics","CarStoppingDistances"},#]&/@{"Descripti
on","ColumnDescriptions"}
Out[69]= {Car stopping distances as a function of speed.,{Speed in miles
per hour.,Stopping distance in feet.}}
```

Continuing the exploration, you see that the first numbers represent the speed in miles per hour, and the second numbers represent the distance in feet.

Note   For more information, add properties as the second argument to ExampleData.

Moving forward in the exercise, you can add the column titles. This distinguishes each data type when you build the dataset (see Figure 4-15).

```
In[70]:= spDataset=Dataset[spData,Background->LightBlue][All,<|#1->1,#2->
2|>]&["Speed in miles per hours","Stopping distance in feet"]
Out[70]=
```

Speed in miles per hours	Stopping distance in feet
4	2
4	10
7	4
7	22
8	16
9	10
10	18
10	26
10	34
11	17
11	28
12	14
12	20
12	24
12	28
13	26
13	34
13	34
13	46
14	26

⊼ ∧ rows 1–20 of **50** ∨ ⊻

Figure 4-15. *CarStoppingDistances dataset*

You have finished the creation of the dataset. This data and the respective column titles can now be exported to a CSV format.

```
In[71]:= Export["Dataset_csv.csv",spDataset,"CSV"]
Out[71]= Dataset_csv.csv
```

If the export is successful, you should have a CSV file in the correct format. For the case of a TSV file, see the following form.

```
In[72]:= Export["Dataset_tsv.tsv",spDataset,"TSV"]
Out[72]= Dataset_tsv.tsv
```

XLS and XLSX Formats

It is worth distinguishing that to export datasets to spreadsheet formats such as XLS or XLSX, you should work the dataset as a list since exporting the dataset directly would result in exporting associations in a single cell, and you are not interested in that. Regarding the second point, since you have the dataset, to extract the values, you use the Normal command, which converts the dataset into a normal expression, followed by extracting the values from the braces with Values.

```
In[73]:= Values@Normal@spDataset
Out[73]={{4,2},{4,10},{7,4},{7,22},{8,16},{9,10},{10,18},{10,26},{10,34},
{11,17},{11,28},{12,14},{12,20},{12,24},{12,28},{13,26},{13,34},{13,34},
{13,46},{14,26},{14,36},{14,60},{14,80},{15,20},{15,26},{15,54},{16,32},
{16,40},{17,32},{17,40},{17,50},{18,42},{18,56},{18,76},{18,84},{19,36},
{19,46},{19,68},{20,32},{20,48},{20,52},{20,56},{20,64},{22,66},{23,54},
{24,70},{24,92},{24,93},{24,120},{25,85}}
```

Now that you have the data, you can add the column titles and export the extracted data from the dataset.

```
In[74]:= colTitles={"Speed in miles per hours","Stopping distance
in feet"};
```

To attach the two lists, let's use Prepend and assign the name exprtData to new values.

```
In[75]:= Short[exprtData=Prepend[%%,colTitles],1]
Out[75]//Short= {{Speed in miles per hours,Stopping distance in feet},{4,2},
{4,10},<<45>>,{24,93},{24,120},{25,85}}
```

You do not define variables to put together this data list and titles. A percentage notation is used to simplify the code. Now that you have complete data, you can export it to an XLS or XLSX format.

```
In[76]:= Export["Stopping_distance_Dataset.xlsx",exprtData,"XLSX"]
Out[76]= Stopping_distance_Dataset.xlsx
```

If you verify the file, you should have something like the dataset created earlier.

JSON Formats

It is also possible to export information to formats such as JSON. The following example creates a JSON structure from an association.

```
In[77]:= Association@{"Name"->"Ellis","Date of birth"->
"1990,01,04","Height"->"180 cm","Favorite color"->"Red","Hobbies"->"Soccer,
Pc gaming, Board games","Social netwoks"->"Twitter, Facebook"};
Export["File_json.json",%,"JSON"]
Out[78]= File_json.json
```

If you open the new JSON file, you see that it has a structure corresponding to a JSON file. It is the same process for the case where you have a nested list, although you can also use the "Rawjson" format when exporting. The idea is that you can export data to JSON formats from associations; as you have seen, the braces and values of an association can be any expression. This leads you to say that more associations can be added, and these can be exported. The vital thing to note is that given the nature of the JSON format of containing braces and values in pairs, it is possible to export data in JSON format from associations. Examining the case for when you have a dataset (see Figure 4-16), proceed as noted here.

```
In[79]:=Association@{"Name"->"Ellis","Date of birth"->
DateObject[{1990,01,04}],"Height"->Quantity[180,"Centimeters"],"Favorite
color"->"Red","Hobbies"->"Soccer, Pc gaming, Board games","Social netwoks"->
"Twitter, Facebook"};
user=Dataset[%]
Out[80]=
```

Name	Ellis
Date of birth	Thu 4 Jan 1990
Height	180 cm
Favorite color	Red
Hobbies	Soccer, Pc gaming, Board games
Social netwoks	Twitter, Facebook

Figure 4-16. *JSON file dataset*

The dataset is built, but in some cases, the dataset may contain quantities or other semantic objects, as in this case, the date and height. So, exporting them would be the same way as before but using the JSON option format, not Rawjson, since this does not allow exporting dataset objects. To use Rawjson, you must convert the semantic objects to strings or numbers.

```
In[81]:= Export["Dataset_json.json",user,"JSON"]
Out[81]= Dataset_json.json
```

If you have a dataset of repeated keys, you can export it to the JSON format (see Figure 4-17).

```
In[82]:= assoc1=<|"Log in Date"->DateObject[{2020,06,29}],"User ID"->
123,"Status"->"Active"|>;
assoc2=<|"Log in Date"->DateObject[{2020,06,28}],"User ID"->122,"Status"->
"Not Active"|>;Dataset[{assoc1,assoc2}]
Export["Dataset2_json.json",%,"JSON"]
Out[83]=
```

Log in Date	User ID	Status
Mon 29 Jun 2020	123	Active
Sun 28 Jun 2020	122	Not Active

Figure 4-17. *User Dataset*

```
Out[84]= Dataset2_json.json
```

To be precise, you can export shapes where the dataset contains complex structures, such as an association of associations. Let's look at the following example, which builds a dataset (see Figure 4-18).

```
In[85]:= assoc3="Player A"->Association["Date"->DateObject[{2020,06,29}],
"User ID"->123,"Status"->"Active"];assoc4="Player B"->Association["Date"->
DateObject[{2020,06,28}],"User ID"->122,"Status"->
"Not Active"];Dataset[{<|assoc3,assoc4|>}]
Out[85]=
```

	Date	User ID	Status
Player A	Mon 29 Jun 2020	123	Active
Player B	Sun 28 Jun 2020	122	Not Active

Figure 4-18. *Tagged dataset*

Subsequently, proceed to export the dataset.

```
In[86]:= Export["Dataset3_json.json",%,"JSON"]
Out[86]= Dataset3_json.json
```

Let's try to better understand how to export in JSON format. When you export information such as a rule list or a single association, the structure of the content in the exported JSON file is through a collection of pairs between braces and values. On the contrary, when you have ordered structures, such as an association of lists and an association of associations, the structure of the content in the JSON file is as an ordered array within the array of the collections of associated pairs between braces and values. Quite the opposite; however, exporting a nested list is already in the form of sorted arrays. To clarify this, the reader can observe how a list of rules is exported through the following code.

```
In[87]:= rules={"apple"->3,"car"->"3","2"->2};
Export["Rules.json",rules,"JSON"]
Out[88]= Rules.json
```

In addition, for a nested list or list of lists.

```
In[89]:= arry=Array[{#1,#2}&,{4,4}]
Export["Array.json",arry,"JSON"]
Out[89]= {{{1,1},{1,2},{1,3},{1,4}},{{2,1},{2,2},{2,3},{2,4}},{{3,1},{3,2},
{3,3},{3,4}},{{4,1},{4,2},{4,3},{4,4}}}
Out[90]= Array.json
```

If the created file is observed, it must contain an array of arrays inside the JSON file.

Content File Objects

It should be concluded that for all the exported files, you can create a content object showing you the properties of the created files. This is done with the ContentObject function, which provides content from a file. Let's use the association's example to create a JSON file to do this.

```
In[91]:= Association@{"Name"->"Ellis","Date of birth"->DateObject[{1990,01,04}],
"Height"->Quantity[180,"Centimeters"],"Favorite color"->"Red","Hobbies"->
"Soccer, Pc gaming, Board games","Social netwoks"->"Twitter, Facebook"};
user=Dataset[%];
jsonFile=Export["Dataset_json_2.json",user,"JSON"];
```

Now, you need to get the path where the file is located with AbsoluteFileName.

```
In[94]:= AbsoluteFileName[jsonFile]
Out[94]= /Users/macosx/Desktop/Dataset_json_2.json
```

Let's now use the file to create the file object type representation. Then, ContentObject is applied to the file object.

```
In[95]:= ContentObject[%]
Out[95]=
```

A content-type object appears (see Figure 4-19).

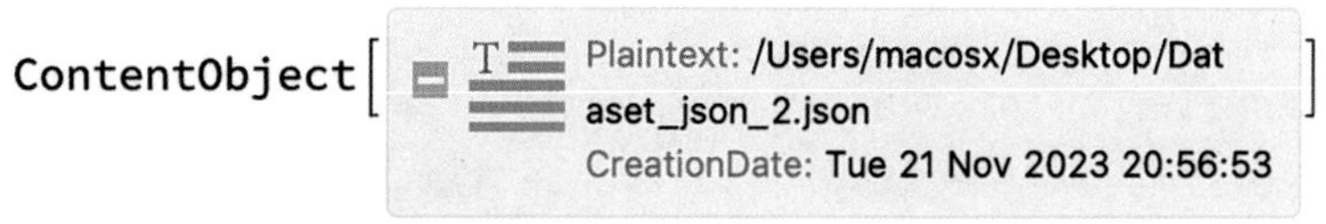

Figure 4-19. *ContentObject for the JSON files created*

Pressing the + icon provides you with the exported file's properties, such as name, size, creation dates, and file localization. You can access the properties programmatically using the following form.

```
In[96]:= ContentObject[%%]["Properties"]
Out[96]= {CreationDate,Plaintext}
```

This can be applied to other exported files.

Searching Files with Wolfram Language

With the Wolfram Language, you can look at the location of the file or files.

The NotebookDirectory command is used to see the path of the notebook directory. It shows the full directory containing the notebook in which you work.

```
In[97]:= NotebookDirectory[]
Out[97]= /Users/macosx/Desktop/
```

Now, SetDirectory is used to set a working directory as the current directory. You can enter the path of the desired directory and establish it as the working directory. However, now set the notebook directory as the new working directory.

```
In[98]:= SetDirectory[NotebookDirectory[]]
Out[98]= /Users/macosx/Desktop
```

With this new directory set, you can locate files in the new directory, the notebook location. Here, the FileNames command lets you explore files in the working directory, which, in this case, is the notebook's directory because it was set up in the previous code.

```
In[99]:= FileNames[]
Out[99]= {Color_table.txt,Grocery_List.csv,Hello_World,Hello_World.
txt,import export.nb,weather.csv}
```

FileNames show all types of files available in the directory. If you have many files in the directory, you can search for a particular file by using FindFile and entering the file's name as a string. The full path of the file is displayed.

```
In[100]:= FindFile["Color_table.txt"]
Out[100]= /Users/macosx/Desktop/Color_Table.txt
```

File extensions can be searched, too.

```
In[101]:= FileNames["*.txt"]
Out[101]= {Color_table.txt,File_text.txt,Hello_World.txt,New_File.txt}
```

Note   Other types of File commands exist; to look for more commands associated with the name file, enter ??File*.

Remember, this is when you set the working directory as the notebook directory. If you have not set a directory previously, Mathematica searches the default directories of your machine, which are the ones shown entering $Path.

Connecting to External Services

Besides export and import capabilities, Mathematica can connect to various external services, like external resources, external connectivity, and database management through external evaluations.

External Connections

With the launch of Mathematica version 13, improvements have been put together, especially in connecting with external services. One notable feature is external evaluators, which enable interaction with various languages such as Julia, Ruby, R, Python, Java, Octave, Node.js, Shell, and SQL. To discover and utilize installed evaluator systems, use FindExternalEvaluators, which scans standard directories for use in any local evaluation.

Executing FindExternalEvaluators[], with no arguments, searches for all available languages installed on your computer. Let's find the version of the Shell evaluator. On macOS, it usually refers to the Bash shell; on Windows, it's typically PowerShell.

```
In[102]:= FindExternalEvaluators["Shell"]//Normal//Print
Out[102] =
<|4ce695dd-ef6a-7006-f30d-b4320329bbd7 → <|System → Shell,
    Version → 3.2.57, Target :→ /bin/bash, Executable :→ /bin/bash,
    Registered → Automatic|>,
```

```
b217afb1-d97f-3cfa-3c52-19ec78df64bc  →  <|System → Shell,
    Version → 3.2.57, Target :→ /bin/sh, Executable :→ /bin/sh,
Registered →Automatic|>,
342330ff-7009-e5ec-c00a-86949f3c0f7a  →  <|System → Shell,
    Version → 5.9, Target :→ /bin/zsh, Executable :→ /bin/zsh,
Registered → Automatic|>|>
```

In this case, the output lists three shell versions: Bash (Bourne Again SHell), Sh (Bourne Shell), and Zsh (Z Shell).

Note   The external language cannot be used if the Registered value is not set to True or Automatic. For troubleshooting, go to the Wolfram documentation page at `https://reference.wolfram.com/language/workflowguide/ConnectingToExternalSoftware.html`.

Once the external evaluator has been registered, it can be used with ExternalEvaluator. You can use ExternalEvaluate by applying the function directly or, in a new cell, by typing '>' to initiate a command line, where a yellow block line appears. Choose your language from a drop-down list on the left icon or input it directly as a string and then the code, as shown in Figure 4-20.

```
ExternalEvaluate["Shell", "echo 'Hello World!'"]
```

```
>|  echo 'Hello, World!'
```

Figure 4-20. *External evaluation for Z shell code using the ExternalEvaluate and the '>' type command block*

Executing the code following prints "Hello World!" using the Z shell. The resulting exit code is 0, signifying success, and is displayed as standard notebook output (see Figure 4-21).

```
In[103]:=
Out[103]=
```

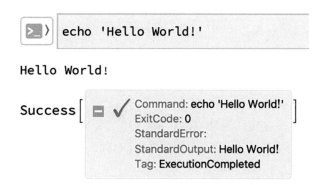

Figure 4-21. *External evaluation using Z shell code Hello World!*

Different prerequisites may be required, such as additional libraries and the language executable, depending on the external language you intend to use. While language cells are handy, ExternalEvaluate offers more programmatic output flexibility.

External Resources

The prior section highlights ExternalEvaluate's role in integrating outer languages in a notebook. Despite this, Mathematica can generate and utilize outer resources like outer functions. Node.js version 21.2.0 was used while creating this book. It can be installed from the official site or approved repositories. In this case, the Homebrew package installer was used. Using Node.js required the zeromq library, installed using npm, as stated in the Wolfram documentation.

Note For detailed info, visit Wolfram documentation. NodeJS for ExternalEvaluate: `https://reference.wolfram.com/language/workflow/ConfigureNodeJSForExternalEvaluate.html`

To automatically identify Node.js, use FindExternalEvaluators["NodeJS"], similar to the shell language process. If successful, Registered shows as Automatic, indicating complete setup. If MissingDependencies appears, Mathematica can't find the necessary dependencies, requiring manual registration. Regardless, it's advised to manually register the external evaluator by adding the executable's path to ensure proper function.

Like in the shell process, to autodetect Node.js, use FindExternalEvaluators["Node JS"]. If Registered shows as Automatic, all setup is done. If MissingDependencies shows, Mathematica lacks needed dependencies, requiring manual registration. Regardless, you should manually register the external evaluator by adding the executable's path to ensure proper function.

```
In[104]:= RegisterExternalEvaluator["NodeJS","/opt/homebrew/bin/node"]
Out[104]= 629ba62a-8d17-e9fe-6cd9-870f94c7933c
```

Then, trying to find it again.

```
In[105]:= FindExternalEvaluators["NodeJS"] // Normal // Print
Out[105]=
<|629ba62a-8d17-e9fe-6cd9-870f94c7933c → <|System → NodeJS,
   Version → 21.2.0, Target :→ /opt/homebrew/bin/node,
   Executable :→ /opt/homebrew/bin/node, Registered → True|>|>
```

The Registered key has a value of True, meaning successful manual registration. To test it, calculate the square root of 25.

```
In[106]:= ExternalEvaluate["NodeJS","Math.sqrt(25)"]
Out[106]= 5
```

With Node.js set, custom functions can be implemented—for instance, a primary function to find the square root of a number.

```
In[107]:=  jsFun1 =ExternalFunction["NodeJS","Math.sqrt"]
Out[107]= ExternalFunction[System : NodeJS Command : Math. sqrt
Session : Automatic ]
```

The outer Node.js system calculates using Math.sqrt. If no external session is manually set, it is automatic. The function is now at hand in the notebook.

```
In[108]:= jsFun1[#]&/@{25,36,49,64}
Out[108]= {5,6,7,8}
```

The Function syntax can vary, but the process is the same; for example, using an arrow function.

```
In[109]:= jsFun2 =
ExternalFunction["NodeJS", "(number) => Math.sqrt(number);"];
jsFun2[#] &/@ {25,36,49,64}
Out[109]= {5,6,7,8}
```

Using the external block is also at hand. Figure 4-22 shows that the node.js function is linked to a default external node.js session.

```
In[111]:=
Out[111]=
```

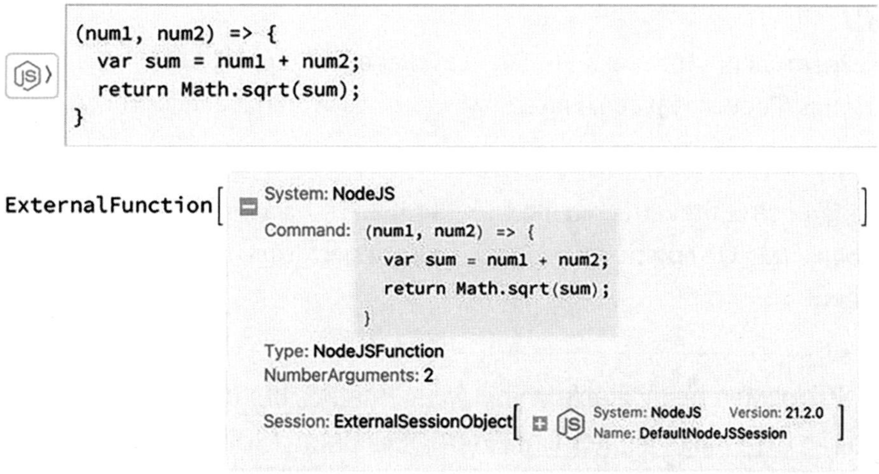

Figure 4-22. *Node.js function to return the square root of the sum of two numbers*

```
In[113]:= %[18,18]
Out[113]= 6
```

Note   To ensure that a function can be called in NodeJS using ExternalFunction, it must be explicitly returned.

To unregister an external evaluator, type the system language and the executable path. In this case, it is the same path used when registered.

```
In[114]:= UnregisterExternalEvaluator["NodeJS","/opt/homebrew/bin/node"]
Out[114]= 629ba62a-8d17-e9fe-6cd9-870f94c7933c
```

Database and File Operations (SQL)

Database and file operations can be performed in Mathematica using external languages like SQL. By leveraging ExternalEvaluate, it is possible to execute SQL queries and work directly with dataset formats.

You can generate a reference object for the database by utilizing a table from the example data folder.

```
In[115]:= DatabaseReference[FindFile["ExampleData/ecommerce-database.
sqlite"]];
Shallow[%]
Out[116]//Shallow=
DatabaseReference[<|Backend → SQLite, Name → /Applications/Mathematica.
app/Contents/Documentation/English/System/ExampleData/ecommerce-database.
sqlite|>]
```

The reference of the retrieved file with FindFile associates the .sqlite local file with the backend SQL engine set as SQLite, which performs operations and data management.

Note   SQL should be available within Mathematica, but check that it appears as a registered external evaluator FindExternalEvaluator["SQL"]. If not, make sure to register the evaluator.

After referencing, view all database table names (see Figure 4-23). Choose a table (offices) (see Figure 4-24) and select territory and city, ordering by territory (see Figure 4-25).

```
In[117]:=
Out[117]=
```

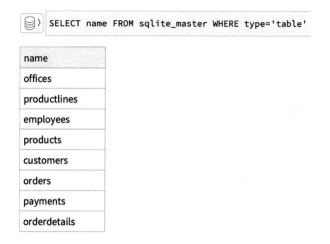

Figure 4-23. *Listing all tables*

In[118]:=
Out[118]=

```
SELECT * FROM offices;
```

officeCode	city	phone	addressLine1	addressLine2	state	country	postalCode	territory
1	San Francisco	+1 650 219 4782	100 Market Street	Suite 300	CA	USA	94080	NA
2	Boston	+1 215 837 0825	1550 Court Place	Suite 102	MA	USA	02107	NA
3	NYC	+1 212 555 3000	523 East 53rd Street	apt. 5A	NY	USA	10022	NA
4	Paris	+33 14 723 4404	43 Rue Jouffroy D'abbans	—	—	France	75017	EMEA
5	Tokyo	+81 33 224 5000	4-1 Kioicho	—	Chiyoda-Ku	Japan	102-8578	Japan
6	Sydney	+61 2 9264 2451	5-11 Wentworth Avenue	Floor #2	—	Australia	NSW 2010	APAC
7	London	+44 20 7877 2041	25 Old Broad Street	Level 7	—	UK	EC2N 1HN	EMEA

Figure 4-24. *Fetching all office data*

In[119]:=
Out[119]=

```
SELECT territory, city FROM offices ORDER BY territory;
```

territory	city
APAC	Sydney
EMEA	Paris
EMEA	London
Japan	Tokyo
NA	San Francisco
NA	Boston
NA	NYC

Figure 4-25. *Sorting offices by territory*

Summary

This chapter explored essential aspects of importing and exporting various file formats, including costume imports. It provides the basics of semantic import, dealing with quantities and large datasets. The chapter also offered a deep dive into data management and the search of content file objects within a notebook. The chapter concluded with a discussion on connecting to external elements, establishing connections, and working with external resources, databases, and files.

CHAPTER 5

Data Visualization

This chapter discusses data visualization in more depth, showing the different ways of visually representing data, using different commands, and creating a range of different types of graphs. It also explains how to customize plots and use predefined plot themes.

Basic Visualization

Data visualization is key for understanding information about data. Visual tools such as 2D plots, contour plots, 3D plots, and time series provide a handy form to view and understand trends and patterns of the data. One of the things about Wolfram Language is that it contains commands that enable you to plot graphs in a simple form. Now, you can better learn how plotting works. Mathematica treats every plot as a graphic object, that is because every graphic is created of primitive elements (points, lines, polygons, geometric figures, etc.), directives (style, shape, size, width, blurriness, etc.), and options (visual modifications, styles, frames, aspects, text, etc.). However, let's focus on the area of 2D and 3D plots.

2D Plots

Simple 2D plots over a specified range are relatively simple to create, as you saw in Chapter 1 with the Plot function. The Wolfram Language gives you accurate control over your plots; for example, you can define the range of your plot's range and many options. For instance, you can add a title to the next plot, a LogPlot, which is a function in a logarithm scale (see Figure 5-1).

```
In[1]:= LogPlot[Log[x]/x,{x,1,20},PlotLabel->"New Log plot"]
Out[1]=
```

© Jalil Villalobos Alva 2024
J. Villalobos Alva, *Beginning Mathematica and Wolfram for Data Science*,
https://doi.org/10.1007/979-8-8688-0348-2_5

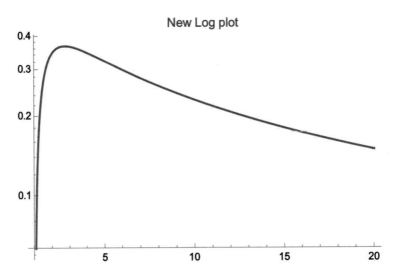

Figure 5-1. *LogPlot*

Figure 5-1 shows that a title has been added.

When plotting points over an interval, the default plot range to show is produced automatically by Mathematica. But with PlotRange, you can override the option and enter a desired range (see Figure 5-2).

```
In[2]:= LogPlot[x+(6/x),{x,1,20},PlotLabel->"New Log
plot",PlotRange->{0,14}]
Out[2]=
```

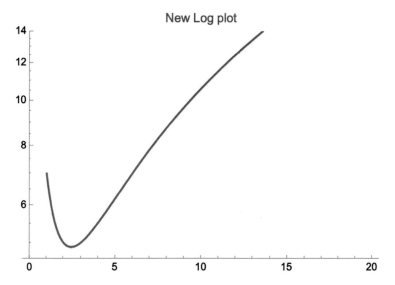

Figure 5-2. *LogPlot of x+(6/x), with custom range*

By selecting All in PlotRange, the y axis increases. Alternatively, you can choose the limits by entering them in the form {y min, y max}. Sometimes, a graphic may not pass through a desired set of coordinates; to force this, AxesOrigin is used (see Figure 5-3). Intersections are written in the form {x,y}, where the coordinates denote the x and y origin points.

```
In[3]:= Plot[Abs[x],{x,-2,2}, AxesOrigin->{0,2}]
Out[3]=
```

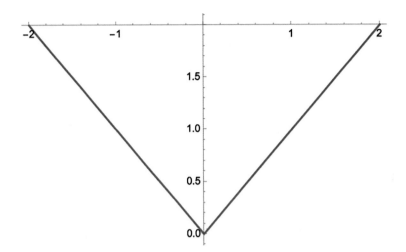

Figure 5-3. *The absolute value of x on origin 0, 2*

AspectRatio is used to control the aspects using their height and width. This option allows you to specify how big or small a graphic can be, calculating the height and width ratio (h/w). However, when using ImageSize to directly select the width and height of a graphic, if you specify the height alone, it is better to set AspectRatio to Full. This ensures proper scaling as the width adjusts accordingly. Both options are shown in Figure 5-4.

```
In[4]:=GraphicsRow[{Plot[Cos[x],{x,0,2\[Pi]},ImageSize->Small],
Plot[Cos[x],{x,0,2\[Pi]},AspectRatio->0.5]}]
Out[4]=
```

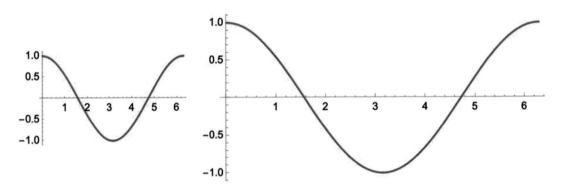

Figure 5-4. *First graphic with ImageSize; second with AspectRatio*

Plotting Data

When plotting graphs, a set of points can be represented in a plot. Data can be plotted with different commands, depending on their purpose. To plot a list of coordinates, ListPlot is used, and the arguments of the plot are represented as x, y coordinates ({x1,y1}, {x2,y2} ...). You can create a list of values and pass them as the arguments. The following example creates a table of values to resemble a hyperbolic cosine, with one step between each point (see Figure 5-5).

```
In[5]:= ListPlot[Table[Cosh[i Degree],{i,1,20}]]
Out[5]=
```

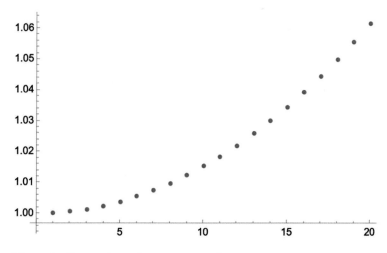

Figure 5-5. *Hyperbolic cosine plot, ranging from 1 to 20*

In this case, you only generate points in {1, y1}, {2, y2}, but you can also plot x and y values. Let's generate the x points with Table and then thread each element of x to a y element and plot (see Figure 5-6) the new set of coordinates.

```
In[6]:= xcoor=Table[i,{i,1,5}];
ycoor={12,5,35,20,55};
coordinates=Thread[{xcoor,ycoor}];
ListPlot[coordinates]
Out[9]=
```

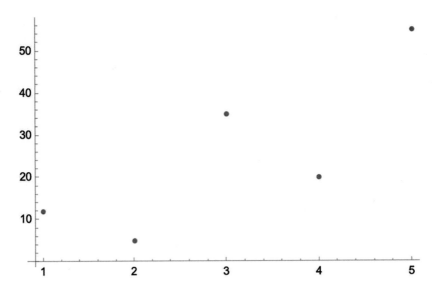

Figure 5-6. *ListPlot of x and y coordinates*

Another useful command is ListLinePlot, which plots points through points by joining them with a line. ListLinePlot (see Figure 5-7) can also plot predefined coordinates. You can show how many points to display to understand how the plot is constructed with the Mesh option.

```
In[10]:= ListLinePlot[coordinates,Mesh->20]
Out[10]=
```

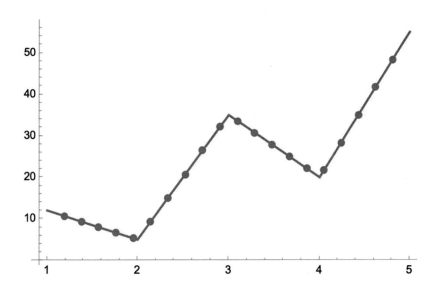

Figure 5-7. *ListLinePlot with mesh option set to 20*

A plot can be represented with different colors and markers. Colors and markers are convenient to distinguish among different plots. To introduce markers, enter the PlotMarkers option followed by the markers symbol. Markers can be special characters or letters; use the special character pallet for a complete list of symbols and characters. By default, different sets are colored differently, but to choose a specific color, use PlotStyle. With PlotStyle the thickness of a line can be changed too, as shown in Figure 5-8.

```
In[11]:=
ListLinePlot[{Table[Cos[i], {i, 0, 2 \[Pi], 0.2}],
  Table[Sin[i], {i, 0, 2 \[Pi], 0.2}]}, PlotMarkers -> {"\[CloverLeaf]", "\
[FilledDownTriangle]"}, PlotStyle -> {Green, Black}]
Out[11]=
```

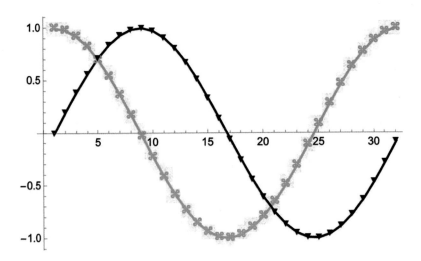

Figure 5-8. *Plots with different marker points*

Another general option is Ticks. With this option, you can modify the indicators on the axes for both x and y. For example, in Figure 5-9, the plot ticks are marked on the x axis; the ticks are –1 and 1. And the y axis is set to automatic (see Figure 5-9).

```
In[12]:= Plot[x^3,{x,-5,5},Ticks->{{-1,0,1},Automatic}]
Out[12]=
```

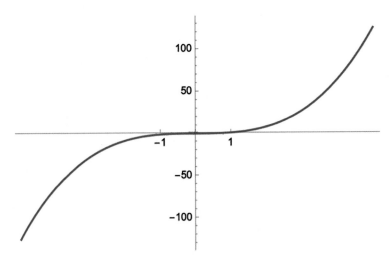

Figure 5-9. *Plots with ticks marked on –1 and 1 for the x axis*

Additionally, plots containing dates can be displayed with DateListPlot. The DateListPlot has the following form, DateListPlot[{v1,v2, ... }, "date specification"]. With DateListPlot, the x axis is converted into a timeline, and the y axis corresponds to the values (v1.v2, ...). Figure 5-10 shows a DateListPlot, starting in June and finishing in November.

```
In[13]:= data1=Table[Power[i,2],{i,0,5}];
data2=Table[Power[i,3],{i,0,5}];
DateListPlot[{data1,data2},{2006,06}]
Out[15]=
```

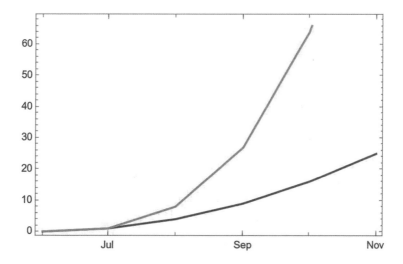

Figure 5-10. *Date plot, starting the plot from June 2006 to November 2006*

Additionally, you can use ListLinePlot or ListPlot to create date plots. Employing the ScalingFunction option with {"Date", Identity} allows a proper scaling along the date axis, for good data visualization over time, as the following code and Figure 5-11 show.

```
In[16]:= data1=Table[{DateObject[{2006,i}],Power[i,2]},{i,3,9}];
data2=Table[{DateObject[{2006,i}],Power[i,3]},{i,3,9}];
ListLinePlot[{data1,data2},ScalingFunctions->{"Date",Identity},PlotStyle->
Automatic,Frame->True,PlotLegends->{"Data 1","Data 2"}]
Out[17]=
```

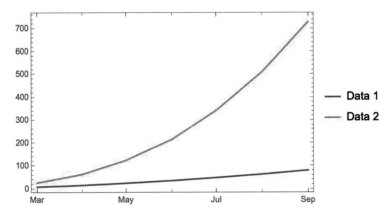

Figure 5-11. *Date plot using ListLinePlot with ScalingFunctions*

Plotting Defined Functions

You can define and plot custom functions (see Figure 5-12). User functions can also be used as arguments for plotting commands. Functions can have a single or multiple variables, as with 3D plots.

```
In[17]:= F[x_]:=Exp[x];
Plot[F[x],{x,-10,10}]
Out[18]=
```

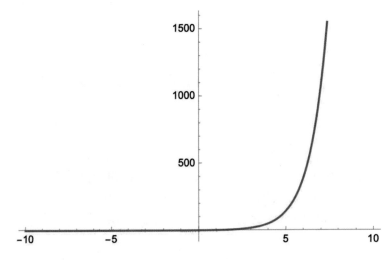

Figure 5-12. *User-defined function for Exp of x*

Also, multiple defined functions are supported. When multiple plots are in the same graphic, each plot is colored differently (see Figure 5-13).

```
In[18]:= X[x_]:=x;Y[y_]:=-Sqrt[y];Z[z_]:=1/z;
Plot[{X[x],Y[x],Z[x]},{x,-10,10}]
Out[19]=
```

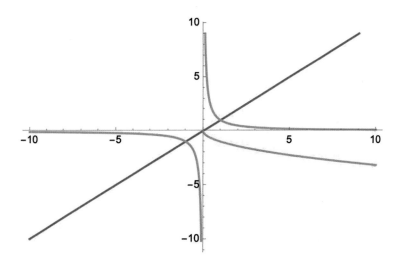

Figure 5-13. *Multiple plots*

Customizing Plots

The Wolfram Language lets users customize plots based on their needs, like adding text, changing color style, adding fill, presenting on tabular frameworks, and so forth. Many commands used in the 2D plots are also preserved in 3D plots. Depending on the graphical representation, options can vary between commands.

Adding Text to Charts

Adding text to charts, like markers and the range of values, can make a chart more informative. Many other elements can be added too.

PlotLabel adds a title to a chart. In addition to this option, there is AxesLabel and PlotLegends. The first allows you to add labels to your axes in the form {"x_label," "y_label"}; the second enables you to add text related to each expression within the graph (see Figure 5-14).

```
In[20]:= Plot[{Abs[x], x^2}, {x, -2, 2}, AxesLabel -> {"x", "y"},
  PlotLegends -> "Expressions"]
Out[20]=
```

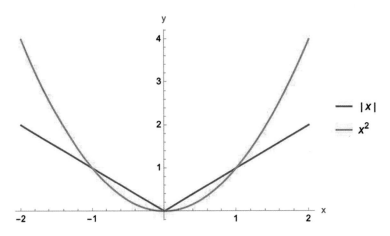

Figure 5-14. *Plots with labeled axes and functions*

You can use Labeled to add costume text expressions on plots (see Figure 5-15). As for the new Mathematica version, passing the cursor over the plot displays the x and y coordinates without creating an explicit tooltip.

```
In[21]:= Labeled[Plot[x^2, {x,-2,2}], "f(x) = "x²,, Left]
Out[21]=
```

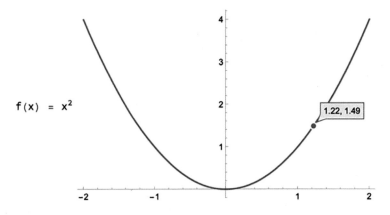

Figure 5-15. *Label placed on the left side of the graphic*

Even with the Labeled command, Tooltips can be constructed. Tooltips display a label tooltip for any expression (see Figure 5-16). Tooltips are displayed when the mouse pointer is passed over the tooltip expression. The difference between Tooltips and PlotLegends is that PlotLegends is an option and not a command.

```
In[22]:= Tooltip[{Plot[x^2,{x,-2,2}]}]
Out[22]= {}
```

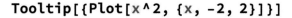

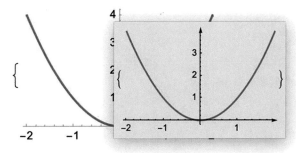

Figure 5-16. *Tooltip created for the plot expression*

When you hover over the entire graph, it shows you the tooltip of the entire graph since you specify it. But you can do it just for the expression of the function (see Figure 5-17).

```
In[23]:= Plot[Tooltip[x^2],{x,-2,2},ImageSize->200]
Out[23]=
```

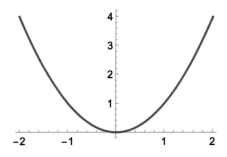

Figure 5-17. *Tooltip for the curve expression*

If you hover over the curve, it shows you the tooltip of x^2; this function also works with the other types of plots. You can add what the tooltip style should look like with the ToolTipStyle option (see Figure 5-18).

```
In[24]:=ListPlot[Tooltip[Range[10], TooltipStyle -> {Bold,Red,
Background -> LightBlue}], ImageSize -> 250]
Out[24]=
```

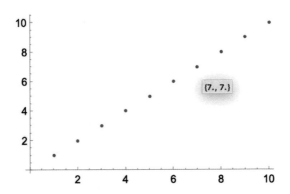

Figure 5-18. *Tooltip for every point plotted*

If you move the cursor to the points, you get the coordinates of the points written in red and the tooltip's background in light blue.

Frame and Grids

Plots can be framed and gridded. The Frame option is used, and to add labels to the frame, use FrameLabel, which receives instructions like AxesLabel (see Figure 5-19).

```
In[25]:= ListPlot[Table[Prime[i],{i,1,10}],Frame->True,FrameLabel->
{"X Framed Axis ","Y Framed Axis"}]
Out[25]=
```

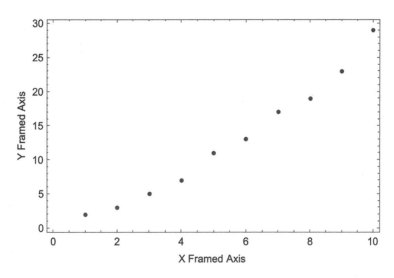

Figure 5-19. *Framed ListPlot*

To add a grid (see Figure 5-20), use the GridLines option.

```
In[26]:= ListPlot[Table[Prime[i],{i,1,10}],GridLines->Automatic,AxesLabel->
{"X Framed Axis ","Y Framed Axis"}]
Out[26]=
```

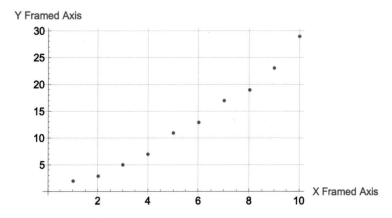

Figure 5-20. *Gridded plot*

To modify the grid style, use the GridLinesStyle option, which can have a particular thickness using Directive (see Figure 5-21).

```
In[27]:= ListPlot[Table[Prime[i], {i, 1, 10}], GridLines -> Automatic,
GridLinesStyle -> Directive[Thickness[0.0002], LightRed]]
Out[27]=
```

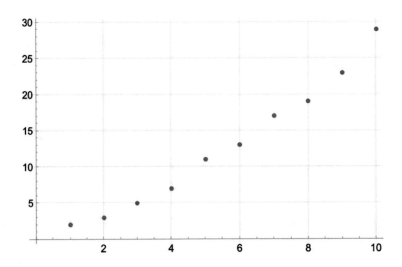

Figure 5-21. *GridLines colored in light red*

Filled Plots

Plots can be filled in various forms—for example, between the x axis, from the bottom and top of a curve (see Figure 5-22).

```
In[28]:= ListLinePlot[Table[Mod[i,2],{i,0,5}],Filling->Bottom]
Out[28]=
```

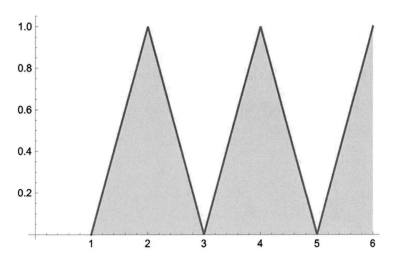

Figure 5-22. *Filled plot from plotted points to the bottom of the axis*

A specified region between curves can also fill them by introducing Filling → {"1st curve" → {"2nd curve"},"2nd curve" → {"3rd curve"}, as shown in Figure 5-23.

```
In[29]:= Plot[{x^2, x^3, x^4},{x,0,5}, Filling->{1->{2}, 2->{3}}]
Out[29]=
```

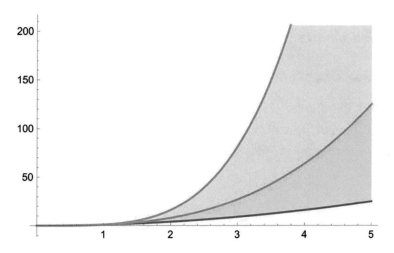

Figure 5-23. *Filled plots*

Filling Patterns and Gradient

The updated version has added new features, such as cross-hatching fillers. This enhancement is used like the standard options illustrated in Figure 5-24.

```
In[30]:= ListLinePlot[Table[Mod[i,2], {i,0,5}], Filling -> Bottom,
FillingStyle -> HatchFilling["Horizontal"]]
Out[30]=
```

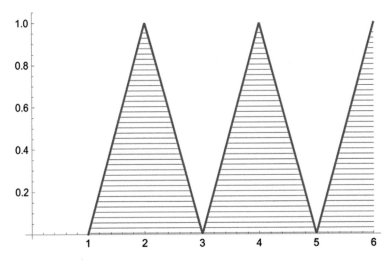

Figure 5-24. *Filled horizontal style*

New function additions are implemented by a style or a pattern, as seen in Figure 5-25.

```
In[31]:= ListLinePlot[Table[Mod[i,2], {i, 0, 5}], Filling -> Bottom,
FillingStyle -> PatternFilling["ChevronLine", ImageScaled[1/20]]]
Out[31]=
```

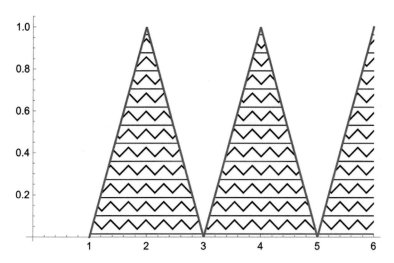

Figure 5-25. *Filled Chevron horizontal line style*

The same applies to shading functions; additions are implemented by the gradient technique, as seen in Figure 5-26.

```
In[32]:= Plot[{x^2,x^3,x^4}, {x,0,5},FillingStyle -> LinearGradientFilling
[{Red,Blue},Top],Filling -> {1->{2},2->{3}}]
Out[32]=
```

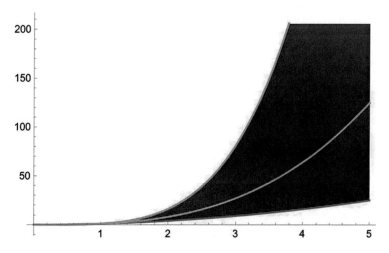

Figure 5-26. *Linear Filled Gradient red, blue, line style*

Combining Plots

To display overlap graphics, there are ways to display the graphs even if they are not of the same type. The following example assigns names to plots without showing the result of each one and finally shows the three graphs. The Show command shows previously defined plots; the arguments are graphic objects followed by options. This is an alternative to doing multiple listable subplots.

```
In[33]:= plot1=Plot[x,{x,0,10},PlotStyle->Red];
plot2=Plot[Cos[x],{x,0,10},PlotStyle->Black];
plot3=ListPlot[Table[Sin[i]+1,{i,1,10}],PlotStyle->Brown];
Show[plot1,plot2,plot3,PlotRange->Automatic]
Out[33]=
```

As shown in Figure 5-27, Show changes the appearance of the graphics; the order in which they are entered is preserved when displayed. Although making the graphics within Show is possible, you can add colors within the Plot command to distinguish the different graphs (see Figure 5-28).

```
In[34]:= Show[Plot[Cos[x],{x,0,10},PlotStyle->Orange],
Plot[Sin[x],{x,0,10},PlotStyle->Purple],PlotRange->Automatic]
Out[34]=
```

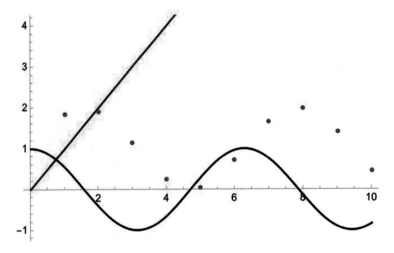

Figure 5-27. *Combined plots shown in the same graphic*

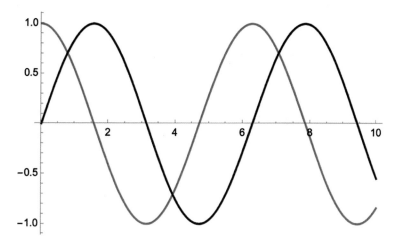

Figure 5-28. *Cosine and Sine plot in the same graphic*

There are several ways to create a list of graphs. You can assign variables to graphs and deploy them as a list.

In[35]:= {Plot1,Plot2,Plot3}
Out[35]=

As seen in Figure 5-29, these three graphs are separated by commas since it is a list.

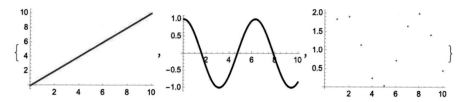

Figure 5-29. *List of three different plots*

Multiple Plots

Multiple plots can be shown in a single output cell. To do this, use the Row command; this command allows the graphs to be displayed horizontally, with each graph on one side of the other (see Figure 5-30). However, Row generally displays expressions in row form, not just graphs.

In[36]:= Row[{plot1,plot2,plot3}]
Out[36]=

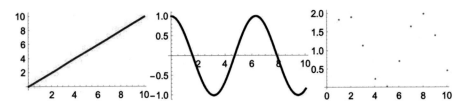

Figure 5-30. *Plots expressed as a row*

By entering a second argument for Row (see Figure 5-31), you have the option to add a separator between the graphs.

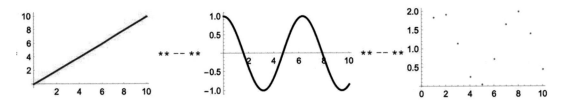

Figure 5-31. *Separator (**--**) added between each plot*

```
In[37]:= Row[{plot1,plot2,plot3},"**--**"]
Out[37]=
```

Alternatively, there is the Column command, which acts similarly to Row but displays expressions or graphs in column form (see Figure 5-32).

```
In[38]:= Column[{plot1,plot2,plot3}]
Out[38]=
```

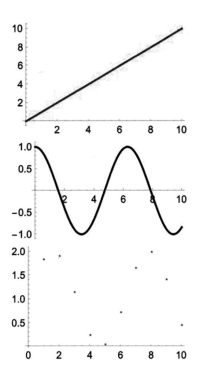

Figure 5-32. *Graphics expressed as a column*

If you look at the following example, it is possible to add frames over the entire chart (see Figure 5-33) for both columns and rows.

```
In[39]:={Column[{plot1,plot2,plot3},Frame-> True],
Row[{plot1,plot2,plot3},Frame->True, FrameMargins->Medium]}
Out[39]=
```

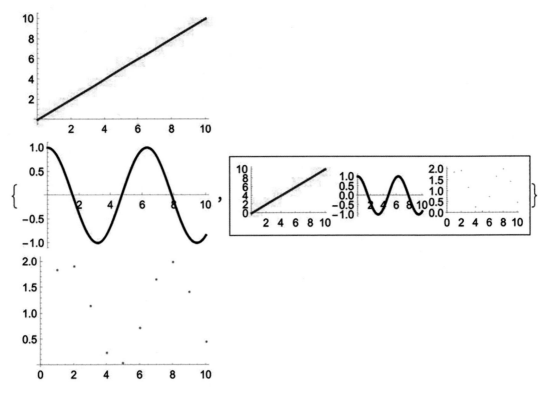

Figure 5-33. *Exhibit of column and row expression for the three plots*

Multiaxis Plots

Since the new version, creating a single graph with multiple coordinate systems into a single pack requires linking the axes with different styles using MultiAxisArrangement. So, the curves connect through the same axis (see Figure 5-34).

```
In[40]:= ListLinePlot[{Table[{x,x^2},{x,0,1,0.1}],Table[{x,x^3}, {x,0,2,0.1}],
Table[{x,x^4},{x,0,3,0.1}]},MultiaxisArrangement-> All]
Out[40]=
```

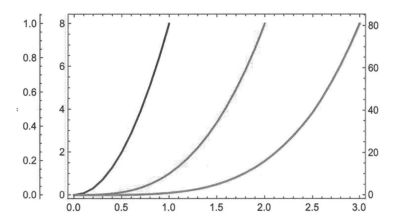

Figure 5-34. *An exhibit of column and row expression for the three plots*

Coloring Plot Grids

Column and Row allow you to customize graphs. There are various ways of changing the color of the frame and adding shading to the graphs (see Figure 5-35).

```
In[41]:= Column[{plot1,plot2,plot3},Frame->True,Background->LightCyan,
FrameStyle->Directive[Black,Dashed],Dividers->All]
Out[41]=
```

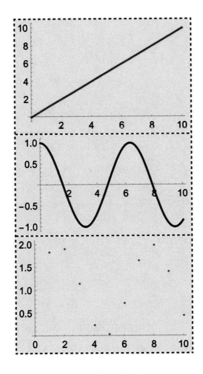

Figure 5-35. *Column graphics with multiple features*

Some options are available depending on whether you use a Row or Column. With Column, there is the option of dividers; in Row, there is no such option, but it is done via a separator, as you saw earlier. Using Table, it is possible to create different shapes on the graphs, either by color or frames, as shown in Figure 5-36.

```
In[42]:= Table[Row[{plot1,plot2,plot3},Frame->True,FrameStyle->Opts],
{Opts,{Thick,Dashed,Dotted}}]
Out[42]=
```

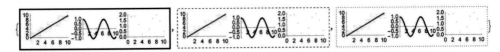

Figure 5-36. *Table of multiple features implemented with the Row command*

Next, let's address the existing alternative using GraphicsRow and GraphicsColumn. Around these commands, there are also options for the image size (see Figure 5-37).

```
In[43]:= {GraphicsRow[{plot1,plot2,plot3},ImageSize->Medium],
GraphicsColumn[{plot1,plot2,plot3},ImageSize->Small]}
Out[43]=
```

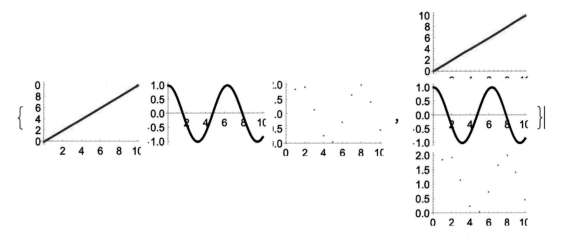

Figure 5-37. *GraphicsRow vs. GraphicsColumn*

GraphicsRow and GraphicsColumn are commands with specific shapes for constructing graphics, whether polygons, lines, dots, and so on. In addition, with Rows and Columns, the graphs are independent. With GraphicsRow or GraphicsColumn, if you select the graph, it is a unique image containing (in this case) the three plots you have made.

Another useful command shows you the graphs as a network, taking up the point stated earlier—if you select the graph, it is a unique image. The following example adds another chart to better illustrate why it's helpful to use GraphicsGrid (see Figure 5-38).

```
In[44]:=plot4=LogLogPlot[Cos[x],{x,0,10},PlotStyle->Yellow];
GraphicsGrid[{{plot1,plot2},{plot3,plot4}},Frame->All,FrameStyle->Purple,
Background->LightCyan]
Out[44]=
```

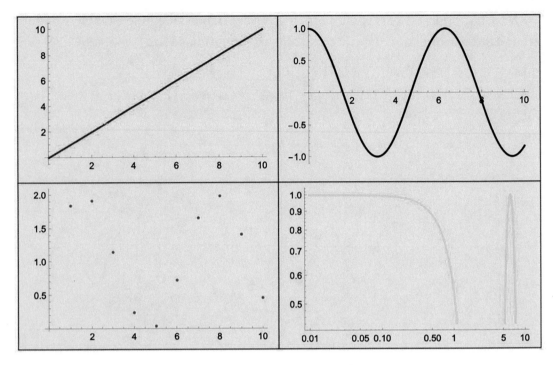

Figure 5-38. *GraphicsGrid showing four different plots*

As shown in Figure 5-38, this shape can help you compactly visualize four graphs at once. Without a doubt, the graphs do not have to be so simple. The options you have seen throughout this chapter can also be added, such as titles and labels on the axes, grid lines and colors, and more, as shown in the following example.

```
In[45]:=
newPlot1=Plot[x,{x,0,10},PlotStyle->{Purple,Thick},PlotLabel->"X"];
newPlot2=Plot[Cos[x],{x,0,10},GridLines->{{-1,0,1},{-1,0,1}},GridLinesSty
le->Directive[Dotted,Blue],PlotLabel->"Cos[x]",ColorFunction->"Rainbow"];
newPlot3=ListPlot[Table[Sin[i]+1,{i,1,10}],Frame->True,FrameLabel->{Style[
"X",Bold],Style["Y",Bold]},PlotStyle->Red,PlotMarkers->"X",PlotLabel->"2D
Scatter Plot"];
newPlot4=LogLogPlot[Cos[x],{x,0,9},Filling->Axis,ColorFunction->
"BlueGreenYellow",PlotRange->{0,1},PlotLabel->"Log Log Plot"];
```

Now that you have the new plots, you can compare them by putting them as a nested list in GraphicsGrid (see Figure 5-39).

```
In[46]:=Labeled[GraphicsGrid[{{newPlot1,newPlot2},{newPlot3,newPlot4}},
Frame->All,Background->White,Spacings->1],Style["Multiple Plots
Box",20,Italic],Top,Frame->True,Background->LightYellow]
Out[46]=
```

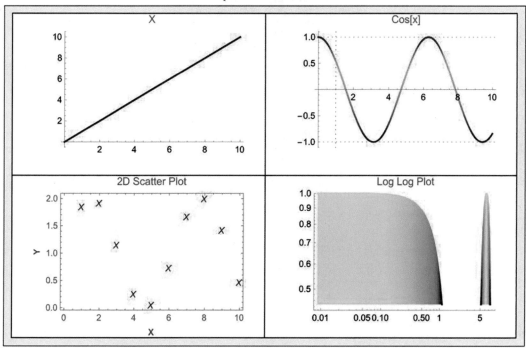

Figure 5-39. *Grid of multiple plots*

This is not restricted to displaying 2D graphs; it also applies to 3D graphs and other types of charts.

Colors Palette

If you are interested in more colors, there is a gamma of various types of colors in Mathematica. For this, go to the menu in Palettes ➤ Color Schemes, as the color palette in Figure 5-40 shows.

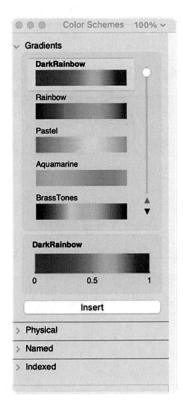

Figure 5-40. *Colors palette*

The tabs that appear are of the colors associated with the different classes. To defer through the colors in the tabs, use the arrows, and the different names of the colors and their color or gradient are displayed. If you want to introduce colors that are not reserved words, then you use the insert button. For example, go to the Gradient tab and click the Insert button, which inserts the function with the chosen color into the notebook.

To illustrate, let's look at the following example. Select the Color BrownCyanTones, insert it with the button, evaluate the expression, and get the result of the ColorDataFunction (see Figure 5-41).

```
In[47]:= ColorData["BrownCyanTones"]
Out[47]=
```

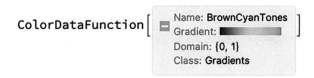

Figure 5-41. *ColorData object*

This gives you a color data object showing the name, color type, class, and domain. Gradient colors are intricate in text and work best with the ColorFunction function. So now that you know the name, you can assign it a color (see Figure 5-42).

```
In[48]:= Plot[x,{x,0,10},ColorFunction->ColorData["BrownCyanTones"]]
Out[48]=
```

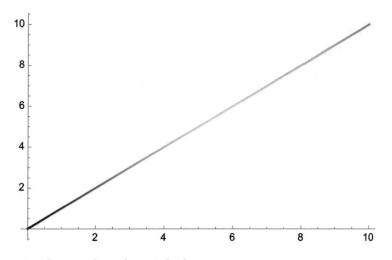

Figure 5-42. *Gradient color of straight line x*

Note   Plain colors are located in the named tab of the palette.

3D Plots

Mathematica can perform various types of 3D graphics, many of which are simple. 3D functions are displayed as surfaces in space. Figure 5-43 presents the example.

```
In[49]:= Plot3D[Sinc[x*8+y^2],{x,-1,2},{y,-1,3},ImageSize->Medium,
PlotPoints->20]
Out[49]=
```

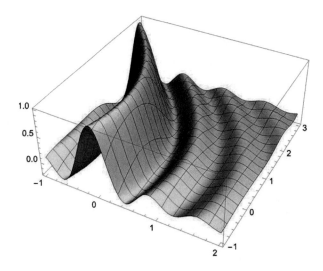

Figure 5-43. *3D plot figure*

Mathematica allows you to observe the graph by moving with the cursor. Hovering over the chart changes the cursor to rotating arrows, which means you can move the chart to observe it from different points. One last observation is that when you press the Ctrl or Cmd key, you can magnify the chart, keeping its position fixed.

Note that the cursor can manipulate 3D graphs so that you can visualize the angle spread graph. Common standard Mathematica displays the graph as a mesh, which can be modified with the Mesh option, as you saw earlier, or by adding more points to evaluate with the PlotPoints option. This increases the number of points in both directions in both x and y. It also serves to improve the quality of the chart.

Customizing 3D Plots

3D graphics can also be customized as 2D graphics (see Figure 5-44) as labels to axes, colors, grids, and so forth. Figure 5-44 shows a 3D plot with the AxesLabel, ColorFunction, and FaceGrids options.

```
In[50]:= Plot3D[Sin[4(x^2+y^2)]/0.5,{x,-0.8,0.8},{y,-0.8,0.8}, AxesLabel->
{"X axis","Y axis","Z axis"},ColorFunction->"Rainbow", FaceGrids->All]
Out[50]=
```

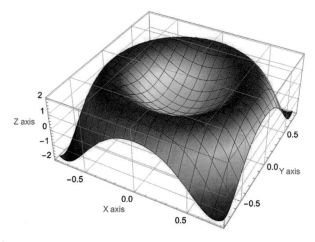

Figure 5-44. *Gridded 3D plot*

Table 5-1 shows general options for 3D graphics.

Table 5-1. *Plot Options*

Option	Instructions
AspectRatio	Height/width ratio
AxesLabel	Add text to axes
PlotStyle	Color, opacity, thickness, etc.
PlotRange	Range of values
PlotLabel	Plot title
Background	Background Color

Customization of graphics depends on how you plan to exhibit them. There is no limit on how graphics are presented. The following example plots a 3D function and colors the background light yellow (see Figure 5-45).

```
In[51]:= Plot3D[Sin[0.9(x^2+y^2)]/0.5,{x,-1,1},{y,-1,1},AxesLabel->
{"X axis","Y axis","Z axis"},FaceGrids->All,ColorFunction->Hue, PlotLabel->
"My 3D Plot",Background->LightYellow,ViewAngle->Pi/7]
Out[51]=
```

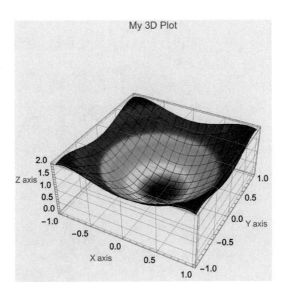

Figure 5-45. *Customized 3D plot*

Hue Color Function and List3D

The Hue color function is a directive that specifies that the values are colored depending on the height they are at. There are three arguments for the Hue color function. The first is for the tone of the color (hue); the second marks the saturation; the third marks the bright one; and the fourth is the opacity. With hue, it is possible to adequately identify the high and low areas from a graph (see Figure 5-46) in the four previous features. You can mark these four different parameters. The hue parameters are in the range of 0 to 1.

```
In[52]:= Plot3D[Sin[0.9(x^2+y^3)]/0.5,{x,-1,1},{y,-1,1}, FaceGrids->
None,ColorFunction -> (Hue[0.5,1,0.6,0.5]&),PlotLabel->Style["My 3D
Plot",Italic,"Arial"], Background->Black]
Out[52]=
```

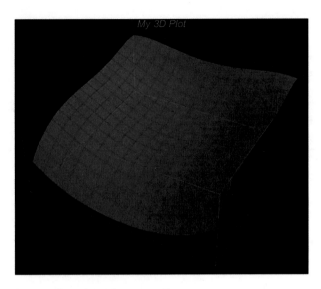

Figure 5-46. *3D plot with colored Hue values*

For 3D scatter plots (see Figure 5-47), you can do it using the same data. With ListPlot3D, the points are joined together to create a surface represented by the height values of each point. With ListPointPlot3D, a scatter plot is generated in 3D points.

```
In[53]:=Row[{ListPlot3D[Table[RandomReal[1,5],{i,5}],ColorFunction->
"SunsetColors",Ticks->None, PlotLegends-> BarLegend[Automatic,
egendMarkerSize->90],ImageSize-> Small,PlotLabel->"ListPlot3D",Filling->
Bottom,BoxRatios-> Automatic] , ListPointPlot3D[Table[RandomReal[1,5],
{i,5}], ColorFunction->"Rainbow", PlotLegends->BarLegend[Automatic,
LegendMarkerSize->90], ImageSize->Small, PlotLabel->" ListPointPlot3D",
Filling->Bottom,BoxStyle->Thick, BoxRatios->{1,1,1}]},Background->Lighter
[Gray,0.80],Frame->True]
Out[53]=
```

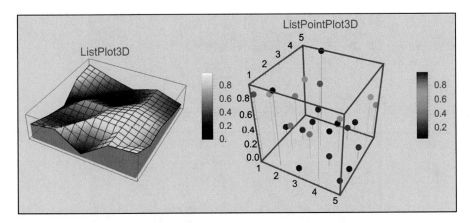

Figure 5-47. *ListPlot3D and ListPointPlot3D for random real numbers*

Contour Plots

One way to visualize a two-variable function is to use a scalar field in which the scalar z = f (x, y) is mapped to the point (x, y). A scalar field can be characterized by its contours (or contour lines) along which the value of f (x, y) is constant. The trace lines of contour line plots or contours can be done using the ContourPlot command, like in the next example.

```
In[54]:= ContourPlot[-((Pi*x)/(3+x^2+y^2)),{x,-5,5},{y,-5,5},ColorFunction-
>"Temperature",PlotLegends->Automatic,FrameLabel->{x,y}]
Out[54]=
```

Figure 5-48 plots a contour plot using the ColorFunction and PlotLegends options. When you use PlotLegends, you specify what type of legends the chart should use; in this case, you use automatic. This shows you the scale of the contours depending on the color of each outline; for example, red is when it is at 0.8 or greater. When you pass the cursor through the contour curves, the value of that curve appears. To label the values of the contour curves in the graph image, add the ContourLabels option and assign the value to true, as shown in Figure 5-49. To add lines that pass through the graph, use the GridLines command, as you saw earlier, or use Mesh. Mesh can be joined with MeshFunction or MeshStyle.

```
In[55]:= ContourPlot[-((Pi*x)/(3+x^2+y^2)), {x,-5,5}, {y,-5,5},
ColorFunction->"DeepSeaColors", PlotLegends-> Automatic, FrameLabel->
```

```
{x,y}, ContourLabels->True, Mesh->{10,10}, MeshStyle->{White},
MeshFunctions-> {#3&}]
Out[55]=
```

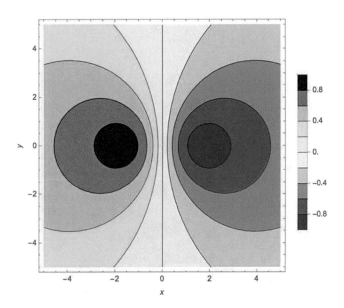

Figure 5-48. *Contour plot for the defined z function*

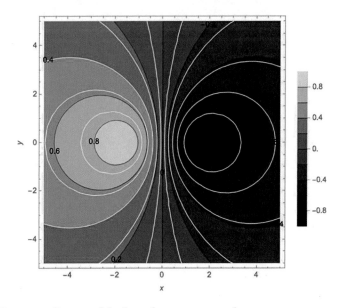

Figure 5-49. *Contour lines added to the contour plot*

To plot data into a contour plot (see Figure 5-50), use ListContourPlot. ListContourPlot creates a contour plot from an array of values shown in heights.

```
In[56]:= ListContourPlot[Table[Exp[x]*Sin[y],{x,0,2,.1},{y,0,2,.1}],
ContourLines->True,Mesh->Full,ContourLabels->True]
Out[56]=
```

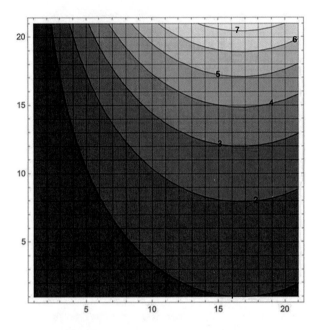

Figure 5-50. *ListContourPlot*

Another plot is DensityPlot (see Figure 5-51). DensityPlot works similarly to ContourPlot.

```
In[57]:= DensityPlot[(Sin[2x]*Cos[3y])/5,{x,0,5},{y,0,5}, ColorFunction->
"SunsetColors", Mesh->Full]
Out[57]=
```

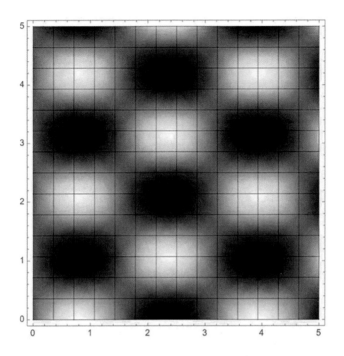

Figure 5-51. *Density plot*

You can plot density plots from data with ListDensityPlot (see Figure 5-52).

```
In[58]:= ListDensityPlot[Table[x/3 + Sin[3 x + y^2], {x, 0, 5, 0.1}, {y, 0,
5, 0.1}],ColorFunction -> "LightTemperatureMap", Mesh -> 10, PlotLegends ->
Placed[Automatic, Left]]
Out[58]=
```

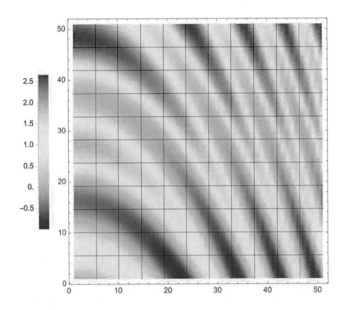

Figure 5-52. *Data represented as a density plot*

3D Plots and 2D Projections

With the Wolfram Language, it is possible to plot functions in 3D and, at the same time, project the contour maps to planes as the axis, as shown in Figure 5-53.

```
In[59]:= Show[Plot3D[(Sin[2 x]*Cos[2 y])/4, {x, 0, 2}, {y, 0, 2},
PlotStyle -> Directive[Opacity[1]], AxesLabel -> {"X axis", "Y axis", "Z
axis"},ColorFunction -> "Rainbow", PlotTheme -> "Marketing"],SliceContourPlo
t3D[(Sin[2 x]*Cos[2 y])/4, {z == -0.15,    z == 0.15}, {x, 0, 2}, {y, 0, 2},
{z, -1, 1}, ColorFunction -> "Rainbow", Boxed -> False],  ViewPoint ->
{1, -1, 1}]
Out[59]=
```

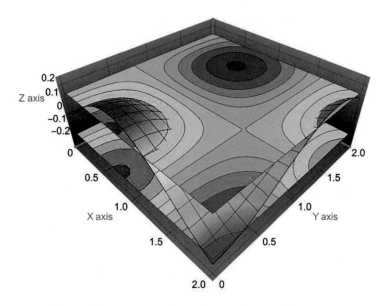

Figure 5-53. *3D plot with contour plots along the xy plane*

Let's discuss what happens in the code. You plot a function in 3D (see Figure 5-53), and to this function, you add color, using the command directive to define the type of opacity, which is set to 1. This is followed by typing the name of the corresponding axes for the x, y, and z axes. The ColorFunction option can help define a function for the color type; in this case, it is Rainbow. The PlotTheme is an option to plot with various themes for visualization. Coming to this point, you move on to the SliceContourPlot3D, which gives you a graph of the function, either on a plane or a surface. you have plotted when z is worth ± 0.15. A cut is made on the xy plane. This occurs when x and y are in the range of 0 to 2, and z is in the range of –1 to 1. In the end, you combine the two graphs with the Show command; you use this command because you would not have the function's graph in 3D only by plotting on its slice contour plot.

Plot Themes

Preconstructed themes can be accessed using the PlotTheme option. You see the autocomplete menu when you add the PlotTheme option, followed by the first apostrophe. Figure 5-54 shows the different themes that exist.

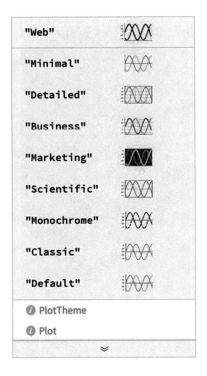

Figure 5-54. *PlotTheme pop-up menu*

PlotTheme supports 3D plots, as shown in Figure 5-55.

```
In[60]:= data=Flatten[Table[{x,y,Sin[10(x^2+y^2)]/10},
{x,-2,2,0.2},{y,-2,2,0.2}],1]; ListPointPlot3D[data,ColorFunction->
"LightTemperatureMap", PlotTheme->"Detailed",ViewPoint->{0,-2,0},
ImageSize->250,PlotLegends->Placed[BarLegend[Automatic, LegendMarkerSize->
90],Left], ImageSize->20]
Out[60]=
```

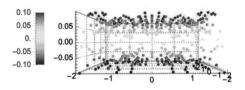

Figure 5-55. *3D scatter plot*

These themes can be used for both 2D and 3D graphics. Now, let's look at another type of theme for a two-dimensional chart (see Figure 5-56).

```
In[61]:= Plot[Cos[x],{x,0,10},PlotLabel->"Cos[x]",PlotTheme-> "Detailed"]
Out[61]= cos(x)
```

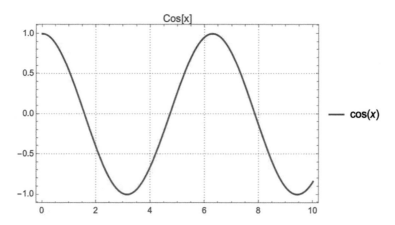

Figure 5-56. *2D plot theme: Detailed*

Let's discuss a characteristic of PlotTheme. Some themes already have functions within these themes. Figure 5-55 shows that the Detailed theme adds frames, plot legends, and grid lines, even though you can add them manually.

It is also notable that other topics can only be used for explanatory and demonstrative purposes—that is, no extra information is needed on the chart, but you need to be able to express the information effectively and concretely, as in the Business and Minimal themes (see Figure 5-57).

```
In[62]:= Table[Plot[Cos[x],{x,0,10},PlotLabel->"Cos[x]",PlotTheme->Pl],{Pl,
{"Business","Minimal"}}]
Out[62]=
```

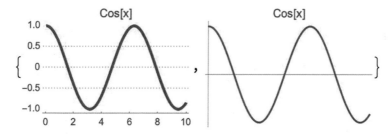

Figure 5-57. *Business and Minimal plot themes*

While there are also topics that show more details, like the Detailed theme you saw earlier, other themes exist, like the Scientific theme, as shown in Figure 5-58. You can add more options, such as ColorFunction and a view, with the ViewProjection option, which allows you a fixed observation point.

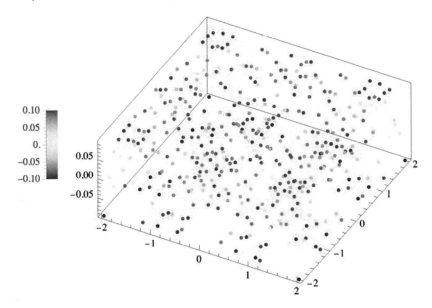

Figure 5-58. *Orthographic point of view*

Note   PlotLegends can work together with ColorFunction, displaying how the colors of the dots transition between blue and red, from lowest to highest.

```
In[63]:= data=Flatten[Table[{x,y,Sin[10(x^2+y^2)]/10},
{x,-2,2,0.2},{y,-2,2,0.2}],1]; ListPointPlot3D[data,ColorFunction->
"LightTemperatureMap",PlotLegends-> Placed[BarLegend[Automatic,
LegendMarkerSize->90],Left], PlotTheme->"Scientific", ViewProjection->
"Orthographic"]
Out[63]=
```

If you want to observe through the coordinate measurements, use the Viewpoint option, which is governed by {x coordinate, y coordinate, z coordinate}. These coordinates are relative to the graph's center, as Figure 5-59 shows.

```
In[64]:= ListPointPlot3D[Data,ColorFunction->"LightTemperatureMap",
PlotLegends->Automatic,PlotTheme->"Scientific", ViewPoint->
{0,0,-2},ImageSize->Medium]
Out[64]=
```

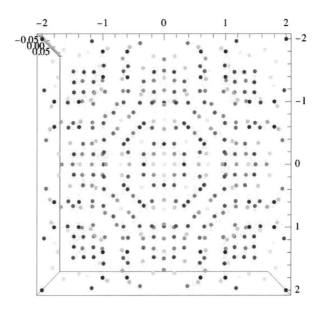

Figure 5-59. *Viewpoint for x and y equal 0 and z equal –2*

Summary

This chapter introduced the basics of data visualization, emphasizing 2D plots, plotting data, and user-defined functions. As progress is made, the section on customizing plots covers text to charts, frames, grids, and filled plots, including further content on fill patterns and gradient filling, followed up by discussing how plot combinations are done, focusing on multiple plots, and coloring plot grids and concentrating on new additions like multi-axes plots. Furthermore, an overview of the color palette was presented, followed by a segmentation of 3D Plots, elaborating on the customization, Hue coloring, and contour plots. Finally, it culminates with an outlook on the variety of plot themes for 3D graphs.

CHAPTER 6

Statistical Data Analysis

This chapter reviews concepts and techniques to analyze with the Wolfram Language, perform a linear adjustment through equations, and implement specialized functions of the Wolfram Language for the same purpose, using statistical functions. The Wolfram Language is a useful tool for statistics and probability. Mathematica has the functions to perform numerical and approximate calculations for descriptive statistics and random distributions, random numbers, and random sampling methods, as you see in this section.

Random Numbers

This section reviews the basic commands to generate random numbers—for the case of integers, real and complex. You see the functions of performing random sampling with replacement and without replacement and, in addition, ensuring that the results are reproducible for random numbers.

To create random numbers, there are several functions to generate random integers and real ones. The RandomInteger function generates entered random numbers; if no arguments are entered in the function, the generation interval is 0 or 1.

```
In[1]:= RandomInteger[]
Out[1]= 0
```

To enter a range, you must define it within the function; for example, between –1 and 1.

```
In[2]:= RandomInteger[{-1,1}]
Out[2]= 1
```

© Jalil Villalobos Alva 2024
J. Villalobos Alva, *Beginning Mathematica and Wolfram for Data Science*,
https://doi.org/10.1007/979-8-8688-0348-2_6

To generate a list of random numbers, you must define how many numbers you want within the list.

```
In[3]:= RandomInteger[{-1,1},7]
Out[3]= {-1,0,1,1,1,1,1}
```

To repeat the numbers, add the form of the list or nested list as a second argument. For example, create a nested list of seven total items in each sublist with four items.

```
In[4]:= RandomInteger[{-10,10},{7,4}]
Out[4]= {{-8,7,7,0},{-4,-8,10,-8},{10,8,-8,0},{-2,-6,8,-10},
{8,-1,-6,-4},{1,4,0,-1},{5,7,9,10}}
```

The function for generating random numbers with a decimal point is called RandomReal. It works similarly to RandomInteger, where the interval is between curly braces.

```
In[5]:= RandomReal[]
Out[5]= 0.020413
```

A command for complex random and prime numbers also exists.

```
In[6]:= RandomComplex[]
Out[6]= 0.727318 +0.998602 I
```

You must define a minimum and maximum interval for random prime numbers—for example, if it is a prime number of the first 100.

```
In[7]:= RandomPrime[{1,100},6]
Out[7]= {89,2,59,71,53,29}
```

This type of function generates pseudorandom numbers so that you can set a seed to generate the numbers. This is done with SeedRandom. With a seed, you can ensure that the starting sequence of random numbers generated is the same to make random outputs reproducible. To set a seed, use the SeedRandom command. The following example sets a seed followed by a sequence of random numbers; once the seed is introduced, the results should be the same for that seed.

```
In[8]:= SeedRandom[6467789];RandomInteger[{-1,1},3]
Out[8]= {0,1,0}
```

The seed must go in the same code block to generate the results. There is the option to choose the method. The following example uses the MersenneTwister method, which generates random numbers. Using another method allows you to generate sequences of different random numbers.

```
In[9]:=SeedRandom[Method->"MersenneTwister"];RandomInteger[{-1,1},{3,3}]
// MatrixForm
Out[9]//MatrixForm
```

$$\begin{pmatrix} -1 & -1 & -1 \\ 0 & 0 & -1 \\ 0 & 0 & 1 \end{pmatrix}$$

The seed enters the function without arguments to return to the original value.

```
In[10]:= SeedRandom[];
```

In addition to introducing a seed, you can create blocks of random numbers in which functions can be used locally and not affect random behavior outside these blocks. This is done with the BlockRandom function.

```
In[11]:= BlockRandom[RandomReal[1]]
Out[11]= 0.774569
```

If you run an algorithm that produces random numbers within the BlockRandom and declare the seed, this should not impact other processes where random numbers are generated outside the BlockRandom. To illustrate, let's look at the example.

```
In[12]:= SeedRandom[121];
{RandomReal[],BlockRandom[RandomReal[]],RandomReal[],RandomReal[]}
Out[13]= {0.994955,0.788549,0.788549,0.957081}
```

As seen, the latter process generated different random numbers

Random Sampling

Use the RandomChoice function to make a sample with a replacement. To select a single item, you write only the list. You set a seed to get the same results.

```
In[14]:= SeedRandom[12345]; ranData=RandomReal[{0,1},10]
Out[15]={0.158069,0.599452,0.656143,0.918006,0.0805897,0.682397,0.638187,
0.431772,0.126333,0.973705}
```

This generated a list of 10 random numbers from 0 to 1, and now you randomly choose an item of these numbers.

```
In[16]:= RandomChoice[ranData]
Out[16]= 0.973705
```

This gives you a single result from the list of 10 items. Similarly, you can choose the number of samples with some elements, with the following form: RandomChoice["data," "number of samples," "several elements"]. You now pick three samples with one element of the ten elements.

```
In[17]:= RandomChoice[ranData,{3,1}]
Out[17]= {{0.126333},{0.431772},{0.973705}}
```

Although, if you want it in the same sample, you only need to specify the number of elements to choose from.

```
In[18]:= RandomChoice[ranData,5]
Out[18]= {0.0805897,0.158069,0.158069,0.0805897,0.973705}
```

To get a sampling without replacement, use RandomSample. This function only chooses a list item from the data list once. To choose, you only specify the number of elements in the sample as the second argument since the first one corresponds to the data list.

```
In[19]:= RandomSample[ranData,9]
Out[19]={0.158069,0.682397,0.431772,0.599452,0.918006,0.638187,0.656143,
0.126333,0.0805897}
```

Looking at the details, you notice that there is no repeated value. Each item in the list is equally likely to be selected in sampling.

In the case that each item in the list has a specific weight associated with it, then to enter those terms, you use the following form of expression, {w1, w2, w3...} → {element1, element2, element3...}; the list of items is associated with a specific weight for replacement sampling. You denote the list of weights and do the sampling by associating the weights and elements.

```
In[20]:=w={0.03`,0.08`,0.22`,0.04`,0.12`,0.3`,0.12`,0.03`,0.04`,0.02`};
RandomChoice[w->ranData,2]
Out[20]= {0.656143,0.638187}
```

They are chosen depending on how each element is assigned a weight. For sampling without replacement, the process is analogous.

```
In[21]:= RandomSample[w->ranData,3]
Out[21]= {0.682397,0.656143,0.599452}
```

Systematic Sampling

To perform a system sampling, you must determine the sample size, M. To get the sample size, you can list the items in the list or get the length of the list. To get started, you create a list of 200 prime numbers.

```
In[22]:= SeedRandom[09876]; rPrime=RandomPrime[{1,100},200];
Length[rPrime]
Out[24]= 200
```

The sample size was already calculated, so you must determine the size of a specific sample; for this case, you want a sample of 20 elements. Once the sample is determined, you calculate the interval of the denoted sampling j; j is calculated through a ratio, the original sample size divided by the total number of elements in the specified sample.

```
In[25]:= j=Length[rPrime]/20
Out[25]= 10
```

This means that the sampling interval for the new sample is from 1 to 10. From here, you select a random number within the interval, and from there, you add j times to choose the next element; that is, for the first element, it is a random h number of the range [1,10], for the second it is h + j, and for the third h + 3j, and so on, until it reaches the size of the original sample.

You chose a random number between 1 and 10.

```
In[26]:= RandomSample[Range[10],1]
Out[26]= {6}
```

The result means that you select from the sixth element. You deploy the list to have a better view of the data.

```
In[27]:= rPrime
Out[27]={7,41,3,7,83,61,41,29,89,5,17,3,41,73,73,67,29,71,23,13,31,19,89,
41,79,19,47,83,13,73,37,67,59,29,13,17,83,43,17,71,89,11,71,23,29,37,89,3,
89,11,41,59,2,37,41,31,59,79,61,13,59,53,53,59,2,43,11,73,41,37,3,31,13,
83,83,3,31,5,37,2,89,23,2,37,23,3,79,17,47,71,79,13,47,13,17,41,71,73,2,
53,29,7,2,7,79,97,83,31,3,43,29,11,37,67,11,41,67,13,23,2,59,53,89,61,29,
19,29,13,11,7,61,71,59,53,5,71,13,43,67,2,73,2,5,67,83,53,11,7,61,71,7,11,
83,59,47,67,17,83,43,53,17,59,11,11,61,2,11,97,2,73,41,7,41,19,41,71,53,3,
3,41,29,5,73,53,79,43,13,19,29,2,73,67,29,41,13,3,43,23,59,89}
```

To get the positions of the items to be selected, it would be the random number for the selection, which is 6, plus n times j until you have 20 elements.

```
In[28]:= Table[6+n*j,{n,0,19}]
Out[28]= {6,16,26,36,46,56,66,76,86,96,106,116,126,136,146,156,166,
176,186,196}
```

Note   Remember that the position index starts from 1 to n elements.

You must choose the positions shown in the previous output. To choose, you use the double square bracket notation.

```
In[29]:= Table[rPrime[[6+n*j]],{n,0,19}]
Out[29]= {61,67,19,17,37,31,43,3,3,41,97,41,19,71,53,67,2,71,43,3}
```

Let's take a closer look at the selected elements, highlighting them in red (here it is plaintext) with the help of MapAt and Style.

```
In[30]:= MapAt[Style[#,FontColor-> ColorData["HTML"]["Red"]]&,
RPrime,{#}&/@{61,67,19,17,37,31,43,3,3,41,97,41,19,71,53,67,2,71,43,3}]
Out[30]={7,41,3,7,83,61,41,29,89,5,17,3,41,73,73,67,29,71,23,13,31,19,89,
41,79,19,47,83,13,73,37,67,59,29,13,17,83,43,17,71,89,11,71,23,29,37,89,3,
89,11,41,59,2,37,41,31,59,79,61,13,59,53,53,59,2,43,11,73,41,37,3,31,13,
83,83,3,31,5,37,2,89,23,2,37,23,3,79,17,47,71,79,13,47,13,17,41,71,73,2,
```

53,29,7,2,7,79,97,83,31,3,43,29,11,37,67,11,41,67,13,23,2,59,53,89,61,29,
19,29,13,11,7,61,71,59,53,5,71,13,43,67,2,73,2,5,67,83,53,11,7,61,71,7,11,
83,59,47,67,17,83,43,53,17,59,11,11,61,2,11,97,2,73,41,7,41,19,41,71,53,3,
3,41,29,5,73,53,79,43,13,19,29,2,73,67,29,41,13,3,43,23,59,89}

As you can see, system sampling does not create a completely random sample. The random selection process comes in the first part when you select the first item to create the new sample. Once the first item is selected, the other selections are from a succession of non-random numbers. Another aspect to consider is the order of the original sample; if the elements are periodic, this can lead to significant variability in the selection of components.

Commons Statistical Measures

Grasping the commonly used statistical formulas is crucial to understanding how the data behaves on a given set of conditions. Descriptive statistics are implemented once data has been collected, and it is one of the first steps in the process of exploratory data analysis, which allows you to find insights into the data collected in terms of discovering patterns, anomalies, trends, seasonality, variations, and so forth.

Exploratory data analysis is a set of techniques to detect characteristics that are not visible at first sight or revealed once the data has been collected. The basic structure of this technique relies on numeric data analysis, graphical representation, and a statistical model. Many reasons to use data exploratory analysis include reviewing for missing data, describing a general and particular idea of the underlying structure, and analyzing for different assumptions associated with the model creation, among many more.

The proposal for such a process was introduced by Jhon Tukey in 1977. To review this technique in more depth, visit the following reference, *Exploratory Data Analysis* (Tukey, J. W. [1977], Vol. 2, pp. 131-160).

Measures of Central Tendency

Given a sample of data, you can calculate the descriptive measures. Central trend measures are those parameters that give you information on the average data values to be studied. The mean, also known as arithmetic mean, is a parameter calculated from the sum of the values of the sample and divided by the sum of the number of elements. The Mean function calculates the average.

```
In[31]:= list1=Table[Prime[i],{i,10}];
"Prime list :"<>ToString@list1
"Mean: "<>ToString@Mean@N@list1
Out[32]= Prime list :{2, 3, 5, 7, 11, 13, 17, 19, 23, 29}
Out[33]= Mean: 12.9
```

Note   The symbol <> is the short notation for StringJoin.

The median is the value that divides the sample into two equal parts; since it is the data's midpoint, the median is the symmetry value relative to the amount of data. The Median function gives you this value.

```
In[34]:= "Median: "<>ToString@Median@list1
Out[34]= Median: 12
```

Mode is the most common value of the sample. You use the Counts command, which gives you the number of occurrences of each item in the list.

```
In[35]:= Counts[list1]
Out[35]= <|2->1,3->1,5->1,7->1,11->1,13->1,17->1,19->1,23->1,29->1|>
```

In this case, the occurrence is 1. There are no repeated values; you can say there is no mode in this data sample.

Measures of Dispersion

Dispersion measurements reveal information on the variability presented in the sample. The range tells you about the interval in which the data varies. This is taken by subtracting the max value and the minimum value. The Max and Min functions return a list's maximum and minimum values.

```
In[36]:= "Range: "<>ToString[Max[list1]-Min[list1]]
Out[36]= Range: 27
```

Variance is a measure obtained by subtracting the mean of each element in the sample. The result is squared, followed by adding the elements together. The summation is divided by the size of the sample. Its function is Variance.

```
In[37]:= "Variance: "<>ToString[N[Variance[list1],3]]
Out[37]= Variance: 81.4
```

Standard deviation is a measurement obtained from the square root of the variance or employing the StandardDeviation function.

```
In[38]:= {"Square root of Variance: " <> ToString[N[Sqrt[Variance[list1]],
2]],"StandardDeviation: " <> ToString[N[StandardDeviation[list1], 2]]}
Out[38]= {Square root of Variance: 9.0,StandardDeviation: 9.0}
```

The standard score, z, is a score that measures how many standard deviations are away from the arithmetic average for each sample element. The mathematical equation is $z = \dfrac{x - \mu}{\sigma}$, where x is the measure, μ the mean, and σ the standard deviation. If z is positive, the element is greater than the mean. When z is negative, it is the opposite case. You determine the z-score for the second item in the list.

```
In[39]:= z=N[(list1[[2]]-Mean@list1)/StandardDeviation@list1,3];
"z score: "<>ToString@z
Out[40]= z score: -1.10
```

This result means that the score for the second element is 1.10 times below average.

Quartile calculation divides data into four equal parts. The lower quartile corresponds to the 25% quartile of the data, while the second quartile is 50%, the third quartile (the upper quartile) is 75%, and the fourth quartile (100%). To calculate the quartiles, you use the Quartiles function, which gives the values of the first, second, and third quartiles.

```
In[41]:= "Quartiles: " <> ToString@Quartiles[list1]
Out[41]= Quartiles: {5, 12, 19}
```

If you want to get a single value, use the Quantile function, followed by the percentile, to be calculated. Then, use the following for calculating the third quartile (75th percentile).

```
In[42]:= Quantile[list1,0.75]
Out[42]= 19
```

To calculate the interquartile range, which is the difference between the upper and lower quartiles, use the InterquartileRange function.

```
In[43]:= InterquartileRange[List1]
Out[43]= 14
```

Statistical Charts

Using charts to display data is a straightforward approach with Mathematica. Many times, studies include various types of information. Mathematica has a repertoire of statistical charts based on users' needs for more visual and understandable presentations.

Bar Charts

Sometimes, when you conduct a statistical study, you can find quantitative and qualitative variables and create a bar graph representation for these variables. A bar graph (see Figure 6-1) is a graphical representation where the number of frequencies of a discrete qualitative variable is displayed on an axis.

```
In[44]:= BarChart[{1,2,3,4},ChartLabels->{"feature 1","feature 2",
"feature 3","feature 4"}]
Out[44]=
```

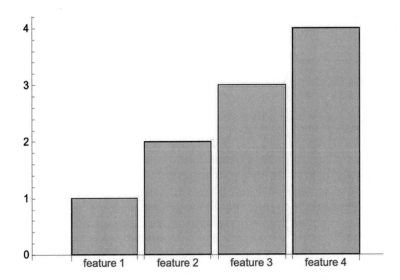

Figure 6-1. *Bar chart*

The different modalities of the qualitative variable are positioned on one of the axes. The other axis shows the value or frequency of each category on a given scale. The feature 2 bar has an associated value of 2. The orientation of the graph can be vertical, where the categories are located on the horizontal axis, and the bars are vertical or horizontal, where the categories are located on the vertical axis. The bars are horizontal (see Figure 6-2).

```
In[45]:= GraphicsRow[{BarChart[{1,2,3,4},ChartLabels->{"feature 1",
"feature 2","feature 3","feature 4"},BarOrigin->Bottom,ChartStyle->
LightBlue],BarChart[{1,2,3,4},ChartLabels->{"feature 1","feature
2","feature 3","feature 4"},BarOrigin->Left,ChartStyle->LightRed]}]
Out[45]=
```

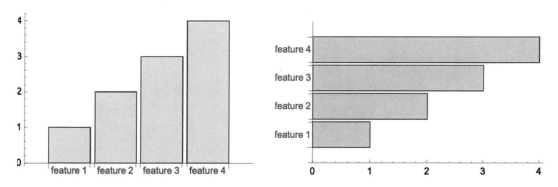

Figure 6-2. *Bottom and left origin bar chart*

Bar graphs can be used to compare magnitudes of different categories and observe how values change according to a fixed variable—for example, each feature. In addition, you can choose how to show the bars, where you show a single series, as shown in the earlier example; grouped, which contains several data series and is represented by a different type of bar; or stacked, where the bar is divided into segments with different colors representing various categories. The percentile layout is displayed on a percentage scale, as shown in Figure 6-3.

```
In[46]:= Labeled[GraphicsGrid[{{BarChart[{{4, 3, 2, 1}, {1, 2, 3}, {3, 5}},
ChartLayout -> "Grouped", ColorFunction -> "SolarColors"], BarChart[{1, 2,
3, 4}, ChartStyle -> LightRed, ChartLayout ->
"Stepped"]}, {BarChart[{{4, 3, 2, 1}, {1, 2, 3}, {6, 5}}, ChartLayout ->
"Stacked"], BarChart[{{4, 3, 2, 1}, {1, 2, 3}, {6, 5}}, ChartLayout ->
```

```
"Percentile", ColorFunction -> "DarkRainbow"]}},
Frame -> All, FrameStyle -> Directive[Black, Dashed], Background ->
LightBlue, ImageSize -> 500], "Bar Charts", Top]
Out[46]=
```

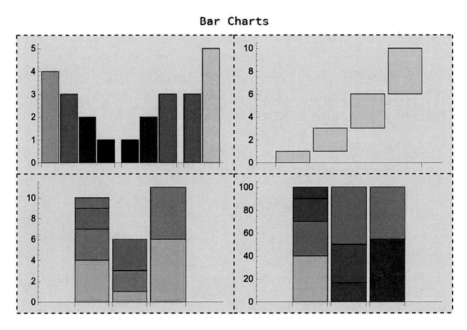

Figure 6-3. *Bar chart grid*

There is also the counterpart to 3D graphics, with BarChart3D (see Figure 6-4).

```
In[47]:= SeedRandom[123];
Labeled[GraphicsGrid[{{BarChart3D[{{4, 3, 2, 1}, {1, 2, 3}, {3, 5}},
ChartLayout -> "Grouped", ColorFunction -> "SolarColors"],
BarChart3D[{1, 2, 3, 4}, ChartStyle -> LightRed, ChartLayout ->
"Stepped"]}, {BarChart3D[RandomReal[1, {10, 5}], ChartLayout -> "Stacked"],
BarChart3D[{{4, 3, 2, 1}, {1, 2, 3}, {6, 5}}, ChartLayout -> "Percentile",
ColorFunction -> "DarkRainbow"]}},  Frame -> All, FrameStyle ->
Directive[Red, Thick],Background -> LightBlue, ImageSize -> 500], "3D Bar
Charts", Top, Frame -> True, Background -> White]
Out[48]=
```

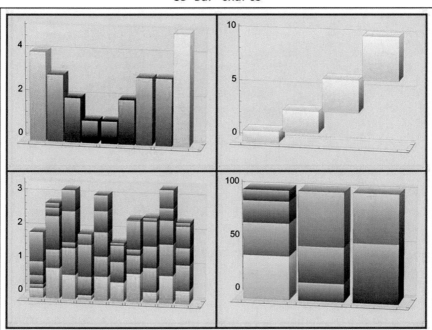

Figure 6-4. *3D bar charts grid*

Histograms

Histograms are a type of visualization that is commonly used in statistical studies. With histograms, you can see how a sample is distributed. Histograms are used to represent the frequencies of a quantitative variable. The variable classes are positioned on the horizontal axis, and the frequencies are on the other axis. The following examples graph a histogram from a population of 50 random values between 0 and 1 and set the number of bins to 10. The second argument for histograms is to define the number of bins (see Figure 6-5).

```
In[49]:= SeedRandom[4322];
hist1=Table[RandomReal[{2,3}],{i,0,20}];
Histogram[hist1,10]
Out[51]=
```

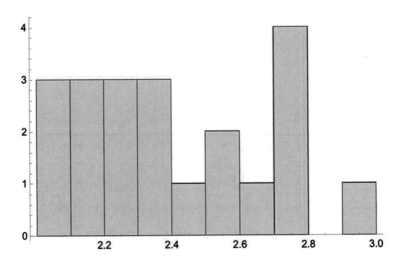

Figure 6-5. *Histogram for random real numbers*

Note   When dealing with charts, if you put the pointer cursor on the graphic, an info tip marks the value.

Just like with bar charts, there are ways to edit the histogram's origin and how the histogram is displayed—stacked or overlapped—as shown in Figure 6-6.

```
In[51]:= hist2=Table[Cos[i],{i,1,20}];
hist3=Table[Sin[i],{i,1,10}];
GraphicsColumn[{Histogram[{hist1,hist2},10,BarOrigin-
>Left,ChartStyle->"Pastel",ChartLegends->{"rand num",
"Cos(x)"}],Histogram[{hist2,hist3},10,ChartLayout->
"Overlapped",ChartStyle->"Pastel",ChartLegends-> {"Cos(x)","Sin(x)
"}],Histogram[{hist2,hist3},10,ChartLayout-> "Stacked",ChartStyle-
>"Pastel",ChartLegends->{"Cos(x)","Sin(x)"}]}]
Out[54]=
```

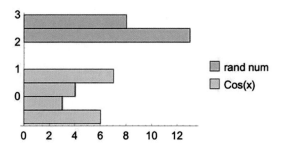

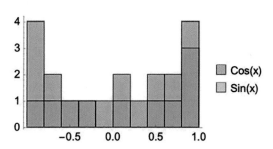

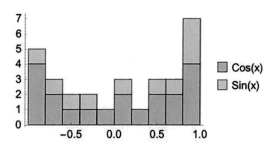

Figure 6-6. *Histogram shapes grid*

With this in mind, you can also graph bidirectional histograms using PairedHistograms. These can be horizontal or vertical orientations and contain two data series whose bars go opposite directions (see Figure 6-7).

```
In[55]:=SeedRandom[123] ;GraphicsRow[{PairedHistogram[{RandomReal[{0,1},20]},
{RandomReal[{0,1},20]},BarOrigin->Left], PairedHistogram[{RandomReal
[{0,1},20]}, {RandomReal[{0,1},20]},10,BarOrigin->Top, ChartStyle->"Pastel"]}]
Out[55]=
```

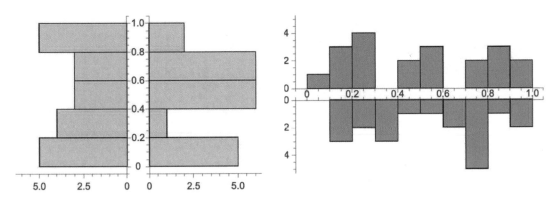

Figure 6-7. *Paired histograms with different origins*

While histograms offer a powerful way to visualize data distribution, you can enhance these visualizations by incorporating various statistical functions directly into the notebook. By default, histograms in the Wolfram Language display data counts within each bin. However, it's often valuable to visualize cumulative distribution functions (CDFs) and probability density functions (PDFs), like the following example and Figure 6-8.

```
In[56]:= (*common options*)
continuousOpts = {Filling -> Axis, Frame -> True, FrameLabel -> {"X", #},
PlotLabel -> "Continuous " <> #} &;
(*Continuous PDF and CDF plots*)
continuousPlots =
 Grid[{{Labeled[Plot[PDF[NormalDistribution[0, 1], x], {x, -3, 3},
Evaluate@continuousOpts["PDF"],  PlotStyle -> Directive[Blue,
Opacity[0.5]]], "PDF", Top],  Labeled[Plot[CDF[NormalDistribution[0,
1], x], {x, -5, 5},  Evaluate@continuousOpts["CDF"], PlotStyle ->
Directive[Red, Thick]], "CDF", Top]}}, Frame -> All]
Out[57]=
```

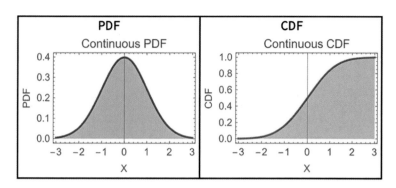

Figure 6-8. *PDF and CDF plots for the standard normal distribution*

The previous code generates the PDF and CDF plots for a continuous distribution, for a standard normal distribution (mean 0, standard deviation 1). It uses the distributions as arguments for the PDF and CDF functions. The plots are labeled accordingly for clarity. Similarly, the process can be done to discrete distributions (see Figure 6-9).

```
In[57]:= (*common options*)
discreteOpts = {ExtentSize -> Full, Frame -> True, FrameLabel -> {"x", #},
PlotLabel -> "Discrete " <> #} &;
(*Discrete PDF and CDF plots*)
discretePlots =  Grid[{{Labeled[ DiscretePlot[PDF[BinomialDistribution
[10, 0.5], x], {x, 0, 10}, Evaluate@discreteOpts["PDF"], PlotStyle ->
Directive[Green, Opacity[0.5]]], "PDF", Top], Labeled[DiscretePlot[CDF
[BinomialDistribution[10, 0.5], x], {x, 0, 10}, Evaluate@discreteOpts["CDF"],
PlotStyle -> Directive[Orange, Thick]], "CDF", Top]}}, Frame -> All]
Out[58]=
```

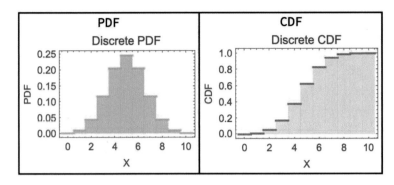

Figure 6-9. *PDF and CDF plots for the binomial distribution with parameters n=10 and p=0.5*

Pie Charts and Sector Charts

Pie charts are circles that are divided into two or more sections. They represent quantitative variables that make up a total; for example, the sector's size is drawn proportional to the value it represents and is expressed in percentages, which only provides relative quantitative information. Pie charts are made with the PieChart command (see Figure 6-10).

```
In[59]:= GraphicsRow[{PieChart[{1,1,1},ChartLegends->{"part a","part b",
"part c"},ChartStyle->{LightRed,LightBlue,LightYellow}], PieChart[{1,1},
ChartLegends->{"part a","part b"},ChartStyle-> "SunsetColors"]}]
Out[59]=
```

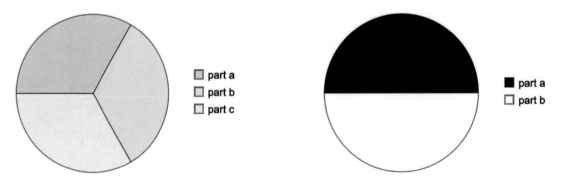

Figure 6-10. *Pie charts*

Sector charts are graphed with the SectorChart command (see Figure 6-11). They are used to compare different data that occur in the same place. They are constructed from the proportional size of x to the value of the radius of y. The dimension in which the quantities are expressed must be the same for all the segments.

```
In[60]:= SectorChart[{{2,1},{1,2}},ChartLegends->{"Sector a","Sector b"},
ChartStyle->{LightRed,LightYellow}]
Out[60]=
```

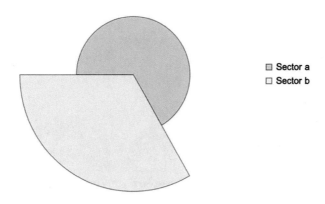

Figure 6-11. *Sector chart*

For each graph seen, there is a corresponding command to create them in 3D, as shown in Figure 6-12.

```
In[61]:=
GraphicsGrid[{{SectorChart3D[{{2, 1, 1}, {3, 1, 2}, {1, 2, 2}},
PlotLabel -> "3D Sector chart",    ChartStyle -> {Red, Blue,
Yellow}],   PieChart3D[{1, 1, 1}, ChartStyle -> "GrayTones",    PlotLabel
-> "3D Pie Chart"]}, {Histogram3D[    Table[{i^3, i^-1}, {i, 20}], 10,
ChartElementFunction -> "GradientScaleCube",    PlotLabel -> "3D
Histogram"], None}}, ImageSize -> 500,  Frame -> True, FrameStyle ->
Directive[Thick, Dotted]]
Out[61]=
```

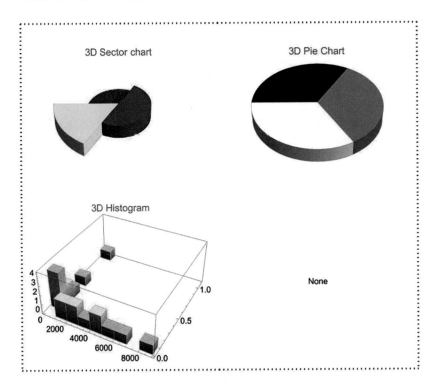

Figure 6-12. *3D grid charts*

Box Plots

The box plot is a way of representing and observing a data distribution. Fundamentally, it highlights aspects of data distribution in one or more series. To graph a box plot, you use the BoxWhiskerChart command (see Figure 6-13).

```
In[62]:= SeedRandom[1234] BoxWhiskerChart[{Table[RandomReal[],{i,0,50}],
Table[RandomReal[],{i,0,50}], Table[RandomReal[],{i,0,15}]},ChartLabels→
{"Chart 1","Chart 2","Chart 3"}]
Out[62]=
```

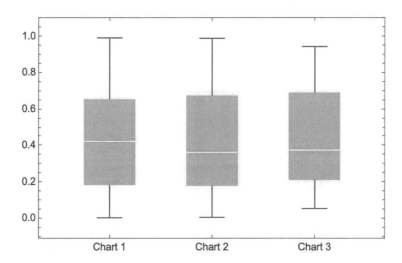

Figure 6-13. *Box plot*

The box is represented by a rectangle that marks the interquartile range of the distribution. The first line from bottom to top marks the value of the first quartile (25%), the line that crosses the box is the median, and the last line that delimits the box is the third quartile (75%). Whiskers are the lines that mark the maximum and minimum values. When passing the mouse cursor over the plot, information about the data is shown; this includes minimum, maximum, median, 75th percentile, and first quartile. Depending on the specification, this can affect the parameters displayed and how (see Figure 6-14).

```
In[62]:= SeedRandom[123];
data = {Table[RandomReal[], {i,0,50}],Table[RandomReal[], {i,0,50}],
Table[RandomReal[], {i,0,15}]};
options = {ImageSize -> Medium, ChartStyle -> "MintColors", FrameStyle ->
Directive[White, 12]};
GraphicsGrid[{{BoxWhiskerChart[data, "Median", PlotLabel -> Style["Median",
White], options], BoxWhiskerChart[data, "Basic", PlotLabel ->
Style["Basic", LightOrange], FrameStyle -> Directive[Orange, 12], options],
BoxWhiskerChart[data, "Notched",
PlotLabel -> Style["Notched", White], options]},
{BoxWhiskerChart[data, "Outliers", PlotLabel -> Style["Outliers",
LightOrange], FrameStyle -> Directive[Orange, 12], options],
BoxWhiskerChart[data, "Mean", PlotLabel -> Style["Mean",
```

```
White], options],BoxWhiskerChart[data, "Diamond", PlotLabel ->
Style["Diamond", LightOrange], FrameStyle -> Directive[Orange, 12],
options]}},FrameTicksStyle -> 18, Frame -> {None, None, {{1, 1} -> True,
{2, 2} -> True, {1, 3} -> True}}, FrameStyle -> Directive[Thick, Red],
Background -> Black]
Out[63]=
```

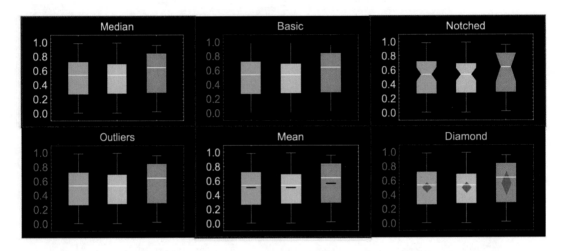

Figure 6-14. *Multiple box plots*

Median is the default specification; it shows the median in the center of the box. Basic is to show only the box. Notches show the confidence interval for the median. Outliers show and mark the atypical points. The mean marks the average of the distribution, and Diamond notes the confidence interval for the mean.

Distribution Chart

A violin diagram is used to visualize the distribution of the data and the probability density. To plot a violin plot (see Figure 6-15), the DistributionChart command is used.

```
In[64]:= DistributionChart[Table[i^Exp[i],{i,0,1,0.01}]]
Out[64]=
```

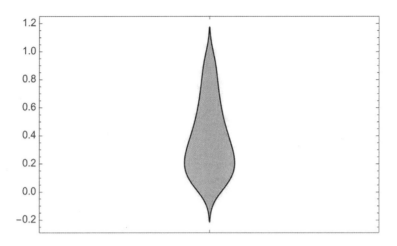

Figure 6-15. *Violin plot*

The graph in the figure combines a box-and-whisker plot and a density plot on each side to show how the data is distributed. DistributionChart has different shapes to graph (see Figure 6-16).

```
In[65]:= GraphicsGrid[{{DistributionChart[Table[i^Exp[i], {i, 0, 2, 0.1}],
ChartElementFunction -> "SmoothDensity", PlotLabel -> "SmoothDensity"],
DistributionChart[Table[i^Exp[i], {i, 1, 2, 0.1}], ChartElementFunction ->
"Density", PlotLabel -> "Density",
FrameStyle -> Directive[Red, 12]]}, {DistributionChart[ Table[i^Exp[i],
{i, 0, 1, 0.09}], ChartElementFunction -> "HistogramDensity", PlotLabel ->
"HistogramDensity", FrameStyle -> Directive[Red, 12]], DistributionChart
[Table[i^Exp[i], {i, 0, 1, 0.0112}], ChartElementFunction -> "PointDensity",
PlotLabel -> "PointDensity"]}}, ImageSize -> Medium, FrameStyle ->
Directive[Thickness[0.02], LightGray], Dividers -> {2 -> Directive[Black,
Dotted], 2 -> Directive[Black, Dotted]}, Frame -> {1 -> False, False}]
Out[65]=
```

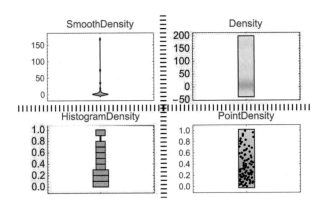

Figure 6-16. *Violin plots in different shapes*

Charts Palette

Another way to add options to charts is through the Chart Element Schemes palette, found within the Palettes menu (Palettes ➤ Chart Element Schemes). This palette is shown in Figure 6-17.

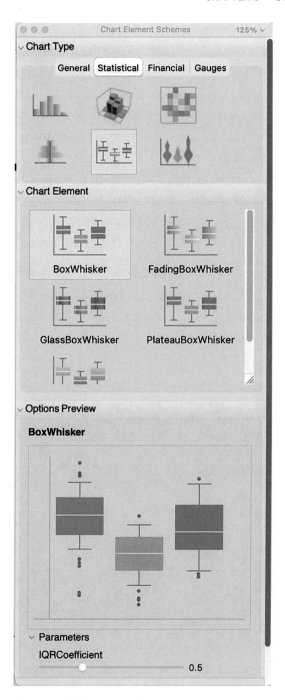

Figure 6-17. *Chart Element Schemes palette*

In the palette, you find three categories. Chart Type is where you choose the type of chart. This contains four tabs: (1) general, where the graphics are found from bar charts, sector, footer, and others; (2) statistical graphs associated with data distributions; (3) financial, associated with charts for financial data; and (4) gauges, which are diagrams of measures. The second category is to choose the shape of the graph with the ChartElementFunction option. The third category is for the preview of the options chosen from the previous categories.

To illustrate this, let's look at the following exercises. First, make the graph of the density of a histogram, and later, modify the shape of the graph with the help of the palette. To graph the density of a histogram, use the DensityHistogram command (see Figure 6-18).

```
In[66]:= DensityHistogram[Flatten[Table[{x^2+y^2,x^2-y^2},
{x,0,2,0.1},{y,0,2,0.1}],1],ChartBaseStyle->Red,ColorFunction->
"SolarColors",Background->Black,FrameStyle->Directive[White,Thick],
FrameLabel->{"X","Y"},ImageSize->300]
Out[66]=
```

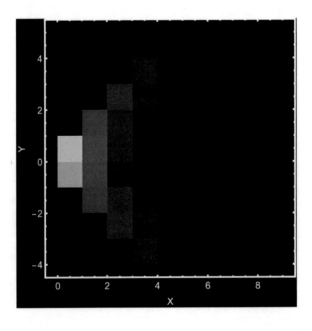

Figure 6-18. *Density histogram*

Once the graph is done, add an option with the pallet head and open the Chart Element Schemes palette. Within the chart type, you click the statistical tab and choose the DensityHistogram chart. Once the chart has been selected, go to Chart Element and select that the type of form is Bubble. Then go to Options Preview to see how the graph would look; if you click Shape, a pop-up menu appears with other shapes; you choose hexagon. Figure 6-19 shows how the preview of the selected chart elements should look.

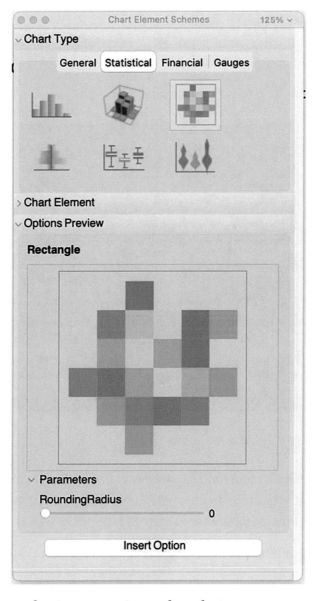

Figure 6-19. *Density histogram options selected*

Once you finish selecting, click the insert button so that it inserts the following code: ChartElementFunction ➤ ChartElementDataFunction ["Bubble", "Shape" ➤ "Hexagon"]. To graph it correctly, add this code as an option and proceed to plot it (see Figure 6-20) to observe the new option added.

```
In[67]:= DensityHistogram[Flatten[Table[{x^2 + y^2, x^2 - y^2}, {x, 0,
2, 0.1}, {y, 0, 2, 0.1}], 1], ChartBaseStyle -> Red, ColorFunction ->
"SolarColors", Background -> Black, FrameStyle -> Directive[White,
Thick], FrameLabel -> {"X", "Y"}, ImageSize -> 300, ChartElementFunction ->
ChartElementDataFunction["Bubble", "Shape" -> "Hexagon"]]
Out[67]=
```

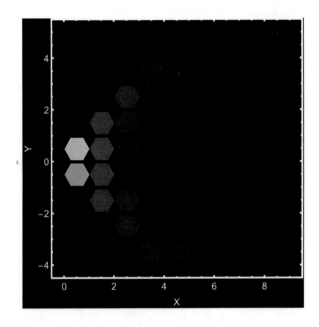

Figure 6-20. *Hexagon density histogram*

The DensityHistogram command allows you to choose how to display the data distribution along the axes; it can be the dimensions, box plots, or histograms if you select the Method type as an option (see Figure 6-21).

```
In[68]:= hist = Flatten[Table[{x^2+y^2,x^2-y^2}, {x,0,2,0.1},
{y,0,2,0.1}],1];
densityHistogram[distAxes_, colFunc_, baseStyle_, plotLabel_,
imgSize_] := DensityHistogram[Hist, Method -> {"DistributionAxes" ->
```

```
distAxes},ColorFunction -> colFunc, ChartBaseStyle -> baseStyle, PlotLabel
-> Style[plotLabel, Bold], ChartLegends -> Automatic,
ChartElementFunction -> ChartElementDataFunction["Bubble", "Shape"
-> "Hexagon"],ImageSize -> imgSize] {MenuView[{densityHistogram
[True, GrayLevel, Directive[FaceForm[Opacity[0.5]], EdgeForm[Red]],
"Density Histogram 1", 200], densityHistogram["Histogram",
Automatic,  Directive[EdgeForm[Thick]], "Density Histogram 2", 200],
densityHistogram["BoxWhisker", "BlueGreenYellow", Automatic, "Density
Histogram 3", 200]}], GraphicsRow[{densityHistogram[True, GrayLevel, Direct
ive[FaceForm[Opacity[0.5]], EdgeForm[Red]],
"Density Histogram 1", 130], densityHistogram["Histogram", Automatic,
Directive[EdgeForm[Thick]], "Density Histogram 2", 130],
densityHistogram["BoxWhisker", "BlueGreenYellow", Automatic, "Density
Histogram 3", 130]}]]}
Out[70]=
```

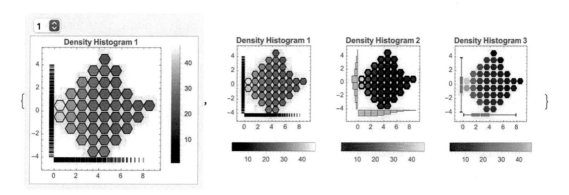

Figure 6-21. *Menu view of the three different method plots*

The plots are shown inside as a menu, so to access the different graphs, you have
to select each graph within the menu. Even so, you show the plots on a small scale
to demonstrate how they should look (see Figure 6-21). The first graph shows the
dimensions of the data distribution along the axes. The second shows the distribution of
the data in the form of histograms, and the third shows the box plots.

Ordinary Least Squares Method

The ordinary least squares method finds the best-fitting line through data points. This method is used to study the relationship between the dependent variable and the independent variable. The process is based on the expression of finding a line of the form y = mx ⊦ b, where x is the independent variable, y is the dependent variable, m is the slope, and b is the y-intercept. The slope and the sorted to origin b are calculated from the following equations.

$$m = \frac{n * \sum(x*y) - \sum x * \sum y}{n * \sum x^2 - |\sum x|^2}$$

$$b = \frac{\sum y * \sum x^2 - \sum x * \sum(x*y)}{n * \sum x^2 - |\sum x|^2}$$

The summation is denoted by the Greek capital letter sigma ($\sum$); n is the amount of data in the sample. The method is calculated for measured data pairs and slope values, and y-intercept sources are calculated to create the best data fit to a line. By substituting in the general equation, you get the equation of the line for the dataset.

To illustrate the method, let's look at the following example using the points for the dependent and the independent variables.

```
In[71]:= data={{-1,10},{0,9},{1,7},{2,5},{3,4},{4,3},{5,0},{7,-1}};
Grid[Transpose[Prepend[data,{"X","Y"}]],Dividers->{2->True,2->
True},Alignment-> Center]
Out[72]=
```

```
X | -1 0 1 2 3 4 5 7
__|_____
Y | 10 9 7 5 4 3 0 -1
```

Next, calculate the data needed to get the slope and y-intercept.

```
In[73]:=n = Length[data];
sumX = Total@data[[All, 1]];
sumY = Total@data[[All, 2]];
sumXY = Total[data[[All, 1]]*data[[All, 2]]];
sumXSqr = Total@(data[[All, 1]]^2);
```

```
m = N@((n*sumXY-sumX*sumY)/n*sumXSqr-Abs[sumX]^2);
b = N@((sumY*sumXSqr-sumX*sumXY)/n*sumXSqr-Abs[sumX]^2);
```

Use the Solve command to solve the equation of the shape y = mx + b. The first argument is the equation, and the second is for the variable to solve. You must use the same double notation to enter the equation since a single equal is for set instruction.

```
In[80]:= Solve[SetPrecision[y==m*x+b,3],y]
Out[80]= {{y->8.47-1.47 x}}
```

This results in the equation of the line being y = 1.47 x + 8.47. Given this equation, you plot the points and the line that best fits these points (see Figure 6-22).

```
In[81]:= Show[Plot[b + m*x,{x,-1,8}, PlotLegends->Placed["Linear Fit: y=-
1.47x+8.47",{0.6,0.8}],PlotRange->Automatic], ListPlot[data, PlotStyle
-> Red]]
Out[81]=
```

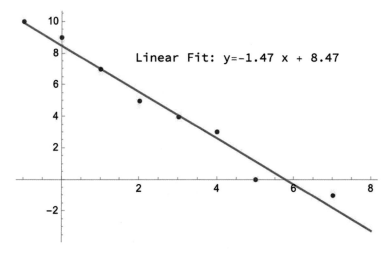

Figure 6-22. *Plot of data and fitted curve*

Having obtained the equation, you observe that this is a model with a negative slope, corroborated by the equation graph shown in blue.

Pearson Coefficient

The measure that tells you that both the points fit the equation is the Pearson correlation coefficient named r. When the points are found with a positive slope, r has a positive value. When the points are negatively sloped, r has a negative value. The coefficient value determines the correct setting, ranging from –1 to 1. When the r value is 1 or –1, it tells you that the points are adjusted exactly to the line. The closer r is to –1 or 1 indicates that there appears to be a linear relationship between the study variables. Otherwise, when r is equal to 0, it tells you that the setting is not correct, and therefore, it can be concluded that there is no apparent linear relationship.

The equation for determining the coefficient is as follows.

$$r = \frac{Cov(x*y)}{\sigma_x \sigma_y},$$

Cov represents the covariance of x, y. The symbols σx and σy represent the standard deviations of x and y.

Now, you proceed to calculate the coefficient r for the created adjustment. For this, you must introduce only the points of x and y, for calculating covariance and standard deviations.

```
In[82]:= r= N@(Covariance@@{data [[All,1]],data [[All,2]]} /
(StandardDeviation@data[[All,1]]*StandardDeviation@data[[All,2]]))
Out[82]= -0.987814
```

The result is close to 1; therefore, the straight is adequately fair to the data. Although it is possible to calculate it through the equation, Mathematica has a function for this calculation. Correlation calculates the coefficient from two lists, so you need to enter only the x data in one list and the data from y in another list.

```
In[83]:= N@Correlation[data[[All,1]],data[[All,2]]]
Out[83]= -0.987814
```

And you get the same result as the previous one.

Linear Fit

Mathematica has functions that specialize in finding the best linear model using LinearModelFit. Given the dataset, you write the LinearModelFit command with the data to work and the variable to write the equation. In addition, you can specify the level of precision for adjustment with WorkingPrecision.

```
In[84]:= model=LinearModelFit[data,x,x,WorkingPrecision->10]
Out[84]= FittedModel[8.473684211-1.466165414 x]
```

The same equation returns to you but with better precision. Within the model, you can access different properties related to the data, the model, and other adjustment parameters, as well as measures of the goodness of the fit, among others. To illustrate this, you see how to do it for the BestFit, BestFitParameters, and Function options, which return the best-fit equation as a list, the best parameters, and model construction for a pure function, respectively.

A critical aspect is that trying to make predictions about a future value using the fitted equation (8.47 – 1.47 x), with values of x outside the range, could generate abnormal values since you have not established whether the relation of the equation outside the range of x is met. Figure 6-23 shows the fitted curve calculations.

```
In[85]:= {"\n" Framed["Best Fit Parameters b and m: " <>
ToString[model["BestFitParameters"]], Background -> LightYellow], "\n"
Framed["Equation: " <> ToString[model["BestFit"]],  Background ->
LightYellow], "\n" Framed["Pure Function:" <> ToString[SetPrecision[model[
"Function"], 3]], Background -> LightYellow], "\n" Framed["r coeficcient:"
<> ToString[r], Background -> LightYellow]}
Out[85]=
```

Figure 6-23. *Fitted parameters, equation, and Pearson coefficient*

Since you have the line that best fits, you should consider whether a relationship exists between x and y. How do you know if the adjustment adequately describes the linear relationship between the x and y variables? To solve this problem, there is the concept of residual.

Model Properties

Residuals can be used as a measure to know how good the fit of the line is to the study points. Residuals are vertical deviations, either positive or negative. A residual point is the difference between the observed value of the dependent variable and the value that predicts the adjustment. To get the residual points, write the FitResiduals property within the model.

```
In[86]:= model["FitResiduals"]
Out[86]= {0.06015038,0.52631579,-0.00751880,-0.54135338,-0.07518797,
0.39097744,-1.14285714,0.78947368}
```

With these points, you can get the residual plot (see Figure 6-24), which is the x variable vs. the residual points.

```
In[87]:= ListPlot[model["FitResiduals"],PlotStyle->{Red,Thick},
PlotLabel->"Residual Plot",AxesLabel-> {Style["X",Bold], Style["residual
points",Bold]},Filling->Axis]
Out[87]=
```

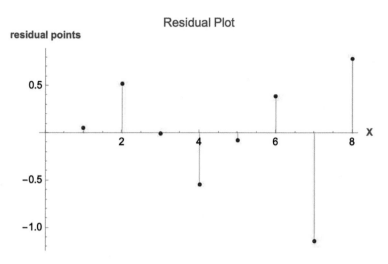

Figure 6-24. *Residual plot of the fitted data*

To show only the observed and predated values for the single prediction, use the SinglePredictionConfidenceIntervalTable option.

```
In[88]:= model["SinglePredictionConfidenceIntervalTable"]
Out[88]=
```

Observed	Predicted	Standard Error	Confidence Interval
10	9.93984962	0.78481739	{8.0194706,11.8602286}
9	8.47368421	0.74856412	{6.6420138,10.3053546}
7	7.00751880	0.72287410	{5.2387096,8.7763280}
5	5.54135338	0.70889670	{3.8067456,7.2759611}
4	4.07518797	0.70732661	{2.3444221,5.8059538}
3	2.60902256	0.71824519	{0.8515399,4.3665052}
0	1.14285714	0.74110068	{-0.6705509,2.9562652}
-1	-1.78947368	0.81811053	{-3.7913180,0.2123707}

In addition to the residual points, you can extract the table from the parameters of the model adjusted with the ParameterTable property.

```
In[89]:= model["ParameterTable"]
Out[89]=
```

	Estimate	Standard Error	t-Statistic	P-Value
1	8.473684211	0.34167121	24.800697	$2.8278226*10^{-7}$
x	-1.466165414	0.094310214	-15.5461996	$4.4832546*10^{-6}$

The coefficients are shown in the table. The first coefficient is the ordinate to the origin, and the coefficient associated with the e variable is the slope. The two coefficients have their respective standard errors. To know the confidence interval for the parameters, you write the ParameterConfidenceIntervalTable property.

```
In[90]:= model["ParameterConfidenceIntervalTable"]
Out[90]=
```

	Estimate	Standard Error	Confidence Interval
1	8.473684211	0.34167121	{7.63764488,9.30972355}
x	-1.466165414	0.094310214	{-1.69693419,-1.23539663}

The default confidence interval is 95%. With these confidence values, you can plot the points inside or outside this range (see Figure 6-25), extracting the values from the predictions and setting the option for the confidence interval to 0.95.

```
In[91]:= model[x];
model["SinglePredictionBands", ConfidenceLevel -> 0.95]; Show[
ListPlot[data, PlotStyle -> Red], Plot[{Model[x],
Model["SinglePredictionBands", ConfidenceLevel -> 0.95]}, {x, -1, 10},
Filling -> {2 -> {1}}], PlotRange -> {Automatic, {-1, 10}}, Frame -> True,
ImageSize -> 400]
Out[92]=
```

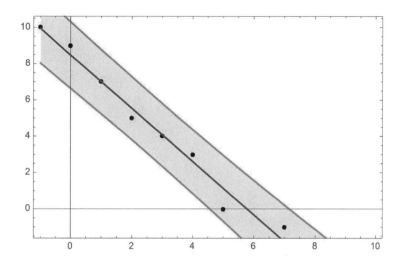

Figure 6-25. *The filled region denotes the 95% confidence interval*

Finally, to obtain the properties related to the sum of the squared errors, you use the ANOVATable property.

```
In[93]:= model["ANOVATable"]
Out[93]=
```

	DF	SS	MS	F-Statistic	P-Value
X	1	107.213346	107.213346	241.68432	$4.48325*10^{-6}$
Error	6	2.6616541	0.44360902		
Total	7	109.8750000			

Summary

This chapter covered the concepts and techniques for conducting statistical analysis using the Wolfram Language and how to perform linear adjustments (least squares, linear fit) through equations and implement specialized statistical functions—demonstrating that the Wolfram Language is an effective statistical tool. In addition, you also view the reference functions available in Mathematica for numerical and approximate calculations of descriptive statistics, random distributions, numbers, and sampling methods.

CHAPTER 7

Data Exploration

This chapter looks at the basics of data management through the Wolfram Data Repository online platform and its use in Mathematica. You also learn how data is viewed inside datasets and how to apply user functions and query commands.

Wolfram Data Repository

The Wolfram Data Repository is a data repository in the cloud. This data repository contains information from different categories, such as computer science, meteorology, agriculture, sports, text and literature education, and many more. Although this repository belongs to Wolfram Research, it is characterized by being in the public domain.

The Wolfram Data Repository consists of computable data selected, structured, and cured for direct use to perform numerical calculations, estimates, analysis, statistics, or demonstrations. The content hosted in this repository is data from many sources, globally known datasets, and publication data. All this information is designed so that any individual can access it globally. The Wolfram Data Repository system provides a data source that, in turn, also enables the storage of new information. The information stored in the repository is designed to directly implement the Wolfram Language.

As you saw in the data import section, you know whether the website is active by receiving an HTTP-type response, as shown in Figure 7-1.

```
In[1]:= URLRead["https://datarepository.wolframcloud.com/"]
Out[1]=
```

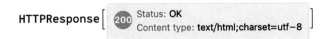

Figure 7-1. *HTTP response object of the Wolfram Data Repository. As you can see, you have received a successful response.*

Wolfram Data Repository Website

To access this website, enter the following URL address in your favorite browser: `https://datarepository.wolframcloud.com`. Figure 7-2 shows the welcome page of the Wolfram Data Repository.

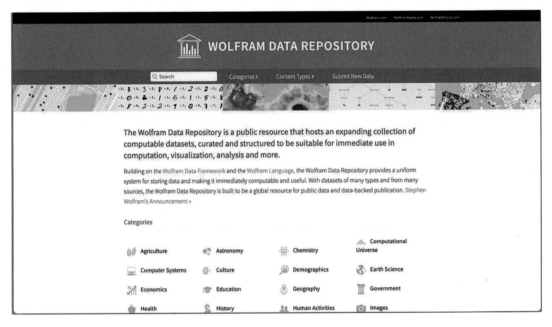

Figure 7-2. *Wolfram Data Repository website*

Note   The images that appear are links that redirect to the dataset associated with that image.

Once the site is loaded, you see a menu of options to navigate the site, either by categories or data type. Within that menu, you find the different categories and data types: text, numerical data, images, and so forth. You also find the contact option, custom searches, and Submit New Data among the menu options. The latter is the option that redirects to another page that displays the instructions for publishing and uploading new data to this repository. Scrolling down, you also see the existing categories and the data types. If so, there is the possibility to browse all resources by clicking the Browse All Resources link (bottom of the web page). To browse categories, you can choose the category from the menu or by clicking the category name at the initial site. Figure 7-3 shows what the site looks like once you have selected a category—in this case, Life Science.

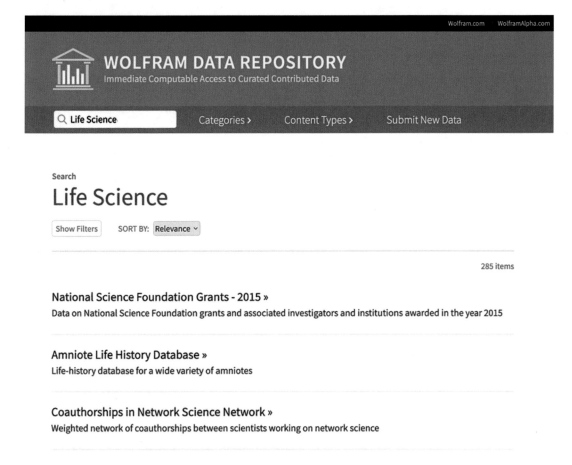

Figure 7-3. *Life Science category of the Wolfram Data Repository*

Note   The same process is for navigating by data type. As new data is added, content is updated regularly.

Selecting a Category

Each category shows the title, the number of elements in that category, and the option to filter the category's contents by the data type. Regarding the content, each sample data type is displayed with its title, a small description of the data it contains, and the different tags associated with that sample data. For example, the image shows Fisher's Irises' known dataset. Once you select a sample dataset, it takes you to the site where the relevant information about that dataset is contained, as shown in Figure 7-4, where the Fisher's Irises dataset is selected.

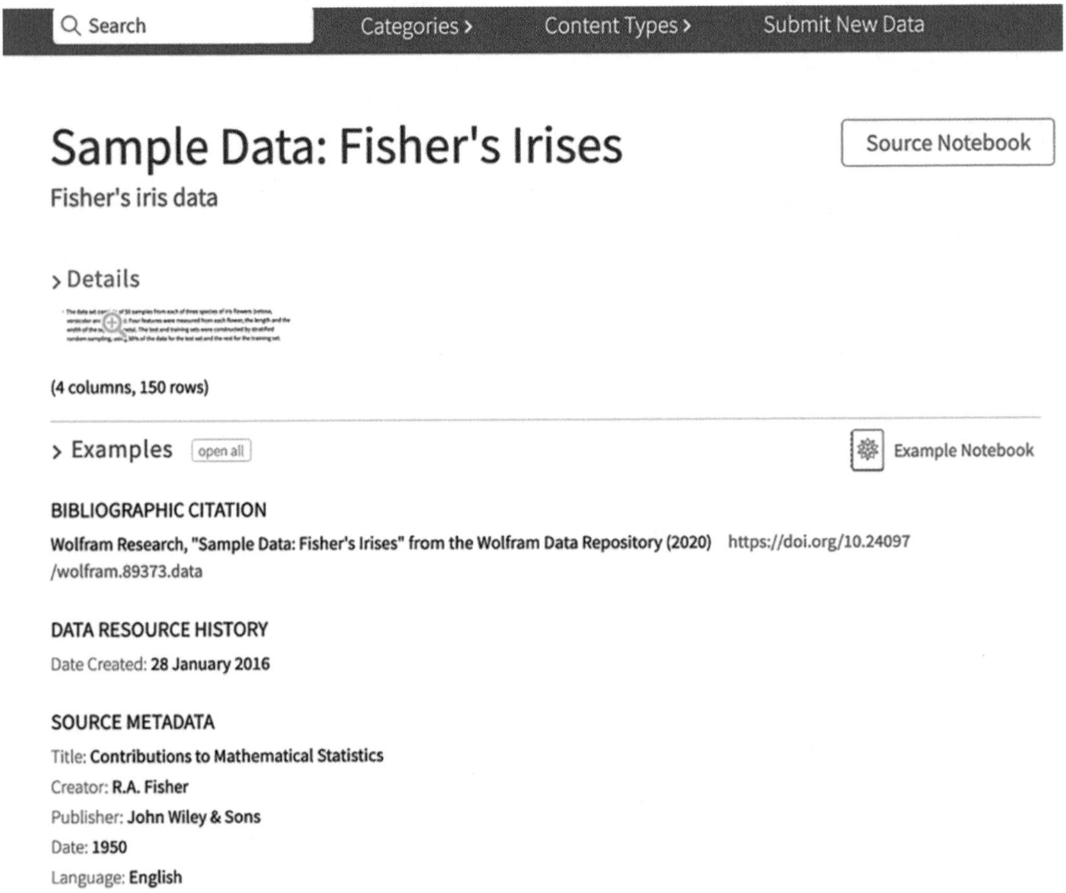

Figure 7-4. *Fisher's Irises dataset*

When a sample dataset is selected, a brief description of the dataset is shown, as well as the different calculations that can be made and different formats to download the data or the notebook. Besides this, it also includes relevant information such as the bibliographic citation, data resource history, and data source. In some instances, the data can be downloaded for different types of formats, such as comma-separated value (CSV), tab-separated value (TSV), JavaScript object notation (JSON), and others. Before starting to download data from the Wolfram Data Repository, it is necessary to have a Wolfram ID. This ID is an account that gives you access to the content of the Wolfram Data Repository in addition to other benefits, such as Wolfram One and Wolfram Alpha. To log in from Mathematica, head to the menu in Help ➤ Sign in, and a window appear like the one in Figure 7-5.

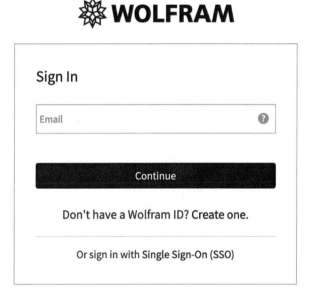

Figure 7-5. *Wolfram Cloud sign-in prompt*

In the new window, you enter your email and password to access the contents of the Wolfram Data Repository from Mathematica.

Extracting Data from the Wolfram Data Repository

Let's start by looking at the information and properties of the Fisher's dataset; for this, you must retrieve the information through a ResourceObject. With ResourceObject (see Figure 7-6), you can now view the different properties of the published data by clicking the plus icon. Detailed information about the data is displayed, such as sample name, type, version, size of the data, and many more.

```
In[2]:= ResourceObject["Sample Data: Fisher's Irises"]
Out[2]=
```

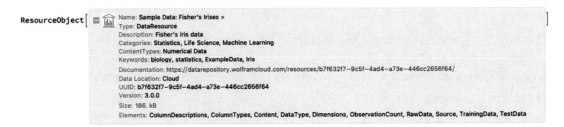

Figure 7-6. *ResourceObject Fisher's Irises*

If you want to look at the properties of the resource object, enter the following code. This code gives you a list of properties that can be accessed and related to the data sample.

```
In[3]:= ResourceObject["Sample Data: Fisher's Irises"]["Properties"]
Out[3]= {AllVersions, AutoUpdate, Categories, ContentElementLocations,
ContentElements, ContentSize, ContentTypes, ContributorInformation,
DatedElementVersions, DefaultContentElement, Description, Details,
Documentation, DocumentationLink, DOI, DownloadedVersion, ExampleNotebook,
ExampleNotebookObject, Format, InformationElements, Keywords,
LatestUpdate, Name, Originator, Properties, PublisherUUID, ReleaseDate,
RepositoryLocation, ResourceLocations, ResourceType, SeeAlso, ShortName,
SourceMetadata, UUID, Version, VersionInformation, VersionsAvailable,
WolframLanguageVersionRequired}
```

Knowing the list of properties related to information, you can now download from Mathematica the exercise notebook of the data sample.

```
In[4]:=ResourceObject["Sample Data: Fisher's Irises"]["ExampleNotebook"]
Out[4]= NotebookObject[Sample Data: Fisher's Irises | Example Notebook]
```

Once you finish evaluating the code, it automatically opens the new notebook. If you want to operate the notebook from the cloud, you can type NotebookObject. This output gives you back a cloud-like object associated with a hyperlink.

```
In[5]:= ResourceObject["Sample Data: Fisher's Irises"]
["ExampleNotebookObject"]
Out[5]= CloudObject[https://www.wolframcloud.com/obj/5e59b79e-d95e-4f6f-
a7c8-f1276ba17be2]
```

If you press the link of the new notebook, it opens the Internet browser and shows you that it is in the Wolfram Cloud. Figure 7-7 shows this.

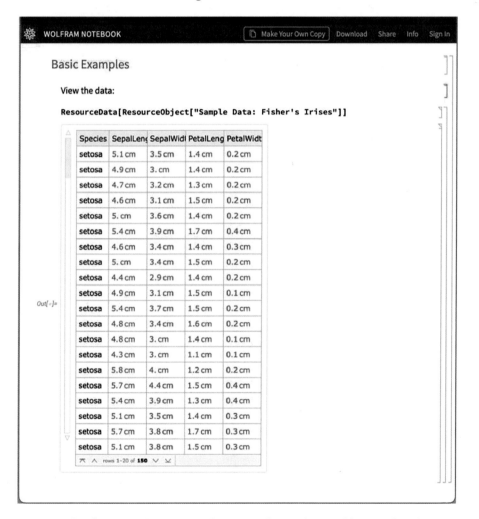

Figure 7-7. *Fisher's Irises data sample, open from the Wolfram Cloud*

To access the original sample data site from Mathematica, enter **Documentation**, which gives you a URL object that you can enter by clicking the double chevron icon.

```
In[6]:= ResourceObject["Sample Data: Fisher's Irises"] ["Documentation"]
Out[6]=URL[https://datarepository.wolframcloud.com/resources/
b7f632f7-9c5f-4ad4-a73e-446cc2656f64/]
```

Accessing Data Inside Mathematica

The same initiative is applied to downloading the data using the ResourceData to the object resource. With ResourceData, you access the contents of the specified resource; in this case, it is the Fisher's Irises data sample (see Figure 7-8).

```
In[7]:= ResourceData[ResourceObject["Sample Data: Fisher's Irises"]]
Out[7]=
```

Species	SepalLength	SepalWidth	PetalLength	PetalWidth
setosa	5.1 cm	3.5 cm	1.4 cm	0.2 cm
setosa	4.9 cm	3. cm	1.4 cm	0.2 cm
setosa	4.7 cm	3.2 cm	1.3 cm	0.2 cm
setosa	4.6 cm	3.1 cm	1.5 cm	0.2 cm
setosa	5. cm	3.6 cm	1.4 cm	0.2 cm
setosa	5.4 cm	3.9 cm	1.7 cm	0.4 cm
setosa	4.6 cm	3.4 cm	1.4 cm	0.3 cm
setosa	5. cm	3.4 cm	1.5 cm	0.2 cm
setosa	4.4 cm	2.9 cm	1.4 cm	0.2 cm
setosa	4.9 cm	3.1 cm	1.5 cm	0.1 cm
setosa	5.4 cm	3.7 cm	1.5 cm	0.2 cm
setosa	4.8 cm	3.4 cm	1.6 cm	0.2 cm
setosa	4.8 cm	3. cm	1.4 cm	0.1 cm
setosa	4.3 cm	3. cm	1.1 cm	0.1 cm
setosa	5.8 cm	4. cm	1.2 cm	0.2 cm
setosa	5.7 cm	4.4 cm	1.5 cm	0.4 cm
setosa	5.4 cm	3.9 cm	1.3 cm	0.4 cm
setosa	5.1 cm	3.5 cm	1.4 cm	0.3 cm
setosa	5.7 cm	3.8 cm	1.7 cm	0.3 cm
setosa	5.1 cm	3.8 cm	1.5 cm	0.3 cm

⊼ ∧ rows 1–20 of **150** ∨ ⊻

Figure 7-8. *Fisher's Irises dataset object*

As shown in Figure 7-8, the returned object is a ResourceData to use with a head of the dataset. Performing a visual inspection of the data sample, you observe that it is a dataset of 150 values containing five columns: Species, SepalLength, SepalWidth, PetalLength, and PetalWidth. If you pay attention, you can see how the values of the SepalLength, SepalWidth, PetalLength, and PetalWidth columns are quantities. Moving further down the entire dataset, the species are divided into three categories: setosa, versicolor, and virginica. If you want to access the information related to the dataset, you must do it through the resource object and retrieve it through a ResourceData form, as shown.

```
In[8]:=ResourceObject["Sample Data: Fisher's Irises"]
["ContentElements"]
Out[8]= {ColumnDescriptions, ColumnTypes, Content, DataType, Dimensions,
ObservationCount, RawData, Source, TrainingData,
TestData}
```

With the ContentElements property, you are accessing the elements of the data sample, which are the ones that appear within the resource object. ContentElements shows you the information associated with the sample data, such as column information, data source, training data, and test data—not to be confused with the properties of the resource object created, as it is not the same since you can construct a resource object for another associated name. To retrieve the information from the ContentElements, you must do it with ResourceData. This command gives you access to the contents of the data sample—in this case, the Fisher's Irises. Now, let's get the data type of the columns.

```
In[9]:= ResourceData[ResourceObject["Sample Data: Fisher's
Irises"],"ColumnTypes"]
Out[9]= {Numeric,Numeric,Numeric,Numeric,Categorical}
```

The second argument of the ResourceData command is the element you are looking for. Running the code mentioned above shows you that there are four data types: three numeric and one categorical. Using a pure function, you can obtain information in a single expression. If you add the Column command, it is possible to have a better view of the information.

```
In[10]:= Column[ResourceData[ResourceObject["Sample Data: Fisher's
Irises"],#]&/@{"ColumnDescriptions","Dimensions","Source"}]
Out[10]= {Sepal length in cm.,Sepal width in cm.,Petal length in cm.,Petal
width in cm.,Species of iris}
{150,4}
Fisher,R.A. "The use of multiple measurements in taxonomic problems"
Annual Eugenics, 7, Part II, 179-188 (1936); also in "Contributions to
Mathematical Statistics" (John Wiley, NY, 1950).
```

This way, you get to know the type of information in the columns, such as dimensions, which are 150 rows per four columns, and the data source.

Data Observation and Querying

This section explains how to observe data inside a dataset. You use the Iris dataset, which has been extracted from the Wolfram Data Repository. Let's start by naming the data sample Fisher; this variable contains the dataset with quantities included.

```
In[11]:= fisher=ResourceData[ResourceObject["Sample Data: Fisher's
Irises"]];
```

In the dataset, the numbers have units and magnitude. Having a dataset, you can perform endless processes, such as grouping the content by the category variable, which is the type of species. (This example accessed the dataset contained in the Fisher's variable.) Let's look at the data that includes each column grouped by species (see Figure 7-9).

```
In[12]:= fisher[GroupBy["Species"]]
Out[12]=
```

	Species	SepalLength	SepalWidth	PetalLength	PetalWidth
setosa	setosa	5.1 cm	3.5 cm	1.4 cm	0.2 cm
	setosa	4.9 cm	3. cm	1.4 cm	0.2 cm
	setosa	4.7 cm	3.2 cm	1.3 cm	0.2 cm
	setosa	4.6 cm	3.1 cm	1.5 cm	0.2 cm
	setosa	5. cm	3.6 cm	1.4 cm	0.2 cm
	50 total ›				
versicolor	versicolor	7. cm	3.2 cm	4.7 cm	1.4 cm
	versicolor	6.4 cm	3.2 cm	4.5 cm	1.5 cm
	versicolor	6.9 cm	3.1 cm	4.9 cm	1.5 cm
	versicolor	5.5 cm	2.3 cm	4. cm	1.3 cm
	versicolor	6.5 cm	2.8 cm	4.6 cm	1.5 cm
	50 total ›				
virginica	virginica	6.3 cm	3.3 cm	6. cm	2.5 cm
	virginica	5.8 cm	2.7 cm	5.1 cm	1.9 cm
	virginica	7.1 cm	3. cm	5.9 cm	2.1 cm
	virginica	6.3 cm	2.9 cm	5.6 cm	1.8 cm
	virginica	6.5 cm	3. cm	5.8 cm	2.2 cm
	50 total ›				

Figure 7-9. *Iris data grouped by species*

Let's look at how the data is divided into three categories: setosa, versicolor, and virginica. Each category contains a number 50 at the end of the Species column of each category. This means that there are 50 more rows in addition to those shown, making a total of 50 for each category, which is 150 rows in total, which matches the number of 150 you review the dimensions of the sample data.

In the meantime, clicking one of the categories shows you the columns for that category alone, as shown in Figure 7-10. The same happens if you select a specific column within a category—it shows only that column for that category; try it to see what happens. There is also the possibility to click any column, and this shows you only the chosen column for the three categories. This means that if you choose SepalLength, for example, you see the contents of that column for the three species, as shown in Figure 7-10.

⊞ › All › All › SepalLength

setosa	5.1 cm	4.9 cm	4.7 cm	4.6 cm	5. cm
	5.4 cm	4.6 cm	5. cm	4.4 cm	4.9 cm
	5.4 cm	4.8 cm	4.8 cm	4.3 cm	5.8 cm
	5.7 cm	5.4 cm	5.1 cm	5.7 cm	5.1 cm
	5.4 cm	5.1 cm	4.6 cm	5.1 cm	4.8 cm
	50 total ›				
versicolor	7. cm	6.4 cm	6.9 cm	5.5 cm	6.5 cm
	5.7 cm	6.3 cm	4.9 cm	6.6 cm	5.2 cm
	5. cm	5.9 cm	6. cm	6.1 cm	5.6 cm
	6.7 cm	5.6 cm	5.8 cm	6.2 cm	5.6 cm
	5.9 cm	6.1 cm	6.3 cm	6.1 cm	6.4 cm
	50 total ›				
virginica	6.3 cm	5.8 cm	7.1 cm	6.3 cm	6.5 cm
	7.6 cm	4.9 cm	7.3 cm	6.7 cm	7.2 cm
	6.5 cm	6.4 cm	6.8 cm	5.7 cm	5.8 cm
	6.4 cm	6.5 cm	7.7 cm	7.7 cm	6. cm
	6.9 cm	5.6 cm	7.7 cm	6.3 cm	6.7 cm
	50 total ›				

Figure 7-10. *SepalLength column selected*

It is possible to group by species and choose only the columns that contain numeric values. This helps if, for example, you want to visually inspect the dataset (see Figure 7-11).

```
In[13]:= Query[GroupBy[ Key["Species"] -> KeyTake[{"SepalLength",
"SepalWidth", "PetalLength",  "PetalWidth"}]]][fisher]
Out[13]=
```

	SepalLength	SepalWidth	PetalLength	PetalWidth
setosa	5.1 cm	3.5 cm	1.4 cm	0.2 cm
	4.9 cm	3. cm	1.4 cm	0.2 cm
	4.7 cm	3.2 cm	1.3 cm	0.2 cm
	4.6 cm	3.1 cm	1.5 cm	0.2 cm
	5. cm	3.6 cm	1.4 cm	0.2 cm
	50 total ›			
versicolor	7. cm	3.2 cm	4.7 cm	1.4 cm
	6.4 cm	3.2 cm	4.5 cm	1.5 cm
	6.9 cm	3.1 cm	4.9 cm	1.5 cm
	5.5 cm	2.3 cm	4. cm	1.3 cm
	6.5 cm	2.8 cm	4.6 cm	1.5 cm
	50 total ›			
virginica	6.3 cm	3.3 cm	6. cm	2.5 cm
	5.8 cm	2.7 cm	5.1 cm	1.9 cm
	7.1 cm	3. cm	5.9 cm	2.1 cm
	6.3 cm	2.9 cm	5.6 cm	1.8 cm
	6.5 cm	3. cm	5.8 cm	2.2 cm
	50 total ›			

Figure 7-11. *Dataset with the species column suppressed*

In the latter code, you use the Key command to access the keys of the species column. Once these keys are accessed, you write a transformation rule so that each extracted key is assigned the associations extracted (KeyTake) from columns (SepalLength, SepalWidth, PetalLength, PetalWidth), then grouped and applied to Fisher's dataset.

If you wanted to count the data elements in Fisher's dataset, you could add an ID column as a label (see Figure 7-12) to list the data it contains. To achieve this, first, create an association with keys and values that go from 1 to the length of the dataset. Then, this instruction is applied to the dataset object Fisher's, which adds the IDs as labels for the rows.

```
In[14]:= Query[AssociationThread[Range[Length@#]→Range[Length@#]]]
[fisher]&[fisher]
Out[14]=
```

	Species	SepalLength	SepalWidth	PetalLength	PetalWidth
1	setosa	5.1 cm	3.5 cm	1.4 cm	0.2 cm
2	setosa	4.9 cm	3. cm	1.4 cm	0.2 cm
3	setosa	4.7 cm	3.2 cm	1.3 cm	0.2 cm
4	setosa	4.6 cm	3.1 cm	1.5 cm	0.2 cm
5	setosa	5. cm	3.6 cm	1.4 cm	0.2 cm
6	setosa	5.4 cm	3.9 cm	1.7 cm	0.4 cm
7	setosa	4.6 cm	3.4 cm	1.4 cm	0.3 cm
8	setosa	5. cm	3.4 cm	1.5 cm	0.2 cm
9	setosa	4.4 cm	2.9 cm	1.4 cm	0.2 cm
10	setosa	4.9 cm	3.1 cm	1.5 cm	0.1 cm
11	setosa	5.4 cm	3.7 cm	1.5 cm	0.2 cm
12	setosa	4.8 cm	3.4 cm	1.6 cm	0.2 cm
13	setosa	4.8 cm	3. cm	1.4 cm	0.1 cm
14	setosa	4.3 cm	3. cm	1.1 cm	0.1 cm
15	setosa	5.8 cm	4. cm	1.2 cm	0.2 cm
16	setosa	5.7 cm	4.4 cm	1.5 cm	0.4 cm
17	setosa	5.4 cm	3.9 cm	1.3 cm	0.4 cm
18	setosa	5.1 cm	3.5 cm	1.4 cm	0.3 cm
19	setosa	5.7 cm	3.8 cm	1.7 cm	0.3 cm
20	setosa	5.1 cm	3.8 cm	1.5 cm	0.3 cm

rows 1–20 of **150**

Figure 7-12. *IDs added to the Fisher's dataset*

If you drag down the bar, you see that the counter reaches 150 elements.

You can use the Counts command if you don't want to add an enumerated column to count the elements (see Figure 7-13).

```
In[15]:= Fisher[Counts,"Species"]
Out[15]=
```

setosa	50
versicolor	50
virginica	50

Figure 7-13. *Counted elements on the dataset*

This results in 50 data belonging to setosa, versicolor, and virginica. If you add them up, you get 150. You can also use the Query command, Query[Counts, "Species"] [Fisher].

Now, let's look at how to get the average of the three categories for each column. It would be possible if you knew the average of SepalLength, SepalWidth, PetalLength, and PetalWidth for the species, setosa, versicolor, and virginica, as exhibited in Figure 7-14.

```
In[16]:=Query[GroupBy[Key["Species"]→KeyTake[{"SepalLength","SepalWidth",
"PetalLength","PetalWidth"}]],Mean][fisher]
Out[16]=
```

	SepalLength	SepalWidth	PetalLength	PetalWidth
setosa	5.006 cm	3.428 cm	1.462 cm	0.246 cm
versicolor	5.936 cm	2.77 cm	4.26 cm	1.326 cm
virginica	6.588 cm	2.974 cm	5.552 cm	2.026 cm

Figure 7-14. *Mean for the four columns, divided by species*

But, if you want to get the average of the columns for all categories, one way to get it would be by applying Mean as a query to the number of columns in the entire dataset (see Figure 7-15).

```
In[17]:= Query[Mean][fisher[[All,2;;5]]]
Out[17]=
```

SepalLength	5.84333 cm
SepalWidth	3.05733 cm
PetalLength	3.758 cm
PetalWidth	1.19933 cm

Figure 7-15. *Average values for the four columns of all species*

Note   The Mean command works with the quantities and returns the average to use as a quantity.

Descriptive Statistics

This section demonstrates how to perform descriptive statistics of the Irises data and computations inside the dataset format and how to create custom grid formats. Let's start by building the function that calculates the maximum, minimum, mean, median, first, and third quartile.

```
In[18]:
stats[data_]:=
{{#[{"Max: ",Max@data}]},
{#[{"Min: ",Min@data}]},
{#[{"Mean: ",Mean@data}]},
{#[{"Median: ",Median@data}]},
{#[{"1st quartile: ",Quantile[data,0.25]}]},
{#[{"3rd quartile: ",Quantile[data,0.75]}]}
}&[Row]
```

Now, apply the created function to each of the columns. This function is to get overall statistics for SepalLength, SepalWidth, PetalLength, and PetalWidth (see Figure 7-16).

```
In[20]:= {{#1,#2,#3,#4},{Fisher[Stats,#1],Fisher[Stats,#2],Fisher[Stats,
#3],Fisher[Stats,#4]}}&["SepalLength","SepalWidth","PetalLength",
"PetalWidth"]//Grid
Out[20]=
```

SepalLength	SepalWidth	PetalLength	PetalWidth
Max:7.9 cm	Max:4.4 cm	Max:6.9 cm	Max:2.5 cm
Min:4.3 cm	Min:2. cm	Min:1. cm	Min:0.1 cm
Mean:5.84333 cm	Mean:3.05733 cm	Mean:3.758 cm	Mean:1.19933 cm
Median:5.8 cm	Median:3. cm	Median:4.35 cm	Median:1.3 cm
1st quartile:5.1 cm	1st quartile:2.8 cm	1st quartile:1.6 cm	1st quartile:0.3 cm
3rd quartile:6.4 cm	3rd quartile:3.3 cm	3rd quartile:5.1 cm	3rd quartile:1.8 cm

Figure 7-16. *Function Stats applied to each column*

This also can be displayed in a compact form in a tab format with TabView (see Figure 7-17).

```
In[21]:= TabView[{#1->Fisher[Stats,#1],#2->Fisher[Stats,#2],#3->
Fisher[Stats,#3],#4->Fisher[Stats,#4]},ControlPlacement-> Left]&
["SepalLength","SepalWidth","PetalLength","PetalWidth"]
Out[21]=
```

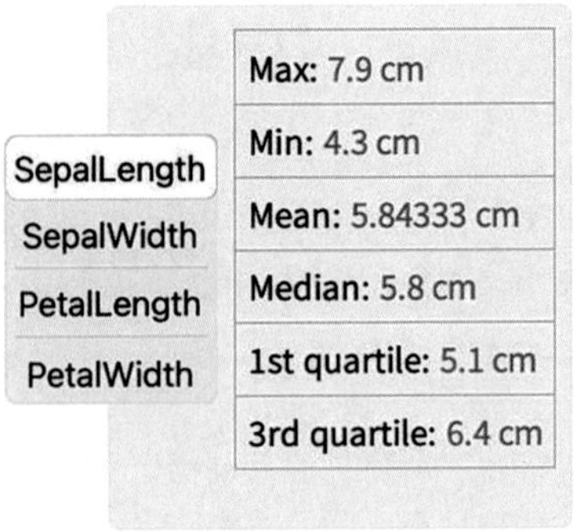

	Max: 7.9 cm
SepalLength	Min: 4.3 cm
SepalWidth	Mean: 5.84333 cm
PetalLength	Median: 5.8 cm
PetalWidth	1st quartile: 5.1 cm
	3rd quartile: 6.4 cm

Figure 7-17. *Tabview format*

With TabView, you create three tabs with the names of each column, which shows the values maximum, minimum, average, median, first, and third quartile; the columns are SepalLength, SepalWidth, PetalLength, and PetalWidth.

Table and Grid Formats

An alternative is to create a table for each species. In this way, you better present the data and thus be able to read it properly. You extract the data by applying the Nest command. With this command, you can specify the number of times a command or function is applied; in this case, you apply it twice.

```
In[22]:= Short[Values[Nest[Normal,fisher,2]]]
{sLall,sWall,pLall,pWall}=%[[All,#]]&/@{2,3,4,5};
Out[22]//Short= {{setosa,5.1cm,3.5cm,1.4cm,0.2cm},{setosa,4.9cm,3.cm,1.4cm,
0.2cm},<<146>>,{virginica,6.2cm,3.4cm,5.4cm,2.3cm},{virginica,5.9cm,3.cm,
5.1cm,1.8cm}}
```

Having the values of all species separated by columns, you create a list instead of a function, where the statistics are displayed according to each column, adding calculations such as variance, standard deviation, skewness, and kurtosis. Then, you assign the calculations in the DescriptiveStats variable.

```
In[23]:={Max[#],Min[#],Median[#],Mean[#],Variance[#],StandardDeviat
ion[#],Skewness[#],Kurtosis[#],Quantile[#,0.25],Quantile[#,.75]}&/@
{sLall,sWall,pLall,pWall};
```

A table (see Figure 7-18) can be created with these calculations and adding the rows and column headings.

```
In[24]:= tableHeads={Style["Sepal Length",#1,ColorData["HTML"]
["Maroon"],#2,#3],Style["Sepal Width",#1,ColorData["HTML"]["YellowGreen"],
#2,#3],Style["Petal Length",#1,ColorData["HTML"]["SteelBlue"],#2,#3],Style
["Petal Width",#1,ColorData["HTML"]["Orange"],#2,#3]}&["Title",Italic,20];
tableRows={Style["Max",#1,#2],Style["Min",#1,#2],Style["Median",#1,#2],
Style["Mean",#1,#2],Style["Variance",#1,#2],Style["Standard\n Deviati
on",#1,#2],Style["Skewness",#1,#2],Style["Kurtosis",#1,#2],Style["1st
quartile",#1,#2],Style["3rd quartile",#1,#2]}&["Text",Italic];TableForm
[descriptiveStats,TableHeadings->{tableHeads,tableRows}]
Out[25]//TableForm=
```

	Max	Min	Median	Mean	Variance	Standard Deviation	Skewness	Kurtosis	1st quartile	3rd quartile
Sepal Length	7.9 cm	4.3 cm	5.8 cm	5.84333 cm	0.685694 cm²	0.828066 cm	0.311753	2.42643	5.1 cm	6.4 cm
Sepal Width	4.4 cm	2. cm	3. cm	3.05733 cm	0.189979 cm²	0.435866 cm	0.315767	3.18098	2.8 cm	3.3 cm
Petal Length	6.9 cm	1. cm	4.35 cm	3.758 cm	3.11628 cm²	1.7653 cm	-0.272128	1.60446	1.6 cm	5.1 cm
Petal Width	2.5 cm	0.1 cm	1.3 cm	1.19933 cm	0.581006 cm²	0.762238 cm	-0.101934	1.66393	0.3 cm	1.8 cm

Figure 7-18. *Table showing descriptive statistics by the four features*

Note that the statistics are calculated with their units, except for skewness and kurtosis, since, by definition, they are dimensionless. However, you can create a better structure from Grid because it is possible to add dividers like a spreadsheet format. To do this, you add the TableRows to the data and then apply a transpose so that each calculated statistic is with its respective name. Subsequently, you add the column titles.

```
In[26]:=
Transpose[Prepend[descriptiveStats,tableRows]];
{" ",Style["Sepal Length",#1, ColorData["HTML"]["Maroon"],#2,#3],
Style["Sepal Width",#1,ColorData["HTML"]["YellowGreen"],#
2,#3],Style["Petal Length",#1, ColorData["HTML"]["SteelBlue"],#2,
#3], Style["Petal Width",#1,ColorData["HTML"]["Orange"],
#2,#3]}&["Title",Italic,20];
newTable=Prepend[%%,%];
```

Next, create the table as a spreadsheet (see Figure 7-19).

```
In[27]:= Grid[newTable,ItemSize->{{None,Scaled[0.11], Scaled[0.11],
Scaled[0.11]}},Background->{{LightGray},None}, Dividers->{{False},
{1,2,3,4,5,6,7,8,9,10,11->True,-2->Blue}}, Alignment->Center]
Out[27]=
```

	Sepal Length	Sepal Width	Petal Length	Petal Width
Max	7.9 cm	4.4 cm	6.9 cm	2.5 cm
Min	4.3 cm	2. cm	1. cm	0.1 cm
Median	5.8 cm	3. cm	4.35 cm	1.3 cm
Mean	5.84333 cm	3.05733 cm	3.758 cm	1.19933 cm
Variance	0.685694 cm^2	0.189979 cm^2	3.11628 cm^2	0.581006 cm^2
Standard Deviation	0.828066 cm	0.435866 cm	1.7653 cm	0.762238 cm
Skewness	0.311753	0.315767	-0.272128	-0.101934
Kurtosis	2.42643	3.18098	1.60446	1.66393
1st quartile	5.1 cm	2.8 cm	1.6 cm	0.3 cm
3rd quartile	6.4 cm	3.3 cm	5.1 cm	1.8 cm

Figure 7-19. *Grid view of the descriptive statistics*

To build the table for each species, you must first separate the dataset by species with the Cases command. You should use Cases since it allows you to work with patterns. First, write the code to extract the raw data. Instead of using Short, use Shallow to suppress the 150 values.

```
In[28]:= Shallow[Values[Nest[Normal,fisher,2]],1]
Out[28]//Shallow= {<<150>>}
```

Create the table for the versicolor species, extract the values for versicolor, and store the values of the columns in the SLVersi, SWVersi, PLVersi, and PWVersi variables.

```
In[29]:= Shallow[Cases[%,{"versicolor",__}],1]
{sLVersi,sWVersi,pLVersi,pWVersi}=%[[All,#]]&/@{2,3,4,5};
Out[29]//Shallow= {<<50>>}
```

Next, repeat the process to calculate the statistics, but instead of the white space, add the name "Versicolor" in the Style text, to distinguish that the table belongs to the versicolor species.

```
In[30]:= tableRows;
{Max[#],Min[#],Median[#],Mean[#],Variance[#],StandardDeviation[#],Skewness
[#],Kurtosis[#],Quantile[#,0.25],Quantile[#,.75]}&/@{sLVersi,sWVersi,
pLVersi,pWVersi};
descriptiveStats2=Prepend[%,%%];
```

```
Transpose[descriptiveStats2];
{Style["Versicolor","Text",Red,Italic,20],Style["Sep
al Length",#1,ColorData["HTML"]["Maroon"],#2,#3],Style["Sepal
Width",#1,ColorData["HTML"]["YellowGreen"],#2,#3],Style["Pet
al Length",#1,ColorData["HTML"]["SteelBlue"],#2,#3],Style["Petal
Width",#1,ColorData["HTML"]["Orange"],#2,#3]}&["Title",Italic,20];
newTable2=Prepend[%%,%];
```

Next, build the table (see Figure 7-20) for the species versicolor.

```
In[31]:= Grid[newTable2,ItemSize-> {{None,Scaled[0.11],Scaled[0.11],
Scaled[0.11]}},Background->{{LightGray},None}, Dividers-> {{False},
{1,2,3,4,5,6,7,8,9,10,11->True,-2->Blue}},Alignment-> Center]
Out[31]=
```

Versicolor	Sepal Length	Sepal Width	Petal Length	Petal Width
Max	7. cm	3.4 cm	5.1 cm	1.8 cm
Min	4.9 cm	2. cm	3. cm	1. cm
Median	5.9 cm	2.8 cm	4.35 cm	1.3 cm
Mean	5.936 cm	2.77 cm	4.26 cm	1.326 cm
Variance	0.266433 cm^2	0.0984694 cm^2	0.220816 cm^2	0.0391061 cm^2
Standard Deviation	0.516171 cm	0.313798 cm	0.469911 cm	0.197753 cm
Skewness	0.10219	-0.351867	-0.588159	-0.0302363
Kurtosis	2.40117	2.55173	2.9256	2.51217
1st quartile	5.6 cm	2.5 cm	4. cm	1.2 cm
3rd quartile	6.3 cm	3. cm	4.6 cm	1.5 cm

Figure 7-20. *Descriptive stats for the versicolor species*

You have only done this for the versicolor species; the same process is performed for each species. For example, if you choose Cases with the other species, you would change the text to the corresponding species.

Dataset Visualization

Having viewed the capabilities of the Wolfram Language to perform descriptive statistics within the dataset, statistical charts can be implemented inside the dataset format, as you see in this fragment.

You can have a better perspective from graphs; you use the dataset format (see Figure 7-21) to display the graphs by their species.

```
In[32]:= fisher[GroupBy["Species"],DistributionChart[#,Plo
tTheme-> "Classic",PlotLabel->"PetalLength cm",GridLines->
Automatic]&,"PetalLength"]
Out[32]=
```

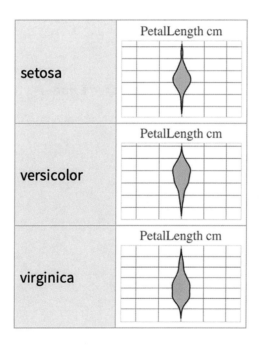

Figure 7-21. *Distribution chart plot*

You can perform the same process but for the box whiskers plot (see Figure 7-22), but choose another column.

```
In[33]:= fisher[GroupBy["Species"],BoxWhiskerChart[#,"Outliers",PlotThe
me-> "Detailed",ChartLabels->Placed[{"SepalLength cm"},Above],BarOrigin->
Right,ChartStyle->Blue]&,"SepalLength"]
Out[33]=
```

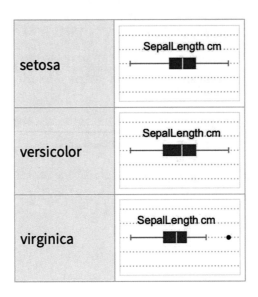

Figure 7-22. *Box whiskers plot*

If the specie is clicked, it amplify the graph (see Figure 7-23).

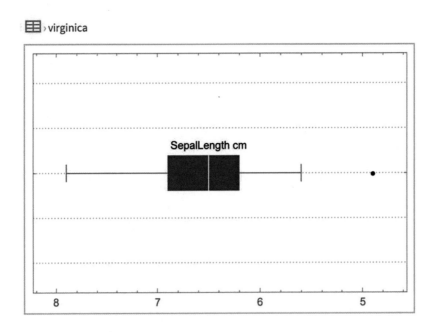

Figure 7-23. *Box whiskers plot for virginica species*

The same applies to histograms. When the graph is extensive, it appears suppressed within the dataset, but you can still select it, as shown in Figure 7-24.

```
In[34]:=fisher[GroupBy["Species"], Labeled[Histogram[#, ColorFunction ->
(Hue[3/5, 2/3, #] &)], {Rotate["Frequency", 90 Degree], "SepalWidth cm"},
{Left, Bottom}] &, "SepalWidth"]
Out[34]=
```

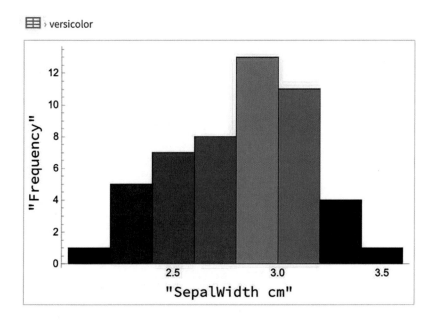

Figure 7-24. *Histogram plot for versicolor*

Here, you show the 3D scatter plots for each species (see Figure 7-25) for sepal length (x) vs. sepal width (y).

```
In[35]:=Fisher[GroupBy["Species"], Labeled[ListPlot[{#, #}], {Rotate["Sepal
width cm", 90 Degree], "Sepal length cm"}, {Left, Bottom}] &,
{"SepalLength","SepalWidth"}]
Out[35]=
```

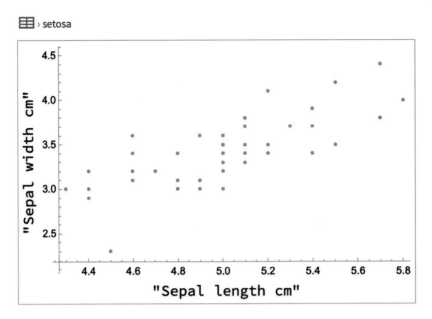

Figure 7-25. *2D scatter plot*

To return to the full dataset, click the dataset icon as with any other.

Data Outside Dataset Format

The truth is that there is also the possibility of extracting the data crudely, as follows. You'll do this to have better data handling. You use the Short command since the list is quite long.

```
In[36]:= Short[ResourceData[ResourceObject["Sample Data: Fisher's
Irises"],"RawData"]]
Out[36]//Short= {<|Species->setosa,SepalLength-
>5.1cm,SepalWidth->3.5cm,PetalLength->1.4cm,PetalWidth-
>0.2cm|>,<|<<1>>|>,<<146>>,<|<<1>>|>,<|<<1>>|>}
```

With the data already extracted, you can get the values with the Values function and convert them to normal expressions.

```
In[37]:= Short[Normal[Values[%]]]
Out[37]//Short= {{setosa,5.1cm,3.5cm,1.4cm,0.2cm},{setosa,4.9cm,3.cm,1.4cm,
0.2cm},<<146>>,{virginica,6.2cm,3.4cm,5.4cm,2.3cm},{virginica,5.9cm,3.cm,
5.1cm,1.8cm}}
```

With the help of MapAt, you can extract the magnitudes of the quantities. The MapAt command lets you choose where to apply the Quantity function. You decided to apply it to all rows with All, but only from columns 2 to 4, which is where the quantities are located.

```
In[38]:= Short[iris=MapAt[QuantityMagnitude,%,{All,2;;5}]]
Out[38]//Short={{setosa,5.1,3.5,1.4,0.2},<<148>>,{virginica,
5.9,3.,5.1,1.8}}
```

Why remove the units if calculations can be made with them? You extract the magnitudes for all quantities because they have the same order of magnitude (cm), so each calculation is in the same units, except if you make conversions or transformations to the data.

2D and 3D Plots

On the other hand, it is easier to manipulate lists with Wolfram Language. Having the data in the form of lists, you now plot the three columns in a box plot and a distribution graph (see Figure 7-26). You only choose the three columns.

```
In[39]:=
Row[{BoxWhiskerChart[{iris[[All, #1]], iris[[All, #2]], iris[[All,
#3]], iris[[All, #4]]}, "Outliers", PlotRange -> Automatic, FrameTicks
-> True, ChartStyle -> "SandyTerrain", PlotLabel -> "All Species",
GridLines -> Automatic, ChartLegends -> Placed[{"SepalLength",
"SepalWidth", "PetalLength", "PetalWidth"}, Bottom], ImageSize -> Small],
DistributionChart[{iris[[All, #1]], iris[[All, #2]], iris[[All, #3]],
iris[[All, #4]]}, PlotRange -> Automatic, FrameTicks -> True, ChartStyle ->
"SouthwestColors", PlotLabel -> "All Species", ChartLegends ->
Placed[{"SepalLength", "SepalWidth", "PetalLength", "PetalWidth"}, Bottom],
PlotTheme -> "Detailed", GridLines -> Automatic, ImageSize -> Small]}] &[2,
3, 4, 5]
Out[39]=
```

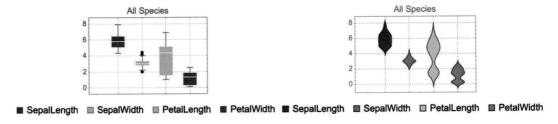

Figure 7-26. *Box whiskers plot and distribution chart for all species*

To improve this, let's graph for each species. You use Cases to separate the list with their respective species (see Figure 7-27).

```
In[40]:= Short[setosa=Cases[iris,{"setosa",__}]];
Short[versi=Cases[iris,{"versicolor",__}]];
Short[virgin=Cases[iris,{"virginica",__}]];
Column@{BoxWhiskerChart[{setosa[[All,#1]],setosa[[All,#2]],setosa[[All,#3]],
setosa[[All,#4]]},"Outliers",PlotRange->Automatic,FrameTicks->True,
ChartStyle->"Rainbow",PlotLabel->"Setosa",ChartLegends->Placed
[{"SepalLength","SepalWidth","PetalLength","PetalWidth"},Bottom],
GridLines->Automatic],BoxWhiskerChart[{versi[[All,#1]],versi[[All,#2]],
versi[[All,#3]],versi[[All,#4]]},"Outliers",PlotRange->Automatic,
FrameTicks->True,ChartStyle->"Rainbow",PlotLabel->"Versicolor",ChartLegends->
Placed[{"SepalLength","SepalWidth","PetalLength","PetalWidth"},Bottom],
GridLines->Automatic],BoxWhiskerChart[{virgin[[All,#1]],virgin[[All,#2]],v
irgin[[All,#3]],virgin[[All,#4]]},"Outliers",PlotRange->Automatic,FrameTicks->
True,ChartStyle->"Rainbow",PlotLabel->"Virginica",ChartLegends-> Placed
[{"SepalLength","SepalWidth","PetalLength","PetalWidth"},Bottom],GridLines->
Automatic]
}&[2,3,4,5]
Out[40]=
```

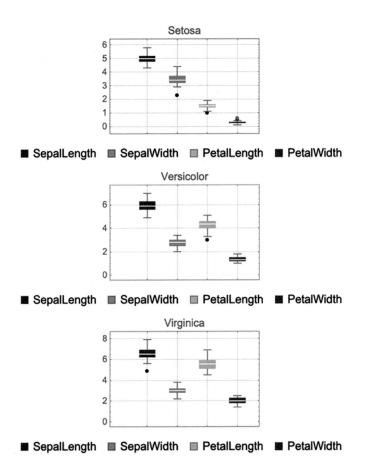

Figure 7-27. *Box whiskers plot for every species with the four features*

In addition, you can join the scatter plots of sepal width vs. sepal length for all species (see Figure 7-28).

```
In[41]:= ListPlot[{setosa[[All, {2, 3}]], versi[[All, {2, 3}]],
virgin[[All, {2, 3}]]}, FrameTicks -> All, Frame -> True,
AspectRatio -> 1, PlotStyle -> {Blue, Red, Green},
FrameLabel -> {Style["Sepal length (cm)", FontSize -> 20],
Style["Sepal width (cm)", FontSize -> 20]}, PlotLegends -> {"Setosa",
"Versicolor", "Virginica"}]
Out[41]=
```

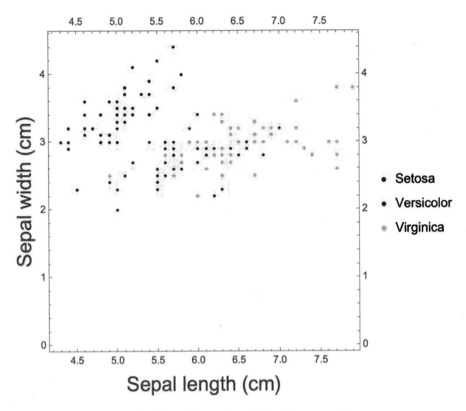

Figure 7-28. *2D scatter plot for all species of the first two features*

Or you can make a 3D scatter plot with three features (see Figure 7-29).

```
In[42]:= ListPointPlot3D[{setosa[[All, {2, 3, 4}]], versi[[All, {2, 3,
4}]], virgin[[All, {2, 3, 4}]]}, Ticks -> All, AspectRatio -> 1,
PlotStyle -> {Blue, Red, Green}, AxesLabel -> {Style["Sepal length cm",
FontSize -> 13], Style["Sepal width cm", FontSize -> 13],
Style["Petal Length cm", FontSize -> 13]}, PlotLegends -> {"Setosa",
"Versicolor", "Virginica"}, PlotTheme -> "Detailed", ViewPoint ->
{0, -3, 3}]
Out[42]=
```

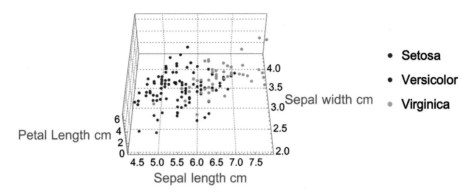

Figure 7-29. *3D scatter plot of three features for every species*

Now, when you have finished working with the resource object, you need to delete it so that the local cache of the resource is removed correctly.

```
In[43]:=Clear[fisher]
DeleteObject[ResourceObject["Sample Data: Fisher's Irises"]]
```

Summary

This chapter explored data exploration using the Wolfram Language. It starts by covering the Wolfram Data Repository, where instructions to navigate the website and select appropriate data categories effortlessly are addressed. The chapter continues to guide by showing how to extract data from the repository, offering insights on accessing, filtering, and observing the data within Mathematica. Additionally, the descriptive statistics section provides the reader with an understanding of table and grid formats. By the end of the chapter, it assists in mastering the visualization of datasets for 2D and 3D plots.

CHAPTER 8

Machine Learning with the Wolfram Language

This chapter introduces the gradient descent algorithm as an optimization method for linear regression; the corresponding computations are shown, as well as the concept of the learning curve of the model. Later, you see how to use the specialized functions of the Wolfram Language for machine learning, such as Predict, Classify, and ClusterClassify, in the case of linear regression, logistic regression, and cluster search. The different objects and results generated by these functions and the metrics to measure the model are shown for these functions. In each case, the parts of the model that are fundamental for the correct construction using the Wolfram Language are explained. This part of the book uses examples of known datasets such as the Fisher's Irises, Boston Homes, and Titanic datasets.

Gradient Descent Algorithm

The gradient descent is an optimization algorithm that finds the minimum of a function through an iterative process. To build the process, the squared error loss function is minimized with the linear model hypothesis of the shape of $(x_j) = \theta_0 + \theta_1 * x_j$, around the point x_j. The following expression gives the loss function.

$$J(\theta) = \frac{1}{2*N} \sum_{j=1}^{N} \left(f(x_j) - y_j \right)^2$$

303

$J(\theta)$ is the cost function, N is the number of observations, $f(x_j)$ is the predicted output for observation j, and y_j is the actual output for observation j. The iterative process of the algorithm consists of calculating the coefficients until convergence is obtained. The following expressions give the coefficients.

$$\theta_0^{i+1} = \theta_0^i - \alpha \left(\frac{1}{N} \sum_{j=1}^{N} \left(\theta_0^i + \theta_1^i * x_j - y_j \right) \right)$$

$$\theta_1^{i+1} = \theta_1^i - \alpha \left(\frac{1}{N} \sum_{j=1}^{N} \left(\theta_0^i + \theta_1^i * x_j - y_j \right) * x_j \right)$$

Here, θ_0^{i+1} and θ_1^{i+1} represent the updated parameters after the $i+1$ th iteration. θ_0^i and θ_1^i indicate their current values at the ith iteration, α is the learning rate, a hyperparameter for updating θ_0 and θ_1, that minimizes error during the learning process. At the same time, N is the total number of dataset observations. x_j and y_j are the jth observations of the independent and dependent variables in the dataset, respectively. The summations are obtained from partial derivatives concerning θ_0 and θ_1. For more mathematical depth about the method and demonstrations, see *Artificial Intelligence: A Modern Approach* by Stuart Russell and Peter Norvig (Prentice Hall, 2010).

Getting the Data

First, you define the data with the RandomReal function and establish a seed. This is to maintain the reproducibility of the data in case of practicing the same example.

```
In[1]:=
SeedRandom[888];
x=RandomReal[{0,1},50];
y=-1-x+0.6*RandomReal[{0,1},50];
```

Therefore, let's observe the data with a 2D scatter plot Figure 8-1.

```
In[4]:= ListPlot[Transpose[{x,y}],AxesLabel->{"X axis","Y
axis"},PlotStyle->Red]
Out[4]=
```

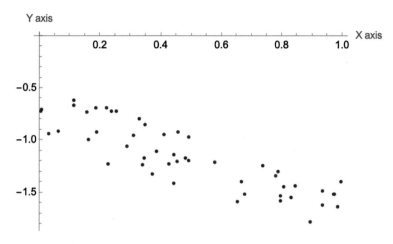

Figure 8-1. *2D scatter plot of the randomly generated data*

Algorithm Implementation

Let's now proceed to implement the algorithm with the Wolfram Language. The algorithm defines the constants, the number of iterations, and the learning rate. Then, you create two lists containing initial values of zero, in which the values of the coefficients for each iteration are stored. Later, you calculate the coefficients through a loop with Table, which does not end until you reach the number of iterations. In this case, you establish several iterations of 250 with a learning rate of 1.

```
In[5]:=
itt=250;(*Number of iterations*)
\[Alpha]=1;(*Learning rate*)
\[Theta]0=Range@@{0,itt};(* Array for values of Theta_0*)
\[Theta]1=Range@@{0,itt};(* Array for values of Theta_1*)
Table[{\[Theta]0[[i+1]]=\[Theta]0[[i]]-\[Alpha]/Length@x* Sum[(\
[Theta]0[[i]]+\[Theta]1[[i]]* x[[j]]-y[[j]]),{j,1,Length@x}];
\[Theta]1[[i+1]]=\[Theta]1[[i]]-\[Alpha]/Length@x*Sum[( \[Theta]0[[i]]+\
[Theta]1[[i]]*x[[j]]- y[[j]])* x[[j]],{j,1,Length@x}];},{i,1,itt}];
```

Since you have determined the calculation of the coefficients, you build the linear adjustment equation by constructing a function and using the coefficient values of the last iteration, which are in the previous position of the lists θ_0 y θ_1.

```
In[10]:= F[X_] := \[Theta]0[[Length@\[Theta]0]] + \[Theta]1[[Length@\
[Theta]1]]*X
```

To know the shape of the best fit, you add the X variable as an argument. This gives you the form $F(X) = \theta_0 + \theta_1 * X$.

```
In[11]:= F[X]
Out[11]= -0.707789-0.923729 X
```

Look at how the line fits the data in Figure 8-2.

```
In[12]:= Show[{Plot[F[X],{X,0,1},PlotStyle->Blue,AxesLabel->{"X axis",
"Y axis"}],ListPlot[Transpose[{x,y}],PlotStyle->Red]}]
Out[12]=
```

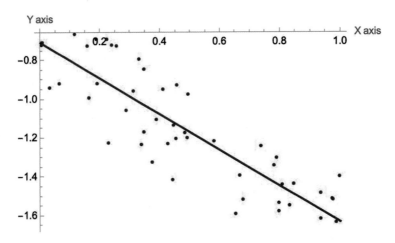

Figure 8-2. *Adjusted line to the data*

Since you have built the linear model, you can make a graphical comparison of the variation of the learning rate with the number of iterations and the loss value given by the function J. But first, you must declare the loss function J. For the summation, you can either use the special symbols of sigma ($\sum$) or write Sum [expr, $\{i, i_{max}\}$].

```
In[13]:= J[Theta0_, Theta1_] := 1/(2*Length[x])* Sum[ (Theta0 +
(Theta1*x[[i]]) - y[[i]])^2, {i, 1, Length@x}]
```

Multiple Alphas

Having seen the previously constructed process, you can repeat the process for different alphas. Following is the graph of loss vs. each interaction for learning rate values of α1=1, α2=0.1, α3=0.01, α4=0.001, and α5=0.001, when repeating the process.

```
In[14]:=\[Alpha]1=Transpose[{Range[0,itt],J[\[Theta]0,\[Theta]1]}];
In[20]:=\[Alpha]2=Transpose[{Range[0,itt],J[\[Theta]0,\[Theta]1]}];
In[26]:=\[Alpha]3=Transpose[{Range[0,itt],J[\[Theta]0,\[Theta]1]}];
In[32]:=\[Alpha]4=Transpose[{Range[0,itt],J[\[Theta]0,\[Theta]1]}];
In[38]:=\[Alpha]5=Transpose[{Range[0,itt],J[\[Theta]0,\[Theta]1]}];
```

Graph with ListLinePlot and visualize the learning curve for different alphas (see Figure 8-3). When changing the alpha value, check how the adjusted line changes.

```
In[39]:=ListLinePlot[{\[Alpha]1,\[Alpha]2,\[Alpha]3,\[Alpha]4,\
[Alpha]5},FrameLabel->{"Number of Iterations","Loss Function"},Frame-
>True,PlotLabel->"Learning Curve",PlotLegends-> SwatchLegend[{Style["\
[Alpha]=1",#],Style["\[Alpha]=0.1",#],Style["\[Alpha]=0.01",#],Style["\
[Alpha]=0.001",#],Style["\[Alpha]=0.0001",#]},LegendLabel->Style["Learning
rate",White],LegendFunction->(Framed[#,RoundingRadius->5,Background-
>Gray]&)]]&[White]
Out[39]=
```

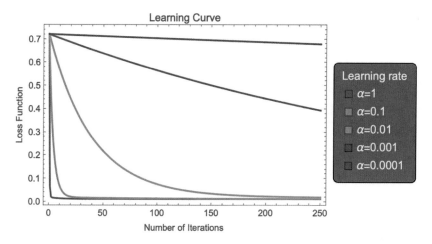

Figure 8-3. *The learning curve for the gradient descent algorithm*

In the previous graph (see Figure 8-3), you can visualize the size of iterations concerning cost and how it varies depending on the alpha value. With a high learning rate, you can cover more ground at each step but risk exceeding the lowest point. To know whether the algorithm works, you must see that each new iteration's loss function is decreasing. The opposite case would indicate that the algorithm is not working correctly; this can be attributed to various factors, such as a code error or an incorrect learning rate value. As the graph shows, adequate alpha values correspond to small values between a scale of 1 to 10^{-4}. It is not necessary to use these exact values; you can use values within this range. Depending on the form of the data, the algorithm may or may not converge with different alpha values as the same for the iteration steps. If you choose minimal alpha values, the algorithm can take a long time to converge, as you can see for alpha values 10^{-3} or 10^{-4}.

Linear Regression

Despite being able to build the algorithms to perform a linear regression, the Wolfram Language has a specialized function for machine learning. In the case of linear regression problems, there is the Predict function. The Predict function can also work with different algorithms, not only regression task algorithms.

Predict Function

The Predict function helps you predict values by creating a predictor function using the training data. It also allows you to choose different learning algorithms, the purpose of which is to predict a numerical, visual, categorical value or a combination. The methods to choose from are decision tree, gradient boosted tree, linear regression, neural network, nearest neighbors, random forest, and Gaussian process. Each method has options within it; the options vary depending on the algorithm chosen to train the predictor function. Let's look at the linear regression method. The input data for Predict can be in the form of a list of rules, associations, or a dataset.

Boston Dataset

Let's look at the first example of loading the Boston Homes data from the Wolfram Data Repository (see Figure 8-4). This dataset contains information about housing in the Boston, Massachusetts, area. For more in-depth information, refer to the article "Hedonic Housing Prices and the Demand for Clean Air," by David Harrison and Daniel Rubinfeld, in the *Journal of Environmental Economics and Management* (1978; 5[1], 81–102. https://doi.org/10.1016/0095-0696(78)90006-2) or *Regression Diagnostics: Identifying Influential Data and Sources of Collinearity: 546* by David Belsley, Edwin Kuh, and Roy Welsch, (Wiley-Interscience, 2013).

```
In[40]:= bstn=ResourceData[ResourceObject["Sample Data: Boston Homes"]]
Out[40]=
```

CRIM	ZN	INDUS	CHAS	NOX	RM	AGE	DIS	RAD	TAX
0.00632	18	2.31	tract does not bound Charles river	0.538 ppm	6.575	65.2	4.09	1	296
0.02731	0	7.07	tract does not bound Charles river	0.469 ppm	6.421	78.9	4.9671	2	242
0.02729	0	7.07	tract does not bound Charles river	0.469 ppm	7.185	61.1	4.9671	2	242
0.03237	0	2.18	tract does not bound Charles river	0.458 ppm	6.998	45.8	6.0622	3	222
0.06905	0	2.18	tract does not bound Charles river	0.458 ppm	7.147	54.2	6.0622	3	222
0.02985	0	2.18	tract does not bound Charles river	0.458 ppm	6.43	58.7	6.0622	3	222
0.08829	12.5	7.87	tract does not bound Charles river	0.524 ppm	6.012	66.6	5.5605	5	311
0.14455	12.5	7.87	tract does not bound Charles river	0.524 ppm	6.172	96.1	5.9505	5	311
0.21124	12.5	7.87	tract does not bound Charles river	0.524 ppm	5.631	100	6.0821	5	311
0.17004	12.5	7.87	tract does not bound Charles river	0.524 ppm	6.004	85.9	6.5921	5	311
0.22489	12.5	7.87	tract does not bound Charles river	0.524 ppm	6.377	94.3	6.3467	5	311
0.11747	12.5	7.87	tract does not bound Charles river	0.524 ppm	6.009	82.9	6.2267	5	311
0.09378	12.5	7.87	tract does not bound Charles river	0.524 ppm	5.889	39	5.4509	5	311
0.62976	0	8.14	tract does not bound Charles river	0.538 ppm	5.949	61.8	4.7075	4	307
0.63796	0	8.14	tract does not bound Charles river	0.538 ppm	6.096	84.5	4.4619	4	307
0.62739	0	8.14	tract does not bound Charles river	0.538 ppm	5.834	56.5	4.4986	4	307
1.05393	0	8.14	tract does not bound Charles river	0.538 ppm	5.935	29.3	4.4986	4	307
0.7842	0	8.14	tract does not bound Charles river	0.538 ppm	5.99	81.7	4.2579	4	307
0.80271	0	8.14	tract does not bound Charles river	0.538 ppm	5.456	36.6	3.7965	4	307
0.7258	0	8.14	tract does not bound Charles river	0.538 ppm	5.727	69.5	3.7965	4	307

rows 1–20 of 506   columns 1–10 of 14

Data not in notebook. Store now

Figure 8-4. *Boston Homes price dataset*

Try using the scroll bars to have a complete view of the dataset. Let's look at the descriptions of the columns and show them in TableForm.

```
In[41]:= ResourceData[ResourceObject["Sample Data: Boston
Homes"],"ColumnDescriptions"]//TableForm
Out[41]//TableForm= Per capita crime rate by town
Proportion of residential land zoned for lots over 25000 square feet
Proportion of non-retail business acres per town
Charles River dummy variable (1 if tract bounds river, 0 otherwise)
Nitrogen oxide concentration (parts per 10 million)
Average number of rooms per dwelling
Proportion of owner-occupied units built prior to 1940
Weighted mean of distances to five Boston employment centers
Index of accessibility to radial highways
Full-value property-tax rater per $10000
Pupil-teacher ratio by town
1000(Bk-0.63)^2 where Bk is the proportion of Black or African-American
residents by town
Lower status of the population (percent)
Median value of owner-occupied homes in $1000s
```

Model Creation

You create a model capable of predicting housing prices in the Boston area through the number of rooms in the dwelling. To achieve this, the columns of interest correspond to RM (average number of rooms per dwelling) and MEDV (median value of owner-occupied homes) since you want to find out if there is a linear relationship between the number of rooms and the price of the house. Applying some common sense, the houses with the most significant number of rooms are more extensive and, therefore, can store more people, increasing the price.

Look at the MEDV and RM scatter plots in Figures 8-5.

```
In[42]:= MEDVvsRM=Transpose[{Normal[bstn[All,"RM"]],Normal[bstn[All,"
MEDV"]]}];
ListPlot[MEDVvsRM,PlotMarkers->"OpenMarkers",Frame->True,FrameLabel->
{Style["RM",Red],Style["MEDV",Red]},GridLines->All,PlotStyle->
Black,ImageSize->Medium]
Out[43]=
```

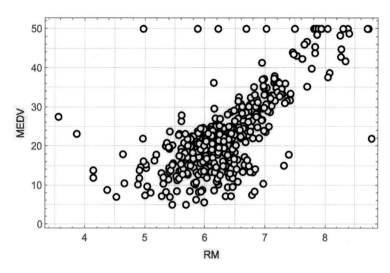

Figure 8-5. *2D scatter plot of MEDV vs. RM*

As seen in Figure 8-5, the house price increases as the average number of rooms increases. This suggests that there is a direct proportional relationship between these two variables. Given what is seen in the graph, let's know the correlation value between these variables. You show this through a correlation matrix by first computing the correlation of the values, assigning the ticks' names, and plotting it with MatrixPlot (see Figure 8-6).

```
In[44]:=correLat=SetPrecision[Correlation[Transpose[{Normal[bstn[All,"RM"]],
Normal[bstn[All,"MEDV"]]}]],2];
xTicks={{1,"RM"},{2,"MEDV"},{1,"RM"},{2,"MEDV"}};
yTicks={{1,"RM"},{2,"MEDV"},{1,"RM"},{2,"MEDV"}};
postionsValues={Text[#1,{0.5,1.5}],Text[#1,{1.5,0.5}],Text[#2,{1.5,1.5}],
Text[#2,{0.5,0.5}]}&[correLat[[1,1]],correLat[[1,2]]];
MatrixPlot[correLat,ColorFunction->"DarkRainbow",FrameTicks->{  xTicks,
yTicks,xTicks,yTicks},Epilog->{White,postionsValues},PlotLegends->
BarLegend[{"DarkRainbow",{0,1}},4],ImageSize->180]
Out[48]=
```

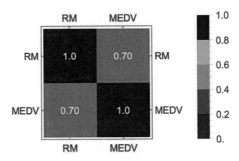

Figure 8-6. *A matrix plot combined with a correlation matrix*

By observing the matrix plot (see Figure 8-6), it can be concluded that there is an excellent linear relationship between RM and MEDV.

Let's now shuffle the dataset randomly and establish a list of rules with Thread because the data to be entered in the predictor function must be as follows: {x → y}—in other terms, input, and target value.

```
In[49]:= newData =  RandomSample[Thread[Normal[bstn[All, "RM"]] ->
Normal[bstn[All, "MEDV"]]]];
```

Once randomly sampled, you select the first 354 elements (70%); this is the training set, and the remaining 152 (30%) is the test set. When splitting, common ratios include 70/30 (training/testing), 80/20, and 60/40. Where the training set is used to train the model and usually the majority of the data. The remaining portion, the test set, is an independent dataset to assess the model performance on unseen data. The choice depends on factors like the size of the dataset and the detailed conditions of the machine-learning task you want to do.

```
In[50]:= {training, test} = {newData[[;; 354]], newData[[355 ;;]]};
```

You train the model, a predictor for the average values of owner-occupied homes (MEDV) as a target. As a method, you choose linear regression. When training a model, specification of the option of training report includes Panel (dynamical updating of the Panel), Print (periodic information including time, training example, best method, current loss), ProgressIndicator (simple progress bar), SimplePanel (dynamic update panel with no plots), and None. Panel is the default option (see Figure 8-7).

```
In[51]:=pF=Predict[training,Method->"LinearRegression",TrainingProgress
Reporting->"Panel"]
Out[51]=
```

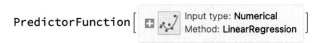

Figure 8-7. *PredictorFunction object of the trained model*

When entering the code, depending on the option added to
TrainingProgressReporting, a progress bar and panel report should appear (see
Figure 8-8). The time of the panel displayed depends on the training time of the model.
To set a specific time for the training, add TimeGoal as an option, which specifies how
long the training should last for the model. Time values are seconds of CPU time—that
is, the number with no units. With units of time (seconds, minutes, and hours), the use
of Quantity command is needed, like TimeGoal ➤ Quantity ["time magnitude," #] & / @
{"Second," "Minute," "Hour"}.

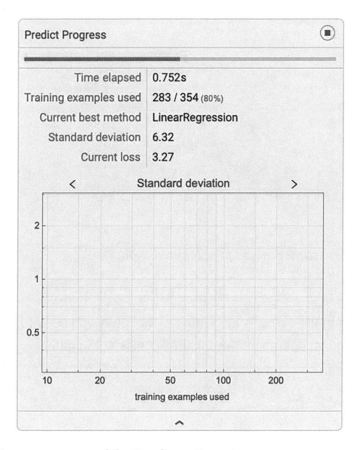

Figure 8-8. *Progress report of the PredictorFunction*

Let's go back to the model. Figure 8-7 shows that the return object is a predictor function (try using Head to verify it). When assigning a name to the predictor function, additional information about the model can be obtained; the command Information is used (see Figure 8-9). The information works for every other expression, not just for machine learning purposes.

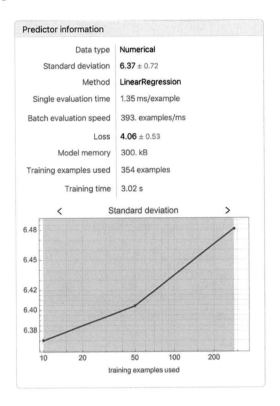

Figure 8-9. *Information report of the trained model*

Note   If you want fixed results involving random data, you need to set the seed before every random operation; this ensures consistent outputs.

```
In[52]:= Information[pF]
Out[52]=
```

The information panel in Figure 8-9 includes data type, root mean squared (StandardDeviation), method, batch evaluation speed, loss, model memory, number of examples for training, and training time. The graphics at the bottom of the panel are for standard deviation, model learning curve, and learning curve for the other algorithms. Hovering the cursor pointer over the numerical parameters shows the confidence intervals and units. If the method's name is correct, it shows the parameters of the linear regression method. Since you did not select a specific optimization algorithm within the LinearRegression method, Mathematica tries to search through the algorithms for the best one (this can be viewed in the learning curve for all algorithms). You see how to access these options further down the line.

Note   Every method used in the predict function has options and suboptions; for full customization, use the Wolfram Language Documentation Center.

Table 8-1 shows the standard options that can be used for model training, as well as their definition and possible values for the training process of a PredictorFunction.

Table 8-1. *Most Common Options for Predict Function*

Option	Definition
Method	AlgorithmPossible values: DecisionTree, GradientBoostedTrees, LinearRegression, NearestNeighbors, RandomForest and GaussianProcess
PerformanceGoal	Performance optimizationPossible values: DirectTraining, Memory, Quality, Speed, TrainingSpeed, Automatic Combination of values supported (PerformanceGoal -> {val1, val2})
RandomSeeding	Seed for the pseudorandom number generatorPossible values: Automatic, "custom seed," Inherited (random seed used in previous computations)
TargetDevice	Specifies a device to perform the training or test processPossible values: CPU or GPU. If a GPU is installed, the automatic target device is the GPU.
TimeGoal	Time spent on the training process
TrainingProgressReporting	Progress reportPossible values: Panel, Print, ProgressIndicator, SimplePanel, None

Model Measurements

Once the model is built, you must observe and analyze the performance of the predictor function in the test set. To carry out this, you must do it within the PredictorMeasurments command. The predictor function goes in the argument (see Figure 8-10), followed by the test set and the property or properties to add. Since the latest version, the final model features predictions are presented instead of just the model of the PredictorMeasurements object.

```
In[53]:= pRM=PredictorMeasurements[pF,test]
Out[53]=
```

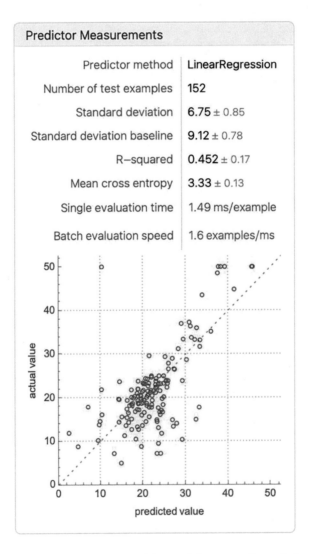

Figure 8-10. *PredictorMeasurements object of the tested model*

The returned object is called PredictorMeasurementsObject. You can add the properties from the PredictorMeasurements command. You can assign a variable to the object to access it more simply. Since the new version of 13, the report is given in the output, so the model report of the test set is suppressed as it returns the same as in Figure 8-10.

```
In[54]:= pRM["Report"];
```

The report in Figure 8-10 shows different parameters, such as the standard deviation and mean cross-entropy. It shows a graph of the model's fit and the current and predicted values. The model is suitable for most cases, except that some outliers still affect performance.

To better understand the precision of the model, let's look at the root mean squared error (RMSE) and RSquared (coefficient of determination) shown in Figure 8-11. To display the associated uncertainties, use the option ComputeUncertainty with True value.

```
In[57]:=Dataset[AssociationMap[pRM[#,ComputeUncertainty-> True]&, {"Standard
Deviation","RSquared"}]]
Out[57]=
```

StandardDeviation	6.8 ± 0.8
RSquared	0.45 ± 0.17

Figure 8-11. *Standard deviation and r-squared values of the linear model*

This gives you a slightly high RMSE value, not an excellent r-squared value. Remember that the r-squared value indicates how good the model is for making predictions. These two values indicate that although there may be a linear relationship between the number of rooms and prices, a linear regression does not necessarily explain this. These observations are also consistent, remembering that you obtained a correlation value of 0.7.

Model Assessment

The graphs made within the model are the model graph and the target variable (ComparisonPlot). To check the distribution of the variance, use the ResidualHistogram function, and to check the residual plot, use ResidualPlot. These are shown in Figure 8-12.

```
In[58]:=pRM[#]&/@{"ResidualHistogram", "ResidualPlot", "ComparisonPlot"} /.
plot_Graphics:>Show[plot,ImageSize->Small]
Out[58]=
```

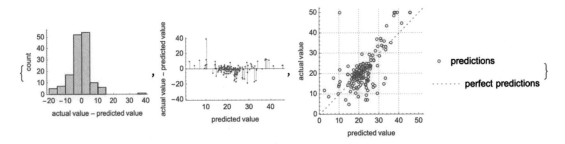

Figure 8-12. *ResidualHistogram, ResidualPlot, and ComparisonPlot*

You write Properties as an argument to find out all the properties of the Predictor Measurements object. These properties can vary between methods.

```
In[59]:= pRM["Properties"]
Out[59]={BatchEvaluationTime,BestPredictedExamples,ComparisonPlot,
EvaluationTime,Examples,FractionVarianceUnexplained,GeometricMeanProbabili
tyDensity,ICEPlots,LeastCertainExamples,Likelihood,LogLikelihood,MeanCross
Entropy,MeanDeviation,MeanSquare,MostCertainExamples,Perplexity,PredictorFu
nction,ProbabilityDensities,ProbabilityDensityHistogram,Properties,Rejectio
nRate,Report,ResidualHistogram,ResidualPlot,Residuals,RSquared,SHAPPlots,SH
APValues,StandardDeviation,StandardDeviationBaseline,TotalSquare,WorstPredi
ctedExamples}
```

If you are not satisfied with the chosen methods or hyperparameters, retraining the model can be done by configuring the new values for the hyperparameters. You access the values of the current method with the help of the Information command and add the properties of Method (shows you the Method used to train the model), method description (description of the Method used), and MethodOption (method options).

```
In[60]:= Information[pF,"MethodOption"]
Out[60]=Method->{LinearRegression,L1Regularization->0,L2Regularization->
1.*10^-6,OptimizationMethod->NormalEquation}
```

You see terms such as L1Regularization, L2Regularization, and OptimizationMethod. The first two terms are associated with regularization methods, and L1 refers to the Lasso regression name and L2 to the Ridge regression name. Regularization is used to minimize the complexity of the model and reduce the variation; it also improves the precision of the model, solving overfitting problems. This is accomplished by adding a penalty to the loss function; this penalty is added to the sum of the absolute value of the coefficient $\lambda_1 * \sum_{i=0}^{N} |\theta_i|$, whereas for L2, it is given by the expression $(\lambda_2 / 2) * \sum_{i=0}^{N} \theta_i^2$, where the function to minimize is the loss function $(1/2) \sum_{i=0}^{N} (y_i - f(\theta, x_i))^2$. For more mathematical depth, refer *Artificial Intelligence: A Modern Approach* by Stuart Russell and Peter Norvig (Prentice Hall, 2010) and *An Introduction to Statistical Learning: With Applications in R* by Gareth James, Trevor Hastie, Robert Tibshirani, and Daniela Witten (Springer, 2017). The third term is which optimization method you want to choose; the existing methods are NormalEquation, StochasticGradientDescent, and OrthanWiseNewton. That said, it must be emphasized that using the vector of coefficients with the L1 and L2 standards is known as an Elastic Net regression model. Elastic Net might be used when there is a correlation in the parameters. For more theory, reference *The Elements of Statistical Learning: Data Mining, Inference, and Prediction* by Trevor Hastie, Robert Tibshirani, and Jerome Friedman (Springer, 2009).

Retraining Model Hyperparameters

As discussed later, let's retrain the model but with the values of L1 → 12, L2 → 100 and the optimization algorithm OptimizationMethod → StochasticGradientDescent, TrainingProgressReporting → None, PerformanceGoal → "Quality," RandomSeeding → 10000, TargetDevice → "CPU."

```
In[61]:= pF2 = Predict[training, Method -> {"LinearRegression",
"L1Regularization" -> 12, "L2Regularization" -> 100, "OptimizationMethod"
-> Automatic}, TrainingProgressReporting -> None, PerformanceGoal ->
"Quality", RandomSeeding -> 10000, TargetDevice -> "CPU"];
```

To see the properties related to an example, type properties after the input data for the PredictorFunction—for instance, PF2["example," "Properties"]. Let's compare the new model's performance by showing the graphs and metrics like before (see Figures 8-13 and 8-14).

Note   Standard deviation refers to the root mean square of the residuals, root mean square error (RMSE).

```
In[62]:= pRM2=PredictorMeasurements[pF2,test];
pRM2[#]&/@{"ResidualHistogram","ResidualPlot","ComparisonPlot"}/.
plot_Graphics:>Show[plot,ImageSize->Small]
Dataset[AssociationMap[pRM2[#,ComputeUncertainty->True]&,{"StandardDeviation",
"RSquared"}]]
Out[63]=
Out[64]=
```

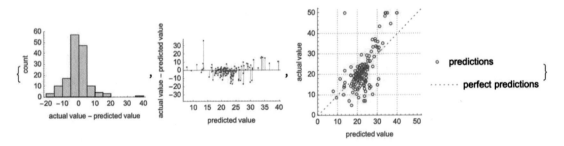

Figure 8-13. *Plots of the retrained model*

StandardDeviation	6.8 ± 0.7
RSquared	0.44 ± 0.15

Figure 8-14. *New values for standard deviation and r-squared*

Observing the graphs and data, you see the model merely decreases to a certain degree; this agrees with the new r-squared value. However, it is still a poor model for making future predictions. The poor performance may be due to the optimization choice, the L1 and L2 parameters. Try to explore different L1 and L2 values for potential improvement.

Logistic Regression

Logistic regression is a technique commonly used in statistics but also used within machine learning. The logistic regression works considering that the values of the response variable only take two values, 0 and 1; this can also be interpreted as a false or true condition. It is a binary classifier that uses a function to predict the probability of whether or not a condition is met, depending on how the model is constructed. Usually, this model type is used for classification since it can provide you with probabilities and classifications since the values of the logistic regression oscillate between two values. In logistic regression, the target variable is a binary variable that contains encoded data. For more information, refer to *Introduction to Data Science: A Python Approach to Concepts, Techniques and Applications* by Laura Igual, Santi Seguí, Jordi Vitrià, Eloi Puertas, Petia Radeva, Oriol Pujol, Sergio Escalera, Francesc Dantí, and Lluis Garrido (Springer, 2017).

Titanic Dataset

For the following example, you use the Titanic dataset, which is a dataset that describes the survival status of the passengers. The variables used are class, age, sex, and survival condition. You load the data directly as a dataset (see Figure 8-15) from the ExampleData and enumerate the rows of the dataset.

Note   This section is constructed using Query language so the reader can understand how to use it more deeply inside datasets.

```
In[65]:= titanic=Query[AssociationThread[Range[Length@#]->Range[Length@#]]]
[ExampleData[{"Dataset","Titanic"}]]&[ExampleData[{"Dataset","Titanic"}]]
Out[65]=
```

	class	age	sex	survived
1	1st	29	female	True
2	1st	1	male	True
3	1st	2	female	False
4	1st	30	male	False
5	1st	25	female	False
6	1st	48	male	True
7	1st	63	female	True
8	1st	39	male	False
9	1st	53	female	True
10	1st	71	male	False
11	1st	47	male	False
12	1st	18	female	True
13	1st	24	female	True
14	1st	26	female	True
15	1st	80	male	True
16	1st	—	male	False
17	1st	24	male	False
18	1st	50	female	True
19	1st	32	female	True
20	1st	36	male	False

rows 1–20 of 1309

Figure 8-15. *New values for Standard deviation and r-squared*

Let's look at the dimensions of the data using the Dimensions command.

```
In[66]:= Dimensions@titanic
Out[66]= {1309,4}
```

Interpreting the result, you see that the dataset comprises 1309 rows and four columns. The dataset has four columns classified by class, age, sex, and survived status. Using the space bar shows that some elements do not register data entry. To see which columns contain missing data, execute the following code by counting the components corresponding to the pattern missing in each column.

```
In[67]:=Query[Count[_Missing],#]@titanic&/@{"class","age","sex","survived"}
Out[67]= {0,263,0,0}
```

This shows 263 missing values within the age column and zero for the others. Let's remove the rows that contain this missing data. First, you extract the row numbers from the missing data by selecting the elements from the age column equal to missing and then extracting the row IDs.

```
In[68]:= Query[Select[#age==Missing[]&]][titanic];
Normal@Keys@%
Out[68]={16,38,41,47,60,70,71,75,81,107,108,109,119,122,126,135,148,153,
158,167,177,180,185,197,205,220,224,236,238,242,255,257,270,278,284,294,
298,319,321,364,383,385,411,470,474,478,484,492,496,525,529,532,582,596,
598,673,681,682,683,706,707,757,758,768,769,776,790,796,799,801,802,803,
805,806,809,813,814,816,817,820,836,843,844,853,855,857,859,866,872,873,
875,877,880,883,887,888,901,902,903,904,919,921,922,923,924,927,928,929,
930,931,932,941,943,945,946,947,949,955,956,957,958,959,962,963,972,974,
977,983,984,985,988,989,990,992,994,995,998,999,1000,1001,1002,1003,1004,
1005,1006,1007,1010,1013,1014,1015,1017,1019,1023,1024,1028,1029,1030,1031,
1033,1034,1035,1036,1037,1038,1039,1040,1042,1043,1044,1045,1053,1054,1055,
1056,1070,1071,1072,1073,1074,1075,1077,1078,1079,1081,1082,1086,1096,1110,
1115,1116,1117,1122,1123,1124,1125,1129,1133,1136,1137,1138,1139,1150,1151,
1152,1155,1156,1160,1163,1164,1165,1167,1168,1169,1171,1173,1174,1175,1176,
1177,1178,1179,1180,1181,1185,1186,1187,1194,1195,1196,1198,1199,1200,1201,
1203,1213,1214,1215,1216,1217,1220,1222,1242,1243,1244,1246,1247,1248,
1250,1251,1254,1256,1263,1269,1283,1284,1285,1292,1293,1294,1298,1303,
1304,1306}
```

These numbers represent the rows containing the age column's missing data. You use the DeleteMissing command to eliminate them, considering there is missing data at level 1. The final dataset is seen in (see Figure 8-16).

```
In[69]:= titanic=DeleteMissing[titanic,1,1]
Out[69]=
```

	class	age	sex	survived
1	1st	29	female	True
2	1st	1	male	True
3	1st	2	female	False
4	1st	30	male	False
5	1st	25	female	False
6	1st	48	male	True
7	1st	63	female	True
8	1st	39	male	False
9	1st	53	female	True
10	1st	71	male	False
11	1st	47	male	False
12	1st	18	female	True
13	1st	24	female	True
14	1st	26	female	True
15	1st	80	male	True
17	1st	24	male	False
18	1st	50	female	True
19	1st	32	female	True
20	1st	36	male	False
21	1st	37	male	True

rows 1–20 of 1046

Figure 8-16. *Titanic dataset without missing values*

To corroborate that there is no missing data, you could apply the same code with counts or by looking at the keys of the removed rows, for example.

```
In[70]:= titanic[Key[16]]
Out[70]= Missing[KeyAbsent,Key[16]]
```

This means that there is no content associated with key number 16. If you want to check all keys, use the row list of the missing data.

Data Exploration

Once you have removed the missing data, you can count the elements of each class, sex, and survival status (see Figure 8-17).

```
In[71]:= Dataset@<|"Class" -> Query[Counts, "class"]@titanic, "Sex"
-> Query[Counts, "sex"]@titanic, "Survival status" -> Query[Counts,
"survived"]@titanic|>
Out[71]=
```

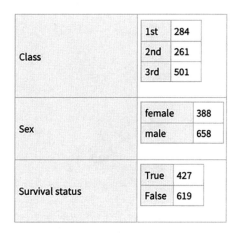

Figure 8-17. *Basic elements count for class, sex, and survival status*

After eliminating the rows with the missing elements, the dataset consists of 284 elements in the first class, 261 in the second class, and 501 in the third class (see Figure 8-18). Also, note that more than half of the registered passengers were male and that there were more deaths than survivors. It is possible to verify this graphically by showing the percentages. The same approach is applied to the column's class and sex.

```
In[72]:= Row[{PieChart[{N@(#[[1]]/Total@#),N@(#[[2]]/Total@#)}&[Counts
[Query[All,"survived"][titanic]]], PlotLabel->Style["Percentage of
survival",#3,#4], ChartLegends-> {"Survived", "Died"}, ImageSize->#1,
ChartStyle->#2,LabelingFunction->(Placed[Row[{SetPrecision[100#,3],"%"}],
"RadialCallout"]&)],
```

```
PieChart[{N@(#[[1]]/Total@#),N@(#[[2]]/Total@#)}&[Counts[Query[All,"sex"]
[titanic]]], PlotLabel->Style["Percentage by sex",#3,#4], ChartLegends->
{"Female", "Male"}, ImageSize->#1,ChartStyle->#2,LabelingFunction->(Placed
[Row[{SetPrecision[100#,3],"%"}],"RadialCallout"]&)],
PieChart[{N@(#[[1]]/Total@#),N@(#[[2]]/Total@#),N@(#[[3]]/Total@#)}&
[Counts[Query[All,"class"][titanic]]], PlotLabel->Style["Percentage by
class",#3,#4], ChartLegends->{"1st", "2nd","3rd"}, ImageSize->
#1,ChartStyle->#2,LabelingFunction->(Placed[Row[{SetPrecision[100#,3],"%"}],
"RadialCallout"]&)]},"----"]&[200,{ColorData[97,20],ColorData[97,13],
ColorData[97,32]},Black,20]
Out[72]=
```

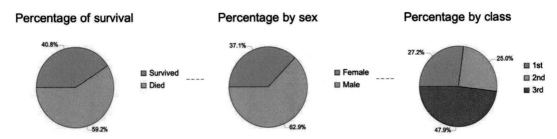

Figure 8-18. *Pie charts for class, sex, and survival status*

This example looks at the survival status of *Titanic* passengers. It builds a model that classifies whether a given class, age, and sex survived and which did not. The features are class, age, and sex; the target is survival status. These variables are the features, which the model then uses to classify whether a class, age, and sex survived, which is the target variable. The dataset is divided into 80% training (837 elements) and 20% test (209 elements). To split the dataset, first do a random sampling; afterward, extract the keys of the IDs and create a new dataset divided by the train and test sets (see Figure 8-19).

```
In[73]:= BlockRandom[SeedRandom[8888];
RandomSample[titanic]];
Keys@Normal@Query[All][%];
{train,test}={%[[1;;837]],%[[838;;1046]]};
dataset=Query[<|"Train"->{Map[Key,train]},"Test"->{Map[Key,test]} |> ]
[titanic]
Out[77]=
```

		class	age	sex	survived
Train	410	2nd	36	male	False
	537	2nd	32	female	True
	874	3rd	42	male	False
	691	3rd	22	male	False
	1021	3rd	21	male	False
	852	3rd	45	female	True
	705	3rd	21	male	False
	743	3rd	45	male	True
	515	2nd	2	male	True
	658	3rd	1	female	True
837 total ›					
Test	1227	3rd	19	male	False
	188	1st	16	female	True
	397	2nd	34	female	True
	944	3rd	37	female	False
	262	1st	35	male	True
	95	1st	4	male	True
	1080	3rd	22	female	True
	918	3rd	39	male	True
	517	2nd	37	male	False
	425	2nd	30	male	False
209 total ›					

Figure 8-19. *Titanic dataset divided by train and test set*

Classify Function

The Classify command is another super function used in the Wolfram Language machine learning scheme. This function can be used in tasks that solve a classification problem. The data that this function accepts are numerical, textual, sound, and image data. This function's input data can be the same as the Predict function {x → y}. However, entering data as a list of elements, an association of elements, or a dataset is also possible. In this case, you introduce it as a dataset.

In this case, you extract the data from the dataset format by specifying that the columns' input (class, age, sex) points to the target (survived). Now, let's build the classifier function (see Figure 8-20) with the following options: Method → {LogisticRegression, L1 → Automatic, L2 → Automatic}. When choosing Automatic, you let Mathematica choose the best combination of L1 and L2 parameters. For the OptimizationMethod, set the StochasticGradientDescent method. And for performance goal set Quality. Finally, you choose a seed with a value of 100,000 and the CPU unit as the target device. The optimization methods for the logistic regression are the limited memory Broyden-Fletcher-Goldfarb-Shanno algorithm, StochasticGradientDescent, and Newton method. These are for estimating the parameters of the logistic function. The rule construction is done from the data inside the dataset using the Query language.

```
In[78]:= cF = Classify[Flatten[Values[Normal[Query["Train", All,
All, {#class, #age, #sex} -> #survived &][dataset]]]], Method ->
{"LogisticRegression", "L1Regularization" -> Automatic,
"L2Regularization" -> Automatic,  "OptimizationMethod" ->
"StochasticGradientDescent"},  PerformanceGoal -> "Quality", RandomSeeding
-> 100000, TargetDevice -> "CPU", TrainingProgressReporting -> None]
Out[78]=
```

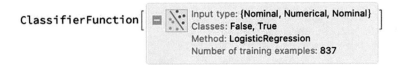

Figure 8-20. *ClassifierFunction object*

After training, like with the Predict function, the Classify function returns a classifier function object (see Figure 8-21) instead of a predictor function. Inspecting the classifier function, you can see the two input data types—nominal and numerical— and the classes, which are the survival status—true or false. The method used (logistic regression) and the number of examples (837). To obtain information on the model, use the Information command. Let's look at the model report.

```
In[79]:= Information[cF]
Out[79]=
```

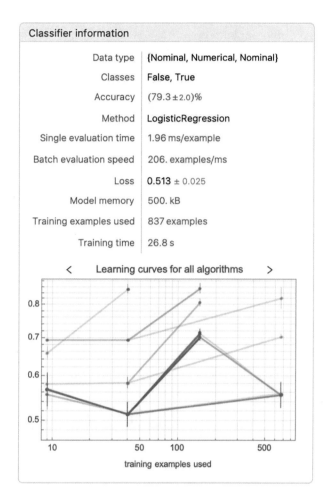

Figure 8-21. *Information about the trained classifier function*

Note   If you click the arrows above the graphs, three plots are shown: Learning curve, accuracy, and Learning curve for all algorithms. If you hover the pointer over the line of the last one, a tooltip appears with the corresponding parameters along with the method used, as shown in Figure 8-22.

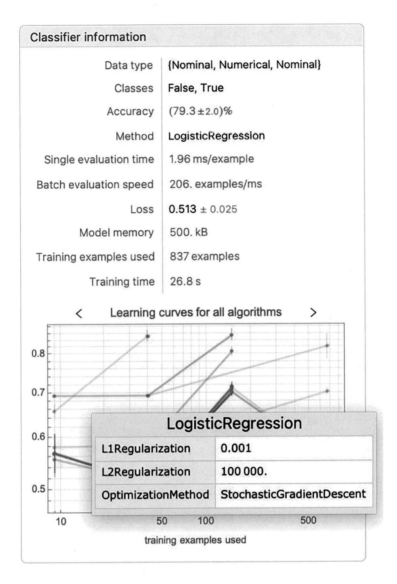

Figure 8-22. *Algorithm specifications tooltip from the method logistic regression*

You see that the model's accuracy is approximately 79%. You also observe by clicking the arrows of the plots that the learning curve and accuracy curve both experience variation at 500 training examples used. To access all the properties of the trained model, add Properties as an option in Information.

```
In[80]:= Information[cF,"Properties"]
Out[80]={AcceptanceThreshold,Accuracy,AnomalyDetector,BatchEvaluationSpeed,
```

BatchEvaluationTime,Calibrated,Classes,ClassNumber,ClassPriors,Evaluation
Time,ExampleNumber,FeatureExtractor,FeatureNames,FeatureNumber,FeatureTypes,
FunctionMemory,FunctionProperties,IndeterminateThreshold,LearningCurve,Max
TrainingMemory,MeanCrossEntropy,Method,MethodDescription,MethodOption,Method
Parameters,MissingSynthesizer,PerformanceGoal,Properties,TrainingClassPriors,
TrainingTime,UtilityFunction}

Note   Depending on the method used, properties may vary.

Let's examine the probabilities for the data: class = 3rd, age = 23, and sex = male. Probability → name or number of class or TopProbabilities → number of most likely classes.

```
In[81]:= cF[{"3rd",23,"male"},{"Probability"->
False,"TopProbabilities"-> 2}]
Out[81]= {0.676982,{False->0.676982,True->0.323018}}
```

The probabilities of the latter example show that the passenger's survival status may be more inclined to the False status.

To see the complete properties of a new classification, type the example followed by Properties. The properties included are Decision (best choice of class according to probabilities and its utility function) and Distribution (categorical distribution object). Probabilities of each class are displayed as associations: ExpectedUtilities (expected probabilities), LogProbabilities (natural logarithm probabilities), Probabilities (all classes), and TopProbabilities (most likely class). This is displayed in the following dataset (see Figure 8-23).

```
In[82]:= Dataset@
AssociationMap[cF[{"3rd",23,"male"},#]
&,{"Decision","Distribution","ExpectedUtilities","LogProbabilities",
"Probabilities","TopProbabilities"}]
Out[82]=
```

Decision	False
Distribution	CategoricalDistribution[Input type: Scalar Categories: False True]
ExpectedUtilities	<| False → 0.676982, True → 0.323018, Indeterminate → 0. |>
LogProbabilities	<| False → −0.39011, True → −1.13005 |>
Probabilities	<| False → 0.676982, True → 0.323018 |>
TopProbabilities	{False → 0.676982, True → 0.323018}

Figure 8-23. Properties for the classifier function of the trained model

---

Note   To check the logarithm result, use the Log command, Log[base, number].

Testing the Model

You now test the model on the test data using the ClassifierMeasurements command, adding the function and the test set as arguments and the uncertainty computation. Like PredictionMeasurement, the output returned shows details about the model (see Figure 8-24).

```
In[83]:= cM = ClassifierMeasurements[cF,Flatten[Values[Normal[Query[
"Test", All, All, {#class, #age, #sex} -> #survived &][dataset]]]],
ComputeUncertainty -> True, RandomSeeding -> 8888]
Out[83]=
```

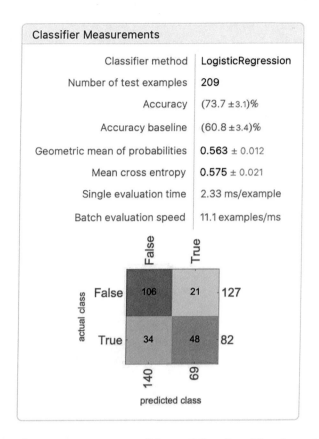

Figure 8-24. ClassifierMeasurements object of the classifier function

The object returned is called a ClassifierMeasurementsObject (see Figure 8-25), which is used to look for the properties of the ClassifierFunction after testing the test set. Just like with the linear regression model, the report of the test set is suppressed as it returns the same as in Figure 8-24.

In[84]:=cM["Report"];

The report in Figure 8-24 shows information such as the number of test examples, the accuracy, and the accuracy baseline, among others. It also shows you the confusion matrix, which shows you the prediction results for the classification model, showing the number of correct and incorrect predictions; these being broken down by class, in this case, return either false or true, which gives you an idea of the errors the model is making and the type of error it is making. It shows you the true positives and true negatives and false positives and false negatives for each class.

Let's look at the graph (confusion matrix) concretely (see Figure 8-25).

```
In[85]:= cM["ConfusionMatrixPlot"]
Out[85]=
```

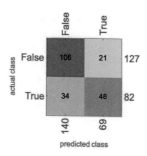

Figure 8-25. *Confusion matrix plot of the tested model*

To get the values of the confusion matrix, use CM["ConfusionMatrix"] or class CM["ConfusionFunction"].

Looking at the plot, you see that the model classified, starting from left to right at the top, 106 examples of false correctly classified, 21 examples of false as true, 34 examples of true as false, and 48 examples of true correctly. To better visualize the performance, look at each class's ROC curves (see Figure 8-26), their respective values, and the Matthews correlation coefficient and AUC values.

```
In[86]:= {cM["ROCCurve"],Dataset@<|{"AUC"->cM["AreaUnderROCCurve"]},
{"MCC"->cM["MatthewsCorrelationCoefficient"]}|>}
Out[86]=
```

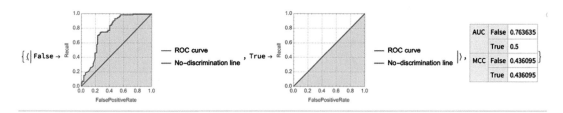

Figure 8-26. *ROC curves for each class, along with AUC and MCC values*

The two classes have different values in the AUC, but comparing the ROC curve; the class False has better classification than the True class. Let's look at which class has worse examples. You can show the less accurate results of the model, which has the highest entropy distribution and mean cross-entropy for each class.

```
In[87]:= cM[{"LeastCertainExamples","ClassMeanCrossEntropy"}]
Out[87]= {{{1st,4,male}->True, {1st,19,male}->False, {1st,22,male}->
False, {1st,24,male}->False, {1st,25,male}->False, {1st,27,male}->
False, {1st,29,male}->False, {1st,30,male}->False, {1st,33,male}->False,
{1st,35,male}->True}, <|False->0.552204,True->0.611137|>}
```

To get the values of the MCC coefficient, use the following properties: FalseDiscoveryRate, FalsePositiveRate, FalseNegativeRate (for each class), FalseNegativeExamples, FalseBegativeNumber (true negatives), FalsePositive and FalsePositiveNumber (true positive). These are shown in a short form here.

```
In[88]:= cM[#] & /@ {"FalseDiscoveryRate", "FalseNegativeRate",
"FalsePositiveRate"}
Out[88]= {<|False->0.242857,True->0.304348|>,<|False->0.165354,True->
0.414634|>,<|False->0.414634,True->0.165354|>}
```

Another way to see if the model behaves consistently in predictions is to look at key metric values like accuracy, recall, F1 score, precision, and the accuracy rejection plot (see Figure 8-27). Let's look at these metrics for the model.

```
In[89]:= cM[{"Accuracy", "Recall", "F1Score",
"Precision",  "AccuracyRejectionPlot"}] // TableForm
Out[89]//TableForm=
```

```
0.736842
<|False → 0.834646, True → 0.585366|>
<|False → 0.794007, True → 0.635762|>
<|False → 0.757143, True → 0.695652|>
```

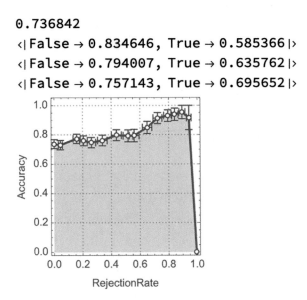

Figure 8-27. *TableForm for the values of Accuracy, Recall, F1Score, Precision, and AccuracyRejectionPlot*

To see related metrics about the accuracy, type the following properties: Accuracy (number of correctly classified examples), AccuracyBaseline (accuracy of predicting the standard class), and AccuracyRejectionPlot (ARC plot, accuracy rejection curve). However, to find information about probability and the predicted class of the test set, use the following properties: DecisionUtilities (value of the utility function for every example in the test set), Probabilities (probabilities for every example in the test set), and ProbabilityHistogram (histogram of class probabilities). Let's look at how the probability behaves by plotting the probability of a passenger's survival status (see Figure 8-28), remembering that the false state means that a passenger did not survive, and True means that a passenger did survive.

```
In[90]:= plotClass[class1_, class2_, class3_, gender_, prob_,
frame_, ticks_,
  imgSize_] := Plot[{cF[{class1, age, gender}, "Probability" ->
prob],    cF[{class2, age, gender}, "Probability" -> prob],    cF[{class3,
age, gender}, "Probability" -> prob]}, {age, 0, 90},   PlotLegends ->
{gender <> " in 1st class",    gender <> " in 2nd class", gender
<> " in 3rd class"},   FrameLabel -> {Style["Age in years", Bold,
15],    Style["Probability", Bold, 15]}, Frame -> frame,   FrameTicks ->
```

```
ticks, GridLines -> {{20, 40, 60, 80}},   ImageSize -> imgSize]

truPlot = {plotClass["1st", "2nd", "3rd", "male", True, True,
All,     Medium],    plotClass["1st", "2nd", "3rd", "female", True, True,
All,     Medium]};
falsePlot = {plotClass["1st", "2nd", "3rd", "male", False, True,
All,     Medium],    plotClass["1st", "2nd", "3rd", "female", False, True,
All, Medium]};
headings = {Style["True class", Black, 20,     FontFamily -> "Arial
Rounded MT"],    Style["False class", Black, 20, FontFamily -> "Arial
Rounded MT"]};

Grid[{{headings[[1]], headings[[2]]}, {truPlot[[1]],    falsePlot[[2]]},
{truPlot[[2]], falsePlot[[1]]}},   Alignment -> {{Center, Center}, {None,
None}},   Dividers -> {False, 1}]
Out[92]=
```

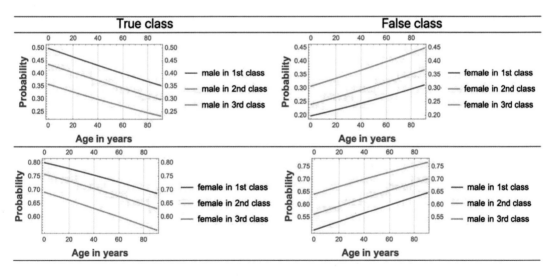

Figure 8-28. *Probabilities of each class, depending on the class, age, and sex*

The graphs shown in Figure 8-30 clearly show that males' probability of survival decreases as age increases, even to hit values below 20% of chance, whether 1st, 2nd, or 3rd class. This is contrary to the probability of survival for females, where it starts with values above 80% of chance and decreases as age increases, too, hitting values above 50% for 1st class.

Data Clustering

The data clustering method is unsupervised learning, as referenced by M. Emre Celebi, and Kemal Aydin in *Unsupervised Learning Algorithms* (Springer, 2018). It is generally used to find structures and characteristics of data clusters, where the points to be observed are divided into diffcrcnt groups by which they are compared based on unique characteristics.

The following example creates a bivariate data series and plot the list of points (see Figure 8-29). To find clusters, there is the Find Clusters command; this command makes a partition of the points according to their similarities.

```
In[93]:= BlockRandom[
SeedRandom[321];
rndPts=Table[{i,RandomReal[{0,1}]},{i,1,450}];]
ListPlot[rndPts,PlotRange->All,PlotStyle->Directive[Thick,Blue],Frame->
True,FrameTicks->All]
Out[93]=
```

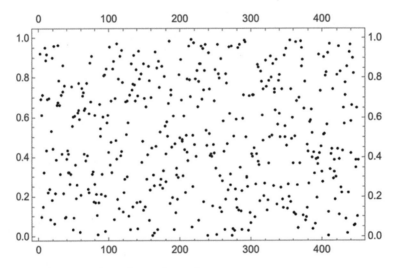

Figure 8-29. *2D scatter plot of random data*

Clusters Identification

The FindClusters function is used to detect partitions within a set of data with similar characteristics. This function gathers the cluster elements into subgroups that the function finds. When you do not add options to the Find Clusters command,

Mathematica automatically sets the cluster identification parameters. Options for other machine learning methods can also be used for this command; for example, PerformanceGoal, Method, and RandomSeeding.

```
In[94]:= clusters=FindClusters[rndPts,PerformanceGoal->"Speed",Method-
>Automatic,DistanceFunction->Automatic,RandomSeeding->1234];
Short[clusters,1]
Out[95]//Short={{{1,0.924416},{8,0.951038},<<162>>,{443,0.824999}},{<<1>>},
{<<1>>}}
```

Let's look at how many clusters were identified. You use the Length command; this way, you obtain the general form of the list.

```
In[96]:= Length[clusters]
Out[96]= 3
```

You see that the result is three. This can be interpreted as follows: the list contains three elements (that is, three sublists), each list represents a cluster, and within each cluster, there is a sublist, which includes the points of each identified cluster. To determine how many elements are included in each cluster, use the Map command and apply the Dimension command at the specification level.

```
In[97]:= Map[Dimensions,clusters,1]
Out[97]= {{165,2},{143,2},{142,2}}
```

This tells you that the first cluster contains 165 elements, the second cluster contains 143 components, and the third cluster contains 142 elements; these are the same number of points you created earlier, totaling 450. Each cluster consists of a two-point coordinate system. The FindClusters command returns the points where it identifies the clusters. Figure 8-30 exhibits the plot of the clusters generated.

```
In[98]:= ListPlot[clusters,PlotStyle->{Red,Blue,Green},PlotLegends->
Automatic,Frame->True,FrameTicks->All,PlotLabel->Style["Cluster Plot",
Italic,20,Black],Prolog-> {LightYellow,Rectangle[Scaled[{0,0}],
Scaled[{1,1}]]}]
Out[98]=
```

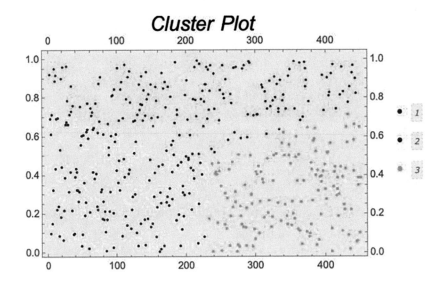

Figure 8-30. *2D scatter plot of the three clusters identified*

Find Clusters automatically colors the clusters. To explicitly establish the number of clusters to search, you add the desired number as the second argument—that is, in the form FindCluster ["points," "a number of clusters"]. In the previous example, you set the method option to automatic. The different methods for finding the clusters are shown here. Agglomerate (which is the algorithm of single linkage clustering), density-based spatial clustering of applications with noise (DBSCAN), NeighborhoodContraction (nearest-neighbor chain algorithm), JarvisPatrick (Jarvis\[Dash]Patrick clustering algorithm), KMeans (k-means clustering), MeanShift (mean-shift clustering), KMedoids (k-medoids partitioning), SpanningTree (minimum spanning tree clustering), Spectral (spectral clustering), and GaussianMixture (Gaussian mixture model).

Choosing a Distance Function

In addition to the method option, there is also the DistanceFunction, which was given the value of Automatic. This option defines how the distance between the points is calculated. In general, when you choose automatic, the square Euclidean distance is used ($\sum (y_i - x_i)^2$). There are also other values for the distance function,

Euclidean distance ($\sum \sqrt{(y_i - x_i)^2}$), Manhattan distance ($\sum |x_i - y_i|$), Chessboard distance, or Chebyshev distance (($|x_i - y_i|$)), among others. Now that you know how the clusters are identified, you want to know the centroid of each one. For this it is necessary to calculate the mean of the points of the clusters. The centroid of a series of points is obtained

from the expression $\left(\mu = \sum \dfrac{x_i}{n} \right)$, which can be interpreted as the average of the points. For

the calculation, you extract the data from each cluster and calculate its arithmetic mean.

```
In[79]:={cluster1Centroid,cluster2Centroid,cluster3Centroid}={N@Mean@
clusters[[1,All]],N@Mean@clusters[[2,All]],N@Mean@clusters[[3,All]]}
Out[79]= {{224.806,0.810328},{105.14,0.331805},{347.514,0.31097}}
```

Let's plot the clusters with their centroids to visualize how the points are classified for each centroid (see Figure 8-31).

```
In[99]:= clusterPlot=ListPlot[clusters,PlotStyle->{Red,Blue,Green},
PlotLegends->{"Cluster 1","Cluster 2","Cluster 3"}];
centroidPlot=ListPlot[{cluster1Centroid,cluster2Centroid,cluster3Centroid},
PlotStyle->Black];
Show[{clusterPlot,centroidPlot},Prolog->{LightYellow,Rectangle[Scaled[{0,0
}],Scaled[{1,1}]]},Frame-> True,FrameTicks-> All,PlotLabel->Style["Cluster
Plot",Italic,20,Black]]
Out[100]=
```

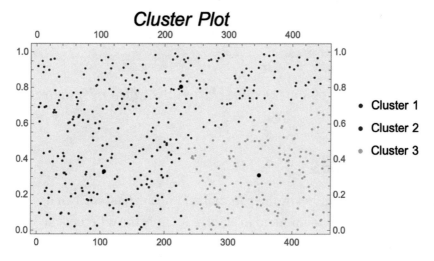

Figure 8-31. *2D scatter plot of the three clusters identified with their respective centroids*

To make sure the first cluster corresponds to the red points, try using ListPlot to plot the points contained in clusters[[1, All]], as well as those in the second cluster (blue) and third cluster (green). Alternatively, you can highlight the area of the centroids by adding the Epilog option to the plot. Epilog is another graphic option like Prolog, but you can use it to highlight the location of the centroid points (see Figure 8-32).

```
In[101]:= Show[{clusterPlot, centroidPlot},  Prolog -> {LightYellow,
Rectangle[Scaled[{0, 0}], Scaled[{1, 1}]]]},  Frame -> True,
FrameTicks -> All, Epilog -> {Opacity[0.2], PointSize[0.1],
Point[cluster1Centroid],   Point[cluster2Centroid],
Point[cluster3Centroid]}]
Out[101]=
```

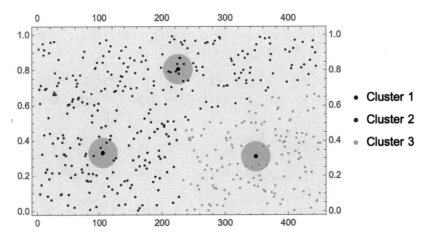

Figure 8-32. *2D scatter plot of the three clusters identified with their respective centroids*

Identifying Classes

Once the clusters are identified by the command FindClusters, you can use the ClusteringComponents command to label or identify the different classes found. You must specify the number of clusters and where to look for the clusters within the ClusteringComponents command since there are several ways to use ClusteringComponents.

```
In[102]:= classes=ClusteringComponents[clusters,3,2,Method->Automatic,
DistanceFunction->Automatic,RandomSeeding-> 1234,PerformanceGoal->"Speed"]
//Shallow
Out[102]={{1,1,1,1,1,1,1,1,1,1,1,1,1,1,1,1,1,1,1,1,1,1,1,1,1,2,1,1,2,1,2,
1,2,2,1,1,1,1,2,1,1,2,1,1,2,1,2,2,2,2,1,1,2,2,1,2,2,2,2,2,2,1,1,2,2,2,2,1,
2,2,2,2,2,2,2,2,2,1,2,2,2,2,2,2,2,2,2,2,2,2,2,2,2,2,2,2,2,2,2,2,2,2,2,2,2,
2,2,2,2,2,2,2,2,2,2,2,2,2,2,2,2,2,2,2,2,2,2,2,2,2,2,2,2,2,2,2,2,2,2,2,2,2,
2,2,2,2,2,2,2,2,2,2,2,2,2,2,2,2,2,2,2,2,2,2,2,2,2},{1,1,1,1,1,1,1,1,1,1,1,1,1,
1,1,1,1,1,1,1,1,1,1,1,1,1,1,1,1,1,1,1,1,1,1,1,1,1,1,1,1,1,1,1,1,1,1,1,1,1,1,
1,1,1,1,1,1,1,1,1,1,1,1,1,1,1,1,1,1,1,1,1,1,1,1,1,1,1,1,1,1,1,1,1,1,1,1,1,1,
1,1,1,1,1,1,1,1,1,1,1,1,1,1,1,1,1,1,3,1,1,3,1,3,1,1,1,1,1,1,1,1,3,1,3,3,1,
3,1,1,3,1,1,1,3,1,3,1,1,1,3,3,1,3,3},{3,3,3,3,3,3,3,3,3,3,3,3,3,3,3,3,3,3,
3,3,3,3,3,3,3,3,3,3,3,3,3,3,3,3,3,3,3,3,3,3,3,3,3,3,3,3,3,3,3,3,3,3,3,3,3,3,
3,3,3,3,3,2,2,3,3,3,3,3,2,3,3,3,3,3,3,3,2,3,3,3,3,3,3,3,3,2,3,3,3,3,3,3,2,
2,2,3,3,3,3,3,3,3,3,3,3,3,3,3,3,3,3,3,3,3,3,3,3,3,3,3,3,3,3,3,3,3,3,3,2,3,
2,3,3,3,3,3,2,3,3,3,3,2,3,3}}
```

In this way, numbers that correspond to the three classes appear. The command only identifies three types of classes; it does not mention what each class means. This is because cluster methods are often performed on unlabeled data, so interpretation is part of the analysis. Let's count how many elements of each class you have.

```
In[103]:= Flatten[classes]//Counts
Out[103]= <|1->174,2->132,3->144|>
```

The command returns that class one contains 174, class two contains 132, and class three contains 144. One point to clarify is why the clusters identified with FindClusters and ClusteringCompnents defer. This is because by setting the automatic option in the distance function, you are telling Mathematica to find the optimal distance function. Depending on the data, one function might gather elements in different forms, as you see later.

K-Means Clustering

Thus far, you have seen how to search for clusters in a generic way. This section focuses on the k-means method. The k-means is a technique to find and classify data groups (k) so that the elements that share similar characteristics are grouped similarly for the opposite case (not similar characteristics). The method calculates the distance between the data for a centroid to distinguish whether the data contain similarities. The elements that have less distance between them is those that share similarities. This technique is an iterative process in which the groups are adjusted until they reach a convergence. The k-means method, a simple algorithm, makes a classification employing specific partitions in different groups, where each point or observation belongs to the group. Clustering is done by minimizing the sum of the distances between each object and the centroid of its group. The k-means clustering technique tries to build the clusters to have the least variation within a group. This is done by minimizing the expression $(C_i) = \sum_{x_j \in C_i} |x_j - \mu_i|^2$, where C_i represents the ith cluster, x_j represents the points, and μ_i represents the centroid of each cluster. The square term of the function is the distance function; the most used is the square Euclidean distance, as in this case.

To learn more about the mathematical foundation behind this technique, consult the reference *An Introduction to Statistical Learning: With Applications in R* by Gareth James, Daniela Witten, Trevor Hastie, and Robert Tibshirani. (1st ed. 2013, Corr. 7th printing 2017 ed.: Springer).

The Fisher's Irises dataset in ExampleData is used in the following example. Recalling the dataset's features, execute the following code.

```
In[104]:= ExampleData[{"Statistics","FisherIris"},"ColumnDescriptions"]
Out[104]= {Sepal length in cm.,Sepal width in cm.,Petal length in cm.,Petal
width in cm.,Species of iris}
```

Let's extract the dataset and assign the variable iris to it.

```
In[105]:= iris=ExampleData[{"Statistics","FisherIris"}];
Short[iris,6]
Out[106]//Short= {{5.1,3.5,1.4,0.2,setosa},{4.9,3.,1.4,0.2,setosa},{4.7,3.2
,1.3,0.2,setosa},{4.6,3.1,1.5,0.2,setosa},{5.,3.6,1.4,0.2,setosa},{5.4,3.9,
1.7,0.4,setosa},{4.6,3.4,1.4,0.3,setosa},<<136>>,{6.8,3.2,5.9,2.3,virginica
},{6.7,3.3,5.7,2.5,virginica},{6.7,3.,5.2,2.3,virginica},{6.3,2.5,5.,1.9,
virginica},{6.5,3.,5.2,2.,virginica},{6.2,3.4,5.4,2.3,virginica},{5.9,3.,
5.1,1.8,virginica}}
```

Dimensionality Reduction

Since the iris dataset consists of four features classified into three species types, you use the PCA method, as this method is used to reduce high-dimensionality problems. In this case, you want to represent these features through two main components. For this, you proceed to standardize the data—that is, they have zero mean and one standard deviation since the variables with larger variance are more likely to affect the PCA.

```
In[107]:= sT=Standardize[iris[[All,{1,2,3,4}]]];(*Showing only the first
4 terms*)
%[[1;;4]]//TableForm
Out[108]//TableForm= -0.897674    1.0156    -1.33575    -1.31105
-1.1392     -0.131539    -1.33575    -1.31105
-1.38073    0.327318     -1.3924     -1.31105
-1.50149    0.0978893    -1.2791     -1.31105
```

There are two ways to do the process, either using the DimensionReduce command or the DimensionReduction command, which are used to reduce the dimensions of the data. The difference between the two is that the first returns the values as a list. The second returns a DimensionReducerFunction (see Figure 8-33) as output, as in the case of Predict and Classify. Both belong to the Wolfram Language special functions for machine learning. For this case, you use the DimensionReduction command. Since you have the data, you introduce the standardized data as arguments, followed by specified target dimensions (2), with the PrincipalComponentAnalysis method. This gives you the DimensionReducerFunction that assigns the name DR.

```
In[109]:= dR=DimensionReduction[sT,2,Method->"PrincipalComponentsAnalysis"]
Out[109]=
```

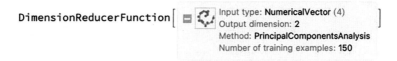

Figure 8-33. *DimensionReductionFunction object*

The properties of the function are "ReducedVectors" (list of reduced vectors), "OriginalData" (deduction from the original data list given the reduced vectors), "ReconstructedData" (data reconstruction by reduction and inversion), "ImputedData" (missing values replaced by imputed ones). You call the standardized data values function, showing the first five. The coordinates x and y are for the principal components 1 and 2, respectively.

```
In[110]:= pCA=dR[sT,"ReducedVectors"]; TableForm[%[[1;;5]],TableHeadings
->{None, {"First principal component","Second Principal component"}},
TableAlignments->Center]
Out[111]//TableForm= First principal component    Second Principal component
2.2647      -0.480027
2.08096      0.674134
2.36423      0.341908
2.29938      0.597395
2.38984     -0.646835
```

This calculates the variance of each component, followed by the total to find the proportion of variance explained. PC1 represents 76% of the data dispersion, and PC2 represents 23%. To obtain the accumulated percentage, you add the variations of each component. To view more depth about the proportion of variation, refer to *An Introduction to Statistical Learning: With Applications in R* by G. James, D. Witten, T. Hastie, and R. Tibshirani (Springer, 2017).

```
In[112]:= Variance@pCA[[All, All]]/Total@Variance@pCA[[All, All]]
// TableForm[#,   TableHeadings -> {{"First PC variation", "Second PC
variation"}, None}] &
Out[112]//TableForm=
First PC variation   | 0.761507
Second PC variation  | 0.238493
```

You look at the plot (see Figure 8-34) of the main components made by the previous process. If you look over the complete iris data from the ExampleData, the first 50 elements correspond to the setosa species, the next 50 to versicolor, and the last 50 to virginica.

```
In[113]:= labels={Style["First principal component", Black, Bold],
Style["Second Principal component",Black,Bold]};ListPlot[{pCA[[1 ;; 50]],
pCA[[51 ;; 100]], pCA[[100 ;; 150]]},PlotLegends->Placed
[{Placeholder["setosa"], Placeholder["versicolor"], Placeholder
["virginica"]}, Right], PlotMarkers -> "OpenMarkers",  GridLines -> All,
Frame -> True, Axes -> False, FrameTicks -> All,  FrameLabel -> labels]
Out[114]=
```

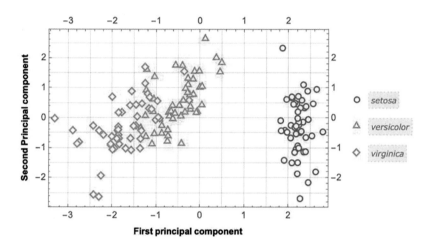

Figure 8-34. *Scatter plot of the two principal components*

Applying K-Means

Now, let's find the clusters with k-means using the Manhattan distance. You assume that the data can be divided into three clusters by specifying to look for three clusters. You know the original data belongs to three species (setosa, versicolor, and virginica). The plot of the clusters is shown here (see Figure 8-35), with their respective centroids. When choosing the k-means method, suboptions can be added, like InitialCentroids. Costum start centroids (a list of centroid coordinates) can be typed, or you can leave the automatic option. To enter the centroids coordinates, you use the following form Method → {"KMeans," InitialCentroids" → {{x1, y1}, {x2,y2}, {x3,y3} ... }}, where x1, y1 represent the centroid of the C1 (cluster 1). Initial centroids are not given to the command FindClusters to keep some randomness.

```
In[115]:= clstr = FindClusters[pCA, 3, Method ->
"KMeans",    DistanceFunction -> SquaredEuclideanDistance,    RandomSeeding
-> 8888];ListPlot[clstr, PlotRange -> All, Frame -> True, AspectRatio ->
0.8,  Axes -> False,  PlotStyle -> {ColorData[97, 1], ColorData[97, 2],
ColorData[97, 3]},  PlotLabel ->    Style["K-
means clustering for K=3", FontFamily -> "Times", Black,    20, Italic],
FrameTicks -> All,  PlotLegends ->   Placed[{Placeholder[Style["Cluster 1",
Bold, Black, 10]],    Placeholder[Style["Cluster 2", Bold, Black, 10]],
Placeholder[Style["Cluster 3", Bold, Black, 10]]}, Right],  PlotMarkers
-> "OpenMarkers", FrameLabel -> labels, GridLines -> All,  Epilog ->
{Opacity[1], PointSize[0.01], Point[Mean@clstr[[1, All]]],    Point[Mean@
clstr[[2, All]]], Point[Mean@clstr[[3, All]]]}]
Out[115]=
```

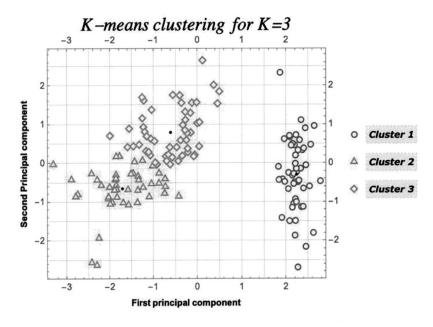

Figure 8-35. *3 clusters identified of the two principal components*

In Figure 8-35, the method identifies the left points as a single cluster (setosa specie), whereas some points between clusters 2 and 3 might be misclassified.

Changing the Distance Function

Changing the DistanceFunction can modify how the clusters are arranged; the following code shows the plot for k = 3 and choosing a different distance function. In the next block of code, the computation of the clusters is made for the same k (3), with a different distance function, and stored into their respective variables. Then, the clusters are plotted (see Figure 8-36) for each of the different distance functions, and finally, they are displayed within a graphic grid.

```
In[116]:= clusteringPlot[distanceName_, distanceFunction_]
:= Module[{clusters, pltTitles, points},  clusters =   FindClusters[pCA,
3, PerformanceGoal -> "Quality",    Method -> "KMeans", DistanceFunction
-> distanceFunction,    RandomSeeding -> 8888]; points = Point[Mean[#]]
& /@ clusters; pltTitles = distanceName; ListPlot[clusters, Frame ->
True, AspectRatio -> 0.8,    PlotMarkers -> "OpenMarkers",    PlotStyle ->
{ColorData[97, 1], ColorData[97, 2],    ColorData[97, 3]}, GridLines ->
All, PlotRange -> Automatic,   ImageSize -> 300, FrameLabel -> labels,
Axes -> False,    FrameTicks -> All, Epilog -> {Opacity@1, PointSize@0.03,
points},    PlotLabel -> Style[pltTitles, Black]]]

eDplt = clusteringPlot["Euclidean Distance", EuclideanDistance];
mhDplt = clusteringPlot["Manhattan Distance", ManhattanDistance];
chDplt = clusteringPlot["Chessboard Distance", ChessboardDistance];
cosDplt = clusteringPlot["Cosine Distance", CosineDistance];

legendsText = {Placeholder[Style["Cluster 1", Bold,
Black, 10]],    Placeholder[Style["Cluster 2", Bold,
Black, 10]], Placeholder[Style["Cluster 3", Bold, Black,
10]]};Labeled[Legended[  GraphicsGrid[{{eDplt, mhDplt},
{chDplt, cosDplt}},Frame->All,Background->White,Spacings->1],
PointLegend[{ColorData[97,1], ColorData[97,2], ColorData[97,3]},
legendsText, LegendMarkers -> "OpenMarkers"]],  Style["K-means clustering
for K=3", FontFamily -> "Times", Black, 20,    Italic], Top]
Out[117]=
```

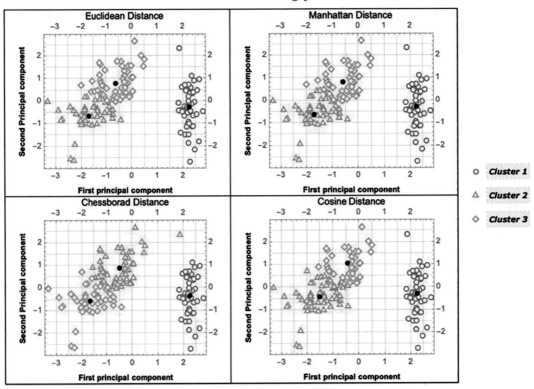

Figure 8-36. *K-means clustering for K = 3, for different distance functions*

The clusters can have different arrangements with different distance functions; one thing to note also is that the cluster's centroids change in each of the subfigures.

Different k's

Having seen that for different distance functions, the clusters can vary, let's now construct the process but with different k's—that is, for k= 2, 3, 4, and 5, as exhibited in Figure 8-37.

```
In[117]:= findKClusters[k_, PCA_] := FindClusters[PCA, k,
PerformanceGoal -> "Speed", Method -> "KMeans",DistanceFunction ->
SquaredEuclideanDistance, RandomSeeding -> 8888];

plotKClusters[k_, clusters_] := ListPlot[clusters, Frame -> True,
```

```
AspectRatio -> 0.8, PlotMarkers -> "OpenMarkers", PlotStyle ->
ColorData[97, "ColorList"][[;; k]], GridLines -> All, PlotRange ->
Automatic, ImageSize -> 260, FrameLabel -> labels, Axes -> False,
FrameTicks -> All, Epilog -> {Opacity@1, PointSize@0.015, Point[Mean
/@ clusters]}, PlotLabel -> Style["K=" <> ToString[k], Black]];

kValues = {2, 3, 4, 5};
kClusters = findKClusters[#, pCA] & /@ kValues;
kPlots = plotKClusters[#, kClusters[[#2]]] & @@@ Transpose[{kValues, Range@
Length@kValues}];

legendsText2 = {Placeholder[Style["Cluster " <> ToString[#], Bold, Black,
10]]} & /@ Range@5;
Labeled[Legended[ GraphicsGrid[Partition[kPlots, 2], Frame ->
All,    Background -> White, Spacings -> 1],   PointLegend[ColorData[97,
"ColorList"][[;; 5]], legendsText2,    LegendMarkers ->
"OpenMarkers"]],  Style["K-means clustering for K=2,3,4,5", FontFamily ->
"Times",    Black, 20, Italic], Top]
Out[120]=
```

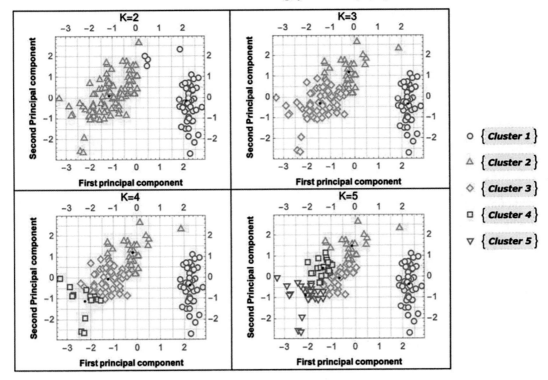

Figure 8-37. *K-means for K from 2 to 5*

The arrangement of the clusters also depends on the number of ks. Complementing with ClusteringComponents, you can count the number of labels registered for a k = 3.

```
In[120]:= ClusteringComponents[clstr,3,2,Method->"KMeans",DistanceFunction
->SquaredEuclideanDistance,RandomSeeding->8888]
Counts[Flatten[%]]
Out[121]={{1,1,1,1,1,1,1,1,1,1,1,1,1,1,1,1,1,1,1,1,1,1,1,1,1,1,1,1,1,1,1,
1,1,1,1,1,1,1,1,1,1,1,1,1,1,1,1,1,1,1},{2,2,2,2,2,2,2,2,2,2,2,2,2,2,2,2,2,2,2,
2,2,2,2,2,2,2,2,2,2,2,2,2,2,2,2,2,2,2,2},{3,3,3,3,2,3,3,3,
3,3,3,3,3,3,3,3,3,3,3,3,3,3,3,3,3,3,3,3,3,3,3,3,3,3,3,2,2,3,2,
3,3,3,3,3,3,2,3,3,2}}
Out[122]= <|1->50,2->51,3->49|>
```

Given a clustering problem, the k-means technique is meant to be used for unlabeled data—that is, data without defined categories. Some factors that can alter the operation of the method include the following.

- The spread, or how far apart the points are. This is reflected if the data contains outliers or are in various scales, which can be erroneously classified as part of a cluster when the opposite is observed visually.

- The dimensionality of the data. Given that more information and features are often added to the model, the number of dimensions grows, leading to the "curse of dimensionality." This type of problem can be solved using data transformation methods, as in the example seen from PCA, but with some restrictions since the PCA method can lose sensitive information on the features.

- The value of k is determined manually, but when there are high-cost function values, it can be interpreted that the intra-cluster variation is high. With low-cost function values, the intra-cluster variation is low. The last two assumptions can also be attributed to the fact that for lower values of k, many observations can be grouped into large individual clusters. For high values of k observations, they can be a proper group.

Cluster Classify

Another command that belongs to the cluster functions is called ClusterClassify (see Figure 8-38). This command works in the same way as Classify does. The following example uses this command to see how the k-means cluster classifies the species based on Sepal length and Sepal width. Split the data into halves when you randomly sample.

```
In[122]:= BlockRandom[
SeedRandom[88888];
RandomSample[iris[[All,{1,2}]]];]
trainingSet=%[[1;;75]];
testSet=%%[[76;;150]];
In[123]:= cC=ClusterClassify[trainigSet,3,Method->"KMeans",
DistanceFunction->Automatic,PerformanceGoal->"Speed",RandomSeeding->8888 ]
Out[123]=
```

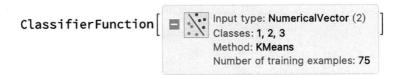

ClassifierFunction[... Input type: NumericalVector (2)
Classes: 1, 2, 3
Method: KMeans
Number of training examples: 75]

Figure 8-38. ClassifierFunction of the cluster classification model

Figure 8-38 shows the details of the cluster classification model. The input vector is a numerical vector, the number of classes (three), the method, and the number of training examples.

Note   To correctly use the k-means method, the number of clusters needs to be specified; otherwise, the command does not execute correctly.

Use the Information command to see the classifier information (see Figure 8-39).

```
In[124]:= Information[cC]
Out[124]=
```

Classifier information	
Data type	NumericalVector (2)
Classes	1, 2, 3
Method	KMeans
Single evaluation time	1.79 ms/example
Batch evaluation speed	228. examples/ms
Model memory	73.9 kB
Training examples used	75 examples
Training time	30.4 ms

Figure 8-39. Classifier information for k-means

More detailed information about the classifier function is shown in Figure 8-39. To get the complete list of properties, type "Properties" as a second argument. Many metrics, such as BatchEvaluationSpeed, BatchEvaluationTime, and TrainingTime, can compare times with different methods.

```
In[125]:= Information[cC,"Properties"]
Out[125]={AcceptanceThreshold,AnomalyDetector,BatchEvaluationSpeed,BatchEv
aluationTime,Calibrated,Classes,ClassNumber,ClassPriors,DistanceFunction,
EvaluationTime,ExampleNumber,FeatureExtractor,FeatureNames,FeatureNumber,
FeatureTypes,FunctionMemory,FunctionProperties,IndeterminateThreshold,
LearningCurve,MaxTrainingMemory,Method,MethodDescription,MethodOption,
MethodParameters,MissingSynthesizer,PerformanceGoal,Properties,Training
ClassPriors,TrainingTime,UtilityFunction}
```

Let's now get the information about the classes identified from the cluster classifier, the number of classes, distance function, feature names, and the training class probabilities.

```
In[126]:=Information[cC,#]&/@{"Classes","ClassNumber","DistanceFunction",
"FeatureNames","TrainingClassPriors"}
Out[126]= {{1,2,3},3,EuclideanDistance,{f1},<|1->0.333333,2->0.293333,
3->0.373333|>}
```

There are three classes: class 1, class 2, and class 3. The distance function used is EuclideanDistance, and the name f1 refers to the numeric vector features. A simple example is chosen by choosing a sepal length of 1 and a sepal width of 2 to show the different properties that can be used when testing the data, shown in the dataset form (see Figure 8-40). The example is first written, followed by the properties Decision (cluster that belongs to the example), Distribution (categorical distribution object for histogram plots), ExpectedUtilities (expected probabilities and indeterminate threshold), LogProbabilities (log probabilities), Probabilities (probabilities of the test data based on classes), and TopProbabilities (best probabilities for the test data).

```
In[127]:=Dataset[AssociationMap[cC[{1,2},#]&,{"Decision","Distribution",
"ExpectedUtilities","LogProbabilities","Probabilities","TopProbabilities"}]]
Out[127]=
```

Decision	3
Distribution	CategoricalDistribution[Input type: **Scalar** Categories: 1 2 3]
ExpectedUtilities	⟨| 1 → 0.0238517, 2 → 2.72758 × 10⁻¹⁶, 3 → 0.976148, Indeterminate → 0. |⟩
LogProbabilities	⟨| 1 → −3.7359, 2 → −35.8379, 3 → −0.0241407 |⟩
Probabilities	⟨| 1 → 0.0238517, 2 → 2.72758 × 10⁻¹⁶, 3 → 0.976148 |⟩
TopProbabilities	{3 → 0.976148}

Figure 8-40. *The dataset of the simple Iris example*

The example belongs to the third cluster and that the associated probability is $3 \rightarrow$ 0.976148. Look at the rest of the data and plot the cluster classification. The classified data plot is shown in Figure 8-41.

```
In[128]:= ListPlot[Pick[testSet,cC[testSet],#]&/@{1,2,3},
PlotMarkers->"OpenMarkers",GridLines->Automatic,PlotLegends->
{Placeholder[Style["Cluster 1",Bold,Black,10]],Placeholder[Style["Cluster
2",Bold,Black,10]],Placeholder[Style["Cluster 3",Bold,Black,10]]},
Frame->True,FrameTicks->All,FrameLabel->{"Sepal Lenght","Sepal Width"}]
Out[128]=
```

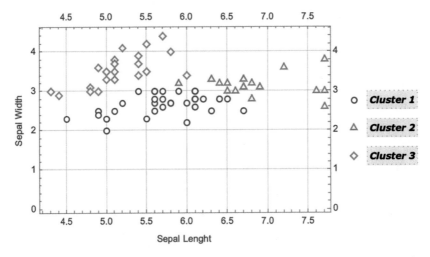

Figure 8-41. *Cluster classification on the example of the iris data for the first two features*

As a complement, a probability restriction for values below an established probability value can be added with IndeterminateThreshold, as depicted in Figure 8-42.

```
In[129]:= ListPlot[Pick[testSet,CC[testSet,IndeterminateThreshold->
0.6],#]&/@{1,2,3,Indeterminate},PlotMarkers-> "OpenMarkers",PlotLegends->
{Placeholder[Style["Cluster 1",Bold,Black,10]],Placeholder[Style["Cluster
2",Bold,Black,10]],Placeholder[Style["Cluster 3",Bold,Black,10]],Placeholder
[Style["Indeterminate",Bold,Black,10]]},Frame->True,FrameTicks->
All,FrameLabel->{"Sepal Lenght","Sepal Width"},GridLines->Automatic]
Out[129]=
```

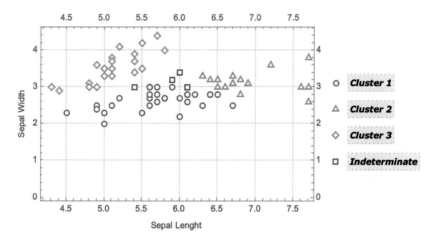

Figure 8-42. *Cluster classification on the example of the iris data for the first two features with a probability restriction*

Summary

The first part of the chapter discussed machine learning, the gradient descent algorithm, and its comprehensive implementation. Then, the linear regression model was introduced by exploring the Boston dataset and the guide to creating, measuring, and refining the created model. This previous process is also carried out for the logistic regression but with the Titanic dataset. As the chapter concluded, you learned about data clustering and k-means clustering.

CHAPTER 9

Neural Networks with the Wolfram Language

This chapter starts with the basic foundations of the neural network framework in the Wolfram Language. The chapter begins with the concepts of layers, how to use the commands for different layers, and the most common layers. You learn how to enter data into the layers by the net port and the different forms of equivalent expression of the layers. This topic is followed by how to distinguish different layers by their symbol. You see that layers can have multiple options that enable them to have various specifications by viewing the concept of a layer in the Wolfram Language scheme, comparing different layers with different purposes, and performing different computations. You also achieve this by looking at the various activation functions supported by the Wolfram Language and inspecting the plots of each function in addition to different syntax forms. Next, you learn about encoders and decoders and how these tools are used to construct a neural network model, depending on the task to be fulfilled. You then learn how these encoders and decoders are used to convert different data types to numeric arrays and how to convert the numeric arrays back to the initial data. You introduce the concept of a container, what it means for the created models, and what types exist. You see how to handle and build containers with different commands and graphically visualize the created model. You see how the Wolfram Neural Net Framework supports MXNet-related operations and how to export a network to the format of the MXNet operation.

© Jalil Villalobos Alva 2024
J. Villalobos Alva, *Beginning Mathematica and Wolfram for Data Science*,
https://doi.org/10.1007/979-8-8688-0348-2_9

Layers

It is necessary to understand that neural networks, in general and in the Wolfram Language, are built from layers. A layer is a term that can be applied to a collection of nodes that operate together at a specific level within the neural network. The layer is an essential and straightforward member for constructing a neural network.

Input Data

The data handled by the layers is of a numeric type and not of another kind. Input variables can be vectors, a unidimensional list, matrixes, a two-dimensional list, arrays, a list of lists, or any other numeric tensor. These input variables can be either features or attributes of the dataset of study, with a known or multidimensional shape. These types of input attributes are associated with the input layer, for which the feature size, in turn, must be equal to the input size of a layer, but not every layer receives the same input and returns the same output; every input varies depending on the type of layer to be used. This definition is one of the most basic ideas in neural networks since they are a crucial component of the whole structure that involves the term neural network. A remark here is to distinguish input from input layer since they do not mean the same.

Linear Layer

A linear layer is the most common and widely used layer in a neural network. To build the simplest layer in the Wolfram Language, use the LinearLayer command.

```
In[1]:= LinearLayer["Input"->1,"Output"->2]
Out[1]=
```

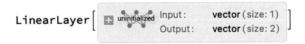

Figure 9-1. *LinearLayer object*

Figure 9-1 represents the LinearLayer object in the Wolfram Language. Clicking the plus icon shows the internal parameters, including details about the layer port's input and output and array rank of the weights and biases of the linear layer, as shown in Figure 9-2.

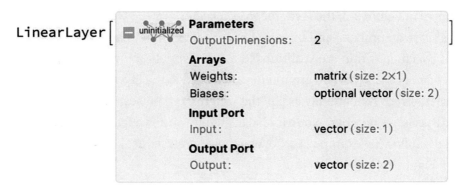

Figure 9-2. *Expanded LinearLayer object*

Each layer has an input port and an output port. Each port has an associated size of what is entering the layer and what is going out. In the latter case, a vector of size one is entering, and the layer returns a vector of size two.

Weights and Biases

The general form of a linear layer is given by the following expression of the dot product **w·x + b**, where **x** is the data vector, **w** represents the matrix of the weights, and **b** is the vector of the biases. Linear layers have other associated names, like fully connected layers, as in the MXnet framework. The input of the layers in the Wolfram Language receives numerical tensors as input—that is, they only act on numerical arrays. To explicitly enter the size of input and output, you write the form of the input port and the output port followed by different options: "Input" or "Output" → {size, Options.}. Options include defining a real number (Real), a vector of form n (single number n), an array ({n1 * n2 * n3} ...), or a NetEncoder, which you see later. Following are some equivalent ways to write layers, as depicted in Figure 9-3.

```
In[2]:= LinearLayer["Input"->{2,"Real"},"Output"->{3,1}]
Out[2]=
```

LinearLayer[uninitialized Input: vector (size: 2)
                           Output: matrix (size: 3×2)]

Figure 9-3. *LinearLayer with different input and output rank arrays*

As shown in Figure 9-3, the layer receives a vector of size two (list of length 2), comprised of real numbers, and the output is a matrix of the shape 3×2. When a real number is specified within the Wolfram Neural Network Framework, it works with the precision of a Real32. When no arguments are added to the layer, the input and output shapes are inferred. To manually assign the weights and biases, write "Weights" → number, "Biases" → number; None is also available for no weights or biases. This is shown in the following example, where weights and biases are set to a fixed value of 1 and 2 (see Figure 9-4).

```
In[3]:= LinearLayer["Input"-> 1,"Output"-> 1,"Weights"-> 1,"Biases"-> 2]
Out[3]=
```

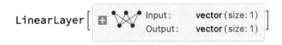

Figure 9-4. *Initialized linear layer, with fixed biases and weights*

Initializing a Layer

Another command allows you to initialize the layer with random values: NetInitialize. So, to establish hold values of weights or biases, you can also use the LearningRateMultipliers option (see Figure 9-5). Besides this, LearningRateMultipliers also mark the rate at which a layer learns during the training phase.

```
In[4]:= NetInitialize[LinearLayer["Input"-> "Real","Output"->
"Real",LearningRateMultipliers->{"Biases"->1}]]
Out[4]=
```

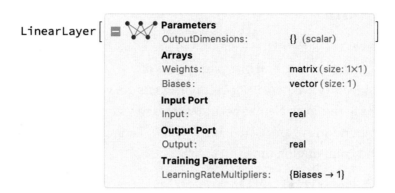

Figure 9-5. *LinearLayer with training parameters*

When a layer is initialized, the uninitialized text disappears. If you observe the properties of the new layer, they appear within the training parameters where fixed biases have been established, and a learning rate has been set. The options for NetInitialize are Method and RandomSeeding. The available methods are Kaiming, Xavier, Orthogonal (orthogonal weights), and Random (weights selection from a distribution). For example, you can use the Xavier initialization sampling from a normal distribution, as seen in Figure 9-6.

```
In[5]:= NetInitialize[LinearLayer["Input"-> "Real","Output"->
"Real",LearningRateMultipliers->{"Biases"->1}],Method->
{"Xavier","Distribution"->"Normal"},RandomSeeding->888]
Out[5]=
```

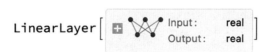

Figure 9-6. *LinearLayer initialized with the Xavier method*

Note   The Option command is recommended to see the options set for a layer.

Despite being able to establish the weights and biases manually, it is advisable to start the layer with random values to maintain a certain level of complexity in the overall structure of a model since, on the contrary, this could have an impact on the creation of a neural network that does not make accurate predictions for non-linear behavior.

Retrieving Data

NetExtract retrieves the value of the weights and biases in the form NetExtract [net, {level1, level2, ...}. The weights and bias parameters of the linear layers are packed in NumericArray objects (see Figure 9-7). This object has the values, dimensions, and type of the values in the layer. NetExtract also serves to extract layers of a network with many layers. NumericArrays are used in the Wolfram Language to reduce memory consumption and computation time.

```
In[6]:= linearL=NetInitialize[LinearLayer[2, "Input"->
1],RandomSeeding->888];
NetExtract[linearL,#]&/@{"Weights","Biases"}//TableForm
Out[7]//TableForm=
```

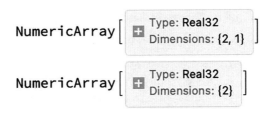

Figure 9-7. *Weights and biases of a linear layer*

With Normal, you convert them to lists.

```
In[8]:=TableForm[SetPrecision[{{Normal[NetExtract[linearL,"Weights"]]},
{Normal[NetExtract[linearL,"Biases"]]}},3],TableHeadings->{{"Weights
->","Biases ->"},None}]
Out[8]//TableForm=
Weights ->      -0.779
0.0435
Biases   ->     0
0
```

For instance, a layer can receive a length of one vector to produce an output vector of size 2.

```
In[9]:= linearL[4]
Out[9]= {-3.11505,0.174007}
```

The layer can only be evaluated when input is introduced in the appropriate shape.

```
In[10]:= linearL[{88,99}]
During evaluation of In[10]:= LinearLayer::invindata1: Data supplied
to port "Input" was a length-2 vector of real numbers, but expected a
length-1 vector.
Out[10]= $Failed
```

The weights and biases are the parameters that the model must learn from, which can be adapted based on the input data that the model receives, which is why it is initialized randomly since if you try to extract these values without initializing, you cannot because they have not been defined.

Layers have the property of being differentiable. It is achieved with NetPortGradient, which can represent the gradient of a net output for a port or a parameter. For example, give the derivative of the output concerning the input for a particular input value.

```
In[11]:= linearL[2,NetPortGradient["Input"]]
Out[11]= {-0.735261}
```

Mean Squared Layer

Until now, you have seen the linear layer, which has various properties. Layers with the icon of a connected rhombus (see Figure 9-8), by contrast, do not contain any learnable parameters, like MeanSquaredLossLayer, AppendLayer, SummationLayer, DotLayer, ContrastiveLossLayer, and SoftmaxLayer, among others.

```
In[12]:= MeanSquaredLossLayer[]
Out[12]=
```

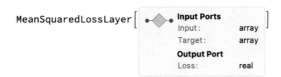

Figure 9-8. *MeanSquaredLossLayer*

MeanSquaredLossLayer[] has more than one input because this layer computes the mean squared loss, which is the following expression $(1/n) \sum (\text{Input - Target})^2$, and has the property that compares two numeric arrays. With the MeanSquaredLossLayer, the input/output ports' dimensions are entered in the same form as a linear layer, and the input and target values are entered as Associations.

```
In[13]:= MeanSquaredLossLayer["Input"->{3, 2},"Target" -> {3, 2}][
Association["Input" -> {{1, 2}, {2, 1}, {3, 2}},  "Target" -> {{2, 2},
{1, 1}, {1, 3}}]]
Out[13]= 1.16667
```

The latter example computes a MeanSquaredLossLayer for input/output dimensions of three rows and two columns or by defining first the layer and then applying the layer to the data.

Note   Use the Matrixform[{{1, 2}, {2, 1}, {3, 2}}] command to verify the matrix shape of the data.

```
In[14]:= lossLayer=MeanSquaredLossLayer["Input"->{3,2},"Target"->{3,2} ];
lossLayer@<|"Input"->{{1,2},{2,1},{3,2}},"Target"->{{2,2},{1,1},{1,3}}|>
Out[15]= 1.16667
```

To get more details about a layer (see Figure 9-9), use the Information command.

```
In[16]:= Information[lossLayer]
Out[16]=
```

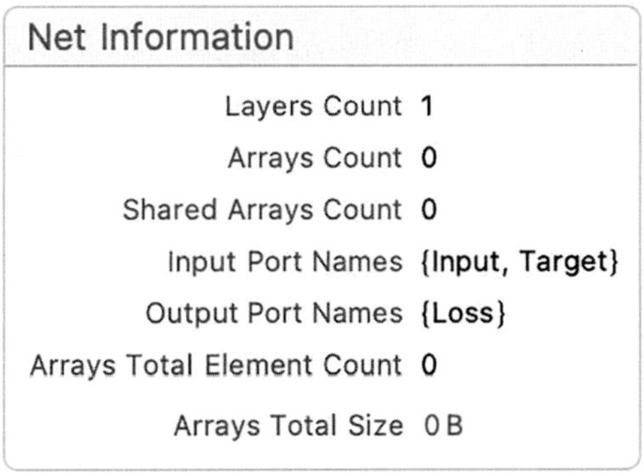

Net Information

Layers Count	1
Arrays Count	0
Shared Arrays Count	0
Input Port Names	{Input, Target}
Output Port Names	{Loss}
Arrays Total Element Count	0
Arrays Total Size	0 B

Figure 9-9. *Information about the loss layer To know the layer options, use the following*

To know the layer options, use the following.

```
In[17]:= MeanSquaredLossLayer["Input"->"Real","Target"->"Real"]//Options
Out[17]= {BatchSize->Automatic,NetEvaluationMode->Test,RandomSeeding->
Automatic,TargetDevice->CPU,WorkingPrecision->Real32}
```

The input port and target port options are similar to that of the linear layer with the different forms, Input → Real, n (a form of a vector n), {n1 × n2 × n3} ... (an array of n dimensions), Varying (a vector or varying form) or a NetEncoder, but with the exception that the input and target must have the exact dimensions. A few forms of layers are shown in Figure 9-10.

```
In[18]:= {MeanSquaredLossLayer["Input"->"Varying","Target"->"Varying"],
MeanSquaredLossLayer["Input"-> NetEncoder["Image"],"Target"-> NetEncoder["I
mage"]],MeanSquaredLossLayer["Input"->1,"Target"->1]}//Dataset
Out[18]=
```

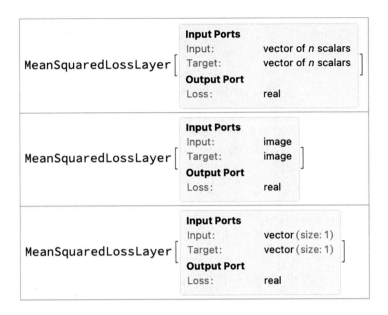

Figure 9-10. *Loss layers with different input and target forms*

Activation Functions

Activation functions are a crucial part of the construction of a neural network. The role of an activation function is to return an output from an established range, given an input. In the Wolfram Language, activation functions are treated as layers. The layer that is frequently used for activation function definition in the Wolfram Language neural net framework is the ElementwiseLayer. With this layer, you can represent layers that can apply a unary function to the input data elements—in other words, a function that receives only one argument. These functions are also known as activation functions. For example, one of the most common functions used is the hyperbolic tangent (Tanh[x]), shown in Figure 9-11.

```
In[19]:= ElementwiseLayer[Tanh[#]&](* Altnernate form
ElementwiseLayer[Tanh]*)
Out[19]=
```

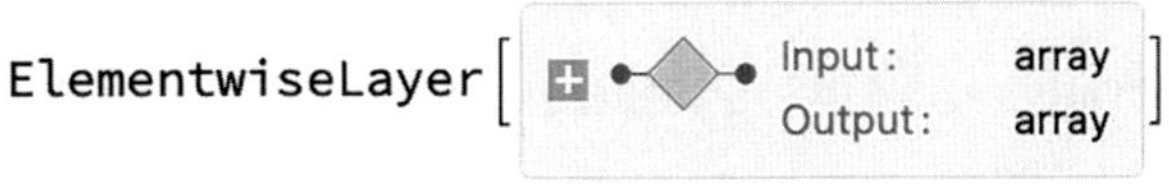

Figure 9-11. *Tanh[x] function layer*

Elementwise layers do not have learnable parameters. The pure function is used because layers cannot receive symbols. If the plus icon is clicked, detailed information about the ports and the parameters with the associated function, Tanh, are shown. Having defined an ElementwiseLayer, it can receive values like the other layers.

```
In[20]:= ElementwiseLayer[Tanh[#]&];
Table[%[i],{i,-5,5}]
Out[21]= {-0.999909,-0.999329,-0.995055,-0.964028,-0.761594,0.,0.761594,
0.964028,0.995055,0.999329,0.999909}
```

When no input or output shape is given, the layer infers the type of data it receives or returns. For instance, by specifying only the input as real, Mathematica infer that the output is real (see Figure 9-12).

```
In[22]:= tanhLayer=ElementwiseLayer[Tanh,"Input"-> "Real"]
Out[22]=
```

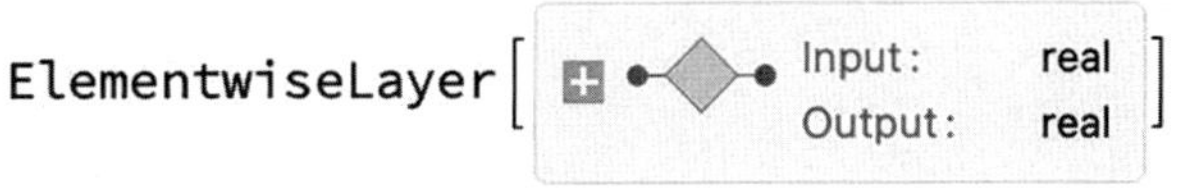

Figure 9-12. *ElementwiseLayer with the same output as the input*

Or, this can be inferred by entering only the output (see Figure 9-13) for a rectified linear unit (ReLU).

```
In[23]:= rampLayer=ElementwiseLayer[Ramp,"Output"-> {1}](*or ElementwiseLay
er["ReLU","Output" -> "Varying"]*)
Out[23]=
```

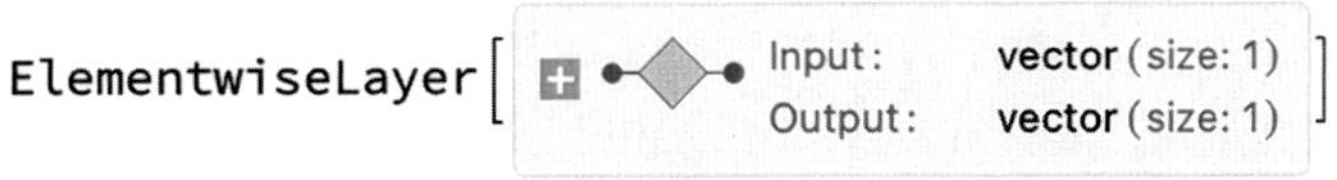

Figure 9-13. *Ramp function or ReLU*

Note   Clicking the plus icon shows the elementwise layer's established function and the layer ports' details.

Every layer in the Wolfram Language can be run through a graphics processor unit (GPU) or a central processing unit (CPU) by specifying the TargetDevice option. It is essential to ensure your computer supports the specified functionality, so if you do not have a GPU, the compulsory target device is the CPU. For example, plot the previously created layers with the TargetDevice on the CPU (see Figure 9-14).

```
In[24]:= GraphicsRow@{Plot[tanhLayer[x, TargetDevice -> "CPU"], {x, -12,
12}, PlotLabel -> "Hiperbolic Tangent", AxesLabel -> {Style["x", Bold,
12], Style["f(x)", Italic]}, PlotStyle -> ColorData[97, 25], Frame ->
True], Plot[rampLayer[x, TargetDevice -> "CPU"], {x, -12, 12}, PlotLabel
-> "ReLU",AxesLabel -> {None, Style["f(x)", Italic]},FrameLabel -> {{None,
None}, {Style["x", Bold, 12], None}}, PlotStyle -> ColorData[97, 25], Frame
-> True]}
Out[24]=
```

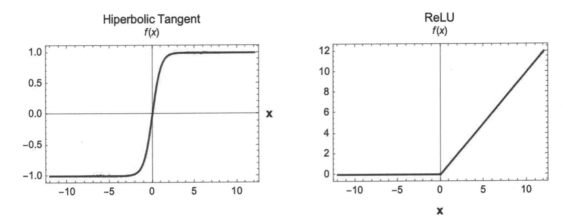

Figure 9-14. *Tanh[x] and Ramp[x] activation functions*

Other functions can be used by their name or Wolfram Language syntax—for instance, the SoftPlus function, as demonstrated in Figure 9-15.

```
In[25]:= GraphicsRow@{Plot[ElementwiseLayer["SoftPlus"][x, TargetDevice
-> "CPU"], {x, -12, 12}, PlotLabel -> "SoftPlus", AxesLabel -> {None,
Style["f(x)", Italic]},FrameLabel -> {{None, None}, {Style["x", Bold, 12],
None}}, PlotStyle -> ColorData[97, 25], Frame -> True], Plot[Log[Exp[x]
+ 1], {x, -12, 12}, PlotLabel -> "Log[Exp[x]+1]", AxesLabel -> {None,
Style["f(x)", Italic]}, FrameLabel -> {{None, None}, {Style["x", Bold, 12],
None}}, PlotStyle -> ColorData[97, 25], Frame -> True]}
Out[25]=
```

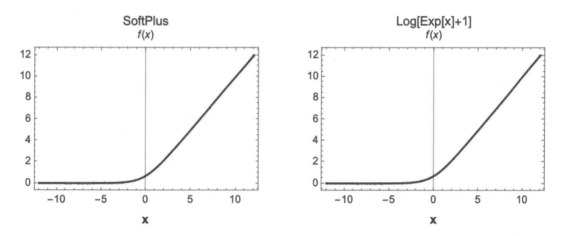

Figure 9-15. *SoftPlus function generated by the associated name and pure function*

Other standard functions are shown in the next plots, such as the scaled exponential linear unit, sigmoid, hard sigmoid, and hard hyperbolic tangent (see Figure 9-16). To view the functions supported, visit the documentation and type ElementwiseLayer in the search box.

```
In[26]:= GraphicsGrid@Partition[Table[If[Or[activation == "Sigmoid",
activation == "HardSigmoid"], Plot[ElementwiseLayer[activation]
[x, TargetDevice -> "CPU"], {x, -10, 10}, FrameLabel -> {Style["x",
Bold], None}, AxesLabel -> {None, Style["f(x)", Italic]}, PlotStyle
-> ColorData[97, 25], Frame -> True, PlotLabel -> activation],
Plot[ElementwiseLayer[activation][x, TargetDevice -> "CPU"], {x, -10, 10},
AxesLabel -> {Style["x", Bold], Style["f(x)", Italic]}, PlotStyle ->
ColorData[97, 25], Frame -> True, PlotLabel -> activation]], {activation,
{"ScaledExponentialLinearUnit", "Sigmoid", "HardSigmoid", "HardTanh"}}], 2]
Out[26]=
```

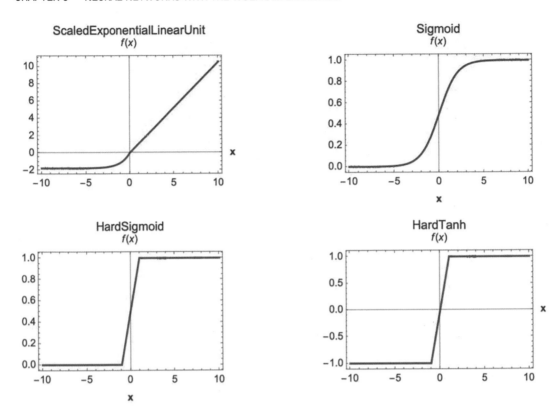

Figure 9-16. *Plot of four different activation functions*

Softmax Layer

SoftmaxLayer is a layer that uses the expression $S(x_i) = \dfrac{Exp(x_i)}{\sum_{j=1}^{n} Exp(x_j)}$, where x represents a vector and x_i the components of the vector. This expression is known as the Softmax function. The functionality of this layer consists of converting a vector to a normalized vector, which consists of values in the range of 0 to 1. This layer is generally used to represent a partition of the classes based on the probabilities of each one, and it is used for tasks that involve classification. The input and output forms in the SoftmaxLayer can be entered as the other common layers except for the shape of "Real."

```
In[27]:= sFL=SoftmaxLayer["Input"-> 4,"Output"-> 4];
```

Now, the layer can be applied to data.

```
In[28]:= SetAccuracy[sFL[{9,8,7,6}],3]
Out[28]= {0.64,0.24,0.09,0.03}
```

The total of the latter equals 1. SoftmaxLayer allows you to specify the level depth of normalization, which is seen in the parameter's properties of the layer. A level of –1 produces the normalization of a flattened list. Also, SoftmaxLayer can receive multidimensional arrays, not just flattened lists.

```
In[29]:= SoftmaxLayer[1,"Input"->{3,2}];
SetPrecision[%[{{7,8},{8,7},{7,8}}],3]//MatrixForm
Out[30]//MatrixForm=
```

$$\begin{pmatrix} 0.212 & 0.422 \\ 0.576 & 0.155 \\ 0.212 & 0.422 \end{pmatrix}$$

Summing the elements of the first columns gives the same for the second column. Another practical layer is called CrossEntropyLossLayer. This layer is widely used as a loss function for classification tasks. This loss layer measures how well the classification model performs. Entering the string Probabilities as an argument of the loss layer computes the cross-entropy loss by comparing the input class probability to the target class probability.

```
In[31]:= CrossEntropyLossLayer["Probabilities","Input"->3 ];
```

Now, the target form is set to the probabilities of the classes; the inputs and targets are entered the same way as with MeansSquaredLoss.

```
In[32]:= %[<|"Input"->{0.2,0.5,0.3},"Target"->{0.3,0.5,0.2}|>]
Out[32]= 1.0702
```

Setting the Binary argument in the layer is used when the probabilities constitute a binary alternative.

```
In[33]:= CrossEntropyLossLayer["Binary","Input"-> 1];
%[<|"Input"-> 0.1,"Target"-> 0.9|>]
Out[34]= 2.08286
```

To summarize the properties of layers in the Wolfram Language, the inputs and outputs of the layers are always scalars and numeric matrixes. Layers are evaluated using lower number precision, such as single-precision numbers. Layers have the property of being differentiable; this helps the model to perform efficient learning since some learning methods go into convex optimization problems. The Wolfram Language has many layers, each with specific functions. To display all the layers within Mathematica, check the documentation or write ?* Layer, which gives you the commands with the word layer associated at the end. Each layer has different behaviors, operations, and parameters, although some may resemble other commands, such as Append and AppendLayer. It is important to know the different layers and what they can do to best use them.

Function Layer

Another recently introduced (version 12.2) and updated (version 13) layer is the FunctionLayer. Unlike the ElementwiseLayer, this layer allows users to apply custom functions that do not come by default in the documentation library. This makes it a flexible tool for more complex operations, where the function to be applied is determined by the user (see Figure 9-17).

```
In[35]:= FunctionLayer[#*4&]
Out[35]=
```

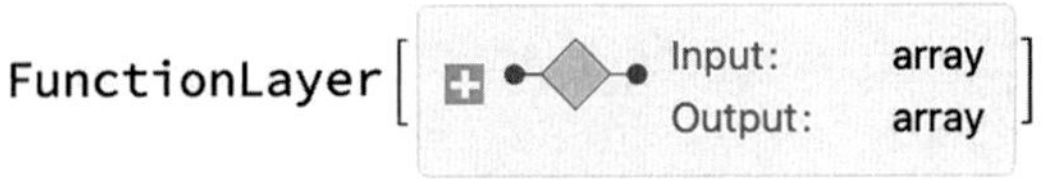

Figure 9-17. *A function layer that multiplies the input (#) by 4, and & is the pure function*

The input and output definitions are similar to the previous layers you have seen. It can be an arbitrary array of input with no shape specification. However, the output shape is determined based on the function used within the layer; for instance, in the previous example, the input is a scalar (represented as a one-element array) and returns a scalar.

```
In[36]:= FunctionLayer[1/(1+Exp[-#])&];
%[{2,-3,4}]
Out[37]= {0.880797,0.0474259,0.982014}
```

With FunctionLayer, built-in functions can also be used instead of user-defined functions, for instance, the logistic sigmoid function, which returns the same as the latter code.

```
In[38]:= FunctionLayer[LogisticSigmoid];
%[{2,-3,4}]
Out[39]= {0.880797,0.0474259,0.982014}
```

A difference between FunctionLayer and ElemewiseLayer is that you can apply a function to each element independently in the first. On the other hand, it performs element-wise operations, ensuring shape consistency.

Encoder and Decoders

Suppose audio, images, or other types of variables are intended to be used. In that case, this type of data needs to be converted into a numeric array to be introduced as input into a layer. This is where encoders and decoders come into play.

Encoder

Layers must have a NetEncoder attached to the input to perform a correct construction. The NetEncoders interpret the image, audio, and data to a numeric value to be used inside a net model. Different names are associated with the encoding type. The most common are Boolean (True or False, encoding as 1 or 0), Characters (string characters as one-hot vector encoding), Class (class labels as integer encoding), Function (custom function encoding), Image (2D image encoding as a rank 3 array), and Image3D (3D image encoding as a rank 4 array). The arguments of the encoder are the name or the name and the corresponding features of the encoder (see Figure 9-18).

```
In[40]:= NetEncoder["Boolean"]
Out[40]=
```

Figure 9-18. *Boolean type NetEncoder To test the encoder, you use the following.*

To test the encoder, you use the following.

```
In[41]:= Print["Booleans:",{%[True],%[False]}]
Out[40]=  Booleans:{1,0}
```

375

A NetEncoder can have classes with different index labels. Like a classification of class X and class Y, this corresponds to an index of the range from 1 to 2 (see Figure 9-19).

```
In[42]:= NetEncoder[{"Class",{"Class X","Class Y"}}]
Out[42]=
```

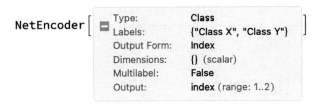

Figure 9-19. *Class type NetEncoder*

```
In[43]:= Print["Classes:", %[Table[RandomChoice[{"Class X", "Class Y"}],
{i, 10}]]]
Out[43]= Classes:{1,1,2,2,2,2,2,1,1,1}
```

The following is used for a unit vector.

```
In[44]:= NetEncoder[{"Class",{"Class X","Class Y","Class Z"},
"UnitVector"}]; Print["Unit Vector:",%[Table[RandomChoice[{"Class X",
"Class Y","Class Z"}],{i,5}]]] Print["MatrixForm:",%%[Table[RandomChoice[{"
Class X","Class Y","Class Z"}],{i,5}]]//MatrixForm[#]&]
Out[47]= Unit Vector:{{0,1,0},{0,1,0},{0,1,0},{1,0,0},{0,0,1}}
```

$$\text{MatrixForm:} \begin{pmatrix} 0 & 0 & 1 \\ 0 & 0 & 1 \\ 0 & 1 & 0 \\ 1 & 0 & 0 \\ 1 & 0 & 0 \end{pmatrix}$$

Depending on the name used inside NetEncoder, properties related to the encoder may vary. This is depicted in the different encoder objects that are created. To attach a NetEncoder to a layer, the encoders are entered at the input port—for example, for an ElementwiseLayer (see Figure 9-20). In this case, the input port of the layer has the name Boolean; the layer recognizes that this is a NetEncoder of a Boolean type. Clicking the name Boolean shows the relevant properties.

```
In[47]:= ElementwiseLayer[Sin,"Input"->NetEncoder["Boolean"]]
Out[47]=
```

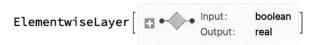

Figure 9-20. *Layer with an encoder attached to the input port*

For a LinearLayer, use the following form.

```
In[48]:= LinearLayer["Input"->NetEncoder[{"Class",{"Class X","Class Y"}}],
"Output"->"Scalar"]
Out[48]=
```

Clicking the input port shows the encoder specifications, as Figure 9-21 shows.

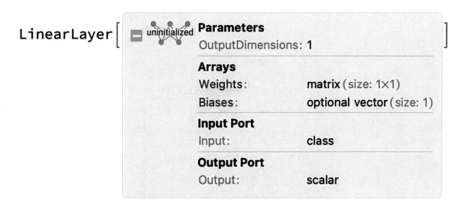

Figure 9-21. *Class encoder attached to a Linear Layer*

A NetEncoder is also used to convert images into numeric matrixes or arrays by specifying the class, the size or width, and height of the output dimensions, and the color space, which can be grayscale, RGB, CMYK, or HSB (hue, saturation, and brightness); for example, encoding an image that produces a 1×28×28 array in grayscale, or 3×28×28 array in an RGB scale (see Figure 9-22), no matter the size of the input image. The first rank of the array represents the color channel, and the other two represent the spatial dimensions.

```
In[49]:= Table[NetEncoder[{"Image",{28,28},"ColorSpace"-> Color}],
{Color,{"Grayscale","RGB"}}]
Out[49]=
```

$$\Big\{\text{NetEncoder}\Big[\; \boxplus \begin{array}{ll} \text{Type:} & \text{Image} \\ \text{Output:} & \textbf{array}\,(\text{size: }1\times28\times28) \end{array} \;\Big], \text{NetEncoder}\Big[\; \boxplus \begin{array}{ll} \text{Type:} & \text{Image} \\ \text{Output:} & \textbf{array}\,(\text{size: }3\times28\times28) \end{array} \;\Big]\Big\}$$

Figure 9-22. *NetEncoders for grayscale and RGB scale images*

Once the encoder has been established, it can be applied to the desired image; then, the encoder creates a numeric matrix with the specified size. Creating a NetEncoder for an image shows relevant properties such as type, input image size, and color space, among others. Applying the encoder generates a matrix in the size previously established.

```
In[50]:=I imgEncoder = NetEncoder[{"Image", {3, 3}, "ColorSpace" ->
"CMYK"}]; Print["Numeric Matrix:", SetPrecision[%[ExampleData[{"TestImage",
"House"}]], 3] // MatrixForm]
Out[50]=
```

$$\begin{pmatrix}
\begin{pmatrix} 0.255 \\ 0.168 \\ 0.255 \end{pmatrix} \begin{pmatrix} 0.145 \\ 0.00392 \\ 0.255 \end{pmatrix} \begin{pmatrix} 0.0784 \\ 0.0116 \\ 0.0274 \end{pmatrix} \\
\begin{pmatrix} 0.153 \\ 0.196 \\ 0.129 \end{pmatrix} \begin{pmatrix} 0.2 \\ 0.31 \\ 0.255 \end{pmatrix} \begin{pmatrix} 0.259 \\ 0.349 \\ 0.306 \end{pmatrix} \\
\begin{pmatrix} 0.047 \\ 0.102 \\ 0.00784 \end{pmatrix} \begin{pmatrix} 0.164 \\ 0.321 \\ 0.164 \end{pmatrix} \begin{pmatrix} 0.262 \\ 0.384 \\ 0.146 \end{pmatrix} \\
\begin{pmatrix} 0.16 \\ 0.262 \\ 0.184 \end{pmatrix} \begin{pmatrix} 0.255 \\ 0.408 \\ 0.478 \end{pmatrix} \begin{pmatrix} 0.325 \\ 0.388 \\ 0.569 \end{pmatrix}
\end{pmatrix}$$

The output generated is a numeric matrix that is now ready to be implemented in a network model. If the input image shape is in a different color space, the encoder reshapes and transforms the image into the established color space. The image used in this example is obtained from the ExampleData[{"TestImage," "House"}].

Pooling Layer

Encoders can be added to the ports of single layers or containers by specifying the encoder to the port—for instance, a PoolingLayer. These layers are used primarily on convolutional neural networks (see Figure 9-23).

```
In[52]:= poolLayer=PoolingLayer[{3,3},{2,2},PaddingSize->0,"Function"->
Max,"Input"-> NetEncoder[{"Image",{3,3},"ColorSpace"-> "CMYK"}](*Or
ImgEncoder*)]
Out[52]=
```

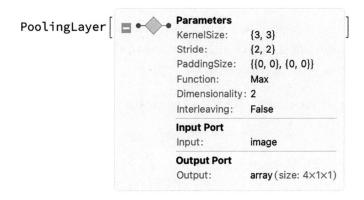

Figure 9-23. *PoolingLayer with a NetEncoder*

The latter layer has a specification for a two-dimensional PoolingLayer with a kernel size of 3×3 and a stride of 2×2, which is the step size between kernel applications. PaddingSize adds elements at the beginning and the end of the input matrix. This is done so that the division between the matrix and kernel sizes is an integer, preventing the loss of information between layers. Function indicates the pooling operation function, which is Max; this calculates the maximum value in each filter patch. It can also compute the mean and total for the average and summation of the filter values, respectively. Sometimes, they might be known as max, average, and sum pooling layers.

```
In[53]:=SetPrecision[poolLayer[ExampleData[{"TestImage","House"}]],3]
//MatrixForm
Out[53]//MatrixForm=
```

$$\begin{pmatrix} (0.255) \\ (0.349) \\ (0.384) \\ (0.569) \end{pmatrix}$$

Decoders

Once the net operations are finished, it return numeric expressions. On the other hand, in some tasks, you do not want numeric expressions, such as in classification tasks where classes can be given as outputs, where the model can tell that a particular object belongs to a class A and another object belongs to a class B, so a vector or numeric array can represent a probability of each class. To convert the numeric arrays into other forms of data, a NetDecoder is used (see Figure 9-24).

```
In[54]:= decoder=NetDecoder[{"Class",CharacterRange["W","Z"]}]
Out[54]=
```

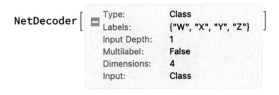

Figure 9-24. *NetDecoder for four different classes*

The dimension of the decoder is equal to class construction. You can apply a vector of probabilities, and the decoder interprets it and tells you the class to which it belongs. It also displays the probabilities of the classes.

```
In[55]:= decoder@{0.3,0.2,0.1,0.4}(*This is the same as Decoder[{0.3,0.2,0.
1,0,4},"Decision"] *)
Out[55]= Z
```

TopDecisions, TopProbabilites, and uncertainty of the probability distribution are displayed as follows.

```
In[56]:= TableForm[{decoder[{0.3, 0.2, 0.1, 0.4},
"TopDecisions" -> 4](*   or {"TopDecisions", 4} the same is for
TopProbabilities*),  decoder[{0.3, 0.2, 0.1, 0.4}, "TopProbabilities"
```

```
-> 4], decoder[{0.3, 0.2, 0.1, 0.4}, "Entropy"]}, TableDirections
-> Column, TableHeadings -> {{Style["TopDecisions", Italic],
Style["TopProbabilities", Italic], Style["Entropy", Italic]},
None}]Out[56]//TableForm=
```

TopDecisions	Z	W	X	Y
TopProbabilities	Z->0.4	W->0.3	X->0.2	Y->0.1
Entropy	1.27985			

Given the list of values, input depth is added to define the class's application level.

```
In[57]:= NetDecoder[{"Class",CharacterRange["X","Z"],"InputDepth"→2}];
```

Applying the decoder to a nested list of values produces the following.

```
In[58]:= TableForm[{%[{{0.1, 0.3, 0.6}, {0.3, 0.4, 0.3}}, "TopDecisions" ->
3](* or {"TopDecisions", 4} the same is for TopProbabilities*), %[{{0.1,
0.3, 0.6}, {0.3, 0.4, 0.3}}, "TopProbabilities" -> 3], %[{{0.1,
0.3, 0.6}, {0.3, 0.4, 0.3}}, "Entropy"]}, TableDirections ->
Column, TableHeadings -> {{Style["TopDecisions", Italic],
Style["TopProbabilities", Italic], Style["Entropy", Italic]}, None}]
Out[58]//TableForm=
```

TopDecisions	Z	Y
	Y	X
	X	Z
	Z->0.6	Y->0.4
TopProbabilities	Y->0.3	X->0.3
	X->0.1	Z->0.3
Entropy	0.897946	1.0889

A decoder is added to the output port of a layer, container, or network model.

```
In[59]:=SoftmaxLayer["Output"→NetDecoder[{"Class",{"X","Y","Z"}}]];
```

Applying the layer to the data produce the probabilities for each class.

```
In[60]:= {%@{1,3,5},%[{1,3,5},"Probabilities"],%[{1,3,5},"Decision"]}
Out[60]= {Z,<|X->0.0158762,Y->0.11731,Z->0.866813|>,Z}
```

Applying Encoder and Decoders

You are ready to implement the whole process of encoding and decoding in Figure 9-25. First, the image is resized by 200 pixels in width to show how the original image looks before encoding.

```
In[61]:= Img=ImageResize[ExampleData[{"TestImage","House"}],200]
Out[61]=
```

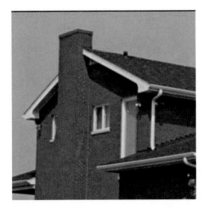

Figure 9-25. *Example image of a house when the encoder and decoder are defined*

```
In[62]:= encoder=NetEncoder[{"Image",{100,100},"ColorSpace"-> "RGB"}];
decoder=NetDecoder[{"Image",ColorSpace-> "Grayscale"}];
```

Then, the encoder is applied to the image, and the decoder is applied to the numeric matrix. The dimensions of the decoded image are checked to see if they match the encoder output dimensions (see Figure 9-26).

```
In[64]:=encoder[img];
decoder[%]
```

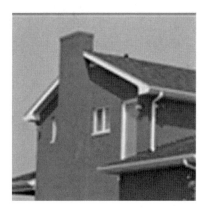

Figure 9-26. *Example of the decoded house*

Figure 9-26 shows that the image has been converted into a grayscale image with new dimensions.

```
In[66]:= ImageDimensions[%]
Out[66]= {100,100}
```

As seen, the picture has been resized. Try to look at the steps in the process, like viewing the numeric matrix and the objects corresponding to the encoder and decoder. Using the encoders and decoders involves the data type you use because every net model receives different inputs and generates different outputs.

NetChains and Graphs

Neural networks consist of different layers, not individual layers on their own. The NetChain command or the NetGraph command is used to construct more complex structures with more than one layer.

Containers

Containers are valuable for properly operating and constructing neural networks in the Wolfram Language. In the Wolfram Language, containers are structures that assemble the infrastructure of the neural network model. Containers can have multiple forms. NetChain is useful for creating linear and non-linear structures' nets. This helps the model to learn non-linear patterns. You can think that each layer in a network has a level of abstraction that detects complex behavior, which could not be recognized if you only worked with one single layer. As a result, you can build networks in a general way, starting from three layers: the input layer, the hidden layer, and the output layer. When there are more than two hidden layers, it is deep learning; for more information, refer to *Introduction to Deep Learning: From Logical Calculus to Artificial Intelligence* by Sandro Skansi (Springer, 2018).

NetChain can join two operations. They can be written as a pure function instead of just the function's name (see Figure 9-27).

```
In[67]:=NetChain[{ElementwiseLayer[LogisticSigmoid@#&],ElementwiseLayer[S
in@#&]}]
Out[67]=
```

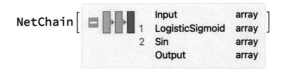

Figure 9-27. *NetChain containing two elementwise layers*

The object returned is a NetChain, and the icon of three colored rectangles appears. This means that the object created (NetChain) or referred to is a net chain and contains layers. If the chain is examined, it shows the input, first (LogisticSigmoid), second (Sin), and output layers. The operations are in order of appearance, so the first layer is applied and then the second. The input and output options of other layers are supported in NetChain, such as a single real number (Real), an integer (Integer), an "n"-length vector, and a multidimensional array (see Figure 9-28).

```
In[68]:= NetInitialize@NetChain[{3,4,12,Tanh},"Input"->1]
Out[68]=
```

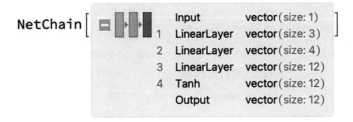

Figure 9-28. *NetChain with multiple layers*

NetChain recognizes the Wolfram Language function names and associates them with their corresponding layers, like 3, 4, and 12. They represent a linear layer with outputs of sizes 3, 4, and 12 (see Figure 9-28). The Tanh function represents the elementwise layer.

Let's append a layer to the chain created with NetAppend (see Figure 9-29) or NetPrepend. Many of the original commands of the Wolfram Language have the same meaning—for example, to delete in a chain would be NetDelete[net_ name, #_of_layer].

```
In[69]:=NetInitialize@NetChain[{1,ElementwiseLayer[LogisticSigmoid@#&]},"In
put"-> 1];
netCH2=NetInitialize@NetAppend[%,{1,ElementwiseLayer[Cos[#]&]}]
Out[70]=
```

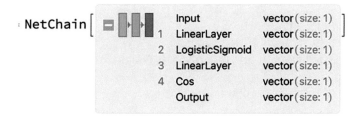

Figure 9-29. *NetChain object with different added layers*

Different options are available when a net is applied to data, such as NetEvaluationMode (mode of evaluation, either train or test), TargetDevice, and WorkingPrecision (numeric precision).

```
In[71]:= netCH2[{{0},{2},{44}},NetEvaluationMode-> "Train",TargetDevice->
"CPU",WorkingPrecision-> "Real64",RandomSeeding-> 8888](*use N@Cos[Sin[Logi
sticSigmoid[{0,2,44}]]] to check results*)
Out[71]= {{0.967873},{0.990894},{1.}}
```

Another form is to enter the explicit names of layers in a chain, which is typed as an association (see Figure 9-30).

```
In[72]:= NetInitialize@NetChain[<|"Linear Layer 1"->LinearLayer[3],
"Ramp"-> Ramp,"Linear Layer 2"->LinearLayer[4],"Logistic"-> ElementwiseLayer
[LogisticSigmoid]|>,"Input"-> 3]
Out[72]=
```

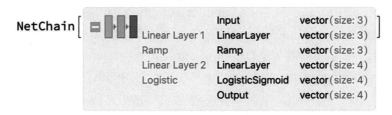

Figure 9-30. *NetChain object with custom layer names*

Inspecting the layer's contents should appear after clicking the layer's name or the layer. If a layer wants to be extracted, then NetExtract is used along with the name of the corresponding layer. The output is suppressed, but the layer should pop out if the semicolon is removed.

```
In[73]:=NetExtract[%,"Logistic"];
```

To extract all of the layers in one line of code, Normal does the job (see Figure 9-31).

```
In[74]:= Normal[netCH2]//Column
Out[74]=
```

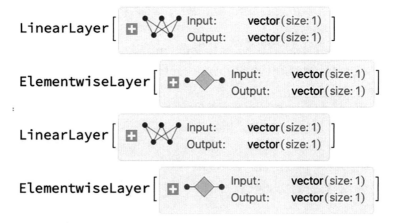

Figure 9-31. *Layers of the NetChain NetCH2*

Multiple Chains

Chains can be joined with a nested chain (see Figure 9-32).

```
In[75]:= chain1=NetChain[{12,SoftmaxLayer[]}];
chain2=NetChain[{1,ElementwiseLayer[Cos[#]&]}];
```

```
nestedChain=NetInitialize@NetChain[{chain1,chain2},"Input"-> 12]
Out[77]=
```

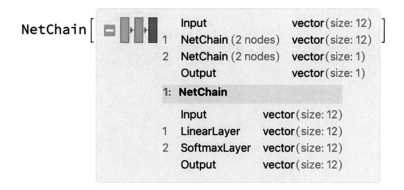

Figure 9-32. *Chain 1 selected of the two chains available*

This chain is divided into two NetChains, each representing a chain. In this case, you see chain1 and chain2, and each chain shows its corresponding nodes. To flatten the chains, use NetFlatten (see Figure 9-33).

```
In[78]:= NetFlatten[nestedChain]
Out[78]=
```

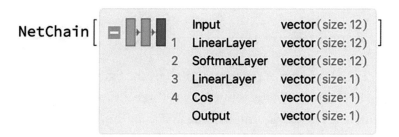

Figure 9-33. *Flattened chain*

NetGraphs

The NetChain command only joins layers in which the output of a layer is connected to the input of the next layer. NetChain does not work in connecting inputs or outputs to other layers; it only works with one layer. To work around this, the use of NetGraph is required. Besides allowing more inputs and layers, NetGraph represents the neural network's structure and process with a graph (see Figure 9-34).

```
In[79]:= NetInitialize@NetGraph[{ LinearLayer["Output"-> 1,"Input"-> 1],
Cos,SummationLayer[]},{}]
Out[79]=
```

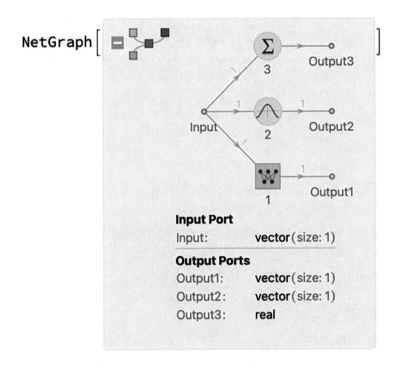

Figure 9-34. *Expanded NetGraph*

The object crafted is a NetGraph, represented by the figure of the connecting squares, as seen in Figure 9-35. The input goes to three different layers, each with its output. NetGraph accepts two arguments: the first is for the layers or chains, and the second is to define the graph vertices or connectivity of the net. For example, the net has three outputs in the latter code because the vertices were not specified. SummationLayer is a layer that sums all the input data.

```
In[80]:= net1=NetInitialize@NetGraph[{ LinearLayer["Output"-> 2,"Input"->
1],Cos,SummationLayer[]},{1-> 2-> 3}]
Out[80]=
```

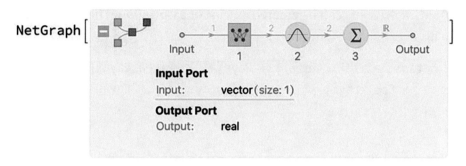

Figure 9-35. *Unidirectional NetGraph*

The vertex notation means that the output of a layer is given to another layer, and so on. In other words, $1 \rightarrow 2 \rightarrow 3$ means that the output of the linear layer is passed to the next layer until it is finally summed up in the last layer with the summation layer (see Figure 9-35), thus preserving the order of appearance of the layers. However, you can alter the order of each vertex. The net can be modified so that outputs can go to other layers of the net, such as 1 to 3 and then to 2 (see Figure 9-36). With NetGraph, layers and chains can be entered as a list or an association. The vertices are typed as a list of rules.

```
In[81]:= net2=NetInitialize@NetGraph[{ LinearLayer["Output"-> 2,"Input"->
1],Cos,SummationLayer[]},{1-> 3->2}]
Out[81]=
```

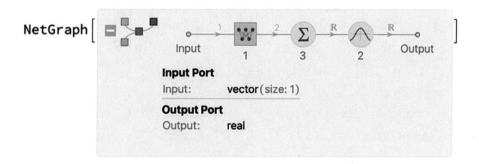

Figure 9-36. *NetGraph structure of Net2*

The inputs and outputs of each layer are marked by a tooltip that appears when passing the cursor over the graph lines or vertices. Because input and output are not specified, NetGraph infers the data type in the input and output port; this is the case for the capital R in the input and output of the layer used, which stands for real.

With NetGraph, layers can be entered as a list or association. The connections are typed as a list of rules (see Figure 9-37).

```
In[82]:= NetInitialize@NetGraph[<|"Layer 1"-> LinearLayer[2,"Input"->
1],"Layer 2"-> Cos,"Layer 3"-> SummationLayer[]|>,{"Layer 2"-> "Layer 1"->
"Layer 3"}]
Out[82]=
```

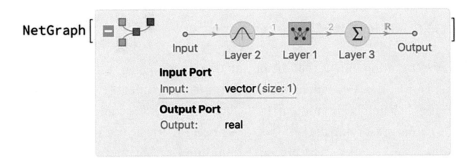

Figure 9-37. *NetGraph initialized with named layers*

It is possible to specify how many inputs and outputs a structure can have from the NetPort command (see Figure 9-38).

```
In[83]:= NetInitialize@ NetGraph[{ LinearLayer[3, "Input" ->
1],  LinearLayer[3, "Input" -> 2], LinearLayer[3, "Input" -> 1] ,
TotalLayer[]}, {NetPort["1st Input"] -> 1, NetPort["2nd Input"] ->
2, NetPort["3rd Input"] -> 3, {1, 2, 3} ->   4}] (*Or NetInitialize@
NetGraph[<|"L1"\[Rule]  LinearLayer[3,"Input"\[Rule] 1],"L2"\[Rule]
LinearLayer[3,"Input"\[Rule] 1], "L3"\[Rule] LinearLayer[3,"Input"\
[Rule] 1] ,"Tot L"\[Rule] TotalLayer[]|>,{NetPort["1st Input"]\
[Rule] "L1", NetPort["2nd Input"]\[Rule] "L2",NetPort["3rd Input"]\
[Rule]"L3",{"L1","L2","L3"} -> "Tot L"}]*)
Out[83]=
```

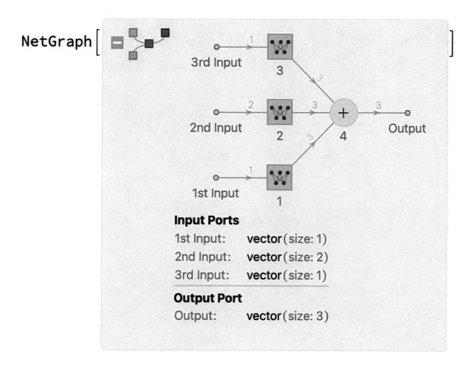

Figure 9-38. *NetGraph with multiple inputs and a single output*

If you have more than one input, each input is entered in the specified port.

```
In[84]:= %[<|"1st Input"-> 32.32,"2nd Input"-> {2,\[Pi]},"3rd Input"-> 1|>]
Out[84]= {82.4758,-42.202,-37.4852}
```

If having more than one output, the results are displayed for every different output (see Figure 9-39).

```
In[85]:= NetInitialize[NetGraph[{LinearLayer[1,"Input"->
1],LinearLayer[1,"Input"-> 1],LinearLayer[1,"Input"-> 1],Ramp,El
ementwiseLayer["ExponentialLinearUnit"],LogisticSigmoid},{1->4->
NetPort["Output1"],2->5-> NetPort["Output2"],3-> 6-> NetPort["Output3"]}],
RandomSeeding->8888] %[{1}]
Out[85]=
```

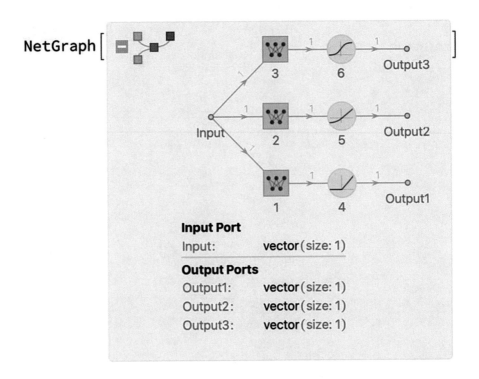

Figure 9-39. *NetGraph with single input and three outputs*

Out[86]= <|Output1->{0.},Output2->{-0.289052},Output3->{0.860635}|>

NetChain containers can be treated as layers with NetGraph (see Figure 9-40). Some layers, such as the CatenateLayer, accept zero arguments.

In[87]:= NetInitialize@NetGraph[{LinearLayer[1,"Input"-> 1], NetChain[{L inearLayer[1,"Input"-> 1], ElementwiseLayer[LogisticSigmoid[#]&]}],NetCh ain[{LinearLayer[1,"Input"-> 1],Ramp}], ElementwiseLayer["ExponentialLin earUnit"],
CatenateLayer[]},{1->4,2->5,3-> 5,4-> 5}]
Out[87]=

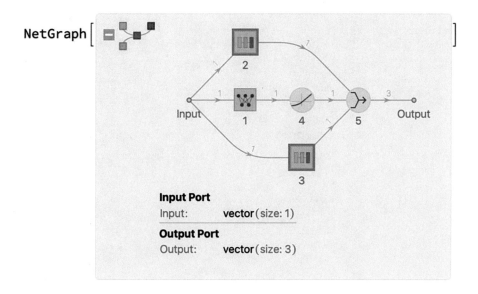

Figure 9-40. *NetGraph with multiple containers*

Clicking the chain or the layer shows the relevant information, and clicking the layer inside a chain gives the information about the layer on the selected chain.

Combining Containers

NetChains, and NetGraphs can be nested to form different structures, as seen in the following example (see Figure 9-41), where a NetGraph and vice versa can follow a NetChain.

```
In[88]:= n1=NetGraph[{1,Ramp,2,LogisticSigmoid},{1-> 2,2-> 3,3-> 4}];
n2=NetChain[{3,SummationLayer[]}];
NetInitialize@NetGraph[{n2,n1},{2-> 1},"Input"-> 22]
Out[90]=
```

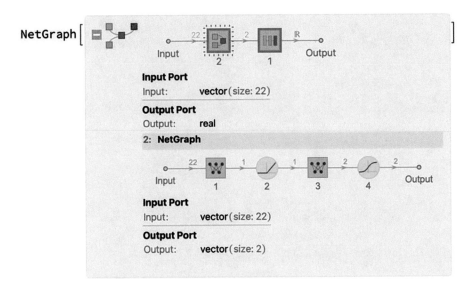

Figure 9-41. *Nested NetGraph and NetChain*

From the graph in Figure 9-40, it is clear that the input goes to the NetGraph, and the output of the NetGraph goes to the NetChain. A NetChain or NetGraph that has not been initialized appears in red. A fundamental quality of the containers (NetChain, NetGraph) is that they can behave as a layer. With this in mind, you can create nested containers involving only NetChains, NetGraphs, or both.

Just as a demonstration, more complex structures can be created with NetGraph, like those in Figure 9-42. Once a network structure is created, properties about every layer or chain can be extracted. For instance, with SummaryGraphic, you can obtain the graphic of the network graph.

```
In[91]:= net = NetInitialize@  NetGraph[{LinearLayer[10], Ramp, 10,
SoftmaxLayer[], TotalLayer[], ThreadingLayer[Times]}, {1 -> 2 -> 3 -> 4,
{1, 2, 3} -> 5, {1, 5} -> 6}, "Input" -> "Real"];
Information[net, "SummaryGraphic"]
Out[92]=
```

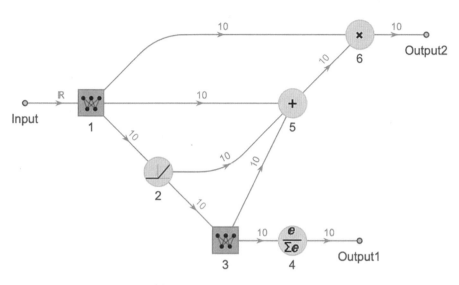

Figure 9-42. *Compound graph net structure*

Network Properties

The properties related to the numeric arrays of the network are Arrays (gives each array in the network), ArraysCount (the number of arrays in the net), ArraysDimensions (dimensions of each array in the net), and ArraysPositionList (position of each array in the net), as depicted in Figure 9-43.

```
In[93]:={Dataset@Information[net,"Arrays"],Dataset@Information[net,"Arrays
Dimensions"],Dataset@Information[net,"ArraysPositionList"]}
Out[93]=
```

1	Biases	NumericArray [Type: Real32 Dimensions: {10}]
1	Weights	NumericArray [Type: Real32 Dimensions: {10, 1}]
3	Biases	NumericArray [Type: Real32 Dimensions: {10}]
3	Weights	NumericArray [Type: Real32 Dimensions: {10, 10}]

1	Biases	{10}
1	Weights	{10, 1}
3	Biases	{10}
3	Weights	{10, 10}

1	Biases
1	Weights
3	Biases
3	Weights

Figure 9-43. *Datasat containing various properties*

Information related to the variable type in the input and output ports are shown with InputPorts and OutputPorts.

```
In[94]:= {Information[net,"InputPorts"],Information[net,"OutputPorts"]}
Out[94]= {<|Input->Real|>,<|Output1->10,Output2->10|>}
```

You can see that the input is a real number, and the net has two output vectors of size 10. The most used properties related to layers are Layers (returns every layer of the net), LayerTypeCounts (number of occurrences of a layer in the net), LayersCount (number of layers in the net), LayersList (a list of all the layers in the net), and LayerTypeCounts (number of occurrences of a layer in the net). Figure 9-44 shows for Layers and LayerTypeCounts.

```
In[95]:=Dataset@{Information[net,"Layers"],Information[net,"LayerType
Counts"]}
Out[95]=
```

{1}	LinearLayer [Input: real / Output: vector(size: 10)]
{2}	ElementwiseLayer [Input: vector(size: 10) / Output: vector(size: 10)]
{3}	LinearLayer [Input: vector(size: 10) / Output: vector(size: 10)]
{4}	SoftmaxLayer [Input: vector(size: 10) / Output: vector(size: 10)]
{5}	TotalLayer [**Input Ports** / Input1: vector(size: 10) / Input2: vector(size: 10) / Input3: vector(size: 10) / **Output Port** / Output: vector(size: 10)]
{6}	ThreadingLayer [**Input Ports** / Input1: vector(size: 10) / Input2: vector(size: 10) / **Output Port** / Output: vector(size: 10)]
LinearLayer	2
ElementwiseLayer	1
SoftmaxLayer	1
TotalLayer	1
ThreadingLayer	1

Figure 9-44. *Information about the layers contained in the symbol Net*

Visualization of the net structure (see Figure 9-45) is achieved with the properties LayersGraph (a graph showing the connectivity of the layers), SummaryGraphics (graphic of the net structure), MXNetNodeGraph (MXNeT raw graph operations), and MXNetNodeGraphPlot (annotated graph of MXNet operations). MXNet is an open-source deep learning framework that supports a variety of programming languages, and one of them is the Wolfram Language. In addition, the Wolfram Neural Network Framework works with MXNet structure as backend support.

In[96]:= Grid[{{Style["Layers Connection",Italic,20,ColorData[105,4]],Style
["NetGraph",Italic,20,ColorData[105,4]]},{Information[net,"LayersGraph"],In
formation[net,"SummaryGraphic"]},{Style["MXNet Layer Graph",Italic,20,Color
Data[105,4]],Style["MXNet Ops Graph",Italic,20,ColorData[105,4]]},{Informat
ion[net,"MXNetNodeGraph"],Information[net,"MXNetNodeGraphPlot"]}},Dividers-
>All,Background-> {{{None,None}},{{Opacity[1,Gray],None}}}]
Out[96]=

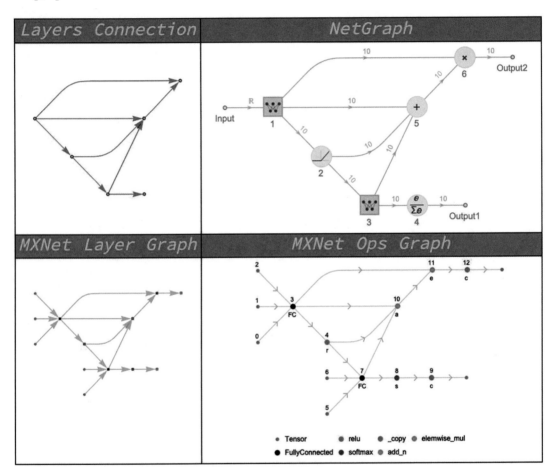

Figure 9-45. *Grid showing multiple graphics*

Passing the cursor pointer over a layer or node in the MXNet symbol graph, a tooltip shows the properties of the MXNet symbols like ID, name, parameters, attributes, and inputs.

Exporting and Importing a Model

Because of the interoperability of the Wolfram Language and MXNet, the Wolfram Language supports the import and export of neural nets, initialized or uninitialized. You create a folder on the desktop with the MXNet Nets name and export the network found in the Net variable.

```
In[97]:= fileDirectory="/Users/macosx/Desktop";
Export[FileNameJoin[{dileDirectory,"MxNet.json"}],net,"MXNet","ArrayPath"->
Automatic,"SaveArrays"-> True]
Out[98]= /Users/macosx/Desktop/MxNet.json
```

Exporting the network to the MXNet format generates two files: a JSON file that stores the topology of the neural network and a file of type .params that contains the required parameters (numeric arrays used in the network) data for the exported architecture; once it has been initialized. With ArrayPath set to Automatic, the params file is saved in the same net folder. Otherwise, it can have a different path. SaveArrays indicate whether the numeric arrays are exported (True) or not (False). Let's check the two files created in the MXNets Nets folder.

```
In[99]:= FileNames[All,File@fileDirectory]
Out[99]= {/Users/macosx/Desktop/MxNet.json,
/Users/macosx/Desktop/MxNet.params}
```

To import an MXNet network, the JSON and params files are recommended to be in the same folder because the Wolfram Language assumes that a certain JSON file matches the pattern of the params file. There are various ways to import a net, including Import[file_name.json, "MXNet"] and Import[file_name.json,{"MXNet," element}] (the same as with .param files). Since version 13, nets are no longer imported as net chains or net graphs but can now be imported as net external objects. However, if you don't intend to use the neural network outside of the Wolfram Language, it's much simpler to store it as a WLNet, which facilitates easier saving and retrieval within the Wolfram Language environment. To export the net to the WLNet format, you can use the following code: Export["file_name.wlnet", <net_symbol or variable_name>]. Then, you can import the net using Import["file_name.wlnet"]

```
In[100]:=Import[FileNameJoin[{fileDirectory,"MxNet.json"}],{"MXNet",
"NetExternalObject"},InputPorts-><|"Input"->{1}|>,"ArrayPath"->None];
```

The latter net was imported with the .params file automatically. To import the net without the parameters, use ArrayPath set to None or set the params file path. Importing the net parameters can be done with a list (ArrayList), the names (ArrayNames), or an association (ArrayAssociation), as shown in Figure 9-46.

```
In[101]:= Row[Dataset[Import[FileNameJoin[{fileDirectory,"MxNet.
json"}],{"MXNet",#}]]&/@{"ArrayAssociation","ArrayList","ArrayNames"}]
Out[101]=
```

1.Biases	NumericArray [Type: Real32 Dimensions: {10}]	NumericArray [Type: Real32 Dimensions: {10}]	
1.Weights	NumericArray [Type: Real32 Dimensions: {10, 1}]	NumericArray [Type: Real32 Dimensions: {10, 1}]	1.Biases 1.Weights
3.Biases	NumericArray [Type: Real32 Dimensions: {10}]	NumericArray [Type: Real32 Dimensions: {10}]	3.Biases 3.Weights
3.Weights	NumericArray [Type: Real32 Dimensions: {10, 10}]	NumericArray [Type: Real32 Dimensions: {10, 10}]	

Figure 9-46. *Different import options of the MXNet format*

The elements of the net to import are InputNames, NetExternalObject, NodeDataset (a dataset of the nodes of the MXNet), NodeGraph (nodes graph of the MXNet), NodeGraphPlot (plot of nodes of the MXNet). The following dataset shows a few options listed before Figure 9-47.

```
In[102]:= {Import[FileNameJoin[{fileDirectory,"MxNet.json"}],{"MXNet","Node
Dataset"}],Import[FileNameJoin[{ileDirectory,"MxNet.json"}],{"MXNet","NodeG
raphPlot"}]}//Row
Out[102]=
```

	op	attrs	inputs
Input	null		
1.Weights	null		
1.Biases	null		
1	FullyConnected	2 total ›	{0, 0, 0}
		3 total ›	
2$0	relu		{3, 0, 0}
3.Weights	null		
3.Biases	null		
3	FullyConnected	2 total ›	{4, 0, 0}
		3 total ›	
4$0	softmax	1 total ›	{7, 0, 0}
Output1	_copy		{8, 0, 0}
5	add_n	1 total ›	{3, 0, 0}
		3 total ›	
6$0	elemwise_mul		{3, 0, 0}
		2 total ›	
Output2	_copy		{11, 0, 0}

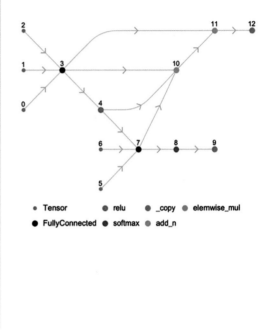

Figure 9-47. *Node dataset and MXNet ops plot*

Some operations between the Wolfram Language and MXNet are not reversible. If you pay attention, the network input, exported to MXNet format, was set as a real number, unlike the network input imported in MXNet format, which marks that the input is an array with specifying dimensions.

When constructing a neural network, there is no restriction on how many net chains or net graphs a net can have. For instance, the following example is a neural network from the Wolfram Neural Net Repository, which has a deeper sense of construction (see Figure 9-48). This net is called CapsNet, which is used to estimate the depth map of an image. To consult the net, enter NetModel["CapsNet Trained on MNIST Data," "DocumentationLink"] for the documentation web page; for the notebook on the Wolfram Cloud, enter NetModel["CapsNet Trained on MNIST Data," "ExampleNotebookObject"] or just ExampleNotebook for the desktop version.

In[103]:= NetModel["CapsNet Trained on MNIST Data"]
Out[103]=

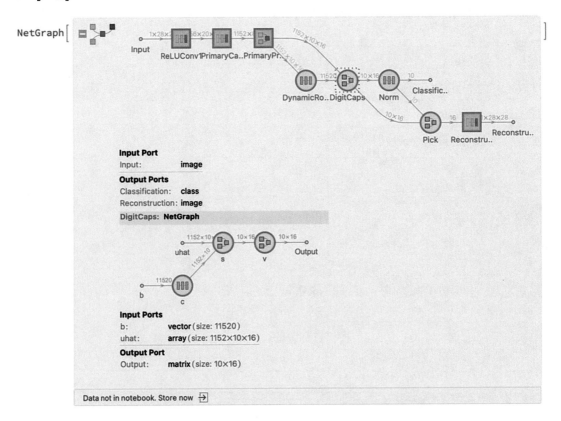

Figure 9-48. *CapsNet neural net model*

Summary

This chapter introduced the neural network scheme in the Wolfram Language and covered basic layers components: data input, weight, and biases. Additionally, the chapter focuses on the encoders and decoders, explaining its structure.

CHAPTER 10

Neural Networks Framework

This chapter explores training a neural network model in the Wolfram Language, how to access the results and the trained network. You review the basic commands to export and import a net model. You end the chapter by exploring the Wolfram Neural Net Repository and reviewing the LeNet network model.

Training a Neural Network

The Wolfram Language contains a very useful command that automates neural network model training. This command is NetTrain. Training a neural network consists of fine-tuning the internal parameters of the neural network. The whole point is that the parameters can be learned during training. This general process is done by an optimization algorithm called gradient descent, which is computed with the backpropagation algorithm.

Data Input

With NetTrain, data can be entered in different forms. First, the net model goes as the first argument, followed by the input → target, {inputs, ...} → {target, ...} or the name of the data or dataset. Once the net model is defined, the next argument is the data, followed by an optional argument of All. The All option creates a NetTrainResultsObject, which shows the NetTrain results panel after the computation and stores all relevant information about the trained model. The options for training the model are entered as the last arguments. Standard options used in layers and containers are available in NetTrain.

© Jalil Villalobos Alva 2024
J. Villalobos Alva, *Beginning Mathematica and Wolfram for Data Science*,
https://doi.org/10.1007/979-8-8688-0348-2_10

The next example uses the perceptron model to build a linear classifier. The data to be classified is shown in the following plot (see Figure 10-1).

```
In[1]:= plt=ListPlot[{{{-1.8,-1.5},{-1,-1.7},{-1.5,-1},{-1,-1},{-0.5,-1.2},
{-1,-0.7}}, {{1,1}, {1.7,1}, {0.5,2}, {0.1,0.3}, {0.5,1}, {0.6,1.3}}},
PlotMarkers->"OpenMarkers",Frame->True,PlotStyle->{Green,Red}]
Out[1]=
```

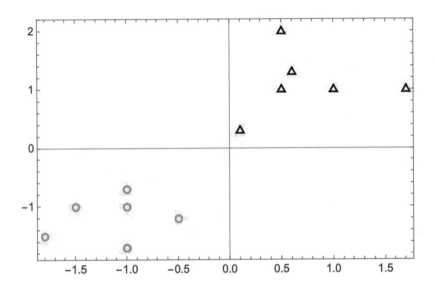

Figure 10-1. *ListPlot showing two different plot points*

Let's define the data, target values, and the training data.

```
In[2]:=data={{-1.8,-1.5},{-1,-1.7},{-1.5,-1},{-1,-1},{-0.5,-1.2},{-1,-0.7},
{1,1},{1.7,1},{0.5,2},{0.1,0.3},{0.5,1},{0.6,1.3}};
target={-1,-1,-1,-1,-1,-1,1,1,1,1,1,1};
trainData=MapThread[#1->]{#2}&,{Standardize[data],target},1];
```

The Standardize function is crucial in the latter code because it normalizes the input data before training the neural network. This step ensures that each feature contributes equally to the learning process during the training phase, preventing any single feature from dominating the others. This process can lead to faster convergence during training and improves the overall performance of the net model. Next, let's define the net model.

```
In[3]:= model=NetChain[{LinearLayer[1,"Input"->2],
ElementwiseLayer[Ramp[#]&]}];
```

Training Phase

Having prepared the data and the model, you proceeded to train the model. Once the training begins, a progress information panel appears with four main results.

- Summary: contains relevant information about the batches, rounds, and time rates

- Data: involves processed data information

- Method: shows the method used, batch size, and device used for training

- Round: the current state of loss value

```
In[6]:=net=NetTrain[model,trainData,All,LearningRate->0.01,
PerformanceGoal->"TrainingSpeed",TrainingProgressReporting->"Panel",
TargetDevice->"CPU", RandomSeeding->88888,WorkingPrecision->"Real64"]
Out[6]=
```

Figure 10-2 shows the loss plot against the training rounds.

NetTrainResultsObject
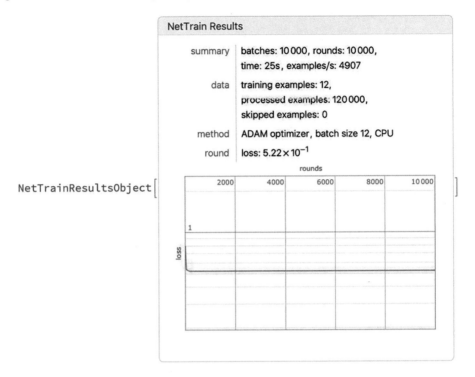

Figure 10-2. *NetTrainResultsObject*

The Adam optimizer is a variant of the Stochastic gradient descent, which you see later. The object generated is called NetTrainResultsObject.

Model Implementation

Once the training is done, getting the trained net and model implementation is as follows in Figure 10-3.

```
In[7]:= trainedNet1=net["TrainedNet"]
Out[7]=
```

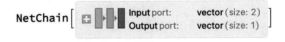

Figure 10-3. *Extracted trained net*

Let's look at how the trained net identifies each point by plotting the boundaries with a density plot (see Figure 10-4).

```
In[8]:= Show[DensityPlot[trainedNet1[{x,y}],{x,-2,2},{y,-3,3},PlotPoints->
50,ColorFunction->(RGBColor[1-#,2*#,1]&)],Plt]
Out[8]=
```

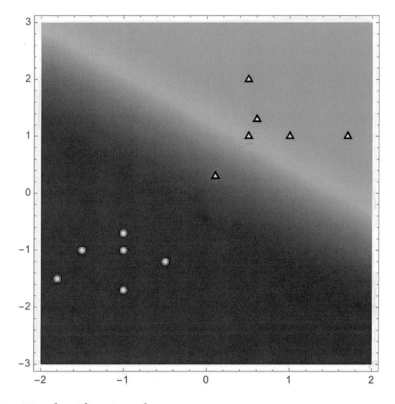

Figure 10-4. *Net classification plot*

The graphic shows that the boundaries are not well defined and that points near zero might be misclassified. This result can be attributed to the ramp function, which gives 0 if it receives any negative number, but for any positive value, it returns that value. This model can still be improved, perhaps by changing the activation function to a hyperbolic tangent to have robust boundaries.

Batch Size and Rounds

If the batch size is not indicated, it has an automatic value, almost always a value of 64 or powers of two. Remember that the batch size indicates the number of examples the model uses in training before updating the internal parameters of the model. The number of batches is the division of the examples within the training dataset by the batch size. The processed examples are the number of rounds (epochs) multiplied by the number of training examples. The batch size is generally chosen to divide the training set's size evenly. The MaxTrainingRounds option determines the number of times the training dataset is passed through during the training phase. When you go through the entire training set just once, it's called an epoch. To better understand this, a batch size of 12 was automatically chosen in the earlier example, which is equal to the number of examples in the training set. This means that it enters a batch of 12/12 -> 1 for epoch or round. Now, the number of epochs was automatically chosen to 10000; this tells you that there are 1 * 10000 batches. Also, the number of processed examples is 12 * (10000), which is equal to 120000. If the batch size does not evenly divide the training set, the final batch has fewer examples than the other batches.

Furthermore, adding a loss function layer to the container or the loss with the LossFunction -> Loss Layer option has the same effect. In this case, you use the MeanSquaredLossLayer as the loss function option, change the activation function to Tanh[x], set the Batchsize to 5, and adjust MaxTrainingRounds to 1000.

```
In[9]:= net2=NetTrain[NetChain[{LinearLayer[1,"Input"->2], ElementwiseLayer
[Tanh[#]&]}],trainData,All,LearningRate->0.01, PerformanceGoal->
"TrainingSpeed",TrainingProgressReporting->"Panel", TargetDevice->
"CPU",RandomSeeding->88888,WorkingPrecision->"Real64", LossFunction->
MeanSquaredLossLayer[],BatchSize->5,MaxTrainingRounds->1000]
Out[9]=
```

Figure 10-5 shows that the loss has dropped considerably.

NetTrainResultsObject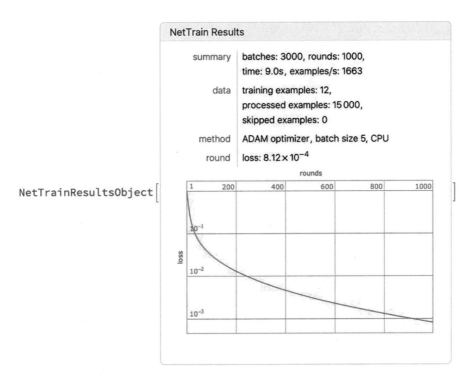

Figure 10-5. *Training results of the Net2*

Let's determine the classification.

```
In[10]:= trainedNet2=net2["TrainedNet"];
Show[DensityPlot[trainedNet2[{x,y}],{x,-2,2},{y,-3,3}, PlotPoints->50,
ColorFunction->(RGBColor[1-#,2*#,1]&)],Plt]
Out[11]=
```

Figure 10-6 shows how the two boundaries are better denoted.

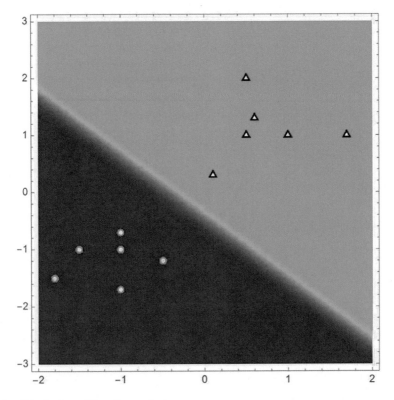

Figure 10-6. *Net2 classification plot*

The previous models represent a prediction of a linear layer, in which this classification is compared with the targets so that the error is less and less.

To obtain the graph that shows the value of the error according to the number of rounds carried out in the training, you do it through the properties of the trained network. You can also see the network model's appearance once the loss function is added.

```
In[12]:= Dataset[{Association["LossPlot"->net2["LossPlot"]],
Association["NetGraph"->net2["TrainingNet"]]}]
Out[12]=
```

Figure 10-7 shows the loss graph as it decreases rapidly according to the number of rounds.

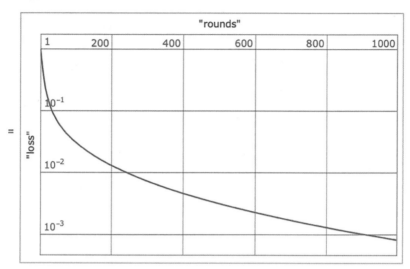

Figure 10-7. *LossPlot contained in the dataset*

To see the network used for training, execute the next code. Mathematica automatically adds a loss function to the neural network (see Figure 10-8) based on the model's layers.

```
In[13]:= net2["TrainingNet"]
Out[13]=
```

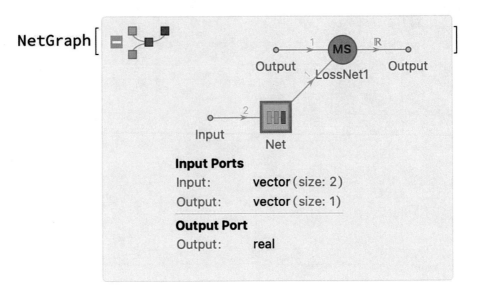

Figure 10-8. *Network model before the training phase*

To see the model's properties, you add the string Properties as an argument.

```
In[14]:= net2["Properties"]
Out[14]= {ArraysLearningRateMultipliers,BatchesPerRound,BatchesPerSecond,Ba
tchLossList,BatchMeasurements,BatchMeasurementsLists,BatchSize,BestValidati
onRound,CheckpointingFiles,ExamplesProcessed,FinalLearningRate,FinalPlots,I
nitialLearningRate,InternalVersionNumber,LossPlot,MeanBatchesPerSecond,Mean
ExamplesPerSecond,NetTrainInputForm,OptimizationMethod,ReasonTrainingStoppe
d,RoundLoss,RoundLossList,RoundMeasurements,RoundMeasurementsLists,RoundPos
itions,SkippedTrainingData,TargetDevice,TotalBatches,TotalRounds,TotalTrain
ingTime,TrainedNet,TrainingExamples,TrainingNet,TrainingUpdateSchedule,Vali
dationExamples,ValidationLoss,ValidationLossList,ValidationMeasurements,Val
idationMeasurementsLists,ValidationPositions}
```

Training Method (NetTrain)

Let's look at the training method for the previous network with OptimizationMethod. Some variants of the gradient descent algorithm are related to batch size. The first one is the stochastic gradient descent (SGD). The SGD takes a single training batch at a time before taking another step. This algorithm goes through the training examples in a stochastic form—without a sequential pattern and only one instance at a time. The second variant is the batch gradient descent, meaning that the batch size is set to the size of the training set. This method utilizes all training examples and makes only one update of the internal parameters. The third variant is the mini-batch gradient descent, which consists of dividing the training set into partitions smaller than the whole dataset to update the model's internal parameters to achieve convergence frequently. To see a mathematical of the SGD and mini-batch SGD, visit the article "Efficient Mini-Batch Training for Stochastic Optimization," by Mu Li, Tong Zhang, Yuqiang Chen, and Alexander J. Smola (2014, August: pp. 661-670; In *Proceedings of the 20th ACM SIGKDD international conference on Knowledge discovery and data mining*).

```
In[15]:= net2["OptimizationMethod"]
Out[15]= {ADAM, Beta1->0.9, Beta2->0.999, Epsilon->1/100000,
GradientClipping->None, L2Regularization->None, LearningRate->0.01,
LearningRateSchedule->None, WeightClipping->None}
```

The method automatically chosen is the Adam optimizer, which uses the SGD method with an adapted learning rate. The other available methods are the RMSProp, SGD, and the SignSGD. Within the available methods, there are also options to indicate the learning rate, when to scale, when to use the L2 regularization, the gradient, and weight clipping.

Measuring Performance

In addition to the methods, you can establish what measures to consider during the training phase. These options depend on the type of loss function used and which is intrinsically related to the task, like classification, regression, and clustering. In the case of MeanSquaredLossLayer or MeanAbsoluteLossLayer, the common option is MeanDeviation, which is the absolute value of the average of the residuals. MeanSquare is the mean square of the residuals, RSquared is the coefficient of determination, and standard deviation is the root mean square of the residuals. After completing the training, the measure appears in the net results (see Figure 10-9). The soft sign activation function is used in this example to try out a different activation function and observe its use.

```
In[16]:= net3 = NetTrain[ NetChain[{LinearLayer[1, "Input" -> 2],
ElementwiseLayer["SoftSign"]}], trainData, All, LearningRate -> 0.01,
PerformanceGoal -> "TrainingSpeed", TrainingProgressReporting -> "Panel",
```

```
TargetDevice -> "CPU", RandomSeeding -> 88888, WorkingPrecision ->
"Real64", Method -> "ADAM", LossFunction -> MeanSquaredLossLayer[],
BatchSize -> 5, MaxTrainingRounds -> 1000, TrainingProgressMeasurements ->
{"MeanDeviation", "MeanSquare", "RSquared", "StandardDeviation"}]
Out[16]=
```

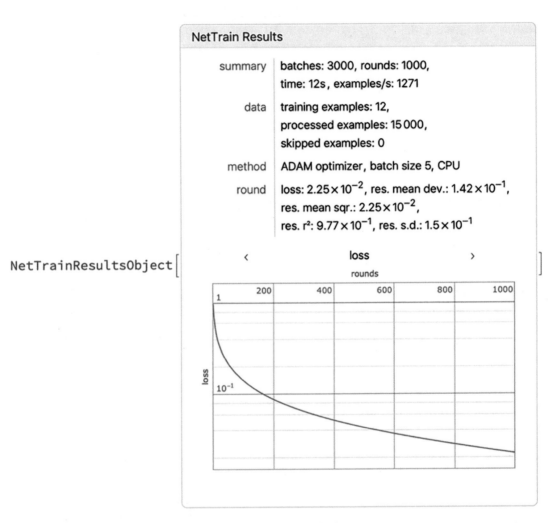

Figure 10-9. *Net results with new measures added*

Model Assessment

To access the values of the measures chosen, use the NetResultsObject. In the case of the training set values, these are found in the properties of RoundLoss (gives the average value of the loss), RoundLossList (returns the average values of the loss during training), RoundMeasurements (the measurements of the training of the last round), and RoundMeasurementsLists (the specified measurements for each round). This result is depicted in Figure 10-10.

```
In[17]:= net3[#]&/@{"RoundMeasurements"}//Dataset[#]&
Out[17]=
```

Loss	0.0224971
MeanDeviation	0.141845
MeanSquare	0.0224971
RSquared	0.977402
StandardDeviation	0.14999

Figure 10-10. *Dataset with the new measures*

To get all the plots, use the FinalPlots option.

```
In[18]:= net3["FinalPlots"]//Dataset;
```

To replicate the plots of the measurements, extract the values of the measurements of each round with RoundMeasurementsLists.

```
In[19]:= measures=net3[#]&/@{"RoundMeasurementsLists"};
Keys[measures]
Out[20]= {{Loss,MeanDeviation,MeanSquare,RSquared,StandardDeviation}}
```

Let's plot the values for each round, starting with Loss and finishing with StandardDeviation. You can also see how the network model makes the classification boundaries (see Figure 10-11).

```
In[21]:= trainedNet3 =
 net3["TrainedNet"]; Grid[{{ListLinePlot[{measures[[1, 1]]
(*Loss*), measures[[1, 2]] (*MeanDeviation*), measures[[1, 3]]
(*MeanSquare*), measures[[1, 4]] (*RSquared*), measures[[1, 5]]
```

```
(*StandardDeviation*)},  PlotStyle -> Table[ColorData[101, i], {i,
1, 5}], Frame -> True, FrameLabel -> {"Number of Rounds", None},
PlotLabel -> "Measurements Plot", GridLines -> All, PlotLegends ->
SwatchLegend[{Style["Loss", #], Style["MD", #], Style["MS", #],
Style["RS", #], Style["STD", #]}, LegendLabel -> Style["Measurements", #],
LegendFunction -> (Framed[#, RoundingRadius -> 5, Background -> LightGray]
&)], ImageSize -> Medium] &[Black], Show[DensityPlot[trainedNet3[{x, y}],
{x, -2, 2}, {y, -3, 3}, PlotPoints -> 50, ColorFunction -> (RGBColor[1 - #,
2*#, 1] &)], plt, ImageSize -> 200]}}]
Out[21]=
```

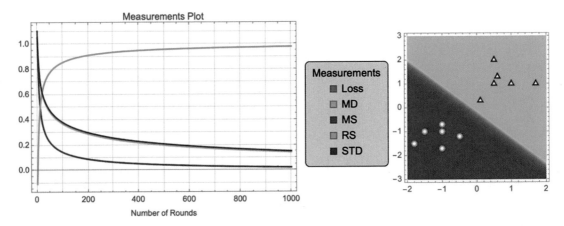

Figure 10-11. *Round measures plot and density plot*

The Loss and MeanSquared have the same values (since the loss is a mean squared error loss function), which is why the two graphics overlap. The mean deviation and standard deviation have similar values but not the same. Three models are constructed, and the activation function changes in each process. Looking at the plots, you see how each function changes how the neural network model learns from the training data. In the previous examples, the graphics were the loss plot for the training process and other measurements related to the means squared loss layer. Make sure to consult the documentation to confirm the measurements' names; remember that not all measurements apply to all loss functions.

In the subsequent section, you see how to generate the loss plot and the validation plot during the training phase to validate that the LeNet model is learning during training and how well the model can perform in data never seen before (validation set).

Exporting a Neural Network

Once a net model has been trained, you can export this trained net to a WLNet format so that the net can be used without the need for training in the future. The export method also works for uninitialized network architectures.

```
In[22]:= Export["/Users/macosx/Desktop/TrainedNet3.
wlnet",net3["TrainedNet"]]
Out[22]= /Users/macosx/Desktop/TrainedNet3.wlnet
```

Importing them back is done precisely as any other file, but imported elements can be specified. Net imports the net model and all initialized arrays; UninitializedNet and ArrayList imports for the numeric array's objects of the linear layers; ArrayAssociation imports for the numeric arrays in association form, and WLVersion is used to see the version of the Wolfram Language used to build the net. The following dataset shows all the options (see Figure 10-12).

```
In[23]:=Dataset@AssociationMap[Import["/Users/macosx/Desktop/TrainedNet3.
wlnet",#]&,{"Net","UninitializedNet","ArrayList","ArrayAssociation",
"WLVersion"}]
Out[23]=
```

Net	NetChain [Input port: vector (size: 2) Output port: vector (size: 1)]
UninitializedNet	NetChain [Input port: vector (size: 2) Output port: vector (size: 1)]
ArrayList	{NumericArray[⊞ Type: Real64 Dimensions: {1, 2}], NumericArray[⊞ Type: Real64 Dimensions: {1}]}
ArrayAssociation	⟨| {1, Weights} → NumericArray[⊞ Type: Real64 Dimensions: {1, 2}], {1, Biases} → NumericArray[⊞ Type: Real64 Dimensions: {1}] |⟩
WLVersion	13.3.0

Figure 10-12. *Dataset with the available import options*

Wolfram Neural Net Repository

The Wolfram Neural Net Repository is a free-access website containing a repertoire of various pre-trained neural network models. The models are categorized by the input and data types, be it audio, image, numeric array, or text. Furthermore, they are also categorized by the kind of task they perform, from audio analysis or regression to classification. The main page of the website is shown in Figure 10-13.

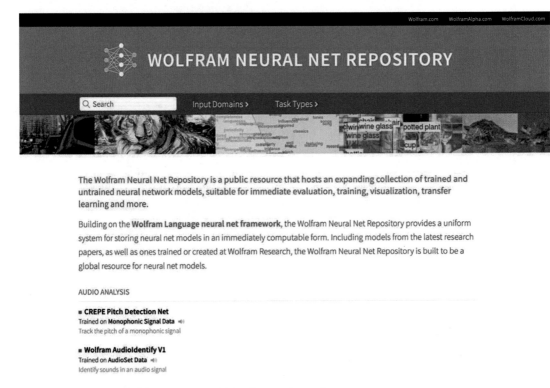

Figure 10-13. *Wolfram Neural Net Repository home page*

Enter `https://resources.wolframcloud.com/NeuralNetRepository/` in your favorite browser to access the web page, or run SystemOpen from Mathematica, which opens the web page in the system's default browser.

Once the site is loaded, net models can be browsed by either input or task. The models in this repository are built in the Wolfram Language, allowing you to use them within Mathematica. This leads to the models being found in a form that can be accessed from Mathematica or the Wolfram Cloud for prompt execution. If you scroll down, you see that the models are structured by name and the data used for training, along with a short description. Such is the case, for example, for the Wolfram AudioIdentify V1 network, which is trained with the AudioSet Data and identifies sounds in audio signals. To browse categories, you can choose the category from the menu. Figure 10-14 shows the site's appearance after an input category is chosen; in this case, the neural networks that receive images as inputs.

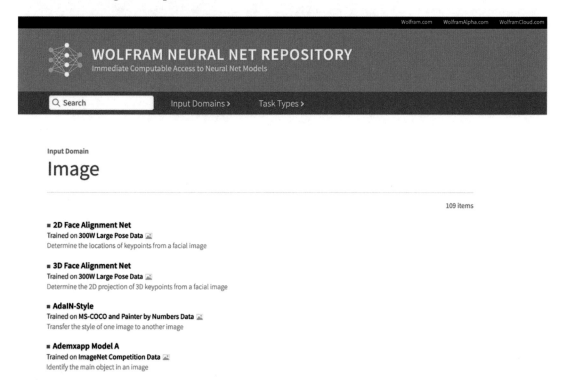

Figure 10-14. *Category site, based on the input image*

Selecting a Neural Net Model

Once a category is chosen, it shows all the net models associated with the selected input category. Like with the Wolfram Data Repository, once the model is selected, it shows relevant information, like in Figure 10-15, where the selected net model is the neural network Wolfram ImageIdentify Net V1.

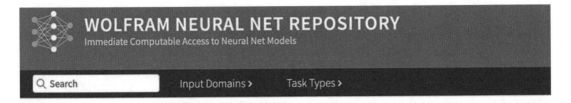

Wolfram ImageIdentify Net V1
Identify the main object in an image

Released in 2017 by Wolfram Research, this net was trained on over 4,000 classes of objects. It is part of the back end for the ImageIdentify function in Wolfram Language 11.1. It was designed to achieve a good balance among classification accuracy, size and evaluation speed.

Number of layers: 232 | Parameter count: 14,713,147 | Trained size: 65 MB |

TRAINING SET INFORMATION

Internal Wolfram ImageIdentify training set, consisting of over 3 million training images and over 4,000 classes of objects (not publicly available).

Examples

> Resource retrieval

> Basic usage

> Feature extraction

> Visualize convolutional weights

> Transfer learning

> Net information

> Export to MXNet

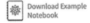 Download Example Notebook

 Open in Wolfram Cloud

Figure 10-15. *Wolfram ImageIdentify Net V1*

It is possible to navigate from the website and download the notebook containing the network model, but it is also possible from Mathematica. In other words, search for network models through ResourceSearch. The example shows the search if you were interested in knowing the models of the networks that contain the word image (see Figure 10-16).

```
In[24]:= ResourceSearch[{"Name"->"Image","ResourceType"-> "NeuralNet"}]
//Dataset[#,MaxItems->{4,3}]&
Out[24]=
```

Name	ResourceType	ResourceObject
Colorful Image Colorization Trained on ImageNet Competition Data	NeuralNet	ResourceObject["Colorful Image Colorization Trained on ImageNet Competition Data"]
ColorNet Image Colorization Trained on ImageNet Competition Data	NeuralNet	ResourceObject["ColorNet Image Colorization Trained on ImageNet Competition Data"]
EfficientNet Trained on ImageNet	NeuralNet	ResourceObject["EfficientNet Trained on ImageNet"]
Wolfram ImageIdentify Net V1	NeuralNet	ResourceObject["Wolfram ImageIdentify Net V1"]

rows 1–4 of 40   columns 1–3 of 6

Figure 10-16. *Resource Dataset*

The dataset shown in Figure 10-16 has only three columns for display purposes, but you can navigate through the entire dataset using the slider. The columns not shown in the image are Description, Location, and DocumentationLink. The last column provides the link that leads to the web model page.

Accessing Inside Mathematica

To access the model architecture, add the object argument; for example, do the following for the Wolfram ImageIdentify Net V1 Network (see Figure 10-17).

```
In[25]:= ResourceSearch[{"Name"->"Wolfram ImageIdentify","ResourceType"->
"NeuralNet"},"Object"]
Out[25]=
```

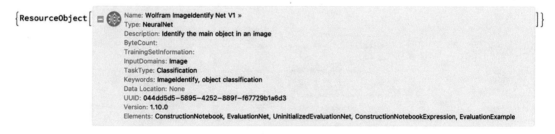

Figure 10-17. *Wolfram ImageIdentify Net V1 resource*

Note   To avoid problems accessing the Wolfram Net Repository from Mathematica, ensure you are logged in to the Wolfram Cloud or your Wolfram account.

The following code is suppressed here to access the pre-trained model, but removing the semicolon returns the NetChain object of the pre-trained neural network.

```
In[26]:= ResourceSearch[{"Name"->"Wolfram ImageIdentify","ResourceType"->
"NeuralNet"},"Object"][[1]]//ResourceData;
Out[26]=
```

Retrieving Relevant Information

Information about the model is accessed from ResourceObject. The following is the relevant information from the ImageIdentify model in a dataset (see Figure 10-18). To see all information in the dataset format, type ResourceObject ["Wolfram ImageIdentify Net V1"][All]//Dataset [#] &.

```
In[27]:= Dataset[AssociationMap[ResourceObject["Wolfram ImageIdentify Net V1"],
{"Name","RepositoryLocation","ResourceType","ContentElements","Version",
"Description","TrainingSetInformation","InputDomains","TaskType","Keywords",
"Attributes","LatestUpdate","DownloadedVersion","Format",
"ContributorInformation","DOI","Originator","ReleaseDate","ShortName",
"WolframLanguageVersionRequired"}]]
Out[27]=
```

Name	Wolfram ImageIdentify Net V1
RepositoryLocation	https://www.wolframcloud.com/obj/resourcesystem/ap...
ResourceType	NeuralNet
ContentElements	{ConstructionNotebook, EvaluationNet, UninitializedEvaluationNet, ConstructionNotebookExpression, EvaluationExample}
Version	1.10.0
Description	Identify the main object in an image
TrainingSetInformation	Internal Wolfram ImageIdentify training set, consisting of over 3 million training images and over 4,000 classes of objects (not publicly available).
InputDomains	Image
TaskType	Classification
Keywords	{ImageIdentify, object classification}
Attributes	{LocalCopyable, CloudCopyable, Multipart}
LatestUpdate	Fri 28 Feb 2020 00:00:00
DownloadedVersion	1.10.0
Format	<| EvaluationNet → WLNet, UninitializedEvaluationNet → WLNet, ConstructionNotebookExpression → NB, EvaluationExample → WXF |>
ContributorInformation	<| PublisherID → Wolfram, DisplayName → Wolfram Research |>
DOI	https://doi.org/10.24097/wolfram.34204.data
Originator	Wolfram Research
ReleaseDate	Mon 20 Feb 2017 16:00:00
ShortName	Wolfram–ImageIdentify–Net–V1
WolframLanguageVersionRequired	11.1

Figure 10-18. *Dataset of some properties of the Wolfram ImageIdentify Net V1*

Here, in a few steps, is the way to access the trained neural network and much relevant information associated with the neural network. It should be noted that the process is also used to find other resources in the Wolfram Cloud or local resources, not only neural networks, since, in general, ResourceSearch looks for an object within the Wolfram Resource System. Such is the case of the neural network models in the Wolfram Neural Net Repository.

LeNet Neural Network

The following example examines a neural network model named LeNet. Despite being able to access the model from a Wolfram resource, as you saw previously, performing operations with networks found in the Wolfram Neural Net Repository with the NetModel command is possible. To get a better idea of how this network is used, let's first look at the description of the network, its name, how it is used, and where it was proposed for the first time.

LeNet Model

The neural network LeNet is a convolutional neuronal network within the deep learning field. The neural network LeNet is recognized as one of the first convolutional networks that promoted deep learning. This network was used for character recognition to identify handwritten digits. Today, architectures are based on LeNet neural network architecture, but you focus on the Wolfram Neural Net Repository version. This architecture consists of four key operations: convolution, non-linearity, subsampling, or pooling and classification. To learn more about the LeNet convolutional neural network, see *Neural Networks and Deep Learning: A Textbook* by Charu C. Aggarwal (Springer, 2018). With NetModel, you can obtain information about the LeNet network that has been previously trained.

```
In[28]:= NetModel["LeNet Trained on MNIST Data",#]&/@{"Details","ShortName"
,"TaskType","SourceMetadata"}//Column
Out[28]= This pioneer work for image classification with convolutional
neural nets was released in 1998. It was developed by Yann LeCun and his
collaborators at AT&T Labs while they experimented with a large range of
machine learning solutions for classification on the MNIST dataset.
```

LeNet-Trained-on-MNIST-Data
{Classification} <|Citation->Y. LeCun, L. Bottou, Y. Bengio, P. Haffner, "Gradient-Based Learning Applied to Document Recognition," Proceedings of the IEEE, 86(11), 2278-2324 (1998),Source->http://yann.lecun.com/exdb/ lenet,Date->DateObject[{1998},Year,Gregorian,-5.]|>

Note   To access all the properties of a model with NetModel, add properties as the second argument—NetModel["LeNet Trained on MNISt Data," "Properties"].

The input this model receives consists of images in grayscale with a size of 28 x 28, and the model's performance is 98.5% on the MNIST dataset.

In[29]:= NetModel["LeNet Trained on MNIST Data",#]&/@{"TrainingSetInformati on","InputDomains","Performance"}//Column
Out[29]= MNIST Database of Handwritten Digits, consisting of 60,000 training and 10,000 test grayscale images of size 28x28.
{Image}
This model achieves 98.5% accuracy on the MNIST dataset.

MINST Dataset

This network is used for rating, just as it appears in TaskType. The digits are in a database known as the MNIST database. The MNIST database is an extensive database of handwritten digits (see Figure 10-19) that contains 60,000 images for training and 10,000 for testing, the latter being used to get a final estimate of how well the neural net model works. To observe the complete dataset, you load it from the Wolfram Data Repository with ResourceData and ImageDimensions to verify that the dimensions of the pictures are 28 x 28 pixels.

In[30]:= (*This is for seven elements randomly sampled, but you can check the whole data set.*)
TableForm[
 SeedRandom[900];
 RandomSample[ResourceData["MNIST", "TrainingData"], 7],
 TableDirections -> Row]

```
Map[ImageDimensions, %[[1 ;; 7, 1]]]
(*Test set : ResourceData["MNIST","TestData"] *)
Out[30]//TableForm=
```

$9 \rightarrow 9$ $5 \rightarrow 5$ $2 \rightarrow 2$ $2 \rightarrow 2$ $6 \rightarrow 6$ $0 \rightarrow 0$ $7 \rightarrow 7$

Figure 10-19. *A random sample of the MNIST training set*

```
Out[31]= {{28,28},{28,28},{28,28},{28,28},{28,28},{28,28},{28,28}}
```

Figure 10-19 shows the images of the digits, the class to which they apply, and the dimensions of each image. You extract the training sets and test sets, which you use later.

```
In[32]:= {trainData,testData}={ResourceData["MNIST","TrainingData"],
ResourceData["MNIST","TestData"] };
```

LeNet Architecture

Let's start by downloading the neural network from the NetModel command, which extracts the model from the Wolfram Neural Net Repository. The next exercise loads the network that has not been trained since you do the training and validation process. It should be noted that the LeNet model in the Wolfram Language is a variation of the original architecture (see Figure 10-20).

```
In[33]:= uninitLeNet=NetModel["LeNet Trained on MNIST Data",
"UninitializedEvaluationNet"](*To work locally with the untrained
model: NetModel["LeNet"]*)
Out[33]=
```

$$
\text{NetChain}\left[\begin{array}{lll}
\blacksquare \text{ uninitialized} & & \text{image} \\
& \text{Input} & \text{array}\,(\text{size: 1×28×28}) \\
1 & \text{ConvolutionLayer} & \text{array}\,(\text{size: 20×24×24}) \\
2 & \text{Ramp} & \text{array}\,(\text{size: 20×24×24}) \\
3 & \text{PoolingLayer} & \text{array}\,(\text{size: 20×12×12}) \\
4 & \text{ConvolutionLayer} & \text{array}\,(\text{size: 50×8×8}) \\
5 & \text{Ramp} & \text{array}\,(\text{size: 50×8×8}) \\
6 & \text{PoolingLayer} & \text{array}\,(\text{size: 50×4×4}) \\
7 & \text{FlattenLayer} & \text{vector}\,(\text{size: 800}) \\
8 & \text{LinearLayer} & \text{vector}\,(\text{size: 500}) \\
9 & \text{Ramp} & \text{vector}\,(\text{size: 500}) \\
10 & \text{LinearLayer} & \text{vector}\,(\text{size: 10}) \\
11 & \text{SoftmaxLayer} & \text{vector}\,(\text{size: 10}) \\
& \text{Output} & \text{class}
\end{array}\right]
$$

Figure 10-20. *LeNet architecture*

The LeNet network in the Wolfram Neural Net Repository is built from 11 layers. The layers that appear in red are layers with learnable parameters: two convolutional layers and two linear layers.

MXNet Framework

With the MXNet framework, let's first visualize the process of this network through the MXNet operation graph (see Figure 10-21).

```
In[34]:= Information[uninitLeNet,"MXNetNodeGraphPlot"]
Out[34]=
```

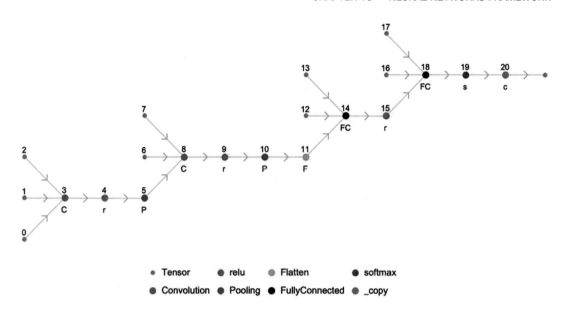

Figure 10-21. *MXNet graph of the LeNet architecture*

LeNet architecture starts at the input with the operation that converts the image to a numeric array, followed by the first operation. This convolution returns a 20-feature map with a rectified linear unit (ReLU) activation function immediately following nodes 3 and 4. Then, the first max-pooling operation (subsampling layers) selects the maximum value in the pooling node 5. Then, the second convolutional operation returns a 50-feature map with a ReLU activation function immediately following nodes 8 and 9. The last convolution operation is followed by another max-pooling operation (node 10), followed by a flattening operation (node 11), which flattens the output of the pooling operation into a single vector. The last pooling operation gives an array of 50*4*4, and the flatten operation returns an 800-vector that is the input of the next operation. Next, you see the first fully connected layer (node 14); the first fully connected layer has a ReLU function (node 15), and the second fully connected layer has the softmax function (node 19). The last fully connected layer can be interpreted as a multilayer perceptron (MLP) that normalizes the output into a probability distribution to indicate the probability of each class. Finally, the tensor is converted to a class with the decoder. Nodes 4, 9, and 15 are the layers for non-linear operations (ReLU), and node 19 applies the softmax function for output classification. In summary, the architecture is as follows: Tensor (input), Convolution, ReLU, Pooling, Convolution, ReLU, Pooling, Flatten, Fully Connected (with ReLU), Fully Connected (with softmax), and Class output.

Preparing LeNet

Since LeNet is a neural network for image classification, an encoder and decoder must be used. The NetEncoder is inserted in the input NetPort, and the NetDecoder is on the output NetPort. Looking into the NetGraph (see Figure 10-22) might be useful in understanding the process inside the Wolfram Language. Clicking the input and output shows the relevant information.

```
In[35]:= NetGraph[uninitLeNet]
Out[35]=
```

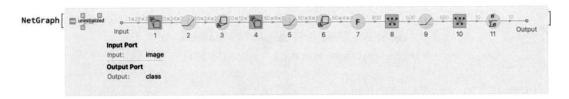

Figure 10-22. *NetGraph of the LeNet model*

You can extract the encoder and decoder to inspect their infrastructure. The encoder receives an image of the dimensions of 28 x 28 of any color space and encodes the image into a color space set to grayscale, returning then an array of the size of 1 x 28 x 28. On the other hand, the decoder is a class decoder that receives a 10-size vector, which tells the probability for the class labels that are 0, 1, 2, 3, 4, 5, 6, 7, 8, and 9.

```
In[36]:={enc=NetExtract[uninitLeNet,"Input"],dec=NetExtract[uninitLeNet,
"Output"]}//Row;
```

First, let's look at how the net model works with NetInitialize; for example, use an image of 0 in the training set.

```
In[37]:= testNet=NetInitialize[uninitLeNet,RandomSeeding->8888];
testNet@trainData[[1,1]](*TrainData[[1,1]] belongs to a zero*)
Out[38]= 9
```

The net returns that the image belongs to class 9, which means that the image is a number 9; clearly, this is wrong. Let's try NetInitialize again but with the different methods available. Writing all, as the second argument to NetInitialize, overwrites any pre-existing learning parameters on the network.

In[39]:= {net1, net2, net3, net4} =   Table[NetInitialize[uninitLe Net, All, Method -> i,   RandomSeeding -> 8888], {i, {"Kaiming", "Xavier", "Orthogonal",   "Identity"}}]; {net1[trainData[[1, 1]]], net2[trainData[[1, 1]]], net3[trainData[[1, 1]]], net4[trainData[[1, 1]]]} Out[40]= {9,9,7,3}

Every net model fails to classify the image in the correct class. This result is because the neural network has not been trained, unlike NetInitialize, which only randomly initializes the learnable parameters without proper training. This is why, with NetInitialize, the model fails to classify the image given correctly. But first, let's establish the network graph to better illustrate the model, as seen in Figure 10-23.

In[41]:= leNet=NetInitialize[NetGraph[<|"LeNet NN" -> uninitLeNet, "LeNet Loss" -> CrossEntropyLossLayer@"Index"|>, {NetPort@"Input" -> "LeNet NN", "LeNet NN" -> NetPort@{"LeNet Loss", "Input"}, NetPort@"Target" -> NetPort@ {"LeNet Loss", "Target"}}], RandomSeeding -> 8888] Out[41]=

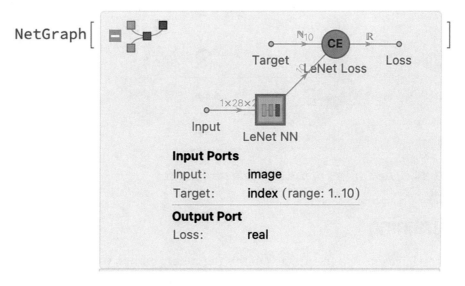

Figure 10-23. *LeNet ready graph*

Before you train the net, you must make the validation set suited for the CrossEntropyLossLayer in the target input because the classes start at 0 and end at 9, and the Index target begins at 1 and goes on. So, the target input needs to be between 1 and 10.

```
In[42]:= trainDts=Dataset@Join[AssociationThread["Input"->#]& /@Keys[train
Data],AssociationThread["Target"-> #]&/@Values[trainData]+1,2];
testDts=Dataset@Join[AssociationThread["Input"->#]& /@Keys[testData],
AssociationThread["Target"-> #]&/@Values[testData]+1,2];
```

The training set and validation set have the form of a dataset. Only four random samples are shown in Figure 10-24.

```
In[44]:= BlockRandom[SeedRandom[999];
{RandomSample[trainDts[[All]],4],RandomSample[testDts[[All]],4]}]
Out[44]=
```

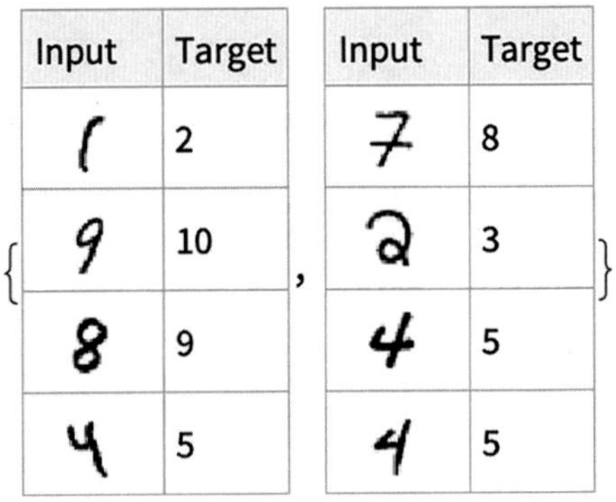

Input	Target	Input	Target
(	2	7	8
9	10	2	3
8	9	4	5
4	5	4	5

Figure 10-24. *The dataset of the training and test set*

LeNet Training

Now that you have grasped the process of this neural net model, you can proceed to train the neural net model. With NetTrain, you gradually modify the learnable parameters of the neural network to reduce the loss. The next training code is set with the options seen in the previous section, but here, you add new options also available for training. The first one is TrainingProgressMeasurements. TrainingProgressMeasurements can specify measures such as accuracy and precision. These are measured during the training phase by round or batch. The ClassAveraging is used to specify to get the macro-average or the micro-average of the measurement specified <|"Measurement" -> "measurement" (Accuracy, RSquared, Recall, MeanSquared, etc.), "ClassAveraging"->"Macro"|>.

The second option is the TrainingStoppingCriterion, which is used to add an early stopping to avoid overfitting during the training phase based on different criteria, such as stopping the training when the validation loss is not improving, measuring the absolute or relative change of a measurement (accuracy, precision, loss, etc.), or stopping the training when the loss or other criteria does not improve after a certain number of rounds <|Criterion->"measurement" (Accuracy, Loss, Recall, etc.), "Patience"-> # of rounds|>.

```
In[45]:= netResults =  NetTrain[leNet, trainDts, All, ValidationSet ->
testDts,   MaxTrainingRounds -> 15, BatchSize -> 2096,   LearningRate ->
Automatic, Method -> "ADAM", TargetDevice -> "CPU",   PerformanceGoal
-> "TrainingMemory", WorkingPrecision -> "Real32",   RandomSeeding
-> 99999,   TrainingProgressMeasurements -> {<|"Measurement" ->
"Accuracy",       "ClassAveraging" -> "Macro"|>,    <|"Measurement"
-> "Precision", "ClassAveraging" -> "Macro"|>    , <|"Measurement"
-> "F1Score", "ClassAveraging" -> "Macro"|>     , <|"Measurement"
-> "Recall", "ClassAveraging" -> "Macro"|>     , <|"Measurement" ->
"ROCCurvePlot", "ClassAveraging" -> "Macro"|>     , <|"Measurement"
-> "ConfusionMatrixPlot",       "ClassAveraging" -> "Macro"|>     },
TrainingStoppingCriterion -> <|"Criterion" -> "Loss", "AbsoluteChange" ->
0.001|>]
Out[45]=
```

The final results of the training phase are depicted in Figure 10-25.

NetTrainResultsObject $\Big[$ 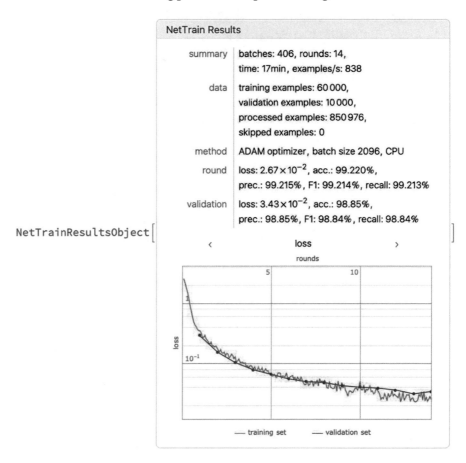 $\Big]$

Figure 10-25. *Net results of LeNet training*

Extracting the trained model and appending the net encoder and decoder is done because the trained net does not come with an encoder and decoder at the input and output ports.

```
In[46]:=NetExtract[netResults["TrainedNet"],"LeNet NN"];
trainedLeNet=NetReplacePart[%,{"Input"->enc,"Output"->dec}];
```

LeNet Model Assesment

The following grid (see Figure 10-26) shows the tracked measurements and plots of the training set. The measurements of the training set are in the RoundMeasurements property. To get the list of the values in each round, use RoundMeasurementsLists.

The performance of the training set is assessed with the round measurements, and the test set is evaluated with the validation measurements. Also, the ROC curves and the confusion matrix plot are shown in both cases.

```
In[48]:= netResults["RoundMeasurements"][[1 ;; 5]];
Normal[netResults["RoundMeasurements"][[6 ;; 7]]];
Grid[{{Style["RoundMeasurements", #1, #2], Style[%[[1, 1]], #1, #2],
        Style[%[[2, 1]], #1, #2]}, {Dataset[%%], %[[1, 2]], %[[2, 2]]}},
Dividers -> Center] &[Bold, FontFamily -> "Alegreya SC"]
Out[50]=
```

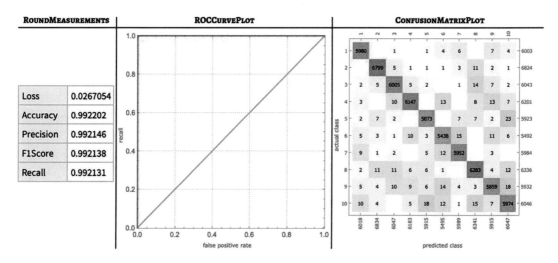

Figure 10-26. *Training set measurements*

To see how the model performed on the validation set (see Figure 10-27), see ValidationMeasurements. To get the list of the values in each round, use ValidationMeasurementsLists.

```
In[51]:= netResults["ValidationMeasurements"][[1 ;; 5]];
Normal[netResults["ValidationMeasurements"][[6 ;; 7]]];
Grid[{{Style["ValidationMeasurements", #1, #2],
Style[%[[1, 1]], #1, #2], Style[%[[2, 1]], #1, #2]}, {Dataset[%%], %[[1,
2]], %[[2, 2]]}}, Dividers -> Center] &[Bold, FontFamily -> "Alegreya SC"]
Out[53]=
```

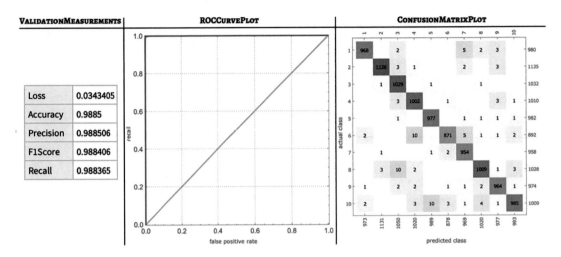

Figure 10-27. *Validation set measurements*

Testing LeNet

Having finished the training and reviewed the round and validation measures, you are now ready to test the trained LeNet neural network with some difficult images to see how it performs (see Figure 10-28).

```
In[54]:=expls=Keys[{testData[[2150]],testData[[3910]],testData[[6115]],test
Data[[6011]],testData[[7834]]}]
Out[54]=
```

$$\{\text{2, 3, 6, 6, 7}\}$$

Figure 10-28. *Difficult examples from the MNIST test set*

The selected images belong to the numbers 2, 3, 6, 5, and 7.

```
In[55]:= trainedLeNet[expls,"TopProbabilities"]
Out[55]= {{2->0.999397},{3->0.999856},{6->0.906024},{6->0.990975},{7->
0.999853}}
```

Write all of the results with the top probabilities with TableForm.

```
In[66]:= TableForm[Transpose@{trainedLeNet[ expls,{"TopDecisions",
2}],TrainedLeNet[ expls,{"TopProbabilities",2}]},TableHeadings->
{Map[ToString,{2,3,6,5,7},1],{"Top Decisions","Top Probabilities "}},
TableAlignments->Center]
Out[66]//TableForm=
      |Top Decisions  Top Probabilities

   ___|_____
   2  |3                 3->0.000580186
      |2                 2->0.999397
      |
   3  |9                 9->0.0000792077
      |3                 3->0.999856
      |
   6  |0                 0->0.0904324
      |6                 6->0.906024
      |
   5  |5                 5->0.00699159
      |6                 6->0.990975
      |
   7  |3                 6->0.990975
      |7                 7->0.999853
```

The trained net has misclassified the image of the number 5 because the top decisions are either a 5 or a 6, being 6 with top probability, which is wrong. Also, you can see the probabilities of the top decisions. Another form to evaluate the trained net in the test set is using NetMeasurements to set the net model, test set, and the interested measure. In the example, the measure of interest is the ConfusionMatrixPlot (see Figure 10-29).

```
In[67]:= NetMeasurements[trainedLeNet,testData,"ConfusionMatrixPlot"]
Out[67]=
```

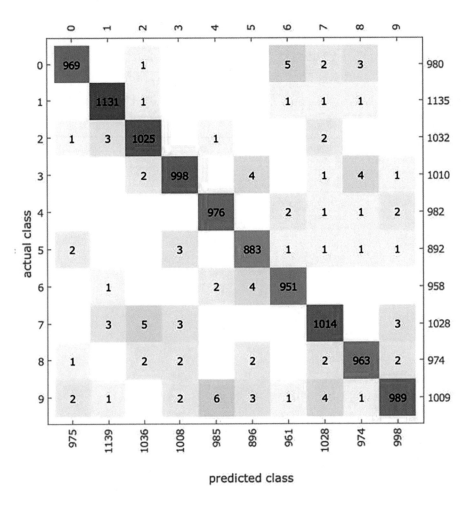

Figure 10-29. *ConfusionMatrixPlot from NetMeasurements*

GPT and LLM Basics

This section explores the neural network GPT models available in the Wolfram Language. You learn the basics of generative pre-trained transformers (GPT), the architecture of some GPT models inside Mathematica, and new LLM (large language model) Mathematica features.

A Brief Overview

GPT is a series of AI models that uses deep learning and transformer architecture to generate human-like text by analyzing preceding text. LLM is a broader category encompassing models trained to understand and generate human-readable text. GPT models fall under the LLM category, representing just one kind of model within the broader LLM framework.

LLM in the Wolfram Language

The Wolfram Language offers several new LLM-based functionalities, including the following.

- Chat Notebooks: a new feature enabling efficient and accessible conversations with LLM (GPT-3, among others) like a traditional Mathematica notebook

- Wolfram Prompt Repository: a collection of useful prompts made by a community for easy access to LLM scope applications

- LLM Function Integration: seamless incorporation of LLM functions within Mathematica

- GPT-1 and GPT-2: available from the Wolfram Neural Net Repository

---

Note   For LLM services in Mathematica, external API access is needed. Ensure your API key is valid; for example, for OpenAI, an active Chat GPT account with billing details is required. Be aware that API costs are separate from their subscription plans and vary based on the model used. Make sure to read OpenAI documentation for pricing and account details.

To connect to OpenAI GPT services, you first need to establish a connection. The most direct path to connect is through the settings or preferences section. Select the AI settings option from there, which shows various tabs related to chat notebooks, services, personas, and tools. The default tab has the general setting for the persona, LLM service, and temperature (model creativity), among other settings. To proceed, go to the Services tab and click Authentication, followed by Connect. This triggers a WolframConnector pop-up that requests the key access, as shown in Figure 10-30.

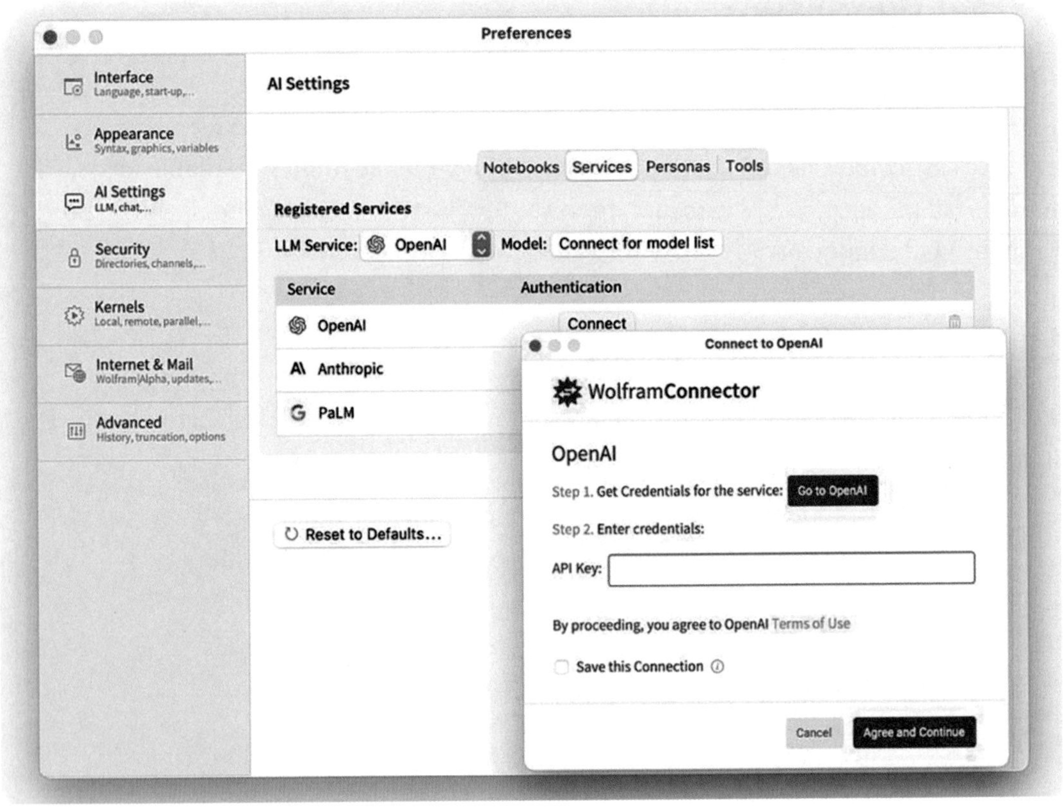

Figure 10-30. *AI settings to connect LLM service from Mathematica*

To get started, enter the key, save it by clicking the checkbox, and agree on the terms of use. Once linked, a checkmark appears under Authentication, like Figure 10-30. If a valid API is not linked, LLM services won't work. To remove the key, click Disconnect and repeat the previous steps.

Note   For quick API and LLM support, visit `https://support.wolfram.com/`

Chat Notebooks

New types of notebooks have been developed apart from regular notebooks. These notebooks are specialized for LLM tasks. These are Chat-Enabled and Chat-Driven Notebooks. To create a new one, go to File ➤ New, then select Chat-Enabled or Chat-

Driven Notebook. By default, chat-enabled use input chat cells with the code assistant persona (sets the LLM's response style), while chat-driven cells use PlainChat (basic dialog, no Wolfram code execution), as seen in Figure 10-31.

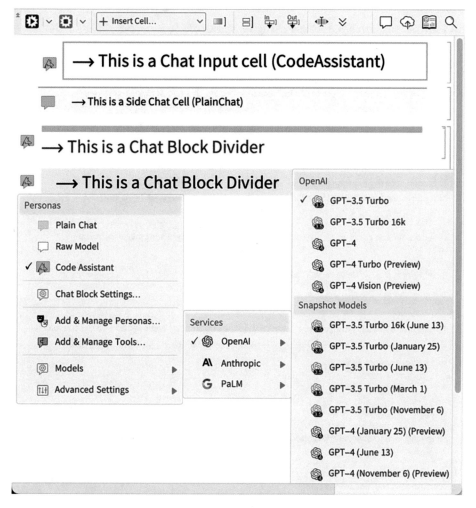

Figure 10-31. *Multiple Chat cells and OpenAI available models*

Apart from the different cells, Figure 10-31 show the various personas and GPT models for use. You can select the one that fits your needs. The base model version used in the following examples is with GPT-3.5 Turbo.

To create a new chat cell, press (') once. Press it twice for a side chat and three times for chat system input. To enable it in a regular notebook, click the chat cell icon in the top right corner (see Figure 10-31). Select "Enable AI chat features" to activate. Select the "Do automatic result analysis" option for LLM tips on output code. Try the example shown in Figure 10-32 to see if everything is working.

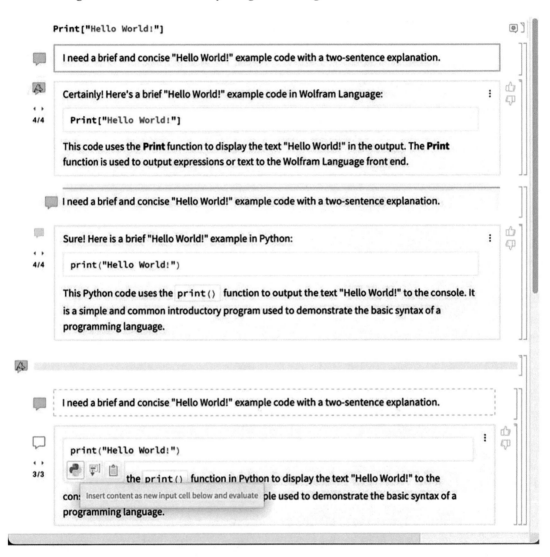

Figure 10-32. *Sample prompt and output for CodeAssistant, PlainChat, and RawModel*

In Figure 10-32, a chat icon is visible in the right cell bracket; this option lets you use LLM with Wolfram code like you use it in Mathematica. The chat history is sequential, and the conversation history output can also be accessed using the chat arrows. Side chat cells or blocks/delimiters separate chats. Distinct personas yield different responses; the CodeAssistant chat implies prompts in Wolfram code, whereas the Plain and RawChat yield output but do not imply that it's related to Wolfram code (unless specified in the prompt), resulting in Python code being used instead. Hovering over the code part allows you to either insert it as a newly evaluated cell, insert it, or copy it.

Note   Keep your prompts concise; always verify the chosen model to avoid unexpected fees since models have different costs based on token count.

Chat cells can rerun the prompt and regenerate the response. But remember that the LLM prompts are not run by Mathematica kernel, so history is saved on the notebook. So, closing the notebook does not erase the conversation.

Wolfram Prompt Repository

The Wolfram Prompt Repository gives you access to a large, curated base of prompts, from LLM prompts, personas, and costume functions. Navigating is similar to other repositories. Select from the accessible sections to find your desired prompts or persona for costume-style conversations. Once a prompt is selected various options are available, like chat samples and how to use it inside Mathematica. The platform further supports uploading, downloading, and utilizing various LLM components, as Figure 10-33 shows.

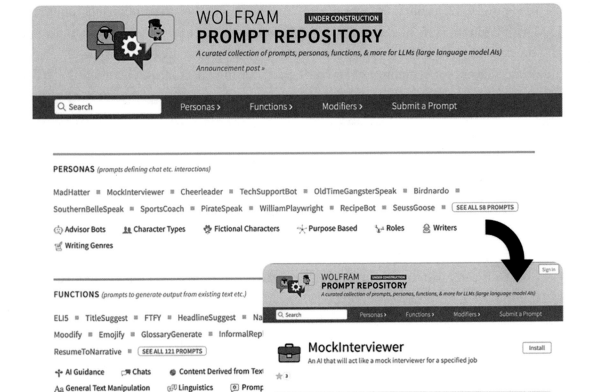

Figure 10-33. *Wolfram Prompt Repository with the MockInterviewer prompt page*

For instance, you can format output with different personas; select the persona from the drop-down menu (see Figure 10-31). To download a persona, go to the Personas tab in the AI setting and install via the prompt repository (see Figure 10-33) or enter the persona URL. Once installed, it should be available as depicted in Figure 10-34; this can also be done via Add & Manage Personas.

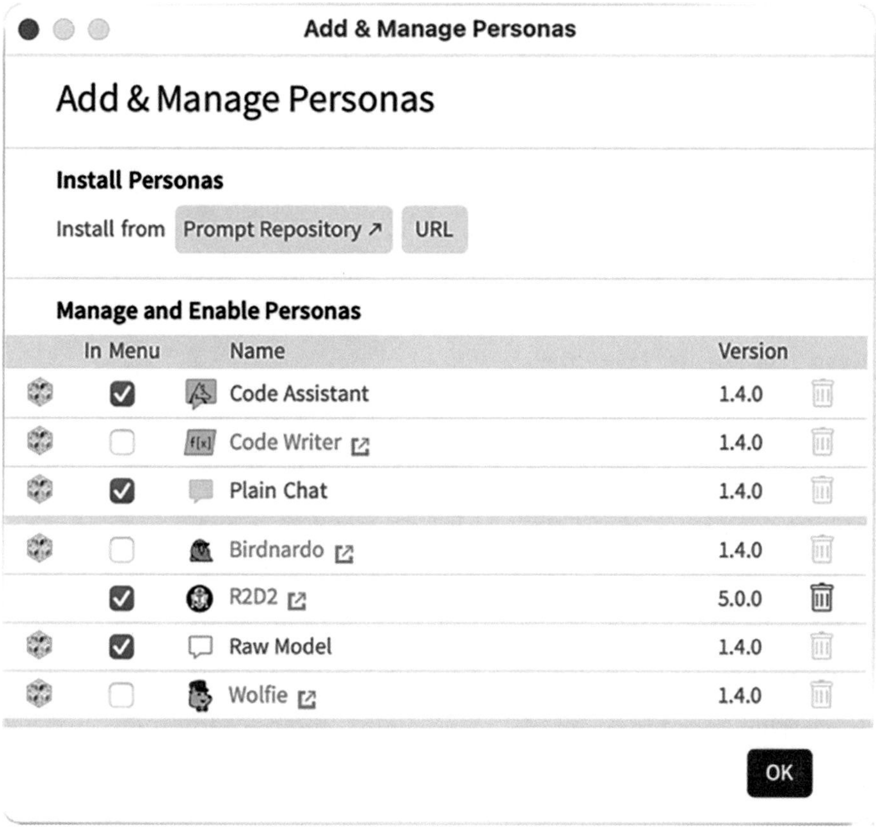

Figure 10-34. *The Add & Manage Personas screen shows the R2D2 persona selected*

Apart from personas, a combination of prompt modifiers can be used. These act on the input or output of a prompt. So, to invoke an input persona, use the character '@persona.' To call for a function input modifier, use '!prompt'; to call an output modifier, use '#param '; input and output modifiers go at the beginning and end of the prompt. To insert parameters to function modifiers, use the vertical bar to separate, like '#prompt|param ' as defined in Figure 10-35.

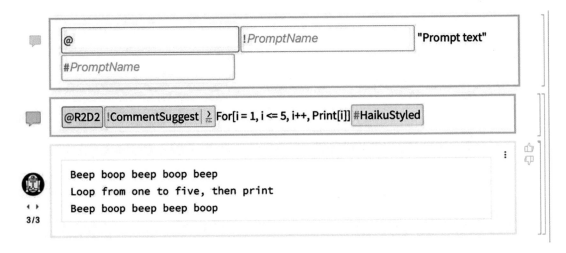

Figure 10-35. *R2D2 code comment in Haiku style*

LLM Functionalities

Chat objects are used along with chat evaluate to manage LLM conversations within
Mathematica. The chat object provides a convenient interface for interacting with the
LLM and managing conversations in a notebook environment. What happens is that
internally, LLM commands work as synthetic functions, which allows the LLM model to
access the Wolfram tools (see Figure 10-36).

```
In[68]:= ChatEvaluate[ ChatObject[], "Break down this code in 3 simple
points?  For[i=1,i<=5,i++,Print[i]", LLMEvaluator -> <|"Prompts" ->
{LLMPrompt["ELI5"]}|>] (*Explain Like I'm Five*)
Out[68]=
```

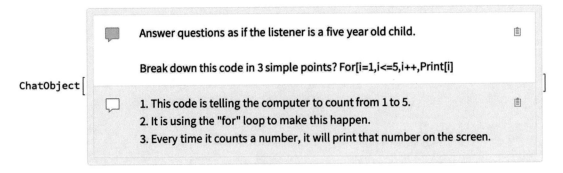

Figure 10-36. *Chatobject for an LLM text prompt*

To retrieve the chat contents and tokens, use the words "Messages" and "Usage".

```
In[69]:=
%["Messages"]
%%["Usage"]
Out[2]= {<|"Role" -> "User", "Content" ->    "Answer questions as if the
listener is a five year old child. Break down this code in 3 simple points?
For[i=1,i<=5,i++,Print[i]",   "Timestamp" ->    DateObject[{2024, 2, 22,
11, 22, 5.627397}, "Instant",     "Gregorian", -6.], "Annotations" -> <|{1,
129} -> "Prompt"|>|>, <|"Role" ->    "Assistant",   "Content" ->
"1. This code is telling the computer to count from 1 to 5.
2. It is using the \"for\" loop to make this happen.
3. Every time it counts a number, it will print that number on the \
screen.", "Timestamp" ->    DateObject[{2024, 2, 22, 11, 22, 6}, "Instant",
"Gregorian", -6.],    "Annotations" -> <|{1, 184} -> "Completion"|>|>}
Out[70]= 92 tokens
```

Like the previous example, you can set a prompt with a specific configuration with LLMConfiguration evaluated with LLMEvaluator, like the base model, temperature, stop tokens, and so forth. It can also be used to generate text (LLMSynthesize), retrieve text (LLMPrompt), or use a template function (LLMFunction), as the following code shows.

```
In[70]:= llmConfig = LLMConfiguration[<|"Prompts" -> LLMPrompt["ELI5"],
"Model" -> "GPT-3.5-Turbo", "Temperature" -> 0.1,  "MaxTokens"
-> 5|>]; LLMSynthesize["Break down this code in 3 simple points?
For[i=1,i<=5,i++,Print[i]", LLMEvaluator -> llmConfig]
Out[71]= Sure! Here's a
```

Note   The default LLM configuration is in $LLMEvaluator but can be overridden.

```
In[72]:= $LLMEvaluator=LLMConfiguration[<|"Prompts"-> LLMPrompt["ELI5"],
"Model"->"GPT-3.5-Turbo", "Temperature"->0.1,"MaxTokens"-> 5|>]
Out[72]= LLMConfiguration[Model: <|Service->Automatic,Name-
>GPT-3.5-Turbo|>]
```

GTP-1 and GPT-2 Models

Besides external LLM services, open models like GPT-1 and GPT-2 are accessible in Mathematica. These models are predecessors to recent GPT models. GPT –1 is one of the initial models trained on a large book dataset, and GPT-2 is an improved version of GPT-1, trained on the WebText dataset. Let's look at some information about GPT-1 and GPT-2; note that the output here is truncated, given the large text.

```
In[72]:= Row[{Short[NetModel[ "GPT Transformer Trained on BookCorpus
Data", #] & /@ {"Details", "ShortName"} // Column, 4],   Short[NetModel[
"GPT2 Transformer Trained on WebText Data", #] & /@ {"Details","ShortName"}
// Column, 4]}]
Out[72]= Released in 2018, this Generative Pre-Training Transformer (GPT)
model is pre-trained in an unsupervised fashion on a large corpus of
English text. This model can be further fine-tuned with additional output
layers to create highly accurate NLP models for a wide range of tasks.
It uses bi-directional causal self-attention, often referred to as a
transformer decoder.
GPT-Transformer-Trained-on-BookCorpus-Data

Released in 2019, this model improves and scales up its predecessor
model. It has a richer vocabulary and uses BPE tokenization on UTF-8
byte sequences and additional normalization at the end of all of the
transformer blocks.
GPT2-Transformer-Trained-on-WebText-Data
```

You can try to retrieve other data, like in the LeNet example. Let's look at model variants and task types examples.

```
In[73]:= NetModel["GPT Transformer Trained on BookCorpus Data", #] & /@
{"ParametersAllowedValues", "Variants"}
NetModel["GPT2 Transformer Trained on WebText Data", #] & /@
{"ParametersAllowedValues", "Variants"}
Out[73]= {<|Task->{FeatureExtraction,LanguageModeling}|>,{{GPT Transformer
Trained on BookCorpus Data,Task->FeatureExtraction},{GPT Transformer
Trained on BookCorpus Data,Task->LanguageModeling}}}
Out[74]= {<|Task->{FeatureExtraction,LanguageModeling},Size-
>{117M,345M,774M}|>,
```

```
{{GPT2 Transformer Trained on WebText Data,Task->FeatureExtraction,Size->117M},
{GPT2 Transformer Trained on WebText Data,Task->FeatureExtraction,Size->345M},
{GPT2 Transformer Trained on WebText Data,Task->FeatureExtraction,Size->774M},
{GPT2 Transformer Trained on WebText Data,Task->LanguageModeling,Size->117M},
{GPT2 Transformer Trained on WebText Data,Task->LanguageModeling,Size->345M},
{GPT2 Transformer Trained on WebText Data,Task->LanguageModeling,Size->774M}}}
```

As seen in the output, variants have different task types and a specific number of parameter sizes, like 117M, 354M, and 774M million parameters. You can pick a model by specifying the parameters, for instance, picking the language-trained model and trying to generate text based on the prediction of the next token (see Figure 10-37).

```
In[75]:= gpt1=NetModel[{"GPT Transformer Trained on BookCorpus
Data","Task"-> "LanguageModeling"}]
gpt2=NetModel[{"GPT2 Transformer Trained on WebText Data","Task"->
"LanguageModeling"}]
Out[75]=
```

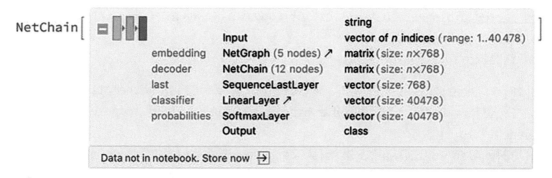

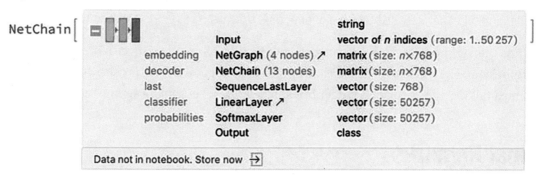

Figure 10-37. *GPT-1 and GPT-2 embedded architectures*

For the token function, the input parameters are the initial text, token count (default 10), and temperature (default 1). In simple terms, this function samples predictions. It attaches each new token to the original string for the fixed token count and returns the initial text plus the generated tokens text.

```
In[76]:= generateText[LLmodel_][initialText_, tokenCount_ :
10, temperature_ : 1] := Fold[StringJoin[#1, LLmodel[#1, {"RandomSample",
"Temperature" -> temperature}]] &, initialText, Range[tokenCount]]
```

Where a token refers to a unit of text that the model reads. It can be as short as one character or as long as one word, like "a" or "app." The model looks at these tokens individually to understand and generate text based on them. So, for GPT-2, BPE tokenization is a method used to break down words into smaller parts.

```
In[77]:= generateText[gpt1]["Alan Turing was a British mathematician
and logician who is considered a pioneer in the field of computer
science.",20,0.5]
Out[77]= Alan Turing was a British mathematician and logician who is
considered a pioneer in the field of computer science.he is a physicist and
is a very good scientist .
 he is also a friend of george w.
```

```
In[78]:= generateText[gpt2]["Alan Turing was a British mathematician
and logician who is considered a pioneer in the field of computer
science.",20,1]
Out[78]= Alan Turing was a British mathematician and logician who is
considered a pioneer in the field of computer science. At the time of his
independence he was selected to pen one of the first (173) contributions to
```

As seen comparing both responses, there is still room for improvement. GPT-1 output seems incoherent with unrelated elements. In contrast, GPT-2 shows more context talking about Turing's career but still lacks clear, complete sentences.

Final Remarks

In summary, the following road map for the general schematics, construction, testing, and implementation of a machine learning or a neural network model within the Wolfram Language scheme are in Figure 10-38.

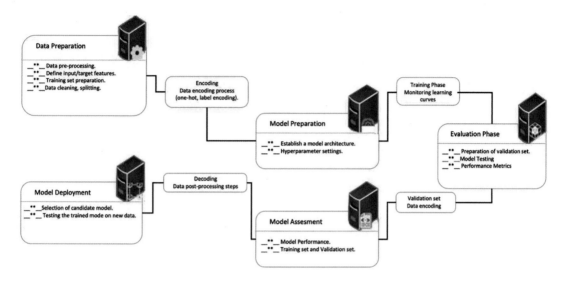

Figure 10-38. *Model overview for training and testing*

The diagram shows a route that can be followed directly; despite this, there may be intermediate points between each process within the route since the route may vary depending on the type of task or problem being solved. However, the route focuses on exposing the important and general points to construct a model using the Wolfram Language. Within the data preparation phase are previous processes, such as data integration, the type of data collected (structured or unstructured), transformations in the data, cleaning in data modules, and so on. So before moving on to the next phase, there must be a pre-processing of the data, to have data ready to be fed to the model.

Model preparation covers aspects such as the choice of the algorithm or the methods to use, depending on the type of learning; establishing or detecting the structure of the model; and defining the characteristics, input parameters, and type of data that is used, whether it be text, sound, numerical data, and tools to be used. All this is linked to a process called feature engineering, whose primary goal is to extract valuable attributes from data. This is needed to move on to the next point, the training phase.

The evaluation phase and model assessment consists of defining the evaluation metrics, which vary according to the task or problem being solved, and preparing the validation used later. The model's output is converted back to a clear, interpretable format at the decoding phase, readying for practical use. At this point, it is necessary to emphasize that the preparation of the model, training, evaluation, and assessment can be an iterative process, including tuning of hyperparameters, adjustments on algorithm techniques, and model configurations such as internal model features. The purpose is to establish the best possible model capable of delivering adequate results and finally reaching the model deployment phase, which defines the model chosen and tested on new data.

Index

M

Printed in the United States
by Baker & Taylor Publisher Services